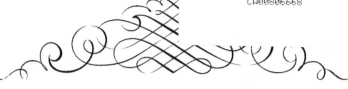

ISBN 978-1-330-02138-5
PIBN 10006027

1 MONTH OF
FREE
READING

at

www.ForgottenBooks.com

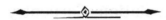

By purchasing this book you are eligible for one month membership to ForgottenBooks.com, giving you unlimited access to our entire collection of over 1,000,000 titles via our web site and mobile apps.

To claim your free month visit:
www.forgottenbooks.com/free6027

orth American Journal

OF 72036

HOMŒOPATHY.

In Certis Unitas.
In Dubiis Libertas.
In Omnibus Caritas.

EDITED BY

GEO. M. DILLOW, M.D.

CLARENCE B. BEEBE, M.D. SIDNEY F. WILCOX, M.D.
MALCOLM LEAL, M.D. EUGENE H. PORTER, M.D.
HENRY M. DEARBORN, M.D. FRED. S. FULTON, M.D.
A. B. NORTON, M.D., Business Manager.

THIRTY-FIFTH YEAR. *THIRD SERIES, VOL. II.*

PUBLISHED BY

THE JOURNAL PUBLISHING CLUB (Limited),

NO. 167 WEST 34TH STREET,

NEW YORK.

—

1887.

JOHN C. RANKIN, JR., PRINTER
34 CORTLANDT ST., NEW YORK

LIST OF CONTRIBUTORS

TO

VOL. XXXV. (VOL. II., SERIES III.)

ALLEN, T. F., M. D., - - - - Original Articles, Editorial, Book Reviews.

BALDWIN, J. G., M. D., - - - - Original Articles.

BARTLETT, CLARENCE, M. D., - - " "

BEEBE, C. E., M.D., - - - - Medical Progress.

BELCHER, GEO. E., M. D., - - - Original Articles.

BETTS, B. F., M. D., - - - - " "

BIGLER, W. H., M. D., - - - - " "

BOYLE, C. C., M. D., - - - - ..

BRINKMAN, M. A., M. D., - - - ..

BROWN, M. BELLE, M. D., - - - " "

BUFFUM, J. H., M. D., - - - - Correspondence.

BULLEL, K. B., M. D., - - - - Original Articles.

BUTLER, WM. M., M. D., - - - " "

CLARK, B. G., M. D., - - - - " "

DANFORTH, L. L., M. D., - - - " "

DEARBORN, H. M., M. D., - - - Original Articles, Book Reviews, Correspondence.

DENNIS, LABAN, M. D., - - - - Original Articles.

DESCHERE, M., M. D., - - - - " "

DILLOW, GEO. M., M. D., - - - Editorials, Book Reviews.

DODS, A. WILSON, M. D., - - - Original Articles.

DOUGHTY, F. E., M. D., - - - " "

DOWLING, J. W., M. D., - - - " "

DOWLING, J. W. JR., M. D., - - .. ..

EMORY, W. J. HUNTER, M. D., - .. ..

FARRINGTON, E. A., M. D., - - .. ..

FOWLER, W. J., M. D., - - - - .. ..

FREER, JAMES A., M. D., - - - " "

FULTON, FRED. S., M. D., - - - Original Articles, Editorials, Book Reviews, Society Reports.

GILCHRIST, J. G., M. D., - - - Original Articles.

GORHAM, GEO. E., M. D., - - - " "

HALLOCK, LEWIS, M. D., - - - " "

HAMAN, WM. A., M. D., - - - Society Reports.

HEARN, R, M. D., - - - - - Correspondence.

HELMUTH, WM. TOD, M. D., - -	Original Articles, Editorials.
HOUGHTON. HENRY C., M. D., - -	" " "
IVINS, HORACE F., M. D., - - -	" "
JACKSON, W. L., M. D., - - - -	Correspondence.
KING, WM. H., M. D., - - - -	Original Articles, Book Reviews, Correspondence.
KNIGHT, S. H., M. D., - - - -	Original Articles.
LAIRD, F. F., M. D., - - - -	" "
LATIMER, WM. C., M. D., - - -	" "
LEAL, MALCOLM, M. D., - - -	Original Articles, Book Reviews, Med. Progress.
LEWIS, GEO. W., M. D., - - - -	Original Articles.
LILIENTHAL, SAMUEL, M. D., - -	Original Articles, Correspondence, Med. Progress.
LINNELL, E. H., M. D., - - -	Original Articles.
MACBRIDE, A. L., M. D., - - -	" "
McDONALD, W. O., M. D., - -	" "
MOFFAT, E. V., M. D., - - - -	" "
MOFFAT, J. L., M. D., - - - -	" "
MORGAN, J. C., M. D., - - - -	" "
NORTON, GEO. S., M. D., - - -	Original Articles, Editorials, Book Reviews.
NOTT, F. J., M. D., - - - - -	Original Articles.
O'CONNOR, J. T., M. D., - - -	Original Articles, Med. Progress.
POPE, A. C., M. D., - - - - -	Correspondence.
PORTER, EUGENE H., M. D., - -	Editorial Comments, News, Book Reviews.
PRICE, ELDRIDGE C., M. D., - -	Original Articles.
RICE, H. E., M. D., - - - -	" "
SCHLEY, J. M., M. D., - - - -	" "
SHERRY, HENRY, M. D., - - - -	" "
TERRY, M. O., M. D., - - - -	" "
THOMAS, CHARLES MONROE, M. D.,	" "
TRITES, W. B., M. D., - - - -	" "
VAN LENNEP, W. B., M. D., - -	" "
WANSTALL, ALFRED, M. D., - -	" "
WARNER, A. G., M. D., - - -	" "
WILCOX, SIDNEY F., M. D., - - -	" " Book Reviews.
WOODWARD, A. W., M. D., - -	" "

INDEX.

Vol. XXXV.   *JANUARY, 1887.*   (Volume II, Third Series.)   No. 1.

North American

JOURNAL OF HOMŒOPATHY.

A TRIBUTE TO THE MEMORY OF THE LATE DR. CARL THEODORE LIEBOLD.*

By WM. TOD HELMUTH, M.D.,

New York.

THE inscrutable ways of Providence are beyond the ken of man, and the mysterious workings of His power cannot be fore-shadowed! Liebold in the evening quietly pursuing the daily routine of his duty; Liebold in the morning dead at his desk! Our minds even now have scarcely recovered from the shock of his sudden demise, and though we are conversant with the fact, and have seen his body resting here in its coffin, we can barely convince ourselves that our friend is no more.

In the short space of time that has been allotted me, it is impossible to do more than portray a brief outline of Dr. Liebold's life, and to collect a few scattered facts regarding his sojourn among us.

Carl Theodore Liebold was born in New-Dietendorf, Thuringen, Prussia, on November 24th, 1831. Of his early youth and manhood nothing is known, save that at the age of twenty he left the father-land and came to America in company with an artist named Grunne-wald. It can readily be understood that; influenced by the erroneous ideas then prevalent throughout Germany regarding the ease of acquiring large possessions in the western parts of our country, he immediately betook himself to those sections and engaged in real estate transactions; and it can also be as easily conceived that the venture was a failure. Discouraged by his want of success, and being a Moravian in his religious belief, he then took up his residence in Bethlehem, Pennsylvania, long famous as a Moravian missionary station. His means were at this time entirely exhausted, but nothing abashed, he sought with his hands (those hands that most of us have seen so steady and so dexterous in surgical manipulations), his daily

---

* Read at the Memorial Services held by the Homœopathic Medical Society of the County of New York, December 9th, 1886.

means of subsistence. We may imagine the feelings of Dr. Liebold during this period of his life, his mind aspiring to higher pursuits, while circumstances compelled him to perform the work of an ordinary laborer ! But persistency was one of the great characteristics of the man. He ever labored for a purpose, which, never revealing to others, he kept steadily before him and by his own unaided exertions toiled sedulously to accomplish. I have myself no doubt that, during these days of anxiety and trial, when youth was strong and hope was high, the profession of medicine was the goal on which he fixed his eyes, to which he, giving no sign, steadily journeyed, and which, as we all know, he successfully attained.

We next hear of him sick in the family of Mr. Henry P. Wolff, then residing in 12th Street, near University Place. Perhaps during his illness or convalescence he had revealed to Mr. Wolff the desires which had always been uppermost in his mind ; however that may be, certain it is that Mr. Wolff called upon Dr. Otto Füllgraff and begged him to find a place for young Liebold, whose sole ambition was the profession of medicine, and who was willing to perform any manner of service to the attainment of that end. This must have been in the winter of 1854. Dr. Füllgraff immediately perceived the capabilities and possibilities in the career of young Liebold, gave him a position, loaned him books, and was instrumental in gaining him admission to the lecture rooms of the medical colleges in this City. Part of these two years, in which Dr. Füllgraff writes me that his industry and economy were untiring and his application and assiduity remarkable, he resided in Williamsburg, but for how long a period I have been unable to ascertain. After two years of hard mental as well as physical labor, having acquired a degree of medical knowledge, having no means of support, and no doubt still in his silent way determined to obtain an honorable medical degree, he repaired to Newark, where he was befriended by Mr. Günther, and where he opened an office. Here for two years he worked by day and by night, economized in every possible manner, saved every penny and, simple as were his wants, deprived himself of many ordinary comforts that he might realize his aspirations for higher instruction and receive a university degree. Any man with health and youth on his side, who fixes a determined mind upon a purpose to be attained, and follows that direction in spite of the obstacles that privation and poverty cast in his way, will certainly be triumphant at the last, and we can imagine the quiet satisfaction of our dear friend when, after his years of struggle, he sat upon the deck of the vessel which was to bear him to his beloved country, and to the revered University of Berlin. Ah ! my friends, most of us who can with a slight modicum of self-denial and restraint obtain the ends we most desire, cannot conceive the high estimation necessarily placed on these good things when they have been acquired by years of labor and self-sacrifice.

Dr. Liebold entered the University of Berlin about the year 1858. According to the regulation of the German universities, the terms of instruction consist of two semesters a year, eight of these semesters being required (namely four years of study), before the degree is conferred. After attending the lectures at Berlin for somewhat over two years and being desirous of completing his education as soon as possible, Dr. Füllgraff received the following letter, which it gives me pleasure to show you, and to read the translation made for me by Dr. Charles McDowell. The letter puts us in possession of facts in his life which are interesting :

My Dear Doctor :

You will indeed be astonished at receiving a letter from me, and still more at the request which it contains. After so many years have passed since I was with you, I come to ask a certificate concerning that time. I am now studying my fifth semester in Berlin, and would like very much to graduate here also. The laws, however, are much more stringent than in America, and eight full semesters are strictly required before one is admitted to the examination. The present Dean of the medical faculty, Prof. Reichert, is, however, very kind to me personally, and upon my asking he promised to use his influence with the Minister to whom I must apply for a remission of time. He also recommended me urgently to procure a certificate from America to the effect that I had there been occupied a long time previously in medical study. He is aware that in England and America, students are required, before receiving a diploma, to have been for several years a student to a practicing physician. Although in the strict meaning of the word I have not been under your especial direction, still it is known to you that I was engaged only in the pursuit of medicine during the entire time that I lived in Williamsburg and Newark and that you considered me your student and I regarded you as my teacher. More than once I have received good advice from you. Therefore, I would kindly request you to prepare for me a certificate covering the years '55 to '58, inclusive. I do not know the exact day on which I (first) called upon you, but it was in the winter of '54 and '55, and it would be the plainest if you would fix the dates from the 1st January, '55, till the 31st December, '58. Please remark therein that through your intercession I was enabled to hear gratis, lectures in the medical college, and that during the last years I so far gained your confidence that I could independently treat patients who were not too extremely ill. However, you will yourself best know how such certificates should be written in order to have force of evidence for an American College, and the very same will answer in my case—for the necessary judicial form it is necessary that the writing be attested by a notary public or a magistrate in a court. My friend Mr. P. Günther will have the goodness to defray the expenses to yourself and I shall not neglect to pay the debt of gratitude on my return to America, which will probably take place about the end of August of next year. Accept in advance my best thanks for your trouble, and in the hope that these lines will find you in the best of health and activity.

Your most obedient,

Berlin, 21–12–'61.   TH. LIEBOLD.

N. B.—Please write the certificate in the English language, and as a member or graduate of the medical college.

Upon the reception of this letter Dr. Füllgraff immediately prepared the requisite document, and having it countersigned by Consul-General Schmidt and Daniel F. Tieman, then the Mayor of New York, forwarded the same. The paper was accepted, and his examinations passed, Dr. Liebold returned to America, bearing not only his degree from the University, but a certificate of attendance upon the cliniques of Baron Von Graefe, who was at that time the most distinguished oculist in Europe. Upon his arrival he again entered the office of Dr. Füllgraff. The clouds of civil war were then rolling over this country ; the American people were arrayed against each other—armies were already in the fields—the carnage had begun and the demands for competent surgeons were urgent, and Dr. Liebold (always a surgeon) immediately sought a position, at once congenial to his tastes and honorable to the union. In this again Dr. Füllgraff became his helper. An incident in this connection is worthy of record. Dr. Füllgraff called upon Prof. John T. Metcalf, of this City, and informed him that a young surgeon just arrived from Berlin desired a position in the medical corps of the army. "What is his name?" inquired Dr. Metcalf. "Dr. Liebold," was the reply. The Professor pondered for a moment and then said : "I know that young doctor. I met him last season at the University of Berlin. As I was not conversant with German, I desired to inspect the list of matriculants to perchance discover a student hailing from America. On that list I found the name Liebold and sought him. The young gentleman was so kind and so courteous in his manner, while he showed me through the University that it will give me pleasure to recommend him." The letter was at once prepared. Seeing this paper, Dr. Van Buren and Surgeon-General Hammond coincided in the recommendation, and in less than forty-eight hours Dr. Theodore Liebold was appointed Resident Surgeon at Point Lookout Hospital. Here at last was a field for his labor, here was the opportunity for the surgeon in theory to become a surgeon in practice, and from every record our friend conducted himself most creditably during this campaign.

Upon referring to the Medical and Surgical History of the War of the Rebellion, I find many records of his skillful surgical performances. In June, 1863, he is recorded as having performed tracheotomy in the case of a severe gun-shot wound, the ball entering behind the left ear and almost entirely cutting away the tongue, filling the trachea with blood.

In August, 1863, he made a secondary exsection of the humerus through the straight incision, with recovery. On July 10th of the same year he removed a large sequestrum from the stump of the left humerus. This case is reported in full and is accompanied with a drawing of the exfoliation, which now stands to the credit of our dead friend in the Army Medical Museum, numbered Specimen 1806. On January 10th, 1863, he reports a case of excision of the head of the radius and of the ulna below the coronoid process through a longitudinal incision. Of this remarkable case, the record tells us, that pronation and supination existed to their fullest extent, and that the motion of the forearm was perfect. On May 20th, 1864, he ligated both ends of the radial artery in the wound with success. On June 8th, of the same year he exsected one and a half inches of the radius and ulna through the longitudinal incision for severe gun-shot wound of the elbow, the patient recovering perfectly. On August 18th, 1864, he made a secondary amputation at the lower third of the left arm, and on February 28th, 1865, he again exsected the caput humeri through a straight incision, with success.

It is unnecessary to go into further details. The surgical skill of Dr. Liebold was acknowledged long before he turned his exclusive attention to ophthalmology.

Upon the close of the war the subject of this memorial returned to New York, and again associated himself with Dr. Füllgraff. It was at this period that an Ophthalmic Clinic was organized in the Bond Street Dispensary, with Dr. Liebold as Surgeon, and it was at this time that he betook himself with zeal toward the exclusive study of that specialty which has since made his name famous.

In the year 1868 the Trustees of the New York Ophthalmic Hospital decided to place that institution under homœopathic treatment, and certain of their number called at the pharmacy of Dr. Henry M. Smith, on Fourth Avenue, to inquire concerning the formation of a surgical staff. Dr. T. F. Allen was then living with Dr. Smith, and the inquirers were referred to him. Dr. Allen himself was then paying especial attention to ophthalmology, and knew of Dr. Liebold's position in the Bond Street Dispensary, and recommended the latter to fill the position as one of the surgeons to the hospital. He accepted, and from that moment, which

was his tide " taken at the flood," his position was assured. It is unnecessary to speak more of the successful career of Dr. Liebold. We all
know it, and details would be needless repetition.

During the next few years of his life our ophthalmic surgeon contributed many articles to the current medical literature of the day.
Among these will be found the following :

1. An article published in the transactions of the American Institute
of Homœopathy, session held in New York, 1867, on "Astringents."

2. An article published in the transactions of the American Institute
of Homœopathy, session held in Boston, 1869, on "Modified Linear
Extraction of Cataract."

3. An article published in the transactions of the American Institute
of Homœopathy, session held in Chicago, 1870, on "Forcible Flexion
of Extremities in Arterial Hemorrhage and Aneurism.

4. State Society, Albany, 1870, "Pyæmic Fever."

5. American Institute of Homœopathy, 1874, Niagara Falls,
"Aquæ Chlorinii and Baryta Iodata in Ophthalmic Practice."

6. American Institute of Homœopathy, 1875, Put-in Bay, "Alumen
Exsiccatum in Ophthalmic Practice."

7. American Institute of Homœopathy, 1877, Lake Chatauqua, "Progressive Myopia in the Schools and its Prevention."

8. State Society, 1878, "Application of Dry Cold in Inflammatory
Diseases."

9. State Society, 1879, " Duboisia as a Mydriaticum."

There are, no doubt, scattered throughout the medical periodicals,
articles of value from his pen, but want of time has prevented their insertion in this place.

Dr. Liebold was a man of few words, but when he spoke "he said
something." I have often remarked in medical and other meetings
the few potent words uttered by Dr. Liebold were always to the point,
and exhibited learning, thought and research.

For my own part, I generally found that I learned something from
intercourse with our friend, and the attention always bestowed upon
his pertinent remarks is evidence that others did likewise.

The chief characteristic of Dr. Liebold was his secretiveness. On
matters concerning himself his silence was remarkable. His most intimate friends—friends who had been in closest contact with him—in
whose houses he was a constant and welcome visitor, and in whose
hospitality he delighted, were, up to the day of his death, entirely ignorant of his personal affairs. His aims and his aspirations were known
to very few. Since his demise his idea of founding a hospital in Berlin, to be conducted on peculiar principles, has been discovered from

an examination of his papers, and from the same source, incidents connected with his previous history and future course have been revealed which have surprised us all. None knew of the charity of this noble man. Few realized the extent of his desires. His religious convictions were an enigma to most of us, and how surprised were the majority of the listeners assembled in this room at his obsequies, to know that he was a faithful and regular communicant of the Moravian Church. Truly he obeyed the injunction, "Let not thy right hand know what thy left hand doeth." Another feature in the character of our friend was his faithfulness in the performance of his duty. Whatever he had to do was done carefully and well. He could not be hurried into slurring over the work he had to do, and always took the requisite time in the performance of each individual item of his duty, no matter how pressing were the other demands upon his time. The patients who waited for him in his parlor would often complain of their long detention, but when they passed to his consulting room, were always pleased with the care and attention bestowed upon their cases. It was this conscientious discharge of his duty that gave rise to the well-known saying, "*That Liebold could never be hurried.*" The brusqueness of his manner with his patients on some occasions was always compensated by the delicacy of his touch, and the steadiness of his hand in the performance of his examinations and surgical operations, which with the nicety of his manipulation, rendered him an operator upon the eye whom few could equal and none surpass.

His quietness of manner in no way precluded the enjoyment of humor, and his cheery voice and hearty laugh at our social meetings will long be remembered by those who were fortunate enough to possess an intimate acquaintance with him.

In the years of my relations with Dr. Liebold I never remember having heard him speak disparagingly of a brother physician. He was lenient to the faults of his friends and generous to their frailties. Without flattery, he was a true friend; without ostentation, he was charitable. He had the courage of his convictions and a self-reliance which was not offensive. What he thought right, he did without flinching, and his high sense of honor was only equalled by his sensitiveness in that regard. In his condition of life his manner of death was a mercy, and his memory will be revered by all who knew him.

> Liebold, my friend, thy spirit took its flight,
> Like flashing meteor in the midst of night.
> Death's angel touched thee with his potent rod,
> And opened wide the paradise of God.

No lingering pain, no grim disease that sears
The founts of life in man's advancing years,
Had bade thee in thy daily life work cease;
The blessed fiat came, "Depart in peace."

Without a word, without a single token,
The silver cord, the golden bowl was broken,
Alone at night thy gentle spirit fled.
Alone at morn, the sun shone on thee—dead.

Thy friends will miss thee in the coming days,
Thy words of counsel and thy quiet ways;
Thy presence long must linger in these halls,
Whose very air thy memory recalls.

The shadowed valley thou hast quickly cross'd,
Here, on the brink, we mourn a friendship lost ;
There, on that other side, we see thee stand,
And smiling, beckon to the heavenly land.

IN MEMORY OF THE LATE DR. CARL THEODORE LIEBOLD.*

By GEORGE E. BELCHER, M.D.,
New York.

IT is meet and proper and in accordance with the promptings of our human nature that we should express some sentiments and declare in this way, if in no other, our estimation of Dr. Liebold as a man and a physician.

I have known him, I may say, intimately for a number of years—twenty years, or thereabouts. His style, manners and conversation always indicated the well-bred gentleman of good birth. In his ways he was reticent, laconic as to speech, habitually retiring and unobstrusive, but occasionally demonstrative; and when so, clearly so. He was a good listener and a close reader, as was readily shown in his conversation and practice. Although at times apparently paying little attention to remarks or suggestions on various subjects, he would evidently ponder over them and frequently, at some time or other, show frankly that they had been heeded and adopted, wholly or in part.

* Read at the Memorial Services held by the Homœopathic Medical Society of the County of New York, December 9th, 1886.

I have always regarded him as a consistent Christian, by his acts and by his words, and by the absence of acts and of the use of words which might have led one to imagine the contrary.

He was kind of heart and benevolent, and he was temperate in all things, yet fond of social life and its genial entertainments.

These and his other good qualities endeared him, as a man, to his friends, and especially to those who knew him well.

As a physician and surgeon, the community are indebted to him for the great good he has done. The whole medical profession has been indebted to him, and has esteemed him highly for the medical and surgical skill exhibited by him, more particularly in the specialty to which he devoted the best of his working days. He was the first physician in the homœopathic school in New York to give his attention to a specialty—adapting his extensive knowledge and scientific acquirements for a short time to general surgery and ophthalmology, and afterwards to the latter exclusively.

His belief in the homœopathic principle of cure was thorough and sincere as to its truth, yet comprehensive and liberal as to its practical scope. He did not disdain a high dilution nor a crude drug, and I have often seen him express delight from the recital of cures following upon the use of remedies selected in accordance with the homœopathic law.

We have lost a true man, a consistent Christian, a good physician, a skillful surgeon and a sound homœopathist—one whose life furnished a good example to those of the rising generation who look forward to be working members of our noble profession.

ORIGINAL ARTICLES IN MEDICINE.

POINTS OF MEDICAL ADVANCE.*

By ELDRIDGE C. PRICE, M.D.,

Baltimore, Md.

I DO not propose—as I have done in some previous reports—to make comparisons between the results of old school treatment and homœopathic treatment; or, in fact, to make comparisons of any kind when I can avoid it. I simply wish to make a record, in so far as my time has allowed, of some of the various occurrences throughout the past year that are of interest and that indicate progress in the

* A revision of the historian's report read at the eighth semi-annual meeting of the Maryland State Institute of Homœopathy, October 21st, 1886.

science and art of medicine, whether it be of one pathy or another, or of no pathy.

Although the amount of progress made in the past year (if there be any way to measure the effects of causes) may be less than that of some previous years, yet there are some points of sufficient interest to record as indicative of the fact that men are working just as hard as ever in the various fields included in the approximate science of medicine, and also in the practical department of the *ars medendi.* Although we do not claim to be sectarians, yet we are most deeply interested in progress. made by the students of science who believe in the principle of similars, and I will, therefore first note such points of interest.

Homœopathy still holds its own in our country, and more. From the report of Dr. B. W. James at the International Homœopathic Convention, and the report of Dr. T. Franklin Smith at the meeting of the American Institute of Homœopathy, come the following :

In the United States, of *practitioners* there are 10,000; 7,345 of whom are alumni from homœopathic colleges.

Of *medical colleges,* 13, with about 1,000 fresh matriculants and 400 graduates annually; of *hospitals,* 51, with 4,000 beds; of *insane asylums,* 3; of *dispensaries,* 48; of *pharmacies,* 33; of *homœopathic journals,* 22; of *national societies,* 5; of *sectional societies,* 2; of *state societies,* 28; of *local societies,* 92; of *medical clubs,* 16.

In all there is a total of 143 homœopathic associations of various kinds in this country.

Dr. James says: "The multiplication of capable specialists in our ranks is much aided by the special training provided in the New York Ophthalmological College and Hospital, which is authorized to confer the diploma of 'Oculi et Auris Chirurgus' upon its students. Our hospitals are receiving large aid both from private donations and from State subventions. Among the latter may be mentioned the assignment to homœopathists of the Westborough Insane Asylum, with $180,000 for its equipment, with the equivalent of about $320,000 in land, buildings, etc., 'making a grand total of $500,000.' The State of Massachusetts 'has also established the Newton General Hospital near Boston, and divided the medical and surgical staff equally between old school and homœopathic physicians. A similar assignment has been made in the Cook County Hospital at Chicago. Providence, Washington and Pittsburgh have corresponding liberality to record from the authorities of their respective States, and the Hahnemann Medical College and Hospital of Philadelphia, the oldest institution of its kind in the country,' has taken 'possession of a new and thoroughly equipped building.'"

$200,000 has lately been given by two homœopathic patrons for the establishment of a homœopathic hospital in Detroit, Mich.

Having given some of the principal points of advance in homœopathic interests, let us enter the broader domain of general art and science as it bears upon the work of the physician, wherein all may meet if they will.

In the field of bacteriology, where so many battles have been waged, we find suggestions of radical changes. The "germ theory," with its friends and enemies, both reasonable and unreasonable, is at last threatened with extinction by an entirely new theory of diseases. The novel suggestions are made by M. Gauthier, a member of the French Academy of Medicine: "The position taken is, that normal, vital action is always attended by the manufacturing of poisons, which, unless eliminated, produce disease." These substances, as I understand it, are somewhat similar to ptomaines, though not identical. The former are supposed to be produced in the body when in perfect health, while the latter are the result of putrefactive changes occurring in the body after death. M. Gauthier "claims to have discovered in the muscular glands five new alkaloids, perfectly defined and crystalizable, which, by experiment, have been found to produce a marked action upon the nervous system, as shown in general weariness, somnolence, and even purging and vomiting. These substances are alkaline bases during life in the tissues, and from their being derived from albuminous matter, are called leucomaines.

"Gauthier's experiments and those of Pettenkofer and Voit, show that some of the vital processes take place without the aid of oxygen, and are due not to combustion, as is the case with the larger part of the vital changes, but to a putrefaction which develops substances called leucomaines, and which, unless speedily eliminated by the excretory organs, produce, by their action upon the nervous system, various forms of disease. A deranged condition of the digestion, the bowels, kidneys or skin by any cause, such as imprudent exposure to cold or heat, intemperance in eating or drinking, or excessive physical or mental fatigue, may so impair their activity as to prevent the rapid elimination of those poisons produced by the vital changes in the tissues, and give rise to diseases more or less violent or varied in their character, according to the conditions of the system.

"Professor Peters, in commenting upon the statement of his colleague, says: 'Can the medical mind hesitate a moment between the parasitic doctrines full of shadowy hypotheses, and this new doctrine, as luminous as it is precise, which explains the phenomena of normal and abnormal life, by life itself in action?' Of course the investigations of Gauthier will be submitted to the careful scrutiny of physiologists and microscopists, who will determine, by renewed and repeated investigations, whether leucomaines exist in the muscular glands, or in sufficient amount to produce the pathological conditions attributed to them. It is very certain that poisons are developed both in animal and vegetable substances, often so subtle as to require the utmost skill in determining them, which not only produce serious disturbances not infrequently fatal to life.' "

Of course the knotty question of what causes abnormal disturbances in the human economy is not yet settled, and it is uncertain when it will be, if ever. The scientific mind may be likened to a great interrogation point. When the "hanger" will be dropped, and the "dot" be evolved into the period, is one of infinity's perpetual vanishing points.

From an hygienic or prophylactic stand-point, it matters little which theory we believe, or whether we believe either; if people observe strictly the rules of hygiene they will keep in health, but if they do not they will be subject to disease. But to the scientific therapeutist the question is full of importance, for upon its approximate decision depends, to a greater or less degree, the mode of the treatment of diseases by the physician of the future, whether he believe in homœopathy or not.

In connection with the leucomaine theory, I extract the following: "Mr. Tait defies the microbe and washes out the abdomen with 'tapwater, warmed by the addition of enough from the boiler. It is full of germs and spores, and small beasts of thirty-four different varieties. '" And yet he claims to have no bad results from such ablutions. He has performed 139 ovariotomies without a single death. A mortality of from three to four per cent. has heretofore been considered as successful as could be expected.

And now I have to record a discovery, which, though previously known to a few, is only recently becoming the property of the many. It is the discovery of the fact that "the kola nut of Guinea. or gara nut of Soudan, the fruit of the steroulia acuminata, cola acuminata of Daniell, has recently assumed a new importance by its remarkable property of antagonizing the effects of alcohol. It has long been known that the kola nut contains caffeine, to which may be attributed the lessened desire for sleep and sense of physical well-being caused by the consumption of it, for which reason it has long been extensively and highly valued throughout a large portion of Africa. Unlike the coffee bean, however, it contains no tannin. It has recently been discovered that when chewed, it antagonizes the effects of alcohol, and constant use of it is said to dissipate the desire, even in old drinkers."

If this discovery be of the importance that its realization would make it, then it is, indeed, a *great* discovery. Proper education of the children of this generation in the knowledge of thorough and true temperance, seconded by the use of this nut in the cases that will not profit by instruction, will in time, we may reasonably hope, produce a nation, nay, a world of temperance people, free from the debasing vice of drunkenness.

Closely allied to this habit is the practice of using tobacco, and for those who *will* smoke, to whom this habit has become a necessity to their happiness, it will be consoling to know that they "may enjoy their pipes or cigars without any fear or being poisoned by nicotine, if they will wet the tobacco with the juice of the water-cress, which will completely destroy its deleterious principles without affecting its aroma."

With the kola nut for drinkers, and the common plantain of our yards and lawns and the water-cress of our cool, shady brooks for tobacco users, the poisonous effects of the use of alcohol and tobacco upon the coming generations of man ought to be so far mitigated as to prove of minimal importance.

It has been discovered that "not a soldier in the Prussian army has died of small-pox since 1875," and this immunity is quite probably "due to the strictness with which vaccination is enforced." The benefits of vaccination have been illustrated many times, both publicly and in private practice. These results are, therefore, the only champion needed in the cause of this prophylactic measure, but yet in the face of well-established facts, we find men who strenuously oppose vaccination. The sincerity of some of these agitators may sometimes be justly questioned. "It is stated by the daily papers that the anti-vaccination crank, who stirred up most of the resistance to vaccination in Chicago and Montreal, on being arrested, was found to have been vaccinated three times within a few weeks."

There are many people in this world continually preaching new doctrines and prescribing new reforms for the good of *other* people, but who are not willing to take their own prescriptions. Spartan broth is what *other people* need, but turtle soup is good enough for them.

Sugar is one of the proximate principles, one of the chemical ingredients of the body, and so thoroughly has it been studied that we might have supposed nothing new could be learned of it; but through the observations of Dr. Vildalosa, of Havana, a new field of usefulness for this substance has been suggested. He "claims that the juice of the sugar cane, either cold or boiled, is an invaluable remedy in phthisis, chronic dysentery and various forms of dyspepsia. He calls the attention of medical men to the fact that the negroes who work on Cuban plantations, exhibit a degree of endurance and health unknown among other classes of laborers. He ascribes this to the fact that they eat the cane and drink the cold and hot juice every day. He gives the following composition of the juice, comparing it with that of woman's milk. He asserts that it acts as a saccharine food in the same manner that cod-liver oil acts as a fatty food:

	Woman's milk.	Juice of cane.
Albuminous substances,	1.5	0.24
Sugar and gum,	11.0	18.47
Mineral substances,	0.4	0.29
Water,	87.1	81.00

He thinks that as soon as the juice of the sugar cane reaches the stomach, it undergoes important changes, giving finally the following results: "1. Those effects produced by all saccharine articles and aromatic condiments (the latter on account of the essential oil it contains) on the economy. 2. The conversion of a certain amount of its sugar into lactic acid, in which form it makes the gastric juice more active, facilitating digestion and improving the appetite. This lactic acid has the further property of dissolving a certain amount of the lime salts contained in other articles of food, thus enabling the organism to assimilate them more easily. 3. The sugar and other alimentary principles of the cane juice are absorbed, and in this way help to build up the body. The following, then, are the author's condensed conclusions: 1. The cane juice is analogous in composition to woman's milk. 2. It stimulates the action of the gastric juice. 3. It contains phosphate of lime in an assimilable form and facilitates the absorption of a large amount of the salts of lime contained in other articles of food."

Dr. Vildalosa is not the first to note the improved condition of the health of the negroes working in sugar cane during the sugar making period, but, so far as I am aware, he is the first to call attention to a possible therapeutic use for the cane juice. In the treatment of phthisis, cases are not infrequently found that cannot tolerate cod-liver oil, even in some of the most palatable emulsions; and even when the palate is satisfied, the stomach will sometimes rebel. May it not be in just such cases that the juice of the sugar cane will supply the needs of the patient without any kind of revulsion on the part of the palate, stomach, or any other organ?

A number of sister cities in the United States may rejoice with Baltimore at the possibility of at last having at command in the not very distant future, the means of rendering our drinking water fit for table use without the necessity of filtration, especially the water supplied during the spring months. "Purification of river water by means of electricity has been undertaken at Roubaix by M. Stoffel. The gist of the process is that the ozone generated by the electrolytic decomposition of the water kills the minute organisms, and oxidizes all organic substances, at the same time precipitating the carbonates in course of dissolution, thus effectively purifying the water."

If proof were wanting that scarlatina and diphtheria are often due to sewer gas, it has lately been obtained by an interesting experiment, *viz.* : "The health authorities of Detroit, Mich., finding the sewerage in a bad condition, with a great mortality from diphtheria, scarlet fever and analogous diseases, went to work vigorously, and put into the two hundred miles of city's sewers 275,000 pounds of sulphate of iron, and burned in the sewer man-holes, under cover, three tons of sulphur, the gas from which was found to pass freely through the whole drainage system of the town. In such close connection with this disinfection that it must be reasonably regarded as its effect, it is reported that there followed a marked diminution in the number of cases of, and deaths from, diphtheria and scarlet fever—in fact, almost a total cessation of those diseases."

From that mine which has furnished the medical profession with some precious gems, other jewels are still being delved. Another new anæsthetic has been discovered. "Lewin obtained from the root of the *Piper methisticum* a semi-fluid resin which he calls ' Alpha Kawa Resin !' Dr. N. A. Randolph, not liking the cumbrous title, suggests that in honor of the discoverer the resin be called Lewinin. When the semi-fluid Lewinin is placed upon the tongue there is a burning sensation with increased salivary secretion, followed by a local numbness which, while extremely superficial, is recognizable for more than an hour. Some pallor of the mucous membrane at the point of application is noticeable. Lewinin is too painfully irritating to apply in practice to the human conjunctiva. The extract will probably be of service in dental practice, as its application certainly mitigates the discomfort of operations on the teeth of those suffering from sensitive dentine. In cases where superficial anæsthesia is required, as in rhinological practice it is superior to cocaine."

In using ether as an anæsthetic, Dr. M. W. Hobbs prefers it warm to cold. He finds that when the temperature is thus raised, ether acts more promptly than when cold (thus requiring less), and it seldom produces either coughing or vomiting. Dr. Hobbs has a special apparatus with which he prepares his ether.

Photography has for some years been enlisted in the cause of medical science and art, but possibly the most delicate methods ever introduced are those lately used to photograph "the retina and the interior of the uterus."

Electricity is also lending its assistance to medicine in a variety of ways. The latest use to which it has been put is the lighting of obscure parts of the body for exploration and operations. It has lately been used in New York "to light up diseased bone which had been drilled by an ingenious instrument called an electro-osteotome. The operation is said to have been successful."

Biology is a branch of general science to which the major part of the correct knowledge of the physician is due. But it is only in very modern times that the importance of investigations in this vast field (with its many sub-divisions), have been assigned their proper and important relative positions by the thinking world. Important discoveries of all kinds are frequently made in one field by workers in another; discoveries are not always anticipated. But of course this is a poor rule to try to follow, for the best and most thorough work is done by specialists in their own departments.

It has been discovered that gray hair will return "to its original color under the use of phosphorized cod-liver oil," although the oil was given for an entirely different purpose. If such a result may always follow the use of this preparation, hair dyes may be permanently shelved, and their bad effects successfully forestalled.

"The *Lancet* says that 'the presence of a heat centre in the brain has apparently been demonstrated by the observations and experiments of Ott, Richet, Aronsohn and Sachs, though its precise position is still open to question.' Exner's observations on the localization of the visual sense support those of Christiani, and are in opposition to those of Munk, Dalton, Ferrier, Luciani and others, for he has found that every part of the cortex of the occipital lobe may be removed without the smallest impairment of the sense of sight."

Regarding the functions of the thyroid gland, I extract the following: "Last year Horsley extirpated the thyroid gland of monkeys and dogs, and obtained results which led him to the conclusion that this organ exercises very important metabolic functions. He believes that the thyroid in some way transforms muciform substances so as to make them available for further purposes in the economy; and he also produces evidence to show that the perfect formation of the blood is furthered by the presence of the same organ. It need hardly be said that Mr. Horsley was not the first to extirpate the thyroid gland from animals, nor was he the first to show that the symptoms thereby resulting belonged to the same category as those of myxœdema, cretinism, and cachexia-strumipriva. But it was his chief care to prove that the loss of the thyroid was the *causa causans* of the symptoms, and the likeness of artificial myxœdema to the other diseases just mentioned was something more than a mere similitude."

"What next?" inquires the New York *Medical Times.* "Teeth have been made to grow upon the tibia by boring into the bone and inserting the tooth, and now we hear that the replacement of a diseased eye by the healthy eye of an animal, has been successfully accomplished."

Two more beliefs that were supposed to be well established facts have recently been seriously disputed. One is the almost proverbial danger of second summers, for teething children, and the other is the contagiousness of leprosy. "The very large mortality among infants, according to the latest census reports, occurs during the first year. The figures presented show that there is, in reality, no such thing as the dreaded second summer." "A physician practicing in China states that leprosy is *not* contagious."

Another statistical report may also be of interest—especially to bachelors : "According to M. Lagneau, the well-known statistician, there is a lower rate of mortality among bachelors under twenty-two years of age than among married men. Above that age the contrary is observed, and married men live longer than bachelors. Among bachelors 38 per 1,000 are criminals, among married men, 18 per 1,000."

It is unnecessary to point the moral.

"The spinning wheel has been prescribed as a cure for insanity. It was introduced into the asylum at Douglas, Isle of Man, as something that might amuse the patients, and they forthwith became so interested in it, and in the idea of contributing to their own support by its use, that the direction of their nervous force was changed, and their condition greatly improved. Experiments are to be tried in other asylums." I will suggest that it is not the spinning wheel, *per se,* to which good results are due, but to a mild and useful occupation which is congenial to the patient and in which he is interested ; it depends upon the principle of properly guiding the mental energy of the patient.

There are, according to the International Congress, which last assembled at Copenhagen, 190,000 physicians in the world, and our charity is broad enough to believe the majority of these men are interested in advancing the welfare of the medical profession to which they belong; at least there are enough men in this fraternity whose good intentions are backed by a force sufficiently strong to compel the attention of their brothers, and fortunately, enough of these brothers recognize the truth unveiled by the van to leaven the whole mass of the profession.

The question of an elevated standard of medical education is still being agitated, and the effect of the prolonged effort is gradually producing good results. The Russian medical colleges are now compelled by law to accept only students having a collegiate education. It is true, this legal enactment is due to the fact that the colleges were overcrowded, but the benefits resulting to the profession and to the laity will, we hope, be all that can be desired.

All the medical colleges in the United States that are recognized as as first-class, are also elevating their educational standards. The Hahnemann of Philadelphia, Pa., has this year inaugurated a compulsory three years' course.

It is a question whether the organization of a new medical college is always an indication of progress, but we will hope that the time is not far distant when no new college will be allowed to open its doors without complying with certain necessary requirements enforced by law. Then a new college will mean much more than it does now. Fortunately the requirements in Japan are sufficiently strict to allow of the organization of as many new colleges as either the public or the profession may demand. This country "has been mapped out into six divisions, and a medical college is to be established in each division." The system of medicine taught in these colleges will, of course, be that of the civilized world generally, and not the collection of superstitions not long since prevalent with the people. According to Hardwicke in his "Medical Education and Practice in All Parts of the World," which was published in 1880, Japan had then but three first-class medical schools (and they were, by no means, thoroughly equipped), only one of which granted degrees; this addition of six new schools, which, of course, will grant degrees, may be called real progress of importance.

In conclusion, I will again refer to the special pathy in which we all have a living faith. Although there are many evidences of the spread of a belief in homœopathy, yet much prejudice against this principle still exists. However difficult it may be for some of our progressive Northern brethren to believe, yet it is a fact that no farther south than our own city of Baltimore are physicians who will not even exchange passing greetings with some of their professional brothers, simply because these brothers happen to acknowledge a belief in, and prescribe drugs according to, homœopathy. And these very men who so condemn what they call arrogant assumption in others, arrogate just as much to themselves, aye, even more, when they say that only men who repudiate homœopathy *openly* (whatever they may *secretly* practice) shall be recognized by *them* as "regular" physicians. Allopathy is a thing of by-gone times, of Hahnemann's days; these gentlemen are not allopaths. "Allopathic" is "bad form," you know; "regular" is proper now.

They claim to be "regular" physicians, but in the meantime all that is "regular" in their methods is the little homœopathy foreshadowed by some of the ancients, and further instilled into their materia medica by Phillips, Ringer, et. al., and they may just as properly be called "allopathic" as "regular," unless they will agree that "regular" applies to legal conformity, in which case this distinctive title becomes the property of every graduate of every legally chartered medical college in good standing. But we must not be uncharitable; our old school brothers probably believe and do the best they know. They have somehow imbibed the opinion that when a man confesses his belief in homœopathy he is thereby rendered incapable of believing in anything else. They believe homœopathy is an absurdity, and, therefore, a man who professes to believe in homœopathy does so either to gull the people or because of some inherent mental deficiency, and he is consequently either a knave or a fool, and is unworthy the respect of honest intelligence. How such a fallacy has arisen it is easy to explain; but why and how it is still accepted by men claiming to be true and just to themselves, it is *not* so easy to explain. Having before us, therefore, the history of the progress of homœopathy, with its defeats and triumphs, from the first proving of *cinchona* to the present time, I think we may, with respect for ourselves, justice to humanity, and due charity for the fallibility of human judgment, uncompromisingly demand as our *right,* that we physicians, who believe in homœopathy, be treated as other members of the medical profession who do *not* believe in homœopathy, and that in all things medical we enjoy "a fair field and no favor." Our demand is not mere "words, words, words," but we mean it, for it is based partly upon a consciousness that we are right, and that we are *sure* we are right, and partly upon a belief in the ultimate of right, of truth. Of course homœopathy has its limitations; but we believe that by whatever name it may be called, this principle is, at least, *based* upon something we call eternal truth. We may be mistaken, but until some better general rule is found for the use of drugs, we will continue to hold this belief.

THERAPEUTICS OF ECZEMA OF THE EAR.*

By W. P. FOWLER, M.D.,
Rochester.

AMONG curable diseases of the ear, a chronic eczema invading the auditory canal is frequently one of the most obstinate. The routinest will stumble in treating this affection, and rarely effect a cure. Each case must be individualized, as it demands treatment peculiarly its own.

At the outset, if an avoidable exciting cause exist, we must remove it ; then resort to such hygienic, constitutional and local measures as seem to be demanded.   He who prescribes the homœopathic remedy and ignores local treatment, will sometimes fail.   On the other hand, the physician who relies upon local treatment to the exclusion of everything else will be disappointed, and his patient doubly so.

Among the avoidable exciting causes may be mentioned : 1st, the habit of picking the ears ; 2d, the use of rancid oils and other irritating substances to relieve ear-ache, and 3d, uncleanliness.

Several cases have come under my notice where picking the ears produced the trouble.   One of these patients, a young lady, seemed to have a morbid propensity in this direction. She used hair-pins, matches, pins, etc., picking and working at her ears until an eczematous eruption was produced.   So strong had the habit become that I almost despaired of breaking her of it. Finally, however, I succeeded, and the eruption quickly disappeared. Irritating substances, such as rancid oils, etc., poured into the auditory canal to soften "ear-wax,"—which, by the way, is seldom present,—and to relieve pain in the ear, may also cause eczema.   There seems to be a fondness for using a mixture of sweet oil and laudanum, and it is, I believe, more frequently employed by the laity than any other remedy to relieve ear-ache.   This oil is oftentimes anything but "sweet;" has perhaps stood in the house for years, and is rancid and unfit for use.   The alcohol of the laudanum adds to the irritating properties of the mixture, which occasionally causes eczema.

Some of the preparations of cosmoline are impure, and when applied to the auditory meatus, excite an eczema.   One preparation of fluid cosmoline that I used made me much trouble, and my patient more.   It produced, in about thirty-six hours, a most beautiful eczema.

Uncleanliness is a frequent cause.   Among the squalid, uncared for children of the very poor, who seem to have a repugnance to the use

*Read before the Homœopathic Medical Society of the State of New York, Sept. 8th, 1886.

of water, eczema of the ear is often encountered in its worst form. The heads of these unfortunates usually swarm with pediculi. To relieve the itching that these parasites produce, vigorous scratching is resorted to, and this, in connection with the filth that is allowed to accumulate, leads to eczema of the scalp. The eruption is then liable to extend to the auricle and auditory canal. When we meet cases of this kind, our first effort, of course, is to enforce habits of cleanliness, rid the head of vermin, and correct such other hygienic errors as may exist.

In chronic suppuration of the middle ear, the discharge is sometimes very acrid, and sets up an eczema of the meatus and auricle. We should direct our efforts to the cure of the primary disease, and the eruption will usually disappear as soon as the discharge ceases.

Among the *predisposing causes* may be mentioned an anæmic and weakened state of the system. Oftentimes the appetite is capricious, and digestion impaired. Heavy eaters are occasionally attacked, but so far as my observation goes, light eaters and the poorly nourished are most frequently the victims. Females who have no strength, no appetite, whose bowels are constipated and whose skin is pale, dry and inactive, are the ones most often affected. Many of them get little or no out-door exercise. Much benefit is usually afforded such patients by a brisk walk every day, and an occasional Turkish bath. A tepid bath, followed by brisk rubbing with a coarse towel, is also of benefit. In fact, it is preferable to the Turkish bath when the patient is much reduced in strength.

Errors in diet must be corrected. Pork, buckwheat, highly seasoned pickles, pies, cakes, etc., I believe to be especially injurious. Among debilitated, nervous female patients we often find a morbid appetite. They frequently refuse to touch good, plain, nutritious food, and crave pastries, strong tea, coffee, and dainties that are but poorly calculated to nourish and support the wasted body.

When a case of chronic eczema of the ear presents itself for treatment, it is advisable to inform the patient that some time will probably be required to effect a cure. If this be not done, he will very likely become discouraged by the tardiness with which relief comes, and discontinue treatment, thus preventing the physician from doing justice to either his patient or himself.

In selecting the homœopathic remedy we can seldom depend upon ear symptoms alone. Concomitant indications must always be taken into account.

Following are the remedies most often curative:

Aconite is occasionally indicated in acute eczema. There is much *heat, redness* and *swelling* of the auricle, which is tender to touch. *Fever, thirst* and *restlessness* are also present.

Arsenicum.—This remedy is the great dependence of old school physicians in the treatment of almost all forms of eczema. That they effect cures with this drug there can be no doubt; but I think it is only when homœopathic to the condition present. It is by no means a cure-all for this disease, though very often called for.

There is itching and *burning* in the affected parts, better during the day and aggravated *after midnight. Warmth relieves.* Moderate redness and swelling are present. In the auditory canal and in the auricle, small vesicles appear. These rupture and discharge their contents. The exudation dries, and with the cast-off epithelium forms small scales. If the eczema is accompanied by suppurative inflammation of the tympanum, the discharge will be very *offensive, acrid,* and *thin.* When *arsenicum* is indicated the patient is usually pale, poorly nourished and easily exhausted, is inclined to be discouraged and melancholy.

Ars. iod.—When *arsenicum* seems indicated, yet gives no relief. There is usually a greater tendency to glandular enlargement than in the purely *arsenicum* cases.

Belladonna.—Of great value in some cases of acute eczema, when the tissues around the auricle become red, swollen, and approach in appearance an erysipelatous condition. The face is flushed, the skin usually *moist* (Acon. dry and hot) and the pain in the ear and head of a throbbing nature. Aggravation is in the afternoon and *evening.* One peculiarity of the disease when *belladonna* is indicated, is the suddenness with which the attack comes on. A recent case illustrates this:

A gentleman, twenty-eight years of age, was attacked with eczema of the ear one week before consulting me; had never suffered from anything of the kind before, and could not account for it in any way. The walls of the meatus and the auricle were dark red, swollen, and sparsely covered with an eczematous eruption. Twelve hours before I saw him, the integument around the auricle began to swell, became red, shining, and tender to touch. The redness and swelling quickly extended to the cheek, scalp, side of the neck and eyelids. Prescribed *belladonna* 3d, and in twenty-four hours was greatly surprised to find the swelling entirely gone and the patient far advanced towards recovery. The eruption persisted in the meatus for several weeks, but was finally cured with other remedies.

Belladonna is not often called for in eczema of the ear, but when called for will give most brilliant results. It should not be overlooked.

Baryta iod.—Chronic cases; subjects are usually thin, *scrofulous, dwarfed children, whose tonsils and cervical glands are enlarged.* They are pale, "pot bellied," and often have a ravenous appetite. The auricle is covered with dirty looking crusts, which, when removed, leave a raw, bleeding surface. Much itching, which scratching does not relieve.

Cal. carb.—In fat, scrofulous children, who have large heads and swollen lymphatic glands. Eczema of the scalp is often present; dentition is difficult. Ear symptoms are not particularly characteristic. There is some itching of the auricle and in the meatus, aggravated in cool air. Behind the ear, on the auricle, and in the canal we find a moist eruption and yellowish crusts.

Calc. iod.—Much the same as *calc. carb.*, only that the discharge from the eczematous surface is *more acrid*, and the tendency to suppuration of the glands greater. Tonsils enlarged.

Croton tig.—One of our most valuable remedies. The diseased surface is greatly congested, and *roughened by numerous vesicles or pustules.* There is much burning and itching, aggravated by rubbing and by warmth. (Ars. relieved by warmth.) Of most use in acute and sub-acute attacks, though chronic cases sometimes yield to it. Does not act well after *rhus.*

Dulcamara.—The skin is inflamed and the eruption vesicular or pustular; oozing of watery fluid; itching, worse in the evening. All the symptoms *are aggravated by a damp, cold change in the weather.*

Graphites.—Very frequently indicated. The integument of the meatus is reddened, more or less dotted with vesicles, which rupture and discharge their transparent, sticky, offensive contents; parts itch much and bleed easily; deep cracks appear behind the auricle, and also just at the entrance of the auditory canal. The eruption frequently extends to the cheek, and backward over the mastoid towards the nape of the neck. Constipation is often present, the stools being in the form of hard balls united by mucous threads. After stool there is much mucus about the anus. It is usually in chronic eczema that *graphites* is called for.

Hepar sulph.—*Extreme sensitiveness of the parts*; even the most careful handling of the ear causes the patient to flinch, as pain is produced by the slightest touch. There is much redness of the walls of the meatus, and an accumulation of thick, whitish, or bloody pus in the canal. On the auricle, and back of the ear over the mastoid, are often found dirty looking crusts; much itching, but patient hesitates to scratch on account of the pain produced. *The slightest abrasion suppurates.* Darting pain in the ears. The pain and itching are aggravated by cold, and relieved by warmth.

Lycopod. has proved curative in some troublesome cases, when the disease was accompanied by dyspepsia with the characteristic lyco-podium symptoms. There was a fine eruption in the canal, some red-ness and itching, relieved by warmth.

Mezereum.—An important remedy. The eruption is vesicular at first, but later it may become pustular. Scabs form,. and *when pressed upon pus escapes from beneath them;* the patient scratches his ears to relieve the *intense itching and burning*, tears off the crusts, and thus leaves a raw, bleeding surface. Aggravation is in the evening and at night ; relief in the dry, open air during the day.

Rhus tox.—Much inflammation, redness and swelling of the auricle and walls of the canal ; eruption vesicular ; *serous, acrid discharge* from the meatus ; itching, changed to burning by scratching ; aggra-vation from change of weather ; relief from warmth.

Sepia.—From this remedy I have obtained most excellent results in several cases of chronic eczema of the ear. The patients were weak, poorly nourished females. There was not much active inflammation of the skin, but a fine eruption, followed by desquamation of minute, bran-like flakes. The itching was *relieved in the open air*, and aggravated by warmth. (Ars. relieved by warmth.)

Sulph. will occasionally effect a cure alone, but more frequently is of value as an intercurrent remedy. Some of the worst cases, in dirty, strumous children, are cured or benefited by it. The ear symp-toms are not characteristic. There is usually much itching, thin, irritat-ing discharge, and dirty, moist crusts. The scalp is often affected as well as the ear. Patient is cross and irritable during the day, and feverish and restless at night ; the feet burn, especially after getting into bed at night; when washed, the child screams and seems to dread the water.

There are quite a number of other remedies that may be of benefit, especially *apis, canth., china mur., kali iod., merc., puls., staph.* and *tellur-ium.*

Local treatment is very important in some cases. Not unfrequently the meatus becomes filled with crusts formed of dried discharge and exfoliated epithelium. Again, the accumulation may be of a thick, cheesy nature. If the passage be not kept clear, a cure can rarely be effected, and the stoppage produces hardness of hearing and annoying tinnitus. But worse than this, the integrity of the membrana tym-pani may be impaired by pressure and irritation produced by contact of the ever-increasing mass. It will thus be seen that eczema of the ear differs from eczema affecting other portions of the surface in that it requires most careful attention lest any organ of special sense be per-manently impaired.

But just here a word of caution will, I think, be in place. There is a tendency on the part of many to overdo the matter of local treatment—cleanliness of the canal, etc. We should always bear in mind that irritation of the parts is to be scrupulously avoided, for to irritate the sensitive surface is to aggravate the disease. If the auditory canal be tolerably clear, my practice is to let it alone, and depend upon the homœopathic remedy, together with hygienic measures, to effect a cure.

When the passage is occluded it must be cleared—but how? Some authorities say, syringe the ear with warm water. Observation of results obtained in many cases by this method forces me to the conclusion that it is usually injurious. Water being of lower specific gravity than the serum of the blood, is greedily taken up by the denuded papillary layer of the skin. As a consequence, swelling of the tissues follows, with pressure on the terminal nerve filaments and much irritation. The disease is thus prolonged. If we raise the specific gravity of the water by adding a little glycerine and chloride of sodium this difficulty is avoided. The solution that I have used contained twelve grains of common salt, and one-half ounce of glycerine to six ounces of water. With this, warmed, the ear should be syringed. In case some of the crusts remain, they can be readily removed with the forceps, or Buck's fenestrated scoop. Instruments, however, should be used with the greatest care, and only when the meatus is illuminated. The crusts should not be torn from the walls of the canal. Syringe the ear until the accumulation has been either removed or thoroughly loosened. In the great majority of cases the syringe will do everything that is required. After drying the canal with absorbent cotton, we can make whatever local application we desire. Of late years I have used either boracic acid, or subnitrate of bismuth, dusting in just enough to whiten the surface.

When the auricle is badly affected, raw and sore, or if deep fissures form behind the ear, I prefer subnitrate of bismuth to any other local application. It protects the denuded surface from the air, absorbs whatever discharge there may be and greatly hastens the cure. It should be freely dusted upon the diseased parts, and into the cracks. We must avoid blowing much of it into the auditory canal, as it is with difficulty removed. Sparingly used, though, it is of great benefit, and does not in any way interfere with the action of homœopathic remedies.

Cosmoline and all oleaginous substances have, as a rule, failed to give me good results. They have seemed to aggravate many cases. Have never found it necessary to use nitrate of silver, tar water, oxide of zinc, and other local applications.

THE STATISTICS OF CROUP AND DIPHTHERIA.*

By W. B. TRITES, M.D.,

Philadelphia.

IT is not the intention of this paper to present statistics of the results of treatment in croup and diphtheria, nor is it written with a desire to provoke a discussion of the already much discussed subject, the identity of these two diseases, but rather to call attention to certain statistics, which, in the writer's opinion, have not received the consideration they deserve, and to draw therefrom certain allowable conclusions, which, he thinks, may be of value in the prevention of diphtheria.

I was first led to compare the death rates of croup and diphtheria in Philadelphia by an article in the Philadelphia *Medical and Surgical Reporter* of August 26th, 1876, giving the results of old school treatment in an epidemic of diphtheria, which had prevailed in the twenty-first ward.† The author claimed to have treated during the epidemic, 1,047 cases, with a loss of but twenty-one. Of those dying, eight were moribund when he was called, and two refused all treatment; deducting these, his death rate was but a fraction over one per cent., a phenominal success in diphtheria. I cannot describe my feelings on reading this article. For a time my faith, in both myself and the system of medicine I profess, was shaken. Can it be possible, I inquired, for the old school to do so much for this terrible scourge, while homœopathy, as applied by me, eliminating all cases which were moribund when first seen, or which refused treatment, showed a loss of from seventeen to eighteen per cent. in about four hundred cases?

I felt sure that the author of the paper had included in his 1,047 cases many which were not diphtheria, for I had myself seen many cases of folliculitis, which, in the alarm of the hour, I had treated as diphtheria, but which were afterward properly diagnosed; but assuming this error, the disparity between our results still remained enormous.

I anxiously began a search for the cause of this great disparity. I found, from the books of the old school, that it could not have been due to the treatment, for he had used the ordinary supporting treatment of milk punch, iron, beef broth and washes. In the reports of

---

*Read before the Pennsylvania Homœpathic Medical Society, Sept. 23d, 1886.

†The twenty-first ward is a rural section of the city, with a population, in 1876, of 18,097 souls. The epidemic referred to began in the spring of 1874, and reached its height in the fall of 1875, during which year one person in every 237 died of the disease.

the Board of Health for 1875 and 1876 the mystery was made plain. I found in these, that, in 1875, seventy-two deaths from diphtheria and thirty-eight deaths from croup had occurred in the twenty-first ward.

In 1876, thirty-nine deaths from diphtheria and twenty-three deaths from croup had occurred.

In 1873 and in 1874, when diphtheria was not prevailing in the ward, the death rate from croup had been four and six, respectively.

Here was beside a high death rate from diphtheria, an unprecedented mortality from croup, and yet, in my practice, I had not seen a single fatal case of croup, but the most of my fatal cases of diphtheria had died from invasion of the larynx.

This explained to me the phenomenal success of my neighbor ; he evidently did not count the death of a patient dying with diphtheritic croup as a loss from diphtheria. This experience led me to believe that membranous croup and diphtheria are often confounded and prepared me to agree with those who adhered to the theory of their identity, in the discussion of the question by the Royal Medical Society in 1879.

Since 1875 I have carefully watched the statistics (of these diseases) in Philadelphia, as well as in other cities, and have been surprised to find how their mortalities keep pace. The average death rate, per week, from diphtheria and croup, in Philadelphia, during the last ten years has been as follows :

	Diphtheria.	*Croup.*		*Diphtheria.*	*Croup.*
1875	12.5	9.6	1880	6.2	5.8
1876	11.6	7.4	1881	8.8	6.0
1877	8.8	6.5	1882	17.9	8.9
1878	8.9	7.4	1883	19.3	9.6
1879	Not Obtained.		1884	13.0	11.1

In this table it will be noted that whenever the death rate from diphtheria is high, the rate from croup also advances, and when that of diphtheria decreases, the rate in croup also lessens. This is especially noticeable in the first six years (of the table) and not so marked afterward, because I think that in the later years the attention of the profession has been aroused to the fact that diphtheria is a frequent cause of croup. If we compare the death rates of these two diseases, week by week, as has been done in these charts,† we will find this correspondence still more manifest, the death rates advancing and declining just as in the table of average weekly mortalities.

---

†Here the writer exhibited ten charts, showing the deaths each week, for ten years, from diphtheria and croup in Philadelphia.

Neither time of season nor atmospheric condition, seems to retard or accelerate one disease beyond the other ; they go hand in hand, through all seasons, in all kinds of weather. In 1875 and 1882, the highest mortality in both diseases was exhibited between the first of October and the last of December.

In 1876 it was highest from the first of January to the first of July, while in 1883 the mortality was frightful, and was distributed evenly over the entire year.

Thus far in my investigation, the statistics seemed to show that the death rate from croup, in any given year, bore a striking similarity to the death rate from diphtheria for that year ; that when the average death rate per week was taken, the same correspondence was seen ; that when charts were made, showing the actual death rate for each week, both croup and diphtheria, the death rates were found to correspond week by week, and finally this similarity was not confined to any particular season, nor dependent upon atmospheric conditions. I thought if I could follow up this examination and compare the results in localities, and should find that the deaths from diphtheria and from croup, occurred not only in the same week, but in the *same localities*, a strong argument would be adduced to prove that, either these diseases were identical, or else that they occurred together. In pursuance of this thought, I made an examination of the weekly returns of deaths by wards, as reported to the health authorities of Philadelphia, and found that when the death rate for any week from diphtheria is high in any ward, the death rate from croup for that ward and week is also high, and *vice versa*. In some years this high mortality was found in the thickly settled and badly constructed portions of the city, other years in the finely built neighborhoods, such as the 15th and 20th wards ; and in other years, in the rural wards, such as the 21st, 22d and 28th wards, but always the peculiarity, that if a high death rate from diphtheria is reported, a high death rate from croup is also reported.

These investigations lead me to think that if the diseases which we call diphtheria and croup are not identical, they are, at least, apt to prevail at the same time, and in the same localities. No one denies the similarity between croup and laryngeal diphtheria, nor is the contagiousness of diphtheria disputed by any considerable number in the profession.

The very obvious lesson to be drawn from these facts, is that patients suffering from croup should be placed under the same restrictions, as to association, the public attendance upon schools, and disinfection, as are required in patients attacked with diphtheria. Yet in the city of Philadelphia, no such quarantine of croup patients is exacted by the authorities, and some physicians, holding to the dual origin and character of the diseases, deride such a suggestion. May not this very fact account for the long continued epidemic of diphtheria in Philadelphia? The following table shows that for over ten years, the death rate from this cause has been in the hundreds.

Table showing the number of deaths each year from Diphtheria and Croup.

	Diphtheria	Croup.		Diphtheria	Croup.
1872	150	..	1879	321	..
1873	110		1880	523	303
1874	179	..	1881	457	317
1875	652	428	1882	933	466
1876	708	386	1883	1006	500
1877	458	338	1884	680	579
1878	464	388	1885	..	..

I am convinced that one cause of this long continued prevalence of diphtheria is due to carelessness, resulting from the widely spread error, among the laity, that it is not contagious, and to the fact that many cases of laryngeal diphtheria are treated under the name of croup, and no effort made to quarantine the patient. I am an advocate of the best sanitary conditions possible for our great city, clean streets, improved pavements and perfected sewer systems. I want every appliance the ingenuity of man can suggest, to prevent the introduction of the germs of diphtheria into our homes, but I believe that in an effort to stamp out diphtheria, it is more important for us to recognize the fact that this disease is often mistaken for croup, than it is for us to build up the most perfect sewers, or to introduce the most efficient traps and other sanitary apparatus.

The State Board of Health should call special attention to the similarity existing between croup and diphtheria, and urge upon school boards and local health boards the necessity of the closest quarantine in every case of croup.

CANNABIS INDICA.—Officinal preparations of *cannabis indica* are very ineffective compared with the fresh drug. The active principle has not yet been isolated. Cannabin tannate has only a slight hypnotic effect, and *cannabinon*, a resinous kind of substance, cannot be regarded as a hypnotic. A dose of 1½ grains was followed by excitement, then collapse and cramps, then peculiar alternating psychical conditions, but no true sleep.—*Lond. Med. Rec.*, Oct., 1886.

ORIGINAL ARTICLES IN SURGERY.

SUPRA-PUBIC LITHOTOMY.*

By CHARLES MONROE THOMAS, M.D.,

Philadelphia.

THE high operation for stone, though steadily growing in favor for the past few years, has quite recently received a more positive impulse through the publication of a large number of interesting cases at the hands of well-known operators. Indeed, in the light of our present experience, it becomes almost a matter of astonishment that this operation should have so long been kept in comparative obscurity.

Its more extended application may, in this country, at least, be traced to the numerous carefully prepared papers and statistics of Charles W. Dulles, William Tod Helmuth and a few others.

During the past three years, however, by far the largest number of cases have been found in the reports of European surgeons, more particularly those on the Continent of Europe, of which the most prominent are Peterson, Trendelenberg, Bergmann and Guyon, and quite recently in England, Sir Henry Thompson, who speaks highly in its praise, and reports seven cases, with one death.

In a discussion at the Congress of German Surgeons in 1886, on a paper by König, of Göttingen, concerning the choice of stone operation, opinions seemed about equally divided between the median and high method, the lateral operation being advocated by very few. Bergmann, of Berlin, reported nineteen supra-pubic lithotomies with but one death, and that not traceable to the operation itself. Trendelenberg gives ten cases, with one death.

The following is a brief report of my experience with the high operation, covering a period of the past twenty months :

CASE I., æt. 67 years. —A patient of Dr. Curtis, of Wilmington. The high section was done on account of a probable sacculation and large size of the stone. The bladder was washed and distended with weak iodine water. The rectum was not inflated. The incision was completed with no difficulty, and the bladder incised on the beak of the silver catheter, which had been used for the injection, a stout thread having first been passed into the fundus to prevent the viscus from sinking below the pubis. The stone was easily reached with the finger, but dislodged with some difficulty from its bed behind and to the left of the prostate. Delivery was then quickly made with for-

*Read before the Pennsylvania Homœopathic Medical Society, September 23d, 1886.

ceps, though the stone proved to be above the average size, weighing three ounces.

An unsuccessful attempt was made to suture the bladder, owing to the thinness of its walls, and its deep seat below the very fat abdominal parietes. The angles of the skin wound were united for a short distance, and a long, large rubber drain introduced into the interior of the bladder and fixed in position by a single silk stitch to the integument. The bladder was now thoroughly washed out from the urethral side, and the soft catheter used for this purpose left in position *a demeure.* The seat of operation was surrounded by masses of absorbent cotton, and the patient placed on his side with hips somewhat elevated. The wound granulated with no untoward symptoms, though slowly, and leaving a fine fistula, which did not close till several months later.

CASE II., æt. 66 years.—High operation was done at patient's request, there being no contra-indication for the perineal incision, except, perhaps, the presence of a very large, hard prostate. In this case, the patient being thin, the distended bladder could be plainly felt and seen above the pubes before the incision of the integument. No staff or catheter was used as a guide in opening the bladder. The vesical wound was closed with a continuous suture of gut, and the abdominal cut united down to the lower angle, when a thick rubber drain was inserted. Inlying catheter was used. Urine appeared at the wound in thirty-six hours, when all the integument stitches were immediately removed, and the edges allowed to gap. The depths of the wound were now freely injected with iodized water every few hours, and the bladder flushed through the inlying catheter at the same time. The urine ceased to appear at the wound after ten days, and healing was complete in five weeks, with no drawbacks. The rectal distension was used here. The stone of the mixed variety weighed five drachms.

*CASE III., æt. 47 years, was a patient of Drs. Childs and McClelland, of Pittsburgh. The *sectis alta* was chosen on account of deep perineal sinuses, fistulæ, etc. Both rectum and bladder were distended. A silver guttered catheter was introduced as an injector and guide, but not used for latter purpose. The course of the operation presented nothing of special interest. Bladder was closed with a combination of the Lembert and continuous stitch. On the fifth day there was a flow from the wound of a clear odorless fluid, the quantity of which was apparently not influenced by the amount of urine in the bladder. This discharge continued more or less profusely for ten days, without causing any complication. Recovery was complete in four weeks. The weight of the calculus was 200 grains.

CASE IV., æt. 70 years, a patient of Dr. David Gardiner, was very feeble and prostrated by long suffering. Had been bed-ridden for several weeks. Urine loaded with pus and exceedingly offensive. The clarified urine showed albumen and tube casts. There was constant

*Reported in *Hahnemannian Monthly* of April, 1886.

desire to urinate, and almost constant stillicidium. By the use of the syringe the bladder could not be made to hold more than three to four ounces. The stone could be grasped by the lithotrite, but owing to the limited size of the bladder, the idea of lithotrity was abandoned and the high operation chosen. On injecting the bladder, instead of the usual hemispherical tumor appearing back of the pubes, a long ovoid enlargement bulged up beneath the thin abdominal walls, well off in the *right iliac* region. The small bladder could be indistinctly felt below the pubis. On incising the bladder, the walls of which were quite thick, the interior was found very small, and holding a little phosphatic stone which was readily removed. On further exploration, the oval iliac swelling proved to be a long diverticulum connected with the bladder; the opening between the two cavities being only large enough to comfortably admit the index finger. This sac also contained a stone larger than the first. Its removal was attended with much difficulty, owing to the small size of the entrance to the diverticulum, and could only be accomplished by crushing it and flooding out the fragments, with the patient rolled on to his face. The fragments collected from the second stone, also phosphatic, weighed 170 grains, the one taken from the bladder proper, 80 grains.

In this case no effort was made to close the bladder. The after-treatment was essentially the same as in Case I. To my surprise, but little immediate shock followed the operation, and no bad symptoms were apparent for twenty-four hours. From that time, however, till his death on the sixth day, his strength gradually failed—the fatal issue seeming to be due to a simple lack of recuperative power. At no time was there any sign of peritonitis or unfavorable inflammation in the wound, or a decreased action of the kidneys. Autopsy was not obtained.

CASE V., æt. 63 years, had had symptoms of stone with vesical blenorrhœa, for several years, but careful explorations by skillful surgeons, had failed to detect a calculus, previous to his application to me. With a short beaked Teevan explorer, I succeeded in touching the stone far to the right of the prostate; and in no position of the pelvis could it be felt in any other location. The examination, though a cautious one, was followed as on the previous explorations by bloody urine. The discharges from the bladder were, and had long been, purulent and offensive. Suspecting encapsulation the high operation was performed, and the stone found imbedded to the right of and between the prostata. Enucleation and extraction were accomplished with but little difficulty. Both bladder and rectum were distended, but no staff guide employed. No stitches were introduced, excepting at the extreme angles of the abdominal section. After-treatment by long large drain as already described. The inlying catheter, not assisting in the drainage, was removed after twenty-four hours, and only introduced at intervals of four to six hours, for the purpose of washing out the bladder. Recovery was uninterrupted, and the case was dismissed healed in twenty-eight days.

REMARKS.—In none of my cases was the peritoneum seen, though in Case III., in seeking for a reason for the free watery flow from the wound, Dr. McClelland, who conducted the after-treatment, suggests the possibility of an unnoticed small wound of the peritoneum as the source. If the character of the cases and the age of the patients be considered (all except one over sixty years), the loss of one case in the five, may, I think, be looked upon as a very fair, if not unusual showing, for *any* form of lithotomy. Indeed, in Cases I., IV. and V., the completion of the operation by any other method than the supra-pubic would have been a matter of difficulty, if not impossibility. In Case I., the stones would almost certainly have had to be crushed through the wound before extraction by the perineum, and in Case IV. I fail to see how the second stone could have been reached at all by the low operation; and in this instance the fatal result cannot well be traced to the method of operation employed.

In the treatment by the *open method*, I have in each instance found that the inlying catheter was practically useless as a drain to the bladder, and in future I should only introduce it when required to flush the organ, as in Case V. When the bladder suture is employed and the closure complete, the more or less constant use of the catheter is, of course, a necessity, and its action is usually all that could be desired.

While the distension of the rectum no doubt tends distinctly to increase the space for operation, I have found it to decidedly interfere with the extraction of the stone, after the bladder is evacuated of its fluid contents, and have been obliged to let off the water from the rectal colpeurynter as soon as the interior of the bladder was exposed.

When the bladder can be distended, I can see no necessity for the use of a guiding staff or *sond a dart*, and did not employ one after my first case.

It appears to me that one of the most important points in the prevention of urinary infiltration and cellulitis is the avoidance of tearing, bruising, or even much manipulation, or fingering of the fat and connective tissue below the abdominal aponeurosis. Clean cutting is just as clearly called for here as in the overlying tissues, and I cannot but express my surprise at the advice given by Sir Henry Thompson in a recent article, to tear the way to the bladder with the finger-nail, after having passed the muscular aponeurosis.

Whatever may be the scope of supra-pubic lithotomy in the future, it appears to me that it is now certainly called for :

First—When the stone is known to be large, say over an inch and a half in any diameter.

Second—In encysted stones.

Third—In sacculated bladder.

Fourth—In all cases, when the perineal space is decidedly encroached upon by pelvic distortions, tumors, etc.

Fifth—In many cases of prostatic enlargement.

Whether in stones of small or medium size, and in young people it will even supplant the median and lateral operations, is a matter which can only be decided from a very much greater experience with the operation than we at present possess.

In simplicity of execution it will certainly compare favorably with any of the cutting operations. The only element in its execution which may be looked upon as dangerous is the risk of wounding the peritoneum, and experience has shown this to be not a theoretical risk; in fact it is certainly at times bound to happen. Quite recently Sonnenburg and Gussenbaur have each reported a case in which the peritoneum was found close in contact, and even adherent to the pubes. Fortunately, however, as to the danger of this mishap, it may be looked upon as comparatively small, for when it has recurred even to the appearance of the bowels in the wound, the cases have almost invariably recovered.

Rupture of the bladder and rectum from over-distension in the preliminary steps to the cutting, are accidents which, though possible and have happened, are easily avoided with ordinary care.

By far the greater number of fatal cases have been the result of post-pubic cellulitis ; the avoidance and combating of which, form now the all absorbing study with those who are interested in perfecting this operation. Whether it be better to attempt by suturing the bladder to prevent the contact of the urine with the wound, or on the other hand, to leave the bladder entirely open and endeavor to lead the urine immediately from the cavity as it enters, is a question difficult to answer at present, though without doubt the method by suture is the ideal one. The proportion of primary union with the suture, though not large, is still sufficiently great to encourage further efforts in this direction. In a publication of forty-one cases of suture collected by Meyer, of Germany, in 1885, primary union resulted in sixteen ; and since then numerous successes have been published by various operators.

The positive advantages of the high operation over any form of the perineal method are, the small amount of primary hemorrhage with which it is attended compared, at least, with the lateral operation; the fact that each layer of tissue, and even the interior of the bladder, is clearly brought to light as well as to touch, while in all other operations the most important part—the deep incision—must be done out of sight, by the sense of touch alone ; the great facility with which the delivery of the stone can be affected; the avoidance of the well-known evils resulting from interference with the bladder-neck and spermatic vesicles.

In cases of very large stones, impacted stones, or when calculi lie in a diverticulum, the high operation is simply above comparison with any other method. Indeed, it would seem that the reduction of peri-vesical cellulitis to a minimum would be the only thing required to establish this as the universal operation for the extraction of stone by incision.

Since the presentation of this paper to the Society, I have removed by the high section an uric acid stone about an inch in diameter, from the bladder of a boy eight years old, a patient of Dr. Snyder, of Ashland, Pa. In this case I met with my first real difficulty, in having to deal with the *peritoneum in close contact with the pubes.* I was fortunately, however, able to push it up, sufficiently to give room for a free incision of the bladder. The bladder was sutured, and united *per primam.* The parietal incision was lightly tamponed with gauze, which was removed on the third day. The boy was up in seven days, and dismissed on the tenth day after the operation.

TREATMENT OF MASTITIS BY REST AND COMPRESSION.*

By M. BELLE BROWN, M.D.,
New York.

MY attention was drawn to the above method of treatment of inflammation of the breast by an article that appeared in the *Medical Record* a little over a year ago. I am well aware that the treatment of mastitis by pressure made by the roller bandage or adhesive straps has long been practiced by many physicians, but the simplicity and ease of application of the method described in this article, led me, in preference to the other methods of applying pressure, to adopt the one therein described. The development of a case of mastitis from that of engorgement, to redness, tenderness, and induration is so familiar to every obstetrician that I will not occupy your time with its unnecessary description. The chief attention of every physician is directed, in these cases of inflammation of the breast, to the prevention of the formation of abscess. The uniform good results that were obtained in the treatment of four cases that came under my care

*Read before the Homœopathic Medical Society County of New York, October, 1886.

during the past year have led me to call your attention to this simple and easy method of applying pressure and averting this troublesome complication. It may be possible that no abscesses would have occurred under any treatment in these cases, and the number is a small one for positive data, but from the fact that they did *not* occur, and one was a case where the woman was scrofulous and said she was subject to "all sorts of gatherings," and whose mastitis was caused by the death of her child, presumably from unhealthy taint, the results are sufficiently good to record in favor of the treatment.

Rest and *Compression.* By rest is meant freedom from rubbing and all unnecessary handling by meddlesome nurses, and nursing; and by compression, equable pressure made over the entire gland by a sufficiently wide bandage passed around the thorax.

I cannot give a better description of applying the bandage than to quote from the article referred to.

The method is as follows: "A piece of strong muslin is used, fourteen or sixteen inches in width, and of sufficient length to reach around the thorax and overlap a few inches. The patient lies on her back with the arms elevated so as to clasp the hands above the head, thus drawing the axillæ well upward. One end of the muslin is slipped through beneath the patient, and the two ends made to overlap exactly as in the application of an abdominal binder. A pad of cotton wadding is placed between the breasts to serve as counter-pressure. The breasts are then pressed upward and toward the sternum by an assistant, and the muslin fastened by pins, which are placed along the middle line about three-quarters of an inch apart. As the pins are put in place, the bandage is drawn tense by about all the force one can comfortably exert through his arms. When the bandage has been fastened, proceeding in this way from above downward, it will usually be found that its upper part is comparatively loose, and a few pins should be removed and reapplied. The bandage should be brought well up against the axillæ, and thus the upper part of the breast will all be included within it. When it is in place a small wad of cotton should be tucked in beneath the folds of the axillæ, above the bandage. This will relieve all feeling of irritation in that location. A strap of muslin may be passed over each shoulder and pinned to the upper edge of the bandage before and behind. This will prevent it from slipping down. All parts of the breasts should be subjected to pressure, for if this be not done, signs of inflammation will appear in the part not compressed. The bandage having been once applied need not be removed until the unpleasant symptoms are entirely gone, but may be tightened as the diminishing size of the breasts will permit.

If only one breast is affected a small hole should be cut with the scissors over the nipple of the sound side, and the child allowed to nurse this breast." The patients on whom I applied the bandage in this way all complained of increased pain and discomfort for several hours, but after that, and at each subsequent tightening they never failed to speak of the relief. An early application of the bandage, before extensive exudation has taken place, will greatly lessen the liability to abcess. Two of the cases received medicine, one *bryonia* and the other *belladonna*, and two of them received none. Those that had no medicine did as well as those that had, thus giving the pre-eminence to the bandage.

THE APPLICATION OF THE PRINCIPLES OF HOMŒOPATHY TO ABDOMINAL SURGERY.*

By B. F. BETTS, M.D.,
Philadelphia.

WHILST the application of the principles of Listerism to abdominal surgery has made it possible to accomplish marvelous results, surgeons are not entirely satisfied, and are striving after improved methods of treatment, in order to protect their patients still more effectually, from the dangers which supervene upon abdominal section. Some of the most successful have discarded the use of germicidal agents, and rely exclusively upon cleanliness as the best safeguard against infection during an operation, and as but little reliance can be placed in the efficacy of opium, quinine or digitalis to combat inflammation, but little medicine is used, either in the preparatory or after treatment of these cases. I have never felt that we were inconsistent or debarred by our faith in homœopathy, from applying the best known principles and practices of surgery, as common property, to strictly operative cases, which are not amenable to medical treatment, yet I rejoice to see that the path which such earnest seekers after truth as Tait, Keith and Bantock have pointed out, enables us to reach a position from which it is possible to apply the principles of our school to abdominal surgery. The attempt to overcome the effects of uncleanliness by the use of a strong germaciticide has always appeared to me like giving powerful medicine to an unfortunate ididvidual in order to keep him from getting sick. The system already impressed by the disease influence, is unable to cope with the additional burden, when it might have been otherwise victorious in the struggle. Yet I have formerly used and still employ antiseptic solutions, when I can-

*Read before the Pennsylvania Homœopathic Medical Society, Sept. 23d, 1886.

not secure perfect cleanliness ; but what I desire is, that we should strive after cleanliness without the necessity for the employment of germicidal solutions within the peritoneal cavity. We can do this better in private hospitals, located and fitted up with proper regard to the sanitary requirements necessary for such cases, than in large public hospitals, contaminated by a vitiated atmosphere.

The toxic effect of germicidal solutions must weigh against the recovery of the patient, and more so in some cases than in others ; and in estimating the amount of strength of the solution that is required in a particular case, to act as a germ destroyer, the susceptibility or idiosyncracy of the patient is not and cannot be taken into account.

This peculiar susceptibility of some patients is strikingly illustrated in the cases of corrosive sublimate poisoning that have been recently reported. Over thirty fatal results from its employment have been published, and it is likely that they represent but a small proportion of the number that have been seriously affected but not published.

Nine deaths have occurred from the use of the solution injected into the vagina or uterus, and one fatal result followed the employment of a *weak* solution as an injection into the vaginal passage. How much more fatal must be the results, should the solution, strong enough to be of use as an antiseptic or a germicidal agent, be unwisely used within the peritoneal cavity during laparotomies.

The carbolic acid solutions are known to interfere with the eliminative action of the kidneys in some cases, and thus endanger recovery, as it is upon a proper action of the emunctories that we must place our main dependence after an abnominal section.

If I have a tumor to remove, the time to operate is not fixed by the size of the mass or the amount of inconvenience it causes the patient, as much as it is by the answer I can give to the question : Is it likely that there will be a time when the action of the patient's skin, kidneys, and intestinal tract will be more satisfactory than at present? The probable result is estimated with far greater accuracy by a knowledge of the general condition of the patient than by the size and condition of the tumor.

With *sulph.*, *lyc.*, *nux vom.*, *bell.*, *sepia*, etc., we are often able to improve this condition, especially if attention is paid to diet, bathing, inunction, etc., until the skin becomes pliable, the urine clearer and the bowels more healthy in their action.

It is considered good practice to proceed with an operation for the extraction of a tumor, whenever it is involved by serious inflammation, for inasmuch as the tumor requires removal at any rate, and peritonitis is as likely to subside after an antiseptic operation as without it, delay only permits the formation of new inflammatory adhesions, to complicate future efforts at extraction, when the patient's life must be again jeopardized. Yet there are times when we cannot proceed with the operation and do it satisfactorily, at such short notice.

Mrs. R. W. P. applied for treatment in July last. She was extremely weak in consequence of loss of rest and profuse menses, and suffered from such marked cerebral anæmia as to cause her to appear confused from the slightest excitement, and she was unable to understand what was said to her or what she read at times : with ringing noises in the head, etc. I diagnosed a cystic tumor of the uterus, with lax attachments. In consequence of over-exertion, within a few days, acute inflammatory symptoms, with a temperature ranging from 103° to 105°, supervened. Her sufferings were intense. The weather was very warm, but as her surroundings were favorable, an immediate operation was proposed. In a short time the extreme pain and acute symptoms were subdued by means of *bell.*, and delay was asked for by her friends until the patient's anæmic condition should improve and arrangements be made for her care and treatment. Since then the anæmia has disappeared under the influence of *china*, and she is feeling better than she has been for a long time ; but of course the tumor remains the same, and is to be operated on soon.

With strict attention to the minutest details in cleanliness, almost any organ of the body may be fearlessly attacked, not excepting the liver, or even the brain, for the system will accommodate itself to severe mutilation without serious inconvenience or delay. The instruments used need not be numerous, and the selection of those that are simple and uncomplicated in their construction is desirable.

Silk-worm gut, immersed in carbolic acid and then washed off in pure dilute alcohol, and kept immersed in the latter fluid until used, along with the needles, answers a good purpose for closing the abdominal incision, after laparotomy. Likewise, the ligatures for the pedicle should be kept immersed in pure water or alcohol until used. Sponges can be cleaned in pure boiled water, for both carbolic and sublimate solutions deprive the peritoneal layer of some of its epithelial covering, hence conduce to the formation of those adhesions between the opposite and contiguous surfaces, which lead to fatal results in some cases.

In the following case carbolic solutions were used :

Mrs. E., æt. 44 years, patient of Dr. E. C. Rembaugh, of this City, did very well after an ovariotomy, on March 9th, 1885, until the 16th, when the sutures were removed from the abdominal incision, and the usual tight dressing was reapplied about the abdomen. Deep-seated pain in the abdomen, with vomiting and obstinate constipation, supervened, until the bowels were moved with an explosive sound within the abdomen, as from the sudden liberation of pent-up accumulations above an occlusion of the intestinal tract. The urine became more scanty ; slimy stools were passed devoid of feces, and the patient succumbed on the 19th. With the experience of the present, the abdominal bandage would have been loosened after the third or fourth day, the bowels moved by enemas of flax and tea, and opium dispensed with entirely, if it were possible to do so.

Great care is needed in the use of sponges within the cavity of the abdomen during an operation, that they do not fret and erode the peritoneum unnecessarily. Such eroded surfaces are very apt to adhere, especially if opium is administered in quantities sufficient to diminish the peristaltic action of the bowels. *Nux vom.*, *bry.* or *sulph.*, by promoting peristalsis, may prove much more beneficial to our patients.

Mrs. R., a patient of Dr. Langer, of this City, was first seen in consultation in July of last year. She suffered from the most intense abdominal pain, with sleeplessness, inability to lie down, and great abdominal soreness. For several years subsequent to the birth of her child, eleven years before, the menses had entirely ceased for three or four months at a time. Recently they had become more regular, but at each period her sufferings were very much intensified. On an examination, an ovarian cyst was found on the right side of the uterus, which deflected the fundus to the left side of the pelvis, and another cyst was found in close proximity to the fundus, but back of it. At the operation, the pedicle of the first tumor was found to consist of the left broad ligament, considerably elongated, whilst the other tumor with a short pedicle had developed from the right ovary. The impaction of the tumors with the uterus accounted for the intense suffering this patient endured for so long a time.

The fluid from the larger cyst was dark, as was also the cyst wall, but devoid of offensive odor. That from the small cyst, which had a very short pedicle, was thicker and of the peculiar pea soup appearance, so often seen when ovarian cysts are evacuated before degenerative changes have taken place from a constriction of the pedicle. This patient had become so accustomed to the use of large doses of morphine that it seemed to have no effect in quieting her after the operation or inducing sleep. It was inert, or worse than useless even, in doses of a grain at a time, for it made her crazy. Diarrhœa set in on the third day, which *rhus* controlled very nicely, and *bell.* given at night enabled her to get a little rest. Under its influence the skin became more active and the urine more copious, and through the whole treatment the kidneys and skin never failed to perform their functional actions satisfactorily. She sat up on the fourteenth day, but it was a long time before she regained control of her nervous system. But it is from the experience of writers, the best part of whose lives has been especially devoted to this work, more than that of my own, that I am led to conclude that there is ground for the belief that the principles of homœopathy can be successfully applied to abdominal surgery.

One of the most successful ovariotomists in the Dominion of Can ada recently declared that after an operation he needed no medicine except when there was vomiting, when he directed the patient to sip hot water, or prescribed *ipecacuanha* in homœopathic doses, preferring the third dilution. He also states that before an operation he avoids purgatives as much as possible. It is by attention to these little details that we turn the balance for or against successful results in many instances. And the truth always leads its votaries to tread a similiar pathway.

———————

MR. PITHIE, Assistant House-Surgeon in the Greenock Infirmary, describes, in the *British Medical Journal*, October 16th, the results of a disaster occurring in the Crarae Quarries, Lochfyneside. "These quarries," he says, "are situated on the side of a hill, and form a large bowl with only a narrow entrance. After an explosion of seven tons of gunpowder, a party of excursionists entered the quarries, but no sooner had they reached the bowl, than they began to stagger and fall in all directions. They all had symptoms of narcotic poisoning, and several died."

———————

THE FIRST EXCISION OF THE SPLEEN IN SPAIN.—Senor Don Dr. Ribera recently performed excision of the spleen on a boy of ten in the Hospital del Niño Jesus in Madrid. This is the first time the operation has been performed in Spain, and unfortunately was followed by a fatal result the next day from shock. Immediately after the operation cyncope came on, and it was with considerable difficulty that the child was revived. It was remarked that the operating theatre, although in one of the most important hospitals in the Spanish metropolis, was badly lighted, and unprovided with a subcutaneous syringe for injecting ether or with a faradisation instrument.—*London Lancet*, December 4th, 1886.

———————

RATIONAL SLEEPING.—Dr. Menli-Hilty proposes to abandon the usual position of sleeping, and to sleep with the head lower than the feet. The habit is to be acquired gradually, and the author claims that it will result in a stimulated and improved circulation, with better nutrition of brain and nerves. Undue congestion of the brain is not to be apprehended, for the typhoid gland acts as a regulator of the distributed blood. The author recommends that the foot of the bed be raised eight inches. He recommends the method as an aid in the treatment of nervous disorders especially depending on anæmia of brain and cord, in infantile chorea epilepsy, mental affections in the first stage of pulmonary diseases, in bronchitis, nausea of pregnancy, varicocele; also in vesical and uterine complaints, hernia, cardiac diseases, and as a preventive against apoplexy.—From *Arch. f. Gesammte Physiologie* and *Lond. Med. Rec.*, October, 1886.

EDITORIAL DEPARTMENT.

The Editors individually assume full responsibility for and are to be credited with all connected with the collection and presentation of matter in their respective departments, but are not responsible for the opinions of contributors.

It is understood that manuscripts sent for consideration have not been previously published, and that after notice of acceptance has been given, will not appear elsewhere except in abstract and with credit to THE NORTH AMERICAN. All rejected manuscripts will be returned to writers. No anonymous or discourteous communications will be printed.

Contributors are respectfully requested to send manuscripts and communicate respecting them directly with the Editors, according to subject, as follows: *Concerning Medicine, 21 West 37th Street; concerning Surgery, 256 West 57th Street; concerning Societies and Hospitals, 121 East 70th Street; concerning News, Personals and Original Miscellany, 461 West 71st Street; concerning Correspondence, 152 West 57th Street.*

Communications to the Editor-in-Chief, *Exchanges* and *New Books* for notice should be addressed to *102 West 43d Street.*

NATURALISTS AND PHYSICIANS.

"**B**ROUSSAIS remarked that 'the real physician is the one who cures; the observation which does not teach the art of healing is not that of a physician, it is that of a naturalist.' There is a wholesome truth in this observation which it would be well for the faculties of our colleges, as well as for those who consider themselves eminently scientific practitioners, to take to heart, and it is this: That neither anatomy nor physiology nor a knowledge of the causes and effects and natural history of disease, neither the botany nor the chemistry of medicaments, nor even skill in diagnosis can make them a master of the art of healing. They constitute the essential equipment of a physician; they do not make him a physician. They define the objects of his craft and fix the limits of its possibilities. He would, to be sure, be helpless without them, but he is worse than helpless with them until he has learned how to use them, how to construct out of them the special art which enables him to cure disease.

"To a certain extent, the tendency of pure pathology has been to diminish faith and create scepticism in the possibilities of therapeutics. It is a common reproach to the teachers of the theory and practice of medicine, that they spend much time and pains in describing the lesions and natural history of diseases, and dismiss the principles and means of cure with few and distrustful words. The reason of this is that pathology only furnishes the object to therapeutics—it does not properly embrace or direct it. The pathologist is essentially a naturalist. He investigates the causes and effects of disease, its onset, progress and terminations. There is nothing, necessarily, in all this that suggests the means of cure. But since pathology has cleared the way, since it has defined and differentiated the effects of many similar causes, and the many causes of similar effects, the progress of the therapeutical art shows that the narrow limitations within which a simple knowledge of pathology would confine the possibilities and means of cure are being constantly enlarged by the independent experimental study of the action of remedial agents."

The preceding quotation we have taken from the late address before the New York Academy of Medicine, delivered by Dr. William H. Draper. Coming from a highly representative physician of the old school, who was introduced as a gentleman " known to erudite men of all classes as a scholar, to his professional brethren as a learned physician, and to his numerous admirers among the public at large as a consummate practitioner," it speaks with authority upon a subject which is of even more vital interest to physicians of the new school. In older physic it notes a period of beginning emergence from the thraldom of pathology over therapeutics. To the adherents of newer physic it serves as a warning to continue their "independent experimental study of the action of remedial agents." Although Hahnemann, nearly one hundred years ago, showed what Dr. Draper now further says, " how the art of healing grows through experimental methods of its own, and how pathology, for the most part, furnishes the objects to therapeutics, and, so to speak, gives the terms of the problems which observation and experiment have to solve," his followers, in the year 1886, have been tending more to the study of medicine, as naturalists, than as pursuers of the art of healing through experimental methods of their own. A glance over the field of work, as shown in our literature during the past year, teaches that now, more than ever, is it necessary to iterate and reiterate the wholesome truths that "pathology does not properly embrace or direct therapeutics;" that " the art of therapeutics has an independent growth of its own,

based upon the experimental study of the effects of remedies;" that
"the art of healing owes its greatest achievements to inductive
methods, " and that only by following induction from independent
experiment can there be an assured future for our true science and art
of healing by the use of drugs.   Standing upon the threshold of a new
year of hope and work, there can be no better guide for us, as a
school, than to bear in mind Dr. Draper's forcible statement of the
logical relation of pathology to the healing art.   The distinction is as
old as Hahnemann, to be sure, but it needs, just now, to be distinctly
realized.   Our own advance will be more conspicuous if we recognize
that, on the one hand, pathology ought not to be undervalued as a
means of making our ends definite and precise, and that, on the other,
it ought not, by undue attention, usurp the very ends for which we
profess to be homœopathic physicians.   And, as a therapeutic school,
we ought steadily to work along the line of therapeutic induction,
according to the rules of therapeutic science, keeping pathology
strictly subordinate to the purpose of homœopathic science, which is
no science at all if not inductive.

Inferring from Dr. Draper's address in full, to which we can give
no more than passing attention, we find much to indicate that homœopathy has accomplished a great mission in the art of healing.   We
have proven, by successful competition, that "the scientific practitioner of the present is often a very poor doctor, and the pure arts-
man, as Plato calls him, may be a very successful one."
More than expectant treatment, which owes its trial indirectly to
homœopathy, by practical abstention and negation we have "exposed
many fallacies, dispelled many delusions, spared much needless
suffering, and saved many lives."   The old traditions of therapeutics
have been exploded, not so much by "revelations in the etiology of
disease and the more exact methods of diagnosis," as by their apparent absurdity, as demonstrated through the practical abandonment of
them by Hahnemann and his followers.   Much longer ago than Dr.
Draper's advent into the world, did Hahnemann, in substance say,
that "polypharmacy is following its victims to the grave, and the test
of a sure aim and intelligent purpose is slowly but surely taking the
place of random shots at imaginary foes."   And now, in these modern

times, when a consummate practitioner and learned physician of the "regular" system of therapeutics confesses that "the art of healing is to-day as empirical an art as it has ever been, but that with the advancing knowledge of disease the empiricism of therapeutics has become more scientific," homœopathy's mission is not yet ended. It needs to adhere still more strictly to the inductive method, not of scientific empiricism, but of its own science and art of therapeutics, to establish still more irrefragably the facts of pure drug experiments, and to faithfully verify our principle, by which, linking together the truly known effects of drugs and the truly observed facts of disease, our aims will become still surer and our purpose even more intelligent. If advance in homœopathic therapeutics can keep even pace with homœopathic progress in material prosperity, there need be no anxiety about the medical system of the future.

NEW YORK SOCIETY WORK.

THAT the interest manifested in societies is a measure of a medical man's interest in his own progress and that of his profession, is one of those truths which go without saying. Attending society meetings, and giving thought as to how societies may be made most effective, however, are more honored in the breach than in the observance, by the majority of medical men. Hence it usually happens that societies gravitate to the management of the few who often have a greater love for power and honor than for the advancement of medical interests, as a whole. The result is that societies have their flow and ebb of usefulness, depending upon the popularity, the earnestness, and the sagacity of the leaders who happen to be in the front. The problem of organizing a society so that personal ambition may be invited, and yet so controlled that only the fittest for engaging and directing the energies of the body of members, for the best results, may rise to the management, does not, as a rule, receive the consideration which the importance of the solution deserves. It is a lamentable observation that societies, like machines, are specially liable to get out of gear.

The history of our New York County Society has been an illustration of the above general observations. It has flowed some at times, and ebbed a great deal at others. Fortunately, of late it has been steadily reaching a flood-tide, and has fairly broken down the barriers of apathy and discontent which have hemmed in its usefulness. Its dignity, as the most numerous body of homœopathic physicians meeting frequently, in the world, is becoming appreciated, and something of a conception of the part which it can and ought to play in the scientific development of homœopathy and in promoting *esprit de corps* is dawning. The plan of vesting the duty of directing in an executive board, the individual members of which lose eligibility for future office from lack of attendance upon its meetings, has resulted not only in quickening interest and developing wiser deliberation, but also in selecting promptly efficient officers. The society has evidently entered upon a higher career of activity which, it is to be hoped, will draw some of the members more frequently from the seclusion of their social clubs to a place where their lights may be seen more by the profession. That it may incite and train good workers, restrain bad workers, and "frame, for the guidance of all alike, a standard of work which will elevate and benefit our art," is the heartiest good-will we can express.

The Society for Medico-Scientific Investigation is another example of well-constructed society machinery. Composed mainly of younger men, through its executive organization it has stimulated effort for the higher class of work. While its ardor for collective investigation has been dampened by a realization of the labor involved in it, which its original study of Hoang-Nan has revealed, it has, nevertheless, called out good individual papers, collected a library, and is on the way to accomplish substantial results in our experimental knowledge of drugs. We look in 1887 for those fruits of original investigation, expressed in the name of the society.

SINGLE EXAMINING BOARDS.

WE regret that the press upon our space will not permit the publication in full of the cogent statement of the Committee on Legislation of the New York State Homœopathic Medical Society. Its reasons for opposing a single State Examining Board should be widely known, in view of the fact that there is a systematic plan throughout the country of getting control of homœopathy through single old school boards of examiners. Homœopathic objections to the scheme are well summed up in the first reason stated : "That the creation of such a board would practically establish a *permanent and powerful medical monopoly* of the licensing franchise, under the immediate control of *one* school of medicine, thereby constituting an exceedingly objectionable form of *class legislation.*" How this would necessarily follow appears clear immediately upon the reading of the explanatory reasons which succeed in logical chain. Our readers are referred for the full text of the Committee's statement to the *Physician's and Surgeon's Investigator* for November, 1886, and to pamphlet reprints.

OUR LOSS IN DR. LIEBOLD.

THE just and true tributes to the memory of Dr. Liebold, paid elsewhere in our columns, can have nothing added to make them more fitting. A loss, not perhaps sufficiently dwelt upon, however, was his knowledge of the application of remedies for the cure of diseases of the eye and ear. Unexcelled as he was as an ophthalmic surgeon, he was *facile princeps* in the art of the physician, in exalting the conservative restoration of medicine before resort to the mutilating and more mechanic art. Only a few weeks before his death, he expressed his still deeper conviction of the truth of the law of homœopathy, and counselled close study of the homœopathic materia medica as the surest way to clinical success. That he had a great store of original information in the homœopathic use of drugs, the product of thorough research, profound thought and extended clinical trial, which has been puffed out like the flame of a candle, is the least consoling reflection in the general sorrow that s̄ felt. Doubtless he had his purpose of putting it in form for survival, but living in and for his work, as he did, the greatest regret must be that, save a few fragments, his work cannot live in our literature.

COMMENTS.

ABUSE OF MEDICAL CHARITY.—Charity reform in the City of New York seems to be progressing backward. Notwithstanding the fact that there are now over forty free dispensaries, in which are treated annually over one-fourth of the population, yet the number of dispensaries is continually increasing. In the earlier days these institutions afforded a wonderful relief to the deserving and suffering poor. Founded in the name and for the sake of true charity, they abounded in good works and gained a merited reputation for genuine benevolence. It was not the custom then to measure the good accomplished by the total number of patients treated in a year, regardless of their condition and necessities. Nor was it thought best then to establish dispensaries simply to benefit colleges, honor hospitals, or glorify particular physicians. There was some attempt made to discriminate between the poor and those who dishonestly endeavored to obtain gratuitous treatment. Cases were investigated and assistance given only where it was deserved. But in these later years a different spirit reigns. That which was originally given for the benefit of the really destitute has been misused and perverted. It is known that fully two-thirds of the patients treated at the dispensaries are able to pay a physician. No investigation of cases is made, but prescriptions are written and medicines given alike to the poor and the rich, the just and the unjust. Managers of hospitals use them to swell the number of patients treated; physicians strive to increase the number that attend their respective clinics; colleges, greedily welcome all who come that they may advertise the abundant material for the use of students. And so this present system, resulting in hypocrisy and continued for gain, besmirches the fair fame of charity, lowers professional standards, fosters medical pauperism, defrauds the younger practicing physicians and makes the very name dispensary a by-word and reproach. The Presbyterian hospital has just decided that it must have an "Out Patient Department." That means, of course, another needless dispensary. No one wants it except the managers of the hospital. Several large and well equipped dispensaries are within a few blocks, and the poor connected with the hospital are already amply cared for. It is evident that the dispensary is simply to act as a "supply" to the hospital, swell its list of patients and enable it to demand larger contributions. If people contributing to the support of some of these institutions were made aware of the perverted use of funds their donations would suddenly cease. It is to be hoped that professional sentiment on this matter will find expression in such a way as to compel a reform. Toleration of abuses has a limit. The man who weakly tolerates a known and flagrant abuse is nearly as guilty as he who commits it.

ALLOPATHIC THERAPEUTIC INSPIRATION.—The *Medical World* has just discovered that *thuja occidentalis* is credited with the remarkable property of causing the disappearance, in a very short time, of all kinds of vegetative and warty growths by its internal administration. For many years this drug has been known and used by the new school. Our "friends the enemy" are only half a century behind in finding out the therapeutical virtues of thuja. The *British Medical Journal* has also contributed its mite to the materia medica. It has found that *liquor hydrargyri perchlor.* is of great use in a diarrhœa of children characterized by frequent watery offensive stools. The writer, Dr. Millard, says : "When the stools are slimy with, it may be, blood streaks, I give liquor hydrargyri perchloridi, 2½ꝫ in two ounces of water, of which a teaspoonful every hour meets the case." In another issue he says : "I did not obtain my information from Dr. Ringer's excellent work but from probably the same source that Dr. Ringer obtained his, of which, to any one that knows, the book contains many traces, *vis.*: from homœopathic treatises." Verily the dry bones are beginning to rattle. Many other so-called discoveries have been made—a long list—all surreptitiously taken from new school literature. The literary thief finds a brother in the medical pirate. Both appropriate the property of others ; both deny the theft and brazenly offer the stolen matter as their own ; both resort to vituperation and slander when exposed, and both receive equal condemnation. The policy of denouncing homœopathy on the one hand, while stealing its methods on the other, does not commend itself as either manly or honest. Our old school brethren in this regard are rapidly getting themselves in that pleasing position popularly known as "between the devil and the deep sea." Adepts as they are at squirming, it is hardly possible for them to wriggle out of this.

A NEW HOSPITAL.—The announcement is made that the authorities of the San Francisco Hahnemann Medical College have secured a suitable building which will be opened at once as a homœopathic hospital. Our friends on the Pacific coast are certainly not laggards. The college is on a solid basis and doing excellent work, and homœopathy is progressing rapidly.

BOOK REVIEWS.

RHEUMATISM : ITS NATURE, ITS PATHOLOGY, AND ITS SUCCESSFUL TREATMENT, by T. J. MacLagan, M.D. Octavo. Illustrated. Vol. IX. of "Wood's Library of Standard Medical Authors" for 1886. New York : Wm. Wood & Co. Pp., 285.

The object of this work is to place rheumatism, its nature and pathology upon a new basis. The treatment was introduced to the profession by the author in 1876, about the same time that German authorities began to advocate a similar course. The author first discusses the varieties, symptoms, duration and seat of rheumatism, devoting several pages to proving its favorite site to be those white fibrous structures of the joints and heart which are subjected to the

greatest mechanical strain,—a point which might be conceded without much argument. The lactic acid theory of the disease is next
discussed, to be condemned mainly upon *a priori* grounds. The
author admits that lactic acid is capable of causing the symptoms peculiar to rheumatism, but holds that it is a product which, while it
may excite the symptoms, is merely co-existent and dependent upon
the action of the real *materies morbi.* His ideas upon this point seem
a trifle involved. Then, upon an analogy between rheumatism and
intermittent fever, which should be equally applicable and quite as
forcible, if the author were endeavoring to prove the intimate relationship of any other two diseases, as, for example, pneumonia or
phthisis and malarial fever, because simply the features common to
nearly all diseased conditions are cited, the author proves conclusively, to his own mind, that rheumatism is a miasmatic disease and dependent upon a miasmatic organism which constitutes the real
materies morbi. The reasoning is as follows : Rheumatism has certain
general analogies to malarial fever ; cinchona compounds cure malarial fever ; salicyl compounds cure rheumatism (the author later,
from his deduced analogy between malarial fever and rheumatism,
concludes that salicin is a germicide) ; therefore rheumatism is malarial in its nature and origin. No clinical facts, experimental proof or
microscopic investigation are adduced to prove the theory. It rests
simply upon an almost puerile analogy and an exuberance of
a priori reasoning.

The stilted explanations and grotesque cut which are necessary to
make the facts fit accurately upon this novel theory is, to say the least,
remarkable. Writers should appreciate that what the medical profession of to-day demands in support of new theories is facts which
have been demonstrated by scientific and original investigation, and
not nicely-elaborated, *a priori* reasonings. Especially should the
old logical fallacy of *circulus in probando* be excluded from forming any
portion of our deductions.

Those chapters which treat of the pathology and general features of
rheumatism, irrespective of the miasmatic theory, are well written and
instructive. We also highly commend the tabulated statement of the
salient points of chapters, and what is to be and has been proved.

In the treatment the author reviews the methods from Sydenham,
in 1666, to the present ; presenting that by venesection, purgatives,
diaphoretics, opium, cinchona, alkalies and, lastly, the salicyl treatment, which he advocates. His plan is to give from ten to thirty
grains of salicin every hour or two hours until the acute pain has subsided, when the dose is to be reduced. The attempt to prove that
salicyl compounds exercise a prophylactic influence over cardiac
complications, in the face of the acknowledgment that such complications do not infrequently occur several days after the treatment has
been effectively started, and the joint inflammation controlled, can
be regarded only as a species of mental gymnastics.

However, if the salicyl treatment will accomplish what the author
claims, the medical profession will be indebted to the author for
his exposition. While the work can scarcely claim to be scientific, it
is certainly interesting in its suggestions.   F.

A TREATISE ON ELECTROLYSIS AND ITS APPLICATIONS TO THERAPEUTICAL AND SURGICAL TREATMENT IN DISEASE, by ROBERT AMORY, A.M., M.D., Fellow of Mass. Med. Society, American Academy of Arts and Sciences, etc., etc. New York : Wm. Wood & Co., Standard Library, 1886.

This is the most complete work on electrolysis that has ever come to our notice. In fact, covering the ground so thoroughly, it would seem that there is nothing left to be said on the subject. The chapter on "The Physics of Electrolysis" comprises all the most recent researches on that subject. The chapters on "The Batteries for Electrolysis" and "Resistance and Diffusion of Electricity" are not only useful to one who practices electrolysis, but to all practicing electro-therapeutics in any form. After the author has devoted considerable space to the destruction of living tissue by electrolysis, he proceeds to treat individually the different diseases for which it is useful, as follows : First, the methods of its application; second, the results which take place in successful operations, describing minutely those which occur in different forms of the same disease; and third, the complications and sequelæ which are liable to arise, and how they should be guarded against.

In fact, the physician who has read this book and thoroughly digested its contents will be capable of successfully practicing electrolysis, and any physician doing such a practice should not be without it.   K.

HANDBOOK OF PRACTICAL MEDICINE, by DR. HERMANN EICHORST. Volume III. Diseases of the Nerves, Muscles and Skin. 157 engravings. Standard Library. Wm. Wood & Co., New York, 1886. Octavo. Pp., 390.

The previous general opinion of Vols. I. and II. is sustained by an examination of the present volume. The manual is compact, well illustrated and valuable for "cramming" and for reference. Its information is exact, full and advanced, the work being preëminently one of facts didactically presented. The treatment is authoritatively laid down and is empirically dogmatic.

THE PHYSICIAN'S VISITING LIST FOR 1887 (36th year). Philadelphia : P. Blakiston, Son & Co.

This handy and well-known pocket book suffices for twenty-five patients per week. It contains a dose table, new remedies for 1886-1887, and other useful information. Its arrangement makes it very convenient, and its size does not bulge the pocket.

CORRESPONDENCE.

HOMŒOPATHY IN ENGLAND.

To the Editor of the NORTH AMERICAN JOURNAL OF HOMŒOPATHY :

The year 1886 is rapidly drawing to a close ; another Christmas day will soon be upon us, and then, after expressing our good wishes for our friends, the New Year will presently open, and again we must " buckle to," and with as much energy and ability as God has given us proceed in the performance of the active duties of life. In medicine, especially in therapeutics, and, above all, in homœopathic therapeutics, these duties are numerous, important and absorbing. To know that homœopathy is true, that it is a life-saving, life-prolonging and illness-shortening truth is a great responsibility. To know that there are thousands of medical prac- titioners around us who, for want of a knowledge of homœopathy, are do- ing infinitely less good to the sick who go to them for relief from the suf- ferings entailed by disease, than they might do did they but appreciate and understand the only way in which medicines can be prescibed in order that the sick may derive the *maximum* of advantage from them ; to know, also, that there are physicians who, for lack of this knowledge, are daily meéting with disappointments and anxieties that ultimately disgust them with the practice of medicine, ought to stimulate us to greater exertions than we have ever yet made to spread a knowledge of the therapeutics originated by Hahnemann and developed by him to so considerable a de- dree of perfection. How to get at these practitioners ; how to induce them to enquire what homœopathy is ; how to persuade them to test its value at the bedside, is a difficulty which has been but partially, very partially, in- deed, surmounted. One more effort is about to be made here ere 1886 has quite passed into history. The twenty-five-guinea prize offered by Major Vaughan-Morgan, the Chairman of the London Homœopathic Hospital, for the best Essay on Homœopathy, has been awarded to Dr. John Davey Hayward, the eldest son of Dr. Hayward of Liverpool, who visited the United States at the first International Homœopathic Conven- tion in 1876. It is now published, and, within a few days, a copy will be posted to every physician and surgeon in the country. Thirteen essays were sent in for the competition, and there was no doubt in the minds of all the adjudicators that the one bearing the motto which, on opening the sealed envelope accompanying the essay, proved to be that adopted by Dr. J. D. Hayward, was far and away the best. In the phraseology of the turf, he " won in a canter, hands down, by several lengths." This pamphlet is as good a presentment of the case for homœopathy as I have seen, and, indeed, better than almost any I remember reading. It will, as I have written, be placed before the entire medical profession in this country within a very short time. What influence it will have it is impossible to say ; whether it will exert any at all is, I am afraid, somewhat doubtful.

The practice of medicine upon the old lines is so much more easy, so much more showy, so much more lucrative than is that arising from homœopathy, that I must confess I do not feel very sanguine as to any great results being achieved by it. That it will have some influence, I do look for ; and, as the perpetual dropping of water will wear through a stone at last, so continually pegging away, never losing an opportunity of demonstrating the uncertainties of habitual prescribing, of pointing out the therapeutic weakness of the teachings of the schools and of setting forth the control, little short of marvellous, which a medicine selected by the method of Hahnemann has upon disease, will eventually make homœopathy the basis of drug-therapeutics throughout the profession. The only danger in front is that of our becoming wearied of " pegging away;" of any of us yielding to the very natural disappointment consequent on seeing the practice arising out of Hahnemann's teaching adopted *en détaille,* instead of the doctrine and materia medica being accepted *en bloc* by the heirs of those who have denounced both the practice and teaching with so much vehemence and persistency throughout the century. *L'homme propose mais c'est le Dieu que dispose.* I for one, cannot believe that such appropriations as have been made from practical homœopathy by Ringer, Brunton, and many others, can be continually repeated without leading intelligent men to homœopathy. For example, Dr. Millard, of Edinburgh, sent a communication to the *British Medical Journal,* lately, testifying to the value of *Liquor Hydrargyri perchlor.* in a certain form of diarrhœa in infants. Dr. Macdonald, of Liverpool, in a letter confirming, from his experience, the observation of Dr. Millard, hinted that the latter had, as he had, derived the " tip " from Ringer. Dr. Millard replied : " I did not obtain my information of the use of *hydrarg. perchlor.* from Dr. Ringer's excellent work, as Dr. Macdonald supposes, but from probably the same source that Dr. Ringer obtained his, of which, to any one who knows, the book contains many traces, *viz.:* from homœopathic treatises." I believe that Ringer and Brunton and men " of that ilk," have done really good work for therapeutics. I wouldn't have done the like for worlds, it is true, simply because I abhor what school boys call " sneaking." But I doubt not that such work was necessary in order to prepare the minds of the members of a profession for the reception of that homœopathy which they have been taught, from their earliest youth, to loathe and detest ; to lead men gently, gradually and silently up to it who were studiously kept, by divers and sundry devices, in entire ignorance of it. This work of preparation is being accomplished, and in order that its full fruition may be obtained we, who know the whole truth, must not allow our efforts to be slackened one jot in proclaiming that truth.

As another means of extending the light of homœopathy, the Homœopathic League which was organized last year is issuing from time to time carefully prepared tracts relating to homœopathy. These are excellent and ought to obtain a wide circulation.

Some little good, I trust, has been done by a discussion which was started last May in *The English Mechanic and World of Science,* in which Dr. Clarke and I took a part. The worst of the matter was, that the opposition to homœopathy was so weak and entirely uninformed. One gentleman—a Bachelor of Medicine and Bachelor of Science— argued that drugs were very valuable and often "magical" in their efforts, and illustrated his assertion by pointing to the power of chlorate of potash to cure stomatitis. He presently added, that he had investigated homœopathy and "found it wanting !"

The London Homœopathic Hospital is prospering without a doubt. Its beds are full. Its funds are increasing—what with legacies and a bazaar, something like £4,000 must have been added to its endowment funds this year, equivalent to an additional income of £160 per annum. The bazaar was a success. It afforded much pleasure to all concerned and added about £1,200 to the resources of the hospital. But what is perhaps more important than anything is that the institution is out of debt ! This I can assure you, is a most singular position for an English hospital "supported by voluntary contributions" to be in. That it is that of the London Homœopathic Hospital is entirely due to the never-tiring energy of those in whose hands its management is placed, in increasing the subscription list and keeping down expenses.

The Hahnemann oration, which is annually delivered at the hospital about the time that the medical schools of the metropolis open, was given this year by Dr. J. H. Clarke, one of our hardest working and most efficient colleagues. I was not able to be present, to my great regret, and as the oration is not yet published, I have only seen an abstract of it, but friends who were there told me that it was a well delivered and excellent address.

Our friends at Birmingham had a capital bazaar last spring, which realized between £1,100 and £1,200. Their hospital is in excellent working order.

At Liverpool, the hospital founded by Mr. Tate is in course of erection, and will, I believe, be opened early next year. An engraving of the elevation published in *The Builder* last summer gives promise of a very handsome structure being devoted to the purposes of a homœopathic hospital.

The British Homœopathic Society revived the annual dinner in commemoration of Hahnemann's birthday this year, and a very pleasant evening we had. Celebrations of this kind are, I think, very useful. They assist in keeping alive that *esprit de corps* which is so essential to united action in any great public effort. They enable men having one common cause at heart to know one another better. They suggest ideas which, after discussion, may prove fruitful in promoting progress. They are eminently productive of good fellowship ; and what is there that tends more to smoothen the rugged path of life than good fellowship ? Aye, and I believe if we had a little more of this good fellowship it would be better for homœopathy too !

It is needless for me to allude to the Convention at Basle. You have heard all about that from Dr. Cowl. It was a first-rate meeting ; I never attended a more delightsome one. Martiny, Lorbacher and Weber did their level best to spoil it, but Hughes was too much for them—they couldn't do it. Martiny and his following were of course absent, but there were two capital fellows from Belgium there all the same—two young and highly educated physicians, who have both the will and the power to work, and in the future will, I doubt not, do good service for homœopathy in their own country. Lorbacher and Weber sulked at home, and then went to the annual meeting of the Central Verein at Frankfort, which, from the report of it that appeared in Lorbacher's journal, was more a burlesque of a medical meeting than anything else. At the close of the Convention it was my privilege to propose the United States as the scene of the next quinquennial meeting, a proposal which met with a heartily unanimous support. The end of five years is a long way ahead, and many things may happen between now and then—aye, and will happen—but meantime as fortunately for us we cannot peer into the future, we may indulge the pleasures of hope ! I propose to hope that I may be there until my being so is rendered impossible. One thing only is certain—it will be a large meeting and a thoroughly good one.

We have lost five of our veterans during this year: that most excellent surgeon, constant friend and thorough-going homœopath, Dr. Dunn: the philosophic, kind and gentle Hagle : that rare good fellow Holland, of Bath, full of fire and energy. I remember hearing him tell the story of his being in the parlor of a country inn, forty years ago, where half-a-dozen Allopaths were present discussing the affairs of the nation in general and those of the profession in particular. The subject of homœopathy cropped up and was there talked of in the fashion usual in those days, when one of them declared that he believed that homœopaths were all "knaves or fools." "You say that in my presence again if you dare," roared out the stentorian voice of Holland. Mr. Allopath repeated his offensive observation, and Holland, without a moment's hesitation, "went for him" and laying hold of the collar of his coat and the seat of his breeches, pitched him across the room against the mirror over the mantel-piece, smashing the glass to atoms ! They didn't worry Holland in Honiton much after that night ! Neville Wood, a reserved and gentlemanly physician, who had done a large amount of patient, steady work at the West End of London during the last forty years, and our earliest homœopathic veterinary surgeon, Moore, whose works in his department have done admirable service, have also passed away at a ripe old age.

Dr. Clarke's account of the state of homœopathy in England during the last five years, at the Basle Convention, and my own remarks on the same topic on that occasion, render it difficult to add anything fresh. I am, however, sure that the number of medical men who practice homœopathy here in England, and admit that they do so, is steadily on the increase. It is so especially in Liverpool, I believe ; and the addition to the muster role of the British Homœopathic Society during the past year afford evi-

dence that such is the fact. While that of those who practice homœopathically more or less, and who declare they do nothing of the sort, is becoming greater than ever. The "boom" you predicted last year has not
occurred yet, but as sure as homœopathy is true it is coming, and when
it comes it will do so with a vengeance !

Finally, let me wish all my friends and brethren in the faith of homœo-
opathy in the United States of America the full enjoyment of a merry
Christmas and a happy New Year.

Yours truly,

ALFRED C. POPE.

Tunbridge Wells, Nov. 27th, 1886.

REPORTS OF SOCIETIES AND HOSPITALS.

HOMŒOPATHIC MEDICAL SOCIETY OF THE COUNTY OF NEW YORK.

The thirtieth annual meeting of the Homœopathic Medical Society of
the County of New York was held in the Reception Room of the New York
Ophthalmic Hospital, corner of Twenty-third Street and Third Avenue,
December 9th, 1886, with President Houghton in the chair.

Seventy-eight members were present.

The minutes of the previous meeting were read and approved.

The following were duly elected members of the society: Dr. C.
Eurich, Dr. James E. Gore, Dr. John Husson, Dr. Abbie H. MacIvor, Dr.
A. H. Rannefeld, Dr. Cornelia Simpson, Dr. Anna C. R. Stevens, Dr. John
J. Sutton, Dr. James W. Harris, Dr. George H. Patcher.

After the withdrawal of Dr. B. G. Clark from nomination as treasurer,
and Dr. George S. Norton from nomination as vice-president, the following
officers were elected for the ensuing year: President, Dr. Clarence E. Beebe;
Vice-President, Dr. F. H. Boynton; Secretary, Dr. A. B. Norton; Treasurer,
Dr. S. H. Vehslage; Librarian, Dr. Charles W. McDowell; Censors, Drs.
Malcolm Leal, F. E. Doughty, S. F. Wilcox, George M. Dillow, H. M.
Dearborn.

The Committee on Drug Proving, Dr. Martin Deschere, Chairman,
reported a paper upon "How to Study Materia Medica," by S. Lilienthal,
in which the doctor contended that the proper method of study was to
keep books upon pathology and symptomatology, in which could be
recorded prominent and corroborated symptoms of different drugs, forming a general registrar of reliable symptoms, to which one could refer.
Also, he advised the keeping of interleaved editions of materia medica,
in which, under each drug, could be recorded the verified symptoms as
they might be found in reading or practice. In that way the doctor
claimed that in a comparatively short time a great amount of valuable
material could be collected.

Dr. George M. Dillow, as Chairman of the Committee on Legislation,
after speaking of the Committee's action regarding the bill to create a
single Board of State Examiners, defeated in the last Legislature, called
attention to the defect which existed in Senate bill 485, also of the last Legislature, in not codifying the laws relating to membership in County medical
societies.

He then read the resolutions adopted at the State Homœopathic Society, held September 7th, 1886, and stated that the Committee had failed of a quorum to consider them. He personally believed that the society should not pass resolutions regarding proposed laws, but should withhold action until the bills, as actually introduced, can be considered. Endorsing bills in advance may be mischièvous, as their wording is important, and new clauses may be added which may entirely alter the meaning of the bills.

Dr. T. Franklin Smith, Treasurer, then reported.

The Secretary, A. B. Norton, reported that the attendance at the meetings during the last year had been larger than at any period in the history of the society; the largest attendance was at the March meeting, when 118 were present. The average attendance was 55 3-10 compared to 47 7-10 the preceding year. Ten regular meetings have been held, and one adjourned. Twenty-eight papers have been presented to the society. The society has 194 members, which is larger than ever before. But one member, Dr. C. Th. Liebold, has died, and but one resigned. With two or three exceptions, the Standing Committees have done their work well.

Dr. A. B. Norton also offered the report of the Executive Committee. The Committee had held nine meetings during the year. The regular routine work had been gone through with, and twice the Committee had supplied material for the following meetings.

Also, certain medical advertising had been investigated and satisfactorily disposed of.

Dr. H. D. Paine then made some remarks upon the character of Dr. C. Th. Liebold, and offered the following resolutions, which were unanimously adopted:

"The New York County Homœopathic Medical Society desires to express its sense of the great loss it has recently sustained by the death of an esteemed associate, Dr. Carl Theodore Liebold, and to put upon record its high estimate of his professional ability and personal worth. Dr. Liebold has lived among us more than twenty years, and by his persistent devotion to his profession, by his consistent life, by his unassuming manners and kindly relations towards his colleagues, he has gained the goodwill of all who knew him. As a skilful practitioner, he has attained an enviable reputation; as a counsellor and teacher, he was sagacious, clear and accurate; as a writer, he was concise and practical. By his erudition, without display, he won the respect of his brethren, while his composed and sympathetic bearing inspired confidence in those who required his services.

"His sudden decease in the midst of a successful and honorable career has stirred the hearts of his surviving colleagues with a profound emotion, and will leave an enduring regret.

"As a testimony of the regard in which his memory is held, it is ordered that this minute be inscribed in the records of the society."

Papers were read and remarks offered upon Dr. Liebold by Drs. Belcher, Helmuth, Wetmore and McMurray.

The committee, consisting of Drs. Allen, Schley and Wilcox, appointed to take suitable action regarding the Laura Franklin Hospital, reported as follows:

Whereas, At the stated monthly meeting of the Homœopathic Society of New York City, held in November, an universal desire was shown to express its appreciation of the establishment of the Laura Franklin Free Hospital for Children; and

Whereas, It has pleased the Delano family, in their liberality, to build and equip in a most perfect manner, sparing no pains or money to make this institution the finest on the continent, and then richly endowing it, placing it thus above the needs and embarrassments that hamper so many similar undertakings; be it therefore

Resolved, That this Society do hereby tender to the Delano family its full appreciation of their benevolence, and also of their confidence in the ability of the Homœopathic School of Medicine to cure and relieve the many diseases to which children are subject; and it is furthermore

Resolved, That the staff, all of whom are active members of this Society, shall work with a perfect *esprit de corps* to show the superiority of this treatment and to demonstrate (*de novo*) by comparative statistics their continued faith in the law of *similia similibus curantur.*

That these resolutions, duly signed by the President and Secretary be forwarded to the Delano family and spread in full in our minutes.

(Signed)   T. F. ALLEN, M.D.
                S. F. WILCOX, M.D.
                J. M. SCHLEY, M.D.

CLARENCE E. BEEBE, M.D., *President.*
A. B. NORTON, M.D., *Secretary.*

After accepting the resignation of Dr. A. W. Lozier, the Society adjourned.

SOUTHERN HOMŒOPATHIC ASSOCIATION.

THE third annual meeting of the Southern Homœopathic Association convened in New Orleans, Dec. 9th, with delegates from nearly every Southern State present. The opening address was delivered by the President, Dr. A. S. Monroe, of Louisville, Ky., in which he reviewed the progress of homœopathy and referred to the oppressive laws against homœopathy which were still in force in some Southern States. Dr. F. H. Orme, of Atlanta, Ga., Chairman of the Committee on Medical Legislation, offered a lengthy report in which the plan of having State Licensing Boards were condemned and in their stead was recommended a fair registration law, allowing any physician to practice after registering his diploma and medical qualifications.

Dr. J. P. Dake, of Nashville, Tenn., offered resolutions in which the withdrawal from the National Board of Health of the funds necessary to prosecute its work, and the imposing of its duties upon the surgeons of the army and navy, were condemned.

The Bureau of Statistics, through its Chairman, Dr. Walter Baily, Jr., of New Orleans, presented some very interesting figures.

At the session held on the 18th, the Bureau of Materia Medica reported. A paper was presented by Dr. Henry, of Montgomery, upon the preparation of the higher attenuations. He held that many of the methods were fanciful and etherial. He recommended individualization in posology as well as in symptomatology. As is usual when the subject of high potencies is touched, a vigorous and rather profitless discussion ensued.

Dr. Geo. M. Ockford, of Lexington, read a paper on " Sanitary Science," reviewing the necessity of its enforcement and the means of rendering dwellings and localities hygienic.

The Bureau of Surgery reported a paper on "Gunshot Wounds of the Spine," by Dr. C. E. Fisher, of Austin, Texas, in which he advocated the propriety of radical operations in extreme cases.

Following this paper was the election of officers, at which Dr. Jos. Jones, of San Antonio, Texas, was made president; Dr. Walter M. Dake, of Nashville, Tenn., First Vice-President; Dr. E. A. Murphy, of New Orleans, Second Vice-President; Dr. C. G. Fellows, of New Orleans, Recording

Secretary; Dr. C. R. Mayer, St. Martinsville, La., Corresponding Secretary ; Dr. J. G. Belden, New Orleans, Treasurer.

At the evening session the report of the Bureau of Surgery was continued.

Dr. E. A. Murphy, of New Orleans, read a paper on "Nephrorraphy." He recommended that in floating kidney a lumbar incision be made and the organ stitched to its rightful place. He cited several cases which had been successfully treated by him after this method.

Dr. W. E. Green presented a paper upon "Excision of the Mammary Gland for Sarcomata."

The third day's session convened with Dr. Walter Baily, Jr., in the chair.

Under the Bureau of Gynæcology, Dr. Jos. Jones, of San Antonio, Tex., presented a paper on "Lacerations of the Perineum," which reviewed the methods of treatment in an able manner.

The Bureau of Pædology considered "Infant Feeding," and discussed the various artificial foods in use.

A reception was given to the Association by Dr. and Mrs. W. H. Holcombe, on Wednesday evening, which was attended by all the members and a few invited guests.

The President announced his appointment of the following Chairmen of the different Bureaus :

Materia Medica and Therapeutics.—W. M. Dake, M.D., of Nashville, Tenn.

Registration and Statistics.—J. H. Henry, M.D., of Montgomery, Ala.

Theory and Practice.—C. R. Mayer, M.D., of St. Martinsville, La.

Surgery.—E. A. Murphy, M.D., of New Orleans.

Diseases of Women and Children.—C. G. Fisher, M.D., of Austin, Texas.

Ophthalmology and Otology.—John M. Foster, M.D., of New Orleans.

Sanitary Science.—Geo. M. Oxford, M.D, of Lexington, Ky.

Legislative Work.—John M. Henry, M.D., of Montgomery, Ala.

Obstetrics.—H. G. Bayliss, M.D., of Knoxville, Tenn.

The closing exercises were held Friday night, at which the President, Dr. A. S. Monroe, of Louisville, Ky., delivered the address, in which he reviewed the medical agnosticism and skepticism of the old school, citing the opinions of eminent authorities as Wunderlich, Magendie, Johnson, editor of the *Medico-Chirurgical Review*, Virchow Niemeyer, O. W. Holmes, etc., as illustrating the want of confidence which the old school feel in their system of medical practice. With some very significant statistics the Doctor then contrasted the results of allopathic and homœopathic prescribing as a practical vindication of the claims made for the superiority of homœopathic therapeutics. The following were some of the more interesting statistics. The table presents the average death loss to number of patients treated by the representatives of the two great schools of medicine :

	Allopathic. Av. Loss.	Homœopathic. Av. Loss.
Boston, 1870, '71 and '72	1735	885
New York, 1870 and '71	1576	848
Philadelphia, '70, '71	1903	1287
New York, '72 '73	2046	1124
Brooklyn, '72, '73	2280	1028
General average	1908	1034

Here also are some hospitals, insane asylums, and almshouse statistics from reliable sources, and gathered from fields where the systems were used side by side:

	Allopathic. Loss.	Homœopathic. Loss.
Albany City Hospital, year ending Sept. '73..	726	533
Brooklyn Hospital, 1883..................	948	800
New York State Insane Asylum..........	649	439
Leipsic hospitals	1273	422
St. Margaret's Hospital, Paris, five years....	1100	705
Denver (Col.) Almshouse................	1003	668

Representing the average results of two years under each form of practice, next comes yellow fever statistics showing the average proportion of death losses during the yellow fever epidemic of 1878 in Southern United States. These statistics represent the mean average of losses as calculated by a commission of yellow fever experts visiting the infected districts immediately after the epidemic: Allopathic, 15.50 per cent. ; homœopathic, 6 per cent.

Dr. J. P. Dake, then delivered an address upon "The State and the Medical Profession," in which he reviewed the legislative attempts to control the practice of medicine, contrasting the results in the United States with England.

The Association then adjourned to meet in New Orleans the second Wednesday in December, 1887, after one of the most profitable meetings ever held by the organization.

RECORD OF MEDICAL PROGRESS.

ADULTERATION OF IODOFORM.—Adulteration of iodoform with picric acid is detected by shaking up with water and filtering. The filtrate should not be yellow, and should give no brownish-red coloration on warming with potassium cyanide.—*Lond. Med. Rec.*, October, 1886.

CONIUM MACULATUM.—Lepage shows that the amount of alkaloid in the root of *conium maculatum* depends on the time of year it is gathered, there being in spring and early summer none in the root, while the rest of the plant may contain it abundantly.—*Lond. Med. Rec.*, October, 1886.

DANGER FROM COCAINE.—Dr. Comanos Bey, of Cairo, reports the case of a patient addicted to morphine, whom he endeavored to cure of the habit by substituting subcutaneous injections of cocaine. The patient was delighted with the change, and soon secretly increased his allowance of cocaine from originally 0.05 grs. three or four times daily to 1-1½ grs. daily. At first unpleasant symptoms from overdoses of cocaine were relieved by small injections of morphine, the patient noting the antagonism between the two. When taking the highest doses he came into a condition similar to delirium tremens, and was then removed to a hospital where, under strict surveillance, he received three daily injections of morphine, and was soon discharged and allowed to resume his morphine habit.—*Berliner Klinische Wochenschrift*, September 20th, 1886.

INCOMPLETE PERICARDIAL SAC—ESCAPE OF HEART INTO LEFT PLUERAL CAVITY.—At a meeting of the Cambridge Medical Society, held October 8th, Dr. Boxall showed the chest organs of a woman who died with symptoms simulating pulmonary thrombosis on the third day after the birth of her third child. The necropsy, however, showed that a peculiar accident had occurred. The pericardium on the lift side was represented only by a sickle-shaped fold attached to the diaphragm and forming a pocket three-quarters of an inch deep. The heart was found lying in immediate contact with the lung, its apex being situated nearly three inches to the left of this pouch, from which it had evidently escaped during a severe attack of vomiting on the second day after delivery. This accident was followed by dyspnœa and collapse, in which the patient died thirty hours later.—*London Lancet*, November 6th, 1886.

TWO CASES OF LUPUS TREATED SUCCESSFULLY WITH IODOFORM.—For the following notes we are indebted to Mr. Guy Tyrril, House Surgeon to the Torbay Hospital, Torquay :

Case I.—Alfred R., aged sixteen, was admitted to the Hospital on February 4th, 1884, suffering from lupus of the nose and lip. The disease had existed for eighteen months, and had already destroyed the lower halves of the alæ of the nose, and almost the whole of the upper lip. The patient was ordered cod-liver oil, and the sore was dressed with an ointment consisting of one drachm of iodoform to one ounce of vaseline, plugs of lint covered with the ointment being inserted into each nostril. The sore immediately began to assume a healthy appearance and healed slowly, but uninterruptedly, and the patient was discharged cured on July 29th.

Case II.—William V., aged sixteen, was admitted on March 13th, 1886, the disease had existed for two years, and extended over nearly the same area, but the lip was not so deeply involved. The same treatment was adopted, and with an equally good result. The patient was discharged cured on August 3d.—*London Lancet*, October 30th, 1886.

IODOL—TETRAIODPYRROL—IN SURGERY.—Dr. Gaetano Mazzoni, of Rome, commends the use of iodol in much the same class of cases as those in which iodoform is now used. Among those benefited by its local use he mentions two cases of diphtheritic inflammation of wounds, and one case of a wound opening into the knee joint. To illustrate its antiseptic properties, portions of brain and intestine were removed from a decomposing cadaver; sprinkled with iodol powder, and exposed to the air and light. In a few days they were found to be superficially hardened, centrally soft, and entirely odorless. In portions exposed in same manner, but without iodol, decomposition proceeded rapidly. It is generally used as powder; but into fistulas and abscesses a solution is injected. This solution is composed of iodol, gramme 1; alcohol, gramme 16 ; glycerin, gramme 34. In abscesses the solution is injected after the evacuation of the pus, and this is repeated as often as pus accumulates. Among the advantages claimed for it are: Mildness of action, absence of odor, harmlessness to the organism, rapidity of excretion, deodorizing power, and its power to prevent scabbing. As objections might be mentioned, its slight solubility in water, and, at present, its high price.—*Berlinere Klinische Wochenschrift*, October 11th, 1886.

DIAGNOSIS OF INFANTILE DISEASES.—Dr. Bradley, in *L'union Méd. du Canada*, gives the following summary of points on the diagnosis of diseases of infants: 1. Congestion of the cheeks, excepting in cases of cachexia and chronic disease, indicates an inflammation or a febrile condition. 2. Congestion of the face, ears, and forehead, of short duration ; strabismus, with febrile reaction ; oscillation of the iris, irregularity of the pupil, with falling of the upper lids, indicates a cerebral affection. 3. A marked degree of emaciation, which progresses gradually, indicates some subacute or chronic affection of a grave character. 4. Bulbar hypertrophy of the fingers and curving of the nails, are signs of cyanosis. 5. Hypertrophy of the spongy portions of the bones indicates rachitis. 6.

The presence between the eyelids of a thick and purulent secretion from the meibomian glands may indicate great prostration of the general powers. 7. Passive congestion of the conjunctival vessels indicates approaching death. 8. Long continued lividity, as well as lividity produced by emotion and excitement, the respiration continuing normal, are indices of a fault in the formation of the heart or the great vessels. 9. A temporary lividity indicates the existence of a grave acute disease, especially of the respiratory organs. 10. The absence of tears in children four months old, or more, suggests a form of disease which will usually be fatal. 11. Piercing and acute cries indicate a severe cerebro-spinal trouble. 12. Irregular muscular movements, which are partly under the control of the will when the child is awake, indicate the existence of chorea. 13. The contraction of the eyebrows, together with a turning of the head and eyes away from the light, is a sign of cephalalgia. 14. When the child holds its hand upon its head, or strives to rest the head upon the bosom of its mother or nurse, it may be suffering from ear disease. 15. When the fingers are carried to the mouth and there is, besides, great agitation apparent, there is probably some abnormal condition of the larynx. 16. The act of scratching or of pinching the nose indicates the presence of worms or of some intestinal trouble. 17. When a child turns its head constantly from one side to the other, there is a suggestion of some obstruction in the larynx. 18. A hoarse and indistinct voice is suggestive of laryngitis. 19. A feeble and plaintive voice indicates abdominal trouble. 20. A slow and intermittent respiration, accompanied with sighs, suggests the presence of cerebral disease. 21. If the respiration be intermittent, but accelerated, there is capillary bronchitis. 22. If the respiration be superficial and accelerated, there is some inflammatory trouble of the larynx and trachea. 23. A strong and sonorous cough suggests spasmodic croup. 23. A hoarse and rough cough is an indication of true croup. 25. When the cough is clear and distinct, there is bronchitis. 26. When the cough is suppressed and painful, there is pneumonia or pleurisy. 27. If the cough be convulsive, it indicates whooping cough. 28. Sometimes a dry and painless cough occurs in the course of typhoid or intermittent fever; in the course of difficult dentition, or an attack of worms. Under these conditions, the cough is often due only to a bronchitis which has been caused by the original disease.—*Lond. Med. Rec.*, October, 1886.

NEWS.

THE University of Berlin is about to add to its Faculty an " Extraordinary Professor." He will lecture on the chemistry of food.

PERSONAL.—Dr. N. L. Macbride announces that hereafter he will confine himself to the practice of ophthalmology and otology.

THE CHOLERA has appeared in South America. It exists in epidemic form in several places in Buenos Ayres and is said to be at Rio Janeiro and in Paraguay.

THE Atlanta physicians having charge of the Free Dispensary do not like to have their medicine ship called a Free Dispensary, so they have christened it the Atlanta Polyclinic.

A MIRACULOUS ESCAPE is the heading of a patent medicine advertisement in many papers. Mrs. Louisa Pike is said to have taken the medicine and escaped death. A great many people have escaped who did not take it.

APPOINTMENT.—Dr. George S. Norton has been appointed to the chair of ophthalmology in the New York Homœopathic Medical College, left vacant by the death of Dr. Liebold.

PRIZE OFFERED.—The French Society for the Prevention of the Abuse of Tobacco, offers a prize of 1,000 francs for the best essay on the effects of tobacco on the health of men of letters, and its influence on the future of French literature.

THE death of J. P. Dake, Jr., of Nashville, Tenn., at the early age of thirty years, is to be deplored. Thoroughly educated, a trained scientist, and devotedly attached to his profession, a bright and promising career was opening before him.

PERSONAL.—The many friends of Dr. Sidney F. Wilcox will be sorry to learn that the genial Doctor has been ill for some time and confined to his bed. We hope that Dr. Wilcox will speedily conquer his sickness and be enabled to again take up his varied duties.

CROTON WATER.—The *Sanitary Era* says: "A recent report by the New York health authorities states that the Croton water shed embraces 239 square miles and has a population of 20,000, with 1,879 dwellings, and as many privies, about as many barn-yards, pig-pens and cesspools, besides cemeteries, slaughter-houses and other sources of contamination, and with no drainage, except by the surface, which conducts it to the aqueduct. Yet the Croton is the best water supply enjoyed by any large city in America or anywhere else."

LONDON HOMŒOPATHIC SCHOOL.—The winter session was opened by the delivery of the Hahnemann oration by Dr. J. H. Clarke. His subject was "The Revolution in Medicine." An interested and appreciative audience listened to the address. Dr. Clarke concluded as follows: "Our work is for truth and justice and light. To all who love justice and are not afraid of truth, we look for help in our endeavor to break down what still remains of the tyranny of darkness in medicine, and to hasten the coming of the perfect day of liberty and light."

ANOTHER OFFICE THIEF.—A well-dressed woman called a short time ago at Dr. Dowling's office and, as he was not in, asked permission to write him a letter in reference to the condition of her sick mother. After she had departed, the gold pen she had used and several other articles were missing from the desk, including some visiting cards, one of which she enclosed in a letter which she wrote to another doctor, thus paving the way to another purloining enterprise. It is the same old trick so often played, generally failing, yet sometimes successful.

PRIMARY MELANOTIC TUMOR OF THE HARD PALATE.—At a recent meeting of the Pathological Society of London, Mr. Treves exhibited a specimen illustrating this lesion, from a woman aged fifty-eight, who was almost edentulous, and who for four years had worn a "false palate," which irritated the front and right side of the palate near the alverlus. In this region a tumor at first appeared of the size of a pea, but rapidly grew. When first seen it was a flat swelling, covered by natural mucous membrane, but very black, or rather mottled in appearance. There was severe pain. With chisel and mallet the portion of the hard palate containing the tumor was successfully removed. It was a large, spindle-celled sarcoma growing from the periosteum ; recurrence of the growth took place after some months. The mucous membrane of the mouth of lower animals was much pigmented, and the present almost, if not quite, unique case seemed to indicate a reversion to a lower type.—*London Lancet*, November 6th, 1886.

A SUCCESS.—The *marche aux fleures* in aid of the Hospital Association of the Hahnemann Medical College of Philadelphia was a decided success. Eleven hundred and fifty tickets had been sold and most of the holders seemed to be present. Bonbons and fruit were sold as well as flowers. Mr. John Hoey sent a wagon-load of flowers from his conservatories at Hollywood, as did Mrs. Childs from Wooton.

FOODS ADULTERATED.—Milk—Addition of water or coloring matter and abstraction of cream. Butter—Substitution of foreign fats and addition of coloring matter. Spices—Addition of starch and other foreign powders; specially true of pepper and mustard. Cream of Tartar—Substitution of starch, gypsum and other cheaper substances. Baking Powders—Alum and other injurious ingredients. Lard—Presence of cheap fats and oils. Olive Oil—Substitution of cheaper oils. Jellies and Preserved Fruits—Substitution of cheaper fruits and addition of coloring matter. Honey—Substitution of cane sugar, glucose and other substances. Molasses—Addition of glucose, presence of tin or other foreign matter. Sugar—glucose, poisonous coloring matter. Maple sugar and syrup, glucose. Confectionery—Terra alba, poisonous coloring matter, fusel oil, arsenical wrappers, etc. Coffee—Mixture of various cheaper substances.

MISTAKES.—The mistakes of life are undoubtedly numerous. Indeed, they are endless. To condense them sufficiently to be briefly stated would seem to be impossible, yet some genius unknown to fame has considered the matter and announced at the conclusion that there are fourteen of them. It may be that some of these mistakes are made by physicians. Here, then, is the list. "It is a great mistake to set up our own standard of right and wrong, and judge people accordingly; to measure the enjoyment of others by our own; to expect uniformity of opinion in this world; to look for judgment and experience in youth; to endeavor to mould all dispositions alike; to yield to immaterial trifles; to look for perfection in our own actions; to worry ourselves and others with what can not be remedied; not to alleviate all that needs alleviation as far as lies in our power; not to make allowances for the infirmities of others; to consider everything impossible that we cannot perform; to believe only what infinite minds can grasp; to expect to be able to understand everything."

WATER TESTING.—The following tests for water are interesting. For hard or soft water: Dissolve a small quantity of good soap in alcohol. Let a few drops fall into a glass of water. If it turns milky, it is hard; if not, it is soft. For earthy matters or alkalies: take litmus paper dipped in vinegar and if, on immersion, the paper returns to its true shade, the water does not contain earthy matter or alkali. If a few drops of syrup be added to water containing earthy matter, it will turn green. For carbolic acid: Take equal parts of water and clear lime water. If combined or free carbonic acid be present a precipitate is seen, to which if a few drops of muriatic acid be added an effervescence commences. For magnesia: Boil the water to a twentieth part of its weight and then drop a few grains of neutral carbonate of ammonia into a glass of it, and a few drops of phosphate of soda. If magnesia be present it will fall to the bottom. For iron: Boil a little nut gall and add to the water. If it turns gray or slate-black, iron is present. (2) Dissolve a little prussiate of potash and if iron is present it will turn blue. For lime: Into a glass of the water put two drops of oxalic acid, and blow upon it. If it gets milky, lime is present. For acid: Take a piece of litmus paper. If it turns red there must be acid. If it precipitates on adding lime water it is carbonic acid. If a blue sugar paper is turned red it is a mineral acid.—*The English Mechanic.*

VOL. XXXV.   *FEBRUARY, 1887.*   (Volume II, Third Series.)   No. 2.

NORTH AMERICAN
JOURNAL OF HOMŒOPATHY.

ORIGINAL ARTICLES IN MEDICINE.

A NEW STUDY OF ARSENICUM ALB.

By A. W. WOODWARD, M.D.,
Chicago, Ill.

THE following cases of poisoning by arsenic are brought to your attention for the purpose of comparing the succession of effects produced by this drug upon many persons.

It will be observed in every instance, while there is a considerable variety of symptoms, there is an orderly progression of phenomena involving the different organs one after another, and this is so uniform when the several provings are compared, we are justified in concluding there is a law governing this evolution of drug effects, which points in this manner to the individuality of this drug.

No. 20. Pauline Philipoff took a large quantity of arsenic by mistake. An hour after, *vomiting came on** which lasted two days. Later she had *feeling of coldness and numbness in extremities.* Cold then reached the forearms and legs, at the same time *great weakness in hands and feet came on,* so that ten days after taking the drug she could not walk without help. She gradually became bedridden, with anæsthesia and muscular atrophy of extremities. * * * *. *Cyclopædia Drug Pathogenesy,* vol. 1, p. 434.

No. 53. A young man who *had been seized with vomiting and purging* two days previous was brought to the hospital while these symptoms continued. His *face was drawn and livid,* eyes not deeply sunken, lips violet and cold, also his nose. Body showed large blue spots, and whole surface was cold. Tongue was icy and covered with bluish coating. Temperature below normal. Matters vomited were green. Patient complained of intense thirst. *Pulse was imperceptible in radial and brachial arteries.* * * *. Arsenic was found in viscera on post-mortem. *Ibid.*

No. 37. *A lad had been vomiting and purging* six hours when seen by physician. He was found *cold, pulseless, restless,* complaining of

*Italics are used for the first symptom of each organ involved.

cramps in upper and lower limbs. Countenance was sunken and neck and chest livid. * * *. On post-mortem, arsenic was found in his body. *Ibid.*

No. 7. A woman took part of a tablespoonful of arsenic. In two hours *became sick at intervals.* In afternoon was found *with cold extremities and almost lifeless. Pulse scarcely perceptible.* Eyes bright, cornea injected. *Intense headache* that was increased by noise and light. Was quite unable to rise without assistance. *Ibid.*

No. 25. A man took ℥ss. of arsenic. *Emesis and catharsis* continued during the night, and gastro-enteric inflammation set in next day. Two days after, *complained of much pain through the system,* and *great itching of the skin.* Tenesmus and *strangury.* * * *. *Ibid.*

No. 17. A young woman took a large quantity of arsenic, *vomiting was induced* and iron was given. *She had some fever* but gradually improved. Eight days afterward *she had severe pains in extremities,* which were swollen. Three days after this she *almost entirely lost power* over *extremities,* and has since continued bedridden. * * *. *Ibid.*

No. 9. A man took some arsenic by mistake, was *seized with vomiting* which continued three days, then the *head felt heavy. Skin was hot* but not dry. *Pulse quickened.* Tongue was dry, epigastrium sensitive. After a remission the symptoms returned and facial expression was dull, eyes fixed, *stupor and slight delirium set in.* He tried to remove the cold cloths on his head. Eyes were injected. Heart beat violently, pulse 85. Restless night, slight delirium but can answer questions. Skin hot and dry. A pustular eruption has developed. Almost complete loss of motion on left side. Sensibility dulled. * * *. *Ibid.*

No. 33. An English nobleman took for a local skin affection 2½ grains 1st trit. arsenicum, twice daily. After three weeks he complained of *dry tongue and thirst,* so great it made him quite ill, this increased, *he had chilly fits and got very pale,* his face was white and pinched, *his pulse weak and quick,* at times irregular, with *extreme prostration.* Eye lids were swollen and puffy. * * *. *Ibid.*

No. 32. Dr. J. J. took arsenicum 3d, drop doses four times daily for six weeks. He lost flesh, *had some acidity and heat of stomach, with thirst,* and *two patches of squamous eruption on malleoli.* * * *. *Ibid.*

No. 31. Took during seven months four grms. arseniate of soda, in gradually increasing doses. *Appetite became excessive,* and he assumed *an embonpoint* quite noticeable to friends. Discontinuance of the drug was followed by emaciation. *Ibid.*

No. 22. W. J. M. after taking 30m. arsenicum, on second day had *colic and burning pains in abdomen,* relieved by loose stool. Severe nausea after drinking cold water. On seventh day pinching pains in abdomen, and desire for stool at unusual hours, it was loose and attended by griping and burning at anus, *ulceration* as from a cold *at commissure of lips. Desire to keep quiet. Ibid.*

No. 11. C. M. Tardieu (one month after first proving), took 4th trit. arsenicum three times daily. On fourth day *considerable soreness of throat*, with aphthæ on each side of fauces, pharynx reddened, continued four or five days. On eighth day *there appeared on chest an eruption* that made him suffer horribly, it began with little red pimples, *obliging him to scratch even to blood.* Eruption extended to arms and back. * * *. *Ibid.*

No. 15. A. W. W. took two grs. 2x trit. arsenicum alb. Immediately *persistent nausea,* followed by *pricking pain over right eye, then neuralgic pains from right shoulder to fingers,* with *numbness* and burning in pharynx. Nausea returns with cold sweat on forehead after exercise. Afterward *sneezing and watery nose.* Was very tired without cause. *Dull headache* one hour after taking drug, thirst, drinking causing nausea, headache continued. Afterward *urinated more freely than usual.* Two hours after, sinking at stomach, cold feet, languor and sleepiness. Waked with neuralgic pains in left temple, was restless and apprehensive. Slight dyspnœa when walking. Three hours after *pulse 90, temperature 99.15°* thirst increased. * * *. *Ibid.*

No. 16. A. H. W. took 5 grs. 2x trit. arsenicum alb. Soon *slight burning in stomach, with eructations,* following which *perspiration* after slight exercise, flatulency after eating and pricking pain in right hip. One hour after, called to stool without relief. *Dull aching in left ulnar nerve,* itching of right knee, soon after, pricking and tingling in various parts *with lachrymation* and shooting pains in occiput. Afterward, eructations, prickling in skin very annoying, causing restlessness *and headache.* Pulse raised four beats. Two hours after taking drug, feels tired and sleepy. After three hours *pulse eighty,* dull occipital headache, with confusion of mind and colicy pains in abdomen. * * * *Ibid.*

Many provings could be given in which the same functions are chiefly involved, but in their records sufficient care has not been taken to note the symptoms in their order of development.

The following description of wholesale poisoning illustrates this :

No. 3. Dr. Feltz had under his care at St. Dennis eighty persons who at one time were poisoned by arsenic. ''Most of these presented similar symptoms. Soon after taking drug, a *sense of weight in epigastrium* and *general malaise,* vomitings occurred one to four hours after taking drug. Several had diarrhœa also. Diarrhœa ceased first, vomiting was frequent with burning in throat, behind sternum and in epigastrium. *Pulse varied between 90 and 110. Skin was dry. Headache severe, with constriction in temples.* Most patients *had noises in ears,* and vertigo. There were extreme *feebleness in legs and prostration,* with severe pains in loins. Urine was normal. On third day these symptoms abated, and in all cases there appeared swelling of eyelids with conjunctivitis. In some the whole face was swollen. Some had urticaria, others herpes or extreme irritation of the skin. On seventh day appetite was still deficient and there still remained some muscular weakness.''—*Cyclopædia Drug Pathogenesy, Vol. I., page 422.*

If we analyze these fourteen provings physiologically, we find the first symptom in every case (including the eighty reported by Dr. Feltz), is manifested upon the alimentary canal and organs of nutrition. From this, as the initial disturbance, the other symptoms develop. In eleven the second system deranged, is the cutaneous, in three, according to the record it may have been either cutaneous or motor. In eight, possibly eleven (not including the indefinite "malaise" of Dr. Feltz cases), the third apparatus disordered is the motor. In every case but one where the symptoms involve the respiratory or circulatory organs, they were the fourth system disturbed. Cerebral symptoms are seen in only four cases, and they are fifth in order of occurrence.

The correctness of this sequence to the involvement of the motor functions is again verified by cases 116, 17 and 20, and by Dr. F.'s report also, in all of them after the subsidence of symptoms of gastro-enteritis, the patients entered the second stage of chronic poisoning, and then suffered chiefly from œdema, eczema, herpes, cutaneous anæsthesia, etc. And after this had subsided in cases 17 and 20 there developed motor paralysis and muscular atrophy.

The significance of this sequence of definite and distinct diseases as a result of this poison, will again be considered.

Granting the various functions of the body may be deranged by this drug in a particular order one after another, you may ask, What practical advantage is to be gained by this knowledge? If you turn again to the records, you find as the influence of the drug extends, and new functions are involved, the old symptoms continually return, and seem to alternate. But if the prover is examined after a few hours (as in the poisonings), while he complains of only one or two symptoms at a time, you find every function in the body is deranged more or less. Hence, while the record shows only a sequence and alternation of symptoms, there really occurs an aggregation of disorders, in which (during the first period of the proving), the functions primarily deranged, are found to be most seriously and prominently affected.

We find, therefore, the succession of effects portrayed in the records *represents a particular combination of organic derangements, which in the aggregate becomes the physiological expression of arsenic.*

Beyond this sequence of effects, there is little. to be learned from these provings, except the symptoms are uniformly of a painful and distressing character. The distinctive arsenic symptoms are too few in number to be a guide in themselves. For this reason, in applying this rule to practice, symptoms will have no bearing except as indicating the progressive development of a chronic disease, which in its course has shown various acute phenomena, one after another, as a new organ became involved.

In acute affections, having no clinical history, this sequence of effects represents the organs which will be found collectively involved (besides the local lesion), and the relative severity of their disturbance.

That there is a limitless variety of diseases in which this combination may be found, is indicated by the variety of special symptoms this drug has produced.

Assuming as fairly proved that the typical action of arsenic is manifested, first and chiefly, upon the digestive organs, and second, on the cutaneous or sensory, and third, on the spinal or motor, and fourth, on the respiratory or circulatory, and fifth, on the brain : in this particular combination and relation one to the other, we ask your attention to the following cases already published, for the purpose of showing that this drug would have been curative under the homœopathic law, regardless of special symptoms, because each case presents this totality of derangements.

CASE I.—*Gastralgia* of a year's standing. Is now thin, weak, pale and haggard, with feeble and slow pulse and flabby tongue ; vomiting of a light yellow, tasteless fluid ; pain in paroxysms of one or two hours' duration, once or twice a day ; pain severe and seemed to go through from the epigastrium to between the shoulders. *Ars.* 3, night and morning, cured soon. Dr. R. Hughes. *Hoyne's Therapeutics.*

CASE II.—*Acute gastritis.* Mrs. H., aged seventy-six. Symptoms : Severe burning pain in epigastrium, followed by vomiting ; indescribable anguish at pit of stomach, with nausea, and almost constant vomiting ; restless, anxious and faint ; pulse thready ; extremities cold ; tongue very red ; intolerable thirst, but even a teaspoonful of water brought on violent retching. *Ars.* 6, relieved in a few hours. Well in two days. Lawrence Newton. *Mon. Hom. Review,* v. 15, p. 209.

CASE III.—*Cholera infantum.* Child, aged eight months, had cholera infantum six weeks ago. Found the child emaciated, eyes sunken, lips blue and dry, great thirst, pulse almost imperceptible. Her food was ejected as often as taken, or it passed through the bowels undigested. Stools dark, mixed with mucus, putrid ; ten copious stools per day, followed by extreme exhaustion. *Ars.* 30, and the white of egg with salt and sugar cured. Dr. Anna Warren. *Hoyne's Therapeutics.*

CASE IV.—D., aged eighteen months, had cholera infantum for four months. Twelve to fifteen stools per day, greenish, watery, and vomiting of a thin, greenish or colorless fluid. Constant fever, dingy, dry skin, pale wan face, insatiate thirst, frequent loose cough, hard tumid belly, extreme emaciation and the general appearance of confirmed marasmus. *Ars.* 3, followed in a week by the 30th, cured. Dr. L. Hallock. *Ibid.*

CASE V.—*Marasmus.* Little girl, one and a half years old, suffers nearly six months with diarrhœa; has now daily twenty to twenty-five watery discharges from the bowels; her abdomen is large and distended. The whole child is emaciated; the skin wrinkled, dry, and of a dirty grayish color; eats very little, but drinks all the time cold water with eagerness; sleeps ·very little; her voice sounds like the voice of a kitten. *Arsen.* 30, in water, two teaspoonfuls every day, improved so far as there were only ten to fifteen stools a day without so bad a smell. The same prescription repeated cured the child. Bojanus, A. H. Z., 80, p. 117.

CASE VI.—*Skin affections.* Two cases of psoriasis guttata, with raised, circular, reddish spots, and covered with scales, especially upon the prominences of knee as well as elbow; anæmia with evident debility were cured with *Ars.* 30. Dr. Ph. Arcularius. *Hoyne's Therapeutics.*

CASE VII.—Girl, aged two, superficial ulcers on legs, surrounded by a somewhat raised pinkish areola. In centre of each was a small, dry, black, slightly depressed scab, from under the edges of which oozed a mixture of thin, light yellow matter and very dark blood. Complained of burning pains in ulcers and had a great desire to scratch round the edges, but disliked to have them exposed to the air. Loss of appetite, general prostration and intense thirst for small quantities of water frequently. *Ars.* 10m. cured. *North American Journal of Homœopathy*, v. 21, p. 105.

CASE VIII.—*Syncope.* Sarah Y., aged nineteen, suffering for six months from chronic diarrhœa; latterly has become so weak that she frequently swooned away, the fainting fits being preceded by nausea and vertigo; muco-aqueous evacuation every few minutes. *Arsen.* 3, thirty minims in half a tumbler of water, one teaspoonful every hour, followed by immediate improvement, and in two days stools became natural. J. C. Burnett, H. W., v. 8, p. 10.

CASE IX.—*Bronchitis.* Elderly person, with profuse, watery, slimy and bloody expectoration, with great difficulty of breathing, thirst and a collapsed state. *China* gave relief for a time. Finally a relapse occurred, with cold extremities, blueness of the skin and tightness of cough, when *ars.* soon restored the expectoration, and the patient was convalescent. Dr. Brewster. *Hoyne's Therapeutics.*

CASE X.—*Hydrothorax.* Woman, aged twenty-seven, affected with yellow leucorrhœa for a week with general dropsy. Face, abdomen, and all the limbs were dropsically swelled. Unable to lie down for an instant—on attempting to do so, such difficulty of breathing came on that she nearly died of strangulation. Yesterday had an attack of weakness, unconsciousness, rattling respiration and cold perspiration, and death seemed imminent. Has frequently recurring cough, with expectoration of blood-streaked mucus, retching and vomiting of food and drink ; has often rigor with goose-skin ; has great thirst, and small, rapid pulse. *Ars.* 6, every six hours, cured. Dr. Haustein. *Ibid.*

CASE XI.—*Dropsy.* Mrs. B., for ten years suffering from general anasarca, especially of the lower limbs ; when the swelling is greatest has nightly fever and restlessness, driving her from place to place ; loose cough in the morning or while lying with the head low ; on going up stairs has to stop often to recover her breath ; during fever constant thirst, drinking often, but little at a time. *Ars.* 40m. one dose cured. Dr. J. G. Gilchrist. *Ibid.*

CASE XII.—*Heart disease.* Man, aged forty, has suffered long with heart disease. The last few days he felt much worse, and one morning he was found almost unconscious in bed. Hippocratic face ; body covered with cold, clammy perspiration ; feet œdematously swollen and cold ; pulse gone ; trembling, irregular motions of the heart ; weak respiration, with scarcely audible voice ; he complains of thirst, weakness, anguish and oppression. *Arsen.,* one of Jenichen's highest potencies, relieved him in ten minutes. Fourteen days afterwards he was again at his business. Landesmann, A. H. Z., 85, 162.

CASE XIII.—*Intermittent fevers.* Chill, without thirst, at ten or eleven A.M. ; shaking chill, felt as though water was running down the back, blue surface, shrunken skin ; burning fever, great thirst, drinking little at a time, but often, marked prostration, dry parched tongue ; little or no sweat, irritable and melancholy. *Ars.* 30 cured. Dr. T. D. Stow. *Hoyne's Therapeutics.*

CASE XIV.—Tertian form, with chills in morning, anticipating. Before chills, diarrhœa ; stools thin and bloody, with burning pain. Chill mixed with heat, accompanied by anguish, thirst, headache, and restlessness. Hot sleep of long duration, with great prostration. Very restless, fear of dying. Sweat not profuse, gradual relief of diarrhœa and pains. *Ars.* 200 every three hours and there was no return of the chill. Dr. A. S. Fisher. *Ibid.*

CASE XV.—*Prosopalgia.* Woman, right side of face daily, from four P.M. to two A.M. Pain, burning, tearing, as though red hot wire were moved through the parts. Shuddering, trembling of limbs ; great anguish ; at last cold perspiration and great prostration. She has a yellow, cachetic tint ; dull eyes, surrounded by dark rings ; is very weak. *Ars.* 3, five drops twice a day, cured. Dr. Payr. *Hoyne's Therapeutics.*

CASE XVI.—*Inflammatory rheumatism.* Miss C. ; face flushed ; dry, hot skin ; pulse ninety-six ; great thirst ; white-coated tongue ; burning pain in knees, ankles, hips ; pains disappear one day, returning the next more severely ; worse at one P.M. ; burning and throbbing pains ; pain and heat without swelling ; thirsty, but drinks little at a time ; water causing nausea, prostration, restlessness, anxiety. B⁄

Arsen. 3, then *arsen.* 6. Cured in a week. L. C. Crowell, H. M., Aug., 1872, p. 47.

CASE XVII.—*Insanity* of malarial origin. Wm. A. Hammond, M.D. (*Quar. Bull. Clin. Soc.*, Oct.), gives the case of a woman of twenty-seven, who had, while living in a highly malarious district, repeated attacks of intermittent fever. December 18th, 1877, without prodromatic symptoms, she suddenly sprang from her seat and ran screaming into the street; after this she was sent to a lunatic asylum, where she remained for about a year in a condition of profound melancholy, with suicidal tendencies and hallucinations of hearing. There was almost constant headache, located mainly in the vertex, flushings of the face and distressing tinnitus aurium. Treatment consisted of $\frac{1}{4}$ grain of morphine before and $\frac{1}{15}$ grain of arsenic after each meal. At present—March 22d—the patient is very much improved, and all the indications point to a complete restoration.

In reviewing these cases, little need be said concerning the first three, as the affection in each corresponds with the primary action of the drug, and the attending symptoms assume their relative prominence, pallor, emaciation or coldness, with considerable restlessness or prostration, and some cardiac weakness.

Cases 4 and 5 illustrate the second stage of the arsenic disease (*vide* provings 11, 17, 20), the gastro-enteritis resulting in marasmus. The indications for remedy being the primary condition plus the marasmus and prostration (doubtless present), and the cough.

In cases 6 and 7, the records are incomplete. A skin affection attended by anæmia or great thirst and debility, leads to the conclusion that the cause is mal-nutrition or gastritis. On such premises only could *arsenic* be useful.

Case 8 shows the succession of disorders peculiar to this drug. First diarrhœa and consequent anæmia, then debility, which increases until syncope results. A cardiac stimulant would not suffice in this case.

Case 9 illustrates the danger of prescribing for present symptoms alone. Had this been a primary affection *china* would have cured. Guided by the symptoms given, it was as well indicated as *arsenic.* Experimentation was necessary here, having no clinical history.

Cases 10, 11 and 12 were probably chronic invalids before respiratory and cardiac symptoms appeared. Without their clinical history a doubt remains whether the guiding symptom was the thirst, or the œdema. *Apis* or *hydrocy. acid* might have done as well.

Cases 13 and 14 were manifestly gastric intermittents.

Cases 15 and 16 were masked intermittents. The gastric symptoms probably ante-dated development of the prosopalgia as well as rheumatism. Without a clinical history in the latter case *aconite* was as well indicated.

Case 17 shows how successfully this drug can be applied, guided solely by pathological indications. Another case in point was a young friend of ours recently cured of severe chorea by drop doses of " Fowler's solution," prescribed by an old school physician, because there was primarily poor assimilation and hyperæsthesia.

While these cases are of limited variety, it is our belief there are no exceptions to this rule for the use of this drug in disease. If any exist, it will be found in Bright's disease. By these provings the renal organs are among the last disturbed, hence *arsenic* will be (as we have found it), only palliative in this affection : for the *arsenic* type comes only as the closing scene in a long history of suffering and debility. It has a much better record in cardiac dropsies, as we have seen.

Doubtless this drug is often required in affections where the clinical history points to other remedies, or in cases that have been saturated with many drugs. In such instances we must be guided solely by the totality of symptoms present. Thus we conclude, when in any disease, whether acute or chronic, we find, besides the local affection, predominant symptoms of the stomach, *with* cutaneous, *and* spinal, *and* respiratory, *and* cerebral phenomena attending in this relative degree and severity, we know *arsenic* is the specific remedy.

THERAPEUTICS OF SPINAL IRRITATION.

By FRANK F. LAIRD, M.D.,

Utica, N. Y.

[*Continued from page 733, Vol. I., Third Series.*]

IODOFORM.—Back of the neck sore, as if bruised. Pain along spine. Spine feels sore, does not want it touched. Pain along right side of dorsal vertebræ. Continued pain in lumbar region, with weakness when straining.

No clinical experience with this remedy has yet been reported. Its symptoms, however, entitle it to consideration.

Lilium tig.—Dull pain in back of neck, with feeling of constriction. Soreness of cervical and occipital muscles, always worse when she has "thirsty spells." Pain in back ; with nausea ; with pain in right ovary. Constant burning in the back. Cold feeling in back, as if cold water was poured upon it. Pain in lower dorsal vertebræ, as if the back would break. Dull, heavy pain in lumbar region. *Pain in sacrum, with a sensation of weight and downward pressure in hypogastrium, worse when standing.*   Pains, aching, drawing or pressive in lumbo-sacral region.   Sensation of pulling upwards and forwards from tip of coccyx.

Depression of spirits ; weeping with fretfulness and fear of some terrible internal disease already seated ; fear of insanity.   *Constant hurried feeling as of imperative duties and utter inability to perform them, with sexual excitement.*

Congestive headache, especially *frontal ;* dull, *hot* or *burning pain* with staggering vertigo and *feeling of an elastic band stretched around from temple to temple.*

Blurred vision, with *heat in eyelids and eyes.*   Dry hacking cough in evening, better in open air.   *Frequent desire to take a long breath with sighing.   Congested,* constricted feeling in chest.   *Severe pain in left mammary gland.   Dull pressive pain in left side of chest, apparently about the heart.   Sharp and quick pain in left side of chest, with fluttering of the heart.*   Feeling as if heart were squeezed in a vise ; or alternately grasped and relaxed.   Slight momentary spasmodic twitchings around heart ; after walking ; often arouses her from sleep.   Palpitation ; Heart's action intermittent, each intermission being followed by a violent throb, causing involuntary catching of the breath with heat and a crowded feeling in head and face.   *Faintness.   All heart symptoms relieved by keeping herself busy.*

Voracious hunger seemingly along spine and up to occiput, not appeased by eating.   *Thirst is a forerunner of severe symptoms.*   Nausea coming and going suddenly ; with sensation of a lump in centre of chest moved down by empty swallowing, but soon returning ; with morning diarrhœa ; with pressure in vagina and pain at top of sacrum.   Distension of stomach and bowels, with flatus.

Pressure in rectum, with almost constant desire for stool.   Bilious morning diarrhœa, "has to go in a hurry."   Pressure on bladder, with frequent irritation, which is followed by smarting and burning in urethra.

Menses scanty ; or normal as to time and quantity, *but flow only when the patient is moving about.   Bearing down, with sensation of heavy weight and pressure in uterine region, as if the whole abdominal contents would press out through the vagina—this dragging being felt even in chest and shoulders ; relieved by pressure of hand against vulva.   Neuralgia of uterus, with great tenderness* of hypogastrium *to touch or jar.   Uterus tender to touch or jar.   Can walk on level surface, but is greatly aggravated when walking on uneven ground.   Bloated feeling in uterine region and all the pelvic organs feel swollen and tender.   Sharp pain in ovarian region, especially left ; neuralgia of ovaries (left)* with burning, stinging, darting pains, accompanied by *severe pains in left mamma.*

One or other ovary (especially left) smells at times of menses. Marked sexual excitement (opp. sepia). *Leucorrhœa ; bright yellow, acrid, excoriating ; leaving a brown stain.*

Pricking sensation at ends of fingers or sensation as of an electric current. Legs ache, especially knees. Burning in palms and soles. *Limbs cold and clammy, worse when excited or nervous.* Cold hands and feet. Frequent faintness, especially in a *warm room* or after *being on the feet* a long time ; with cold sweat on back of hands and on feet. *The pains all occupy small spots as if produced by hard pressure with the ends of the fingers.*

Worse walking, yet pains so much worse after ceasing to walk that he must walk again. Sleep restless and unrefreshing.

Aggravation.—*From 5 P.M. to 8 A.M.; from loss of self-control; standing still.*

Amelioration.—During the day ; from fresh air ; *from keeping busy;* in warm room.

In spinal irritation, *dependent upon ovarian and uterine troubles* (*especially* [anteversion), *lilium tig.* is a grand remedy. Slow in its action, the drug *seldom manifests its curative influence under two weeks,* and hence should not be hastily discarded, as is too often the case. It closely resembles *sepia,* but can be readily distinguished by its conditions and concomitants.

Lobelia inflata.—Burning pain in back as if in posterior wall of stomach. Pain about third, fourth and fifth dorsal vertebræ. Extreme tenderness over sacrum ; cannot bear slightest touch ; cries out if an attempt is made to examine the parts ; sits up in bed, bending forward.

Dull, heavy pain passing around the forehead, from one temple to the other, on a line immediately above the eyebrows.

Sensation as of a foreign body in throat impeding respiration. Inclination to sigh or take a deep breath. Spasmodic asthma. *Extremely difficult breathing caused by a strong constriction at middle of chest.* Constriction of larynx. Pressure as from a foreign substance or morsel of food along whole course of æsophagus, worse below larynx, with *twisting* peristaltic from thence downward to pit of stomach ; feeling of a plug from pit of stomach to spine.

Increase of saliva. Feeling of great weakness in the stomach and qualmishness. An indescribable feeling about stomach compounded of nausea, pain, heat, oppression and excessive uneasiness, accompanying the symptoms of the respiratory organs. *Nausea; with deathly pale face; in the morning, better after a drink of cold water; with cold sweat on head, especially face,* with ineffectual efforts to vomit.

Urine deposits a rosy red sediment, with crystals of uric acid.
Prickling sensation through whole body, even to fingers and toes.
Amelioration.—Nearly all symptoms disappear in the evening.

We occasionally meet with asthma associated with spinal irritation in the upper dorsal region and uterine derangements. In these cases, the Indian tobacco is often very efficient.

Lycopodium.—Involuntary stretching of the neck, now forward, now backward. *Stiffness and tensive pain in neck and occiput; pressure in a small spot in nape.* Head constantly tends to sink forward from paresis of cervical muscles, with dizziness. Drawing pain in outer cervical muscles, extending to shoulders and elbows. Pain as from a sprain in nape of neck, with sensitiveness to touch. Burning, pressing and drawing in the back. Violently pressive pains in the back, sometimes over its whole extent, sometimes in one place, as though one's fist were pressed against the lower vertebræ, when it was accompanied by a similar pressure on the lower extremity of the sternum, so that he was obliged to hold his breath (while sitting and writing in the morning). Sticking stitches in back on breathing. *The first dorsal and lumbar vertebræ are painful on touch and motion.* Involuntary approximation of scapulæ backward, alternating with contraction of pectoral muscles forward. *Burning as from glowing coals between the scapulæ ;* also drawing.

Pain in small of back ; so violent that it draws the chest together with pressure in stomach and constriction in abdomen ; as if the flesh were loosened ; *so violent that she was unable to move, on rising from bed in morning (during menses). Drawing* and *pressure in small of back.*

Depression of spirits. Anxiety and apprehensiveness, as if in pit of stomach. Great fear ; of frightful images which her fancy conjures up ; *when left alone,* yet often desires solitude; *anthropophobia. Very irritable, fretful, obstinate. Alternation of merry and melancholy mood.* Indifference. *Distraction of mind ; can neither comprehend nor remember what he has read ; loss of ideas, cannot express himself, selects wrong words and syllables ; makes mistakes in writing, spells words wrongly, adds or omits letters, uses wrong words* (patient is *conscious* of these mistakes, hence a *functional* trouble). *Mental effort causes stupefaction of the head, with vanishing of thought and,* sometimes, nausea.

Great confusion of head with difficulty in collecting thoughts. *Vertigo ; in a hot room ; when drinking ; when sleeping ; in the morning when and after rising ;* when rising from a seat ; with stupefaction, reeling, nausea and hot face ; when she sees anything turning. Has for an hour a sensation as though her body was turning. Involuntary nodding of head, now to right, now to left. Heaviness, heat and confusion in the head.

Headache—(1) *General*—*If she did not eat during the ravenous hunger, had headache which was relieved by eating.* Headache; *after breakfast;* on stooping, shaking or turning the head; with stupefaction, heat of face and hands; like a clang through the head as from the snapping of a piano-string; as if head would be forced asunder and as if brain were swashing to and fro, worse when walking, ascending steps and rising from stooping; *painful pressure, worse reading and when lying down; throbbing in brain on leaning head backward,* also *after every paroxysm of coughing;* balancing and jerking in head; feels every step in her head when walking.   (2) *Frontal*—Alternating contraction and relaxation of skin of forehead, causing opening and closing of eyelids. Pressing asunder in forehead and above eyes extending to top of head with nausea and trembling of limbs; dull pain as if forehead was compressed from both sides; *pressive pain with heat of head* and face and often with vertigo and stupefaction of head; violent throbbing in evening, then tensive and extending across occiput to nape of neck. Forehead very painful to touch.   (3) *Temporal*—*Pressure and pressive pains in temples, as if screwed together. With cough, shattering as from a shock in temples and in chest.*   (4) *Parietal*—External headache, left side, extending to ear and teeth, worse in evening and intolerably aggravated by reading, writing and by slightest pressure. Drawing on right side extending down into neck.   (5) *Vertex*—*Pressive pain on top of head.*   (6) Occiput—Dull heaviness; burning pain in both occipital eminences; occiput fills with blood after stooping. Throbbing, pressure and tearing in occiput. A violent shock extending from back up towards vertex, compelling her to hold the head, while sitting (after eating to satisfy).   (7) External Head—Painful tension in scalp just above forehead with painful drawing about root of nose. Contracted sensation in scalp with feeling as if hair would be pulled up. Takes cold in head very easily; a little cold air causes cutting in the scalp. *Aggravation;* from physical or mental exertion; from stooping; from heat of a warm room or the bed; from 4 to 8 P. M.

Amelioration—From cool, open air; from lying down; from uncovering the head.

Photophobia; *evening light blinds very much; can see nothing on the table. Hemiopia; only sees left half of an object distinctly. Black spots before the eyes;* also veil and flickering. *Vision weak; is unable to distinguish small objects as well as formerly.*

Over-sensitive hearing with roaring in ears. *Smell extremely sensitive;* even odor of hyacinths nauseates. *Fan-like motion of alæ nasi.*

Yellowish-gray or *pale sickly color of the face.*

Dryness of mouth and tongue without thirst; mouth and tongue sensitive as if burnt ; vesicles on tip of the tongue feeling scalded and raw.

Feeling as if a ball rose from below up into throat. Cough, dry day and night with painfulness in region of stomach ; cough hurts and causes throbbing in head. Dyspnœa as if chest were constricted by cramp. Constriction of chest in region of false ribs, almost taking away the breath. *Dull aching pain all over the lungs as if they had been overworked, with feeling of constriction of chest as from a tight waistcoat.* Pressure and heaviness on chest as from a weight, obliging deep breathing. Palpitation ; *nearly every evening in bed ; after eating,* pulse accelerated. "Wind gurgles under apex of heart in left hypochondrium, with oppressed breathing " (Morgan).

Taste ; sour ; bitter ; fatty ; *sour* (or bitter) *taste to all food. Excessive appetite ; the more he eats, the more he wants. Hunger, but a small quantity fills him up ; constant feeling of satiety ; if he eats "his fill," has an unpleasant distressed feeling in liver. Eructations ; acid ; incomplete burning eructations which only rise into pharynx where they cause burning for several hours ; frequent belching without relief.* HICCOUGH. *Heartburn.* Nausea ; in pharynx and stomach; in morning, fasting ; with accumulation of water in the mouth ; *almost constant nausea. Feeling of tension beneath the stomach as if everything were too tight.* Fullness in stomach and bowels ; *pit of stomach sensitive to contact or tight clothing. Constriction and cramp in stomach. Pressure and heaviness in stomach as if distended ; in evening,* after eating only a little. MUST *sleep* after *eating.* Cannot digest fresh vegetables or leguminosa.

Hepatic region painful to touch ; sore pressive pain in region of liver on breathing. Gurgling in left side of upper abdomen. Sensation as though something heavy were lying in left side of abdomen. Flatulent distension of abdomen ; incarcerate flatus with continuous rumbling and rolling in abdomen, pressing upward toward chest and downward upon rectum and bladder. *The abdomen, especially the epigastric region, is sensitive to pressure, cannot bear the clothes tight. Pains across hypogastrium from right to left.*

Rectum contracted and protrudes during hard stool. Constipation ; stools dry and hard, or *first part lumpy, second soft;* feeling as if much remained unpassed (Nux) or great distress in rectum ; ineffectual urging *from contraction of anus.*

Severe backache, relieved by passing urine. Frequent desire to urinate. *Red sand in the urine.* Profuse watery urine. Strangury, retention, incontinence, cystospasm with symptoms characteristic of the drug.

" *Spinal* irritation due to excessive sexual indulgence is well met by *lycopodium* when the sexual desire is depressed and there are violent pains in the back, with dyspeptic symptoms and constipation" (Hoyne).

Drawing, tearing pains in all the limbs. Crawling and falling asleep in arms, hands and feet. *Great weakness of limbs.* Cramps in calves at night ; *profuse fetid foot sweat with burning of the soles* (Dr. D. A. Gorton) ; *one foot hot, the other cold,* or *cold sweaty feet (Calc. C.); cramp in toes when walking.* The whole body feels bruised (*Am*). *Affects especially right side.*

Great prostration with feeling of utter powerlessness. Desire for open air. Involuntary alternate extension and contraction of muscles. Emaciation.

Yawning and sleepiness during the day. Sleep restless; at ease in no position, must get up and walk; *cries or laughs in sleep,* starts ; with frequent waking; *falls asleep late* and awakes unrefreshed ; *hungry when awaking.* Dreams anxious, frightful.

Aggravation—ALL SYMPTOMS FROM 4 TO 8 P. M.; on lying down ; while sitting ; after eating ; moistening the parts ; on beginning to move ; on alternate days.

Amelioration—After 8 P. M. ; from continued motion ; from cold ; from warm food and drink.

Lycopodium presents a fine picture of *general* neurasthenia of which the irritation of the spine is but a part. *Brain-fag* stands out in bold colors. The drug ably meets those old, obstinate cases which Allopathy has painted over with iron, arsenic and quinine until tired Nature has uttered her protest. The *aggravation from 4 to 8 P. M., together with the head and gastro-intestinal symptoms,* is always the guide to its successful choice. *Red sand may* be present in the urine, but its absence *is by no means a counter indication.*

Natrum Chlorinatum—" Dr. R. T. Cooper (*British Journal of Homœopathy,* 1872), has found this remedy, in the first attenuation, of great service for debilitated women suffering from leucorrhœa, prolapsus uteri or metrorrhagia, accompanied by inter-scapular and vertebral neuralgia" (Minton).

Natrum mur.—Stiffness of nape of neck with pain. Cervical muscles painful on touch and when turning the head. *Sticking and stitches in back of neck, at night. Painfulness of the spine when lying*

down, aggravated by lying on the back. Tension, pressure and drawing
pains in spine. Burning smarting on uppermost dorsal vertebræ. In
small of back; *paralyzed feeling in the morning on rising ; violent pulsation ; pain as if broken.* Dull, bruised pain in coccyx and right
zygoma.

*Melancholy, depressed, sad and weeping ; consolation aggravates.
Terrible sadness during menses. Irritability. Absence of mind.
Anthropophobia. Likes to dwell on past unpleasant occurrences.*

Bursting headaches, especially frontal. *Worse in morning when
waking,* from reading, writing and talking and better from gentle
exercise—*generally disappear about noon.* Stitches as with knives in
occiput. Scalp sensitive.

*Dimness of sight, eyes give out when using them; letters and stitches
run together.*

Yellow color of face which *shines as if greasy.* Cough. Tension
in chest. Palpitation. Fluttering of the heart with a weak faint feeling, worse lying down. Irregular intermissions of heart and pulse
beat, worse lying on left side. Spasmodic stricture of œsophagus.

Mapped tongue. Taste ; *bitter;* salty; *lost. Violent thirst with dry
sticky mouth, worse in evening. Lids crack.* Craving for salt ; bitter
things. *Aversion; to bread of which she was once very fond;* to coffee.
Nausea and water brash. Cardialgia, pains coming on soon after eating and terminating when digestion is completed. Stitches and tension
in hepatic region. Abdomen distended; rumbling and incarceration
of flatus.

*Sensation of contraction in the rectum during stool; hard feces evac-
uated first with the greatest exertion that causes tearing in the anus so that
it bleeds and pains as if sore;* afterward thin stools also are passed ;
constipation every other day. Stools *hard, dry and crumbling. Stools
irregular, sometimes two or three passages per day, at other times no stool
for days;* alternation of constipation and diarrhœa. *The mental condition varies with the degree of constipation.*

Urine ; *pale, watery ;* yellow, turbid, with brick-dust sediment.
Involuntary urination while walking, coughing or laughing. Frequent micturition. *Cutting* (and burning) *in urethra after urination.*

*Menses late and scanty. Dysmenorrhœa with convulsions. Prolap-
sus uteri with aching in lumbar region, better lying on the back, with cutting in urethra after micturition. Pushing and bearing down in genitals
every morning, has to sit down to prevent prolapsus; feels weakest mornings in bed.* Leucorrhœa profuse, greenish, worse while walking.
Uterine cramps with burning and cutting in groins.

Drawing pains in thighs, knees and legs. *Feeling as if hamstrings were too short.* Cold feet. *Marked emaciation. Easily fatigued. Takes cold easily.*

Sleepy during day ; sleepless at night. *Dreams of robbers in the house.*

"*Natrum muriaticum* meets those cases which are attended with morning headache ; constipation with sensation of contraction of the anus; palpitation of the heart; white-coated or mapped-tongue; longing for salt; and especially when after great bodily exertion an itching nettle rash appears." (Hoyne.)

(*To be continued.*)

THE PATHOLOGY OF CROUPOUS PSEUDO-MEMBRANES.*

By JOHN C. MORGAN, M.D.,
Philadelphia.

THERE are general resemblances between pseudo-membranous formations, wherever found ; yet diversity of subjacent and contiguous tissues gives rise to characteristic differences, while the diverse functions of the parts involved widely separate them with regard to clinical symptoms and results. Fibrinous exudation, containing living leucocytes, which mostly die, becoming pus globules sooner or later, is the leading feature, when acute. When chronic, other conditions prevail, which are in their nature mainly cicatricial, sometimes ulcerative; for instance, within the uterine and rectal cavities. The general appellation of these is, "croupous membranes," and the attendant inflammation "croupous inflammation." The pseudo-membranes of mucous surfaces will be here mainly discussed, with the reasons and causes of such formations. The preliminary thought in all is, that a croupous formation is not the simple phenomenon of exudation, which it is often supposed to be, but is a complex fact requiring careful and analytical study for its comprehension, and also for its proper treatment, since a false method must inevitably tend to failure and often to death. The first maxim in medicine should be to do no harm, and we look chiefly to pathology to guide us in its fulfillment. Positive therapeutics is a more remote problem, where Hahnemann becomes master.

We will first briefly consider what may be *seen*, in gross and under the microscope. The gross appearance is that of a membrane, in masses of varied size and shape, moulded by the containing organ, of

*Read before the Pennsylvania State Homœopathic Medical Society, Sept. 23d, 1886.

diverse tints, from grayish white to yellowish, sometimes bloody at
the surfaces of separation. I shall here ask attention to the microscopical examination of two cases of my own, made with simple " teasing"
of the membranous product, pressure under the cover-glass, and observation with a quarter-inch objective, and eyepieces Nos. 1 and 2 ;
one, of membranous expectoration of subacute croup ; and one of
chronic membranous dysmenorrhœa.

CASE I. —L. S., a little girl seven years old, had a catarrh of the respiratory passages during several weeks, croup supervening, and finally proving fatal, despite the evacuation, with muco-purulent catarrh,
of much of the pseudo-membrane, in chunky pieces, during many
days.
    A fragment of this product, being teased into a thin layer, and ex-
amined, showed only fibres, closely interlaced, and inclosing myriads
of leucocytes, otherwise called white blood globules, emigrants from
the congested blood vessels of the air-tubes, and now known to us as
"pus corpuscles," all of which names, however, as now known, are
held to mean one and the same thing, differing only in numbers and
in circumstances.   Only a few epithelial cells were found, mostly isolated.

CASE II.—Mrs. B., aged forty years, from whom I removed a
mucous polypus, several years previous had had, since her last confinement, some ten years before, subinvolution of the uterus, with
menorrhagia, and very painful periods ; and during the intervals, great
inflammatory soreness, and on examination with the speculum, livid
redness of the uterus and vagina, hyperplastic enlargement of the
former, and a foul, gray, purulent. irritating leucorrhœa.
    In my judgment, every such case is to be suspected of a croupous
or membranous nature, and she was, therefore, instructed to save
everything evacuated at the next menstrual period.   I found therein a
complete cast of the corpus uteri, the pseudo-membranous quality of
which was easily proved, to the disgust and even alarm of the patient.
It was internally smooth, externally shaggy.   The microscopical examination showed, of course, an abundance of red blood globules, in
and around the membranous material ; the latter was composed of
fibres of coagulated fibrine, inclosing numerous leucocytes, or, we
will say, globules.

    In both of my cases, from the respiratory and the uterine mucous
membrane, the structure of the morbid product was the same, composed essentially of fibres and pus-cells ; with red blood globules,
when connected with menstruation.   In none was the mucous membrane itself examined ; in all, therefore, the separated product only
was observed.   The lack, however, is well supplied by other investigators, who have made thin sections of the diseased parts—post-mor-

tem—extending from healthy tissues, to and through the lesions, including all the transitional elements, enabling us to clearly perceive the steps of the morbid changes in the organs themselves, as well as the nature of the adventitious substance.

This membrane constitutes the objective point of all empirical treatment, and in pseudo-membranous croup of the trachea, it is described by Wagner (*Gen. Path.*, page 263) under the name "croup membrane," and he states that it "shows a remarkably great resistance to heat and all chemical reagents" (rather discouraging news for the empirics).

This "croup membrane" closely resembles all fibrinous exudations, but its peculiarity is that it is not a mere pouring out of fibrine and leucocytes upon the free surface of the mucous epithelium ; but it "has its origin in a peculiar metamorphosis of the epithelium itself" ; so that it *takes the place* of the epithelium, which is there partially wanting in consequence.

In the *normal* processes of epithelial nutrition and metamorphosis, the cells are rapidly formed, and soon die by change into mucus proper, developing the albuminoid principle called *mucin ;* new or young cells, however, being first formed, take the place of those about to be thus degenerated, metamorphosed, or dissolved. This normal change of the epithelial cells is called mucous degeneration, or rather, "mucous metamorphosis."

When, however, croup membrane is formed, this normal change of the cells is supplanted by a totally different one ; this mucous degeneration and solution. and the reproduction of young epithelial cells, both cease, and a new and morbid change occurs in them, called "croupous metamorphosis," whilst beneath this the basement tissue becomes practically little less than an ulcer. Thus, the origin and character of the lesions, in the several localities whose product I examined, and in all such cases, become clear, viz.: superficial ulceration, covered with metamorphosed epithelium, destitute of life and of cellular structure, but, as a fibrino-purulent cover, adhering to the ulcerated surface. How it can be separated, and how a normal epithelium can be restored, is then the question ; but some other points must be first considered, viz.: the mode of development and the progressive microscopic appearances of this croupous metamorphosis of the epithelium, together with the etiology of this process.

According to Wagner, it shows, in the first place, an increase in quantity in the protoplasm of the epithelial cells, with a consequent enlargement of them. Next, there appear in the protoplasm minute coagulations, at many points $\frac{1}{100}$ of a millimeter, or less, in size, and as they increase in number they advance from the periphery towards the centre of the cell. The effort at normal young cell formation is occasionally still seen also in the enlargement and division of the nucleus, as is usual in health.

Between these points of intro-cellular coagulation, the remaining liquid protoplasm disappears, the cell-wall is seen, brighter or darker, according to the direction of the light falling upon it, and the general effect is to give such cells a porous or indented look ; and it is now that they become, as previously intimated, "strikingly resistant."

This change in the cells goes on, however, until the last of the liquid protoplasm disappears ; the cell-wall is contracted irregularly, forming pores, and toothed outlines, fusing with those of adjacent cells, these being, however, artificially separable, as by maceration of the membrane in "Müller's fluid." This being effected, the process, in all its stages, can be studied in the separated elements, each showing its own degree of the metamorphosis called "croupous." During its progress, of course, the nuclei gradually disappear. Still others of these cells are invaded by emigrated white blood globules, and these become pus-cells, to the number, sometimes, of half a dozen in a single one of the epithelial elements.

Such is croupous metamorphosis, and such is the origin of the dense, resistant, fibrino-puruloid pseudo-membrane with which we have to do. As before said, however, and notwithstanding this demonstrated mode of development within the individual cells, the *completed* membrane, in gross, and even by microscopic examination *without* the artificial cell separation just described, cannot be distinguished from any ordinary fibrinous exudation, with its usual fibrillation, with its entanglement of white cells, and of the serum of the blood. By way of emphasis, I will quote Wagner again : "Croupous exudation, on account of its similarity with fibrinous exudation, is in many ways confounded with it, but, from its nature and origin, is entirely distinct from it" ; yet he says repeatedly, it "resembles coagulated fibrine," as I have myself, also, demonstrated above ; and we may, therefore, fancy, at least, that, after all, the protoplasm of the altered cells has itself gradually undergone a *change to fibrinous fluid*, in order to suffer such a metamorphosis. At all events, all clinical considerations must begin by recognizing the *cellular origin* of all croupous pseudo-membranes, and the folly of treating it as a mere fibrinous effusion upon a free surface must be now evident.

Diphtheria furnishes a pseudo-membrane, very similar to other croupous membranes, but produces also an *interstitial* deposit, the so-called "pure diphtheritic exudation," to wit, an infiltration of the mucous membrane and subjacent tissues with white globules, and particularly with free nuclei, tending to strangulation and sloughing. Indeed, this infiltration is widely extended in the body generally, in the viscera, etc., doubtless causing general toxic effects. In addition, the micrococcus, the microbe of so many low morbid states, and even of some healthy organs, as the mouth, throat, etc., is found in the superficial strata of the membrane, as well as in internal parts. Still farther, according to Lœffler's recent researches, occur the peculiar bacilli observed by Klebs and himself, and which he regards as the only *specific* microbe of diphtheria. It is found in the deeper strata of the pseudo-membrane.

The very latest portion only of this product that is found immediately overlaying the engorged vessels, in fatal cases, and probably deposited subsequent to the true croupous metamorphosis of all the epithelium, consists of diffuse fibrinous exudation, pure and simple, according to the same authority.

These traits distinguish diphtheria from simple "membranous croup" of the larynx, trachea, etc.; the frequent albuminuria, and the systemic infection are also wanting in the latter. Finally, it should be remembered that pure croup, according to Wagner, presents, in the greater number of fatal cases, an extension of membrane upwards to the soft palate (recalling the key note of *bromine*, false membrane extending upwards from the larynx), together with muco-purulent catarrh of the bronchi.

En passant, it must be noted that not all pseudo-membranes are croupous. Thus, ulcers of the intestines, having no epithelium, may have passed beyond the possibility of that metamorphosis, yet produce a fibrinous exudation, entangling cells and other *débris*, as shown under the microscope.

Returning to the purely croupous pseudo-membranes, we are led to ask why the epithelial cells of all or any of the mucous membranes, not alone the respiratory, should ever suffer the characteristic fibrine-like metamorphosis of their protoplasm, above described. This etiological question bears on that of a reasonable therapy.

We may, in seeking a reply, interrogate the blood-vessels, the blood itself, and the forces of the circulation ; also the lymphatics, the nerves, etc.

First, the *blood vessels*. These, in the initial inflammation, are, of course, arterially and actively distended. Later, and along with the diminution of the fever heat, as in all other active diseases, the minute veins show a greater participation, as we find illustrated in conjunctivitis and in pharyngitis, the color becoming darker. Coincidently, all sorts of exudation more easily occur, through their mechanical distention, and so we have swelling.

Second, the *blood itself.* Here we find great possibilities as to fibrinous formations. The reaction of normal blood is decidedly *alkaline ;* yet, from what we know of the action of the liver upon digested starch and sugar, producing glycogen, or animal dextrine, which goes everywhere with the blood ; and remembring that the mere splitting of a molecule of glycogen produces two molecules of lactic acid ; that this is a normal result of muscular irritation, as in normal activity, partial alteration of the blood in this respect is not surprising with the conditions existing, during active disease. Rheumatic hepatitis likewise seems capable of it. It is certain that alkalinity opposes fibrinous coagulation, whilst acidity, however slight, tends to promote it. Since, according to Brown–Sequard, fibrine is also a special product of muscular activity, this body may be chemically affected at its very source, or in patients who are abnormally active.

In still another particular, may the blood itself contribute to fibrinous metamorphosis. Polli and Virchow have shown that fibrine, in the lymph, exists in a form which does not readily and spontaneously coagulate and even when this does not take place, the clot is soft and diffluent. In the blood, a part of the fibrine normally exists in the same form, and has been distinguished by Denis, by the name of "dissolved fibrine," this does not, when removed from the body, spontaneously coagulate, but adding the Epsom salt—the sulphate of magnesia—causes it to do so. Thus, without the presence of any free acid at all, lactic or other, we find that the introduction of a *saline* substance is capable of promoting the fibrinous metamorphosis. That this particular salt may, therefore, be pathologically homœopathic to this process, will, of course occur to everyone in our ranks, upon the mere mention of it. Tests are, however, yet lacking.

The remainder of the fibrine is spontaneously coagulable when at rest, when exposed to the air, or when mechanically entangled ; and this is called, by way of distinction, "concrete fibrine." The two forms, as combined in the blood, form a total within the body, called by Denis and Schmidt, *plasmine*, in opposition to all the other albuminoid matter of the blood liquor, which receives the name, *serine.* This double fibrine is, furthermore, *wholly* coagulated by an excess of chloride of sodium. In croupous pneumonia, and other acute diseases, as all know, there is a disappearance of chlorides from the urine, whils there is increase of the same in the expectoration. How far this local accumulation of the chlorides may promote the croupous metamorphosis, is certainly worthy of thought.

These facts, also, raise the same question as arose in reference to the magnesium sulphate, viz.: Is the sodium chloride pathologically homœopathic to croupous diseases?

It may be objected that all these are "too similiar," that is, that they are "identical," and hence not truly homœopathic. If so, a sufficient variation may be found, perhaps, as to the sodium salt, in the bromide, or the iodide, or the bicarbonate, which is, besides not without a record of empirical success in pseudo-membranous croup, or the biborate, likewise valued in membranous dysmenorrhœa, or if we think of a potassium chloride, the *kali carb.*, which has done good work in both maladies, or *kali caust.*, which has also done something. Of the magnesium salts, the soluble citrate may be worthy of particular consideration ; and as to lactic acid, its sodium and potassium salts may be mentioned—uniting the indications for these bases with its own, that is, if they do not materially subvert each other. The ammonium salts also deserve a good word. Again, if the sulphuric acid of the magnesium sulphate, and not the base, be thought of as the coagulant, then its sodium, lime and potassium salts may be found suitable. The latter two find place in Schüssler's croup system. All of which, however, in the view of a sound and conservative homœopathy, must await the proof to be furnished by experiments upon healthy human bodies. And we are obliged, of course, to extend the same query to lactic acid, for the same reasons first given.

Whatever in medicine, or diet, or musular exercise, or irritation, can cause the accumulation of either of these bodies in the blood*, should be regarded with suspicion, lest it prove a dangerous factor of fibrinous, and of croupous diseases, simple or diphtheritic, acute or chronic, tracheal or uterine, etc. (and possibly, in that other and fatal affection, heart-clot).

Third, the *blood momentum* has normally, a large share in preserving the fibrinous principles in fluid form, and also in preventing exudation, thus in two ways opposing pseudo-membranous formations. Everything which in the least degree diminishes the force of the circulation, therefore—even the obstruction produced by spasmodic croup —may be of grave significance, and for this same reason, a too rapid cessation of fever is most undesirable also, and may often be a legitimate ground for apprehension, whilst a sudden weakening of the

---

*See Burnett on "Supersalinity of the Blood."

heart by material doses of *aconite* or *veratrum vir.*, may prove lethal in this way.

Any loss of arterial force—arterial obstruction in particular—has a tendency, also, wherever arterial *anastomosis* is anatomically deficient, as in the spleen, and in the cortex of the brain, in operations after ligating every vessel, to promote hæmorrhage, and often, surprisingly soon, of which the result is often, in spleen or brain, an apopletic blood-clot, called in the former organ a "hæmorrhagic infarction." This is explained by the known violent reflux of the venous blood, whenever and wherever the arterial *vis a tergo*, both direct and anastomotic, happens to be withdrawn. There is an added possibility in all diseases where antiphlogistic measures are abusively pushed. It is also a fair question whether a like effect may not occur, without extravasation, at all, of red blood globules ; that is, with fibrinous globules, not globule hæmorrhage. The significance of this mechanical agency, however, I would expect to appear more in the corporeal uterine circulation than in the tracheal ; and in the chronic membranous dysmenorrhœa, as well as in the acute forms, the arterial system of the womb being greatly isolated, like a segument of the spleen.

Fourth, and coincidently, deficiency of (blood and body) heat, as after the subsidence of a high fever, may help on the degeneration. Fever, if moderate, is often conservative.

Fifth, the function of the lymphatic system in relation to pseudo-membranes is sometimes very conspicuous. In diphtheria, the glandular swellings sometimes become enormous—a point of distinction from simple membranous croup. Still, even in the latter, this system cannot play an indifferent part, as its subjacent relations with both the epithelium and the capillaries show.

Both the blood vessels and the lymphatics have an ultimate structure of connective tissue, and their endothelial lining consists simply of flattened and oblong connective tissue cells. In the capillaries, these cells are disposed with their edges closely together, only excepting points where their individual outline is incomplete, and it is, at these incomplete points, clearly visible under the microscope only when the vessel is distended, that the emigration of white blood globules from the blood-vessels is so easily observed. The excess of blood-liquor, containing the fibrine excrement of the tissues also escapes, and all these are at once carried off by the lymphatics, if not disabled, but are detained in situ, if the channels be impaired.

The beginnings of the lymphatics are two-fold, and their endo-thelium is here always so sparse, as to form only spaces of connective tissue, not vessels, at all, until they have advanced somewhat towards

the common centre, when the vessels became perfect and are completely lined, like the blood-vessels with endothelial cells. Thus their
beginnings are admirably adapted to the absorption of all exudations. These beginnings are : 1, just beneath the mucous capillaries,
to which they thus form a half-sheath, the mucous epithelial cells
forming the roof of the same ; and 2, minute extensions of these lymphatic spaces, reaching up between the capillaries, touch the under
surfaces of the epithelial cells of the mucous membrane. The lower
half-sheath of the capillaries formed by these lymphatic or connective
tissue spaces, are now seen to surround the individual blood-vessels,
and are, therefore, called "perivascular spaces." In the brain, they
envelop the whole vessel, and are regarded as of great importance. In
the mucous membrane, they cannot be unimportant, particularly as to
a proper *drainage* of the tissues. Every superficial or deep swelling
depends very much upon the filling up of the lymphatic or connective tissue spaces.

Inflammation, as in croup, causes excessive accumulation of the
materials poured out above and below the vessels, and the perivascular lymph-spaces have, in their own way, as much to contend with as
the mucous epithelium. Failing to remove all these accumulations,
swelling, obstruction, stasis, result—drainage is incomplete—fibrine
excrement remains in the tissues, with venosity from pressure, also, to
confuse their nutrition. At the same time, the extension of the inflammation to the connective tissue itself must, by multiplying its own
cells, exaggerate this obstructive interference. According to Wagner,
the lymphatics, in inflammation, are either dilated and filled with these
products, viz. : "pus, fat, detritus," and occasionally with fibrinous
coagula ; or, on the other hand, owing to the outside compression, the
lymphatics have often been found progressively collapsed, the lymph
stream becoming slower and slower, and then ceasing entirely ; tissue
drainage in that direction ceasing also. Simultaneously, the distended
venous capillaries cease to do their part as absorbents, whilst the
secretory cells fail to do theirs, in the proper metamorphosis and final
evacuation of the materials brought to them.

Sixth, the venous system must be included among the factors of
croupous metamorphosis. I will not retread this well-beaten track to
any great extent, but only remind you that it is foremost in causing
spasmodic symptoms, not only in tracheal croup, but in membranous
dysmenorrhœa, dysentery, etc. ; and, besides this, that in all cell-life, of
which these are abnormal illustrations, the trophic, or tissue-formative
nerves, have an undoubted function. A familiar instance is seen in
ulcerations of the cornea, due to paresis of the ciliary nerves. That a

like paresis, or some other perversion of the tracheal or uterine or other trophic nerves may contribute to the croupous metamorphosis, by negation, at least, of their normal preventive activity, is more than likely. Excessive medication is naturally hurtful in the presence of such paresis.

Seventh, and lastly, the cell-life itself, in abnormal action, or inaction, is obviously the nearest of all the facts in causation of the croupous metamorphosis. Why should the living cells, which normally resist and resent all intrusion of improper materials, and assure the elaboration of normal products only, fail, in so grave a manner, to perform these duties ? There are two parts to the reply : on the one hand, we must say that all the above-named causes of abnormal pabulum may co-operate to *overwhelm* their normal conservatism ; and, on the other hand, their own dynamic conditions may be defective—and this, in several ways ; by constitutional taint, inherited or acquired, or by paresis of the trophic nerves, as just mentioned ; through either or both of these agencies, the elective matter-exchanges, which are their chief function, cease to be effected, and they can thus become the passive victims of even the ordinary access of the blood-liquor, fibrine and all.

Put all these possibilities and facts together, and we may the more intelligently give answer to the final question : What is the *natural history* of croupous pseudo-membranes ?

Recall, if you please, what was first said as to the formation within the affected epithelial cells, of minute opaque particles at the periphery, where the fibrinoid alteration first takes place, and how this may be proved by macerating the tissues in Müller's fluid, whereby the elements are caused to fall apart, and may be separately studied in every stage of the change ; and how this formation gradually advances to the centre of the cell, obscuring the nucleus, and finally replacing all the ordinary or normal protoplasm which it previously contained. Then, compare this with the normal procedures, and thus learn what has to take place, in either the acute or the chronic form, before the mucous membrane can return to a state of health.

Normally the epithelial cells continuously and also rapidly grow, multiply, die and disappear. They mature and then undergo the "mucous metamorphosis ;" in other words, they become chemically transformed, particularly as to their protoplasm, into a new form of albuminoid body, called mucus, the basis of which is *mucin.* Thus they are successively liquefied, and mingled with cast-off individual epithelia, and with emigrated white globules, here called " mucous corpuscles;" and, thereafter, the whole is disposed of as the ordinary secretion of the part.

Now, the croupous ruin of even the superficial epithelia of a given space must be separated by the interference of the subjacent and youngest cells, which having thus far escaped the process, are still vital and active, the part undergoing a kind of cicatrization, indeed, very much like healing under a scab.

The croupous cells, however, being virtually necrosed, a more extreme involvement, extending to the deeper layers, removes the barrier to free emigration of white blood globules (leucocytes) from the distended vessels; consequently, these are copiously effused from the vessels, depleting them and promoting their restoration. The white globules themselves become pus-cells; and, in short, there is now suppuration beneath the croupous epithelium, which duly separates as a slough, sometimes *en masse*, sometimes piece-meal.

At the same time, every remaining normal cell in the deepest layers, and in the surrounding region, being stimulated by the neighboring inflammation, is growing, multiplying, forming mucus, and thus helping to undermine and cast off the pseudo-membrane, and to reform the normal tissue.

What can Nature do in this corrective process? Nature can and must do everything, and will, if we but content ourselves with *aiding her in these processes*, and avoiding impatient and impertinent interference with her, by over-drugging and by other excesses, which can only aggravate. Croupous pneumonia, once believed to be incurable, without the most heroic measures of depletion, counter-irritation, expectorants, anodynes, etc., is now known to be, when simply reversed, *self-limited*. What a thought for the doctor about to lose his head in the presence of a case of croupous laryngo-tracheitis!

Certain observations at the seashore during the past summer, have inspired the query with me, are not the majority of fatal cases of the latter disease actually killed by kindly meant heroic doctoring? One little girl I saw, with the red cicatrix of a laryngotomy done in June last, and after only twenty-four hours of allopathic medication. I could not refrain from believing, as I still do, that nothing but the drugs and other active and aggravating expedients used made the operation necessary. Just at this time, I was called to a precisely similar case, to which Dr. J. R. Tantum, of Wilmington, Delaware, was also a witness. The child recovered gradually, quietly and perfectly, within three weeks, after very conservative homœopathic medication, based upon the reflection that the other case got well when her physician had doubtless, after opening the larynx, recovered his

senses sufficiently to suspend active measures, and to reasonably depend on nature for the resolution of the inflammation, and the normal
separation of the pseudo-membrane. In my own case, this separation
was duly announced by a choking and swallowing spell, followed by
entire and permanent abolition of all signs of croup. The only remedies used, aside from two doses of *cham.*, which acted adversely, were
the three old stagers, given as Hahnemann would give them, viz.:
aconite in the fifteenth centesimal dilution, *spongia*ᵐ, and *hepar sul-
phuris*ᵐ. There may be no drug substance beyond the eleventh centesimal dilution. This is a pathological, not a clinical paper, and I
submit to that decision if you will, but thereby I must strongly emphasize one more question, viz.: Is not acute membranous croup normally
self-limited?

The chronic forms, I am sure, are subject to parallel reasoning,
only remembering that Hahnemann has taught us that all chronic diseases are such by virtue of an added factor, opposing the natural
tendency to health, viz.: some chronic miasm ; to the reality of which,
as I have argued elsewhere, modern pathology has given weighty
testimony.

As to the bearing of the foregoing remarks upon "croupous pneumonia," and upon that form of Bright's disease known as "croupous
nephritis," no detailed discussion can be indulged in at this time, and
this paper would be thereby unjustifiably extended. That question
may, however, be raised with propriety, in closing, and left for the reflection of thinking physicians.

ORIGINAL ARTICLES IN SURGERY.

CASES OF EMPYEMA, WITH SOME SUGGESTIONS AS TO TREATMENT.

By W. O. McDONALD, M.D.,
New York.

CASE I. The first case in the order of time was that of a young man
nineteen years old, in 1881. He appeared to have suffered from
malarial fever, contracted by rowing on some fresh water lake. Pleuritis, as a sequence of catching cold after prolonged muscular effort, was
followed by empyema of the left side. Aspiration was first performed
on March 19th, 1881, and it was repeated at intervals, until some
four hundred ounces of pus were taken away. On July 8th an aperture
was made in the chest, on a line with the anterior border of the axillary space, and about one inch of the seventh rib was exsected. The
pleural cavity was washed out with weak carbolized water for about a
month, when the aperture having closed, he left the city.

He has reported for the completion of the record. He is five feet eight and a quarter inches high, and his weight 150 pounds. Before his illness it had gone up to 160 pounds ; but since, he has never surpassed 155 pounds. Formerly quite a prominent athlete, a competitor in five and ten mile contests, he has been since obliged to confine himself to races of one hundred yards or thereabouts, but he claims to be among the best in these. His appetite, digestion and nutrition, are very good.

The apex impulse of the heart is normal in location. The shoulders are even. There is some flatness—want of rotundity—of the left side of the chest, in the vicinity of the scar left by the section. He has neither cough nor palpitation, and, excepting the shortness of breath alluded to above, he does not feel that his health or physical capacity have been impaired.

Aspiration was unduly repeated in this case beyond a doubt, but my previous experience had not rendered me sanguine, and I was slow to adopt operative measures.

There are points in the management of empyema in regard to which practitioners still differ, and I am not prepared to settle certain mooted questions, even for my own guidance ; but I must own to a certain feeling of dissatisfaction, when I hear men, whose professional position entitles them to a certain degree of respect, urge, at this date, that they consider aspiration to be an adequate and ample remedy for this disease. I am quite well aware that cases of cure of pyothorax by aspiration do occur not so infrequently in children, and also every now and then in adults. I say cure with a qualification. In my opinion, no case of this affection should be considered as cured until after the lapse of from one to two years.

There are certain sequelæ of pyothorax that prevent the recovery of the sufferers, perhaps after the pus has gone from the chest. The more common of these are perforation and discharge of the pus through the chest wall; perforation and discharge through the lung substance ; encapsulation of pus, followed by caseous change, and this later by abscess ; excessive and progressive production of fibrinous exudation, leading to adhesive pleurisy; and, finally, phthisis.

Let it be understood that I am objecting to the application of aspiration as a sufficient and competent remedy for the disease, to be employed alone, and to be pushed until time or the death of the patient demonstrates its futility.

Aspiration employed to settle the diagnosis; used to remove enough of the fluid to render anæsthesia safer ; or undertaken to tide the patient over some time of stress or danger; under such circumstances the process is invaluable.

Aspiration by itself, and alone, is a slow acting remedy, and it certainly favors the development of the complications specified above. Let no man feel safe from perforation of lung tissue because he is regularly and periodically extracting all the pus from the pleura that the patient can permit, because in just such a case I have seen perforation and discharge by the bronchial tubes.

The prolonged use of aspiration necessitates the equally prolonged stay of pus in the pleura. The instrument can never take all the fluid ; can never exhaust the quantity present. Finally, there must be a quantity left, for which the most favorable fate will be incapsulation. In a certain proportion of cases the encapsulated mass suppurates at a later date, and discharges into the thorax, abdomen, or through the chest wall.

The longer the pus remains in the pleura the greater the quantity of fibrinous material exuded, and an extensive fibrinous exudation is apt to end in either fibrous phthisis or in great contraction and deformity of the chest, and still more remotely in the formation of a cavity with rigid walls, that, while they will not permit the expansion of the lung, at the same time are unable to approximate the bony walls of the thorax, thus perpetuating the condition indefinitely.

CASE II. My next case was that of a girl ten years old, in 1882. The empyema developing as the sequence of scarlatina, located in the right side, and with it there were so much congestion and œdema of the lower part of the chest wall that it was pronounced to be abscess of the liver by one physician who was called to see her.

A permanent operation was made on February 2d, 1882, and was kept open for something over two months by repeated washing and the use of an oakum plug. A piece of the sixth rib was excised in the axillary line.

This patient presents more deformity than any other of the series. The shoulders are nearly even, the left scapula is "wrung out," probably on account of rotation of the bodies of the vertebræ, but the flattening of the right side of the chest is very moderate.

As far as concerns the child's health, it is a perfect recovery. She is tall for her age, but her nutrition is good. She is fleshy and strong, and a good runner, showing that her breathing capacity is above the average. Formerly prone to attacks of bronchial catarrh, since the operation she has had none. In the judgment of her mother, she suffers from nothing that can be attributed to the disease or to the treatment.

The only comment I have to make on this record is that the prognosis is stated by authors to be particularly bad when empyema appears as a sequence of scarlatina.

CASE III. My next case was one of a man who was thirty-four years old, in 1884. Early in May he fell through the floor of a burning house, lodging when he had gone through to the waist. In the fall he broke one or two of his ribs on the left side, probably the fourth and fifth, near the nipple. No doubt the fragments penetrated the lung, as he had hæmoptysis and pneumo-thorax at once; pneumonia followed; later he presented pneumo-hydro-thorax probably, and pneumo-pyo-thorax certainly.

On May 17th and 28th aspiration obtained air only, but on the 31st, pus being drawn out, the chest wall was perforated in the seventh space in the left axillary line ; but as the ribs did not approach one another the rib was not exsected. Before the operation was performed he had passed into a typhoid state, and after it he did not improve at once. Soon he developed a phlebitis of the veins of the left leg, inner side, the redness and swelling finally extending from the foot to the groin. After the phlebitis yielded he began to gain rapidly, and the chest opening closed in about one month after it was made. The washing out process caused so much cough and disturbance that it was discontinued.

Early in 1886, when overhauled, the result was as follows: Appetite and digestion are good ; nutrition rather too good, as he has become bulky, weighing two hundred and thirty pounds with a height of five feet and eleven inches. He is able to attend to business, which takes him out of doors much of the time, but his breath is short. He cannot hurry or run, and he is forced to go up stairs slowly. His weight is thirty pounds greater than before his illness. He has not been sick in any way since he convalesced, but the accident and its sequences have impaired his vitality to a much greater degree than in any other one of the series. But he claims that his general want of physical capacity is due largely to the varicose veins that have appeared in his left leg from the phlebitis, and that the swelling and weakness of the limb and the cramp of the muscles are greater hindrances than the shortness of breath resulting from the thoracic lesions.

His chest is not deformed ; the shoulders are even. There is flatness of the chest near the scar, but he appears to possess a fine amount of thoracic expansion. He presents no other thoracic symptoms or disturbances.

I find, upon inquiry, that the long-continued washing out of the cavity, after the evacuation of the pus, is practiced by the majority of operators and insisted on by some as a protective against septic infection, and as favoring the discharge of pus contained in pockets or depots. Loomis, however, condemns it, and says it has caused a fatal issue in three of his cases. In some of mine it caused so much cough that I was forced to give it up after a time. I am at present of the opinion that the prolonged use of injections into the cavity of the pleura will be found to be unnecessary if the peroxide solution is used after the fashion indicated in the histories of the next two cases.

Case IV. The fourth patient was a young man twenty-four years old, in 1885. His illness began with pneumonia, both sides, excited by prolonged exposure to cold wind after severe skating rink exercise. An alarming state of collapse came on after the crisis ; from this he happened to have been rescued by free alcoholic stimulation; and while resolution was progressing favorably in his right side, and probably in the left as well. fluid began to accumulate in the left pleural cavity. Typhoid symptoms came on rapidly, and as aspiration furnished pus, the chest wall was opened on April 20th, 1885,. some three-fourths of an inch of the ninth rib being exsected in the left axillary line. It was observed that there was an unusual amount of fibrinous material both in the pus which flowed forth and on the surface of the pleura. The pus, which was somewhat peculiar in odor, became very fœtid ; the shreds of fibrine discharged changed in tint, grew darker, blue, green, almost black ; the fibrine on the pleural surface, as seen through the aperture, presented similar tints, and it became evident that gangrene was impending. The carbolized water used in washing out the cavity exercised no good effect. The patient's general condition changed for the worse ; the typhoid state returned in a pronounced degree.

The solution of hydrogen peroxide was now tried as an injection into the pleural sac with an effect that was simply marvelous. The odor, which had become offensive beyond the power of words to describe, was promptly extinguished, and the production of pus was stopped. The intense interest of this dramatic situation was such as can only be appreciated by a participant. Here was a cavity pouring forth its horrible pus, the odor of which contaminated the whole house every time the plug was removed, nauseating the attendants, lay and professional; disgusting to all but the patient, who had passed into such a state of insensibility that he could hardly be roused to swallow, having lost all power of expression of suffering, and certainly consigned, in the minds of all who saw him, to a speedy death as a happy release from the existing misery. To have this tide of disaster stayed, to have this foul spring quenched, this stinking cavern sweetened, simply by the use of a few spoonfuls of a clean liquid, known to the druggist from whom it was obtained only as "a hair wash used to make dizzy blondes," was a result so near to the miracles that it only needed suitable change of time and scene to have caused the one responsible to be burned as a sorcerer or revered as a demi-god.

Owing, doubtless, to the great extent of the pus-producing surface, and to the impossibility of applying the solution to the whole of it at once, both discharge and odor returned to a slight extent in some twenty-four hours, but the repetition of the injection corrected them promptly, and for the next week or ten days it was needful to repeat the use of the solution at intervals of from twenty-four to thirty-six hours. I was present in this case as the consultant and operator, but my work was practically done when the hydrogen peroxide solution was first used. Both the foul odor and the pus production were stopped by the use of the agent.

The aperture closed in thirty-eight days after it was made, and the patient convalesced without let or hindrance.

This young man is five feet and eight and a half inches high; his weight is 154 pounds. His appetite, digestion, nutrition and development are all excellent. His ability to endure fatigue is shown by many long trips on the bicycle; on one day he got over nearly ninety miles and was in no way exhausted at the end of it. He is not sensitive to changes in the weather; he has no pulmonary symptoms, and he is not short-winded; in fact he is not aware that he has been damaged in any way by the experiences referred to above.

There is no retraction of the chest. There is some flatness in the vicinity of the scar, but the left shoulder is a trifle the higher.

I am not able to point out any organ or function as having suffered or been impaired by this empyema or the means adopted for its cure.

When the solution of hydrogen peroxide is brought in contact with pus it produces a yeast-like effervescence, with apparently a great production of free gas, and if the mixture is made in a cavity this yeasty fluid is apt to boil out of the aperture with much fuss and bubble. The solution used by me was stated to have been originally twelve per cent., but it is evident that it becomes much weaker in time. However, to guard against possible accident in this case, it was diluted with three parts of water, and thus used, it produced no evident disturbance.

In the *Medical News* of November 30th, 1886, a report is presented, taken from the *Lancet*, October 9th, 1886, of what is styled a fatal result of peroxide of hydrogen injections. The report originated with a Norwegian surgeon, but the death occurred from the use of the peroxide solution in a fistula about one and a half inches long, the remnant left after two months of an exsection of the ninth and tenth ribs for an empyema. Death followed in some ten minutes after the seventh injection was made. But even by this report, "the cause of death was, therefore, by no means clear." We do not know whether the solution was strongly charged with gas; whether there was an abundant opportunity for the escape of gas and fluid externally; whether the death was due to the solution, to the gas, or to the method of administration of the injection.

In a discussion on this subject, a surgeon stated that he had injected, through a perforation in the chest, in a case of empyema, a solution of the mercuric bichloride in preference to the hydrogen peroxide, because he was afraid of the bad effects of the rapid discharge of gas which would ensue if the latter agent were used. It probably never occurred to him that he was resorting to an agent which is known to be much more noxious; that he could not tell how much of his bichloride he would leave in the chest, exposing his patient to the possibility of mercurial poisoning, or that he could so dilute the peroxide solution as to get all its good effects without producing the rapid, abundant, and possibly dangerous ebullition within the pleura.

CASE V. The last case was one of a girl seven years old, in 1886, in which I was called as a consultant. She sickened in May, beginning with chills, fever and general indisposition, attributed to malaria, which progressed, until in June she suffered from an attack of prostration so severe as to warrant the fear that she would perish. She rallied, however, and the case dragged along with chilliness at times, fever, sweats and pronounced emaciation, until, in the latter part of September, when, coming under the charge of another physician, the true nature of the case was recognized.

It was then found that the right side of the thorax was greatly distended, with a special bulge in the vicinity of the anterior extremities of the third and fourth ribs, right side. After aspirating twice to reduce the amount of pus, a perforation was made in the chest wall, a section being cut from the fifth rib in the right mammillary line, the pleural cavity was washed out and the peroxide solution injected. The production of pus ceased promptly and the aperture closed in ten days.

In some two weeks' time fever and general disturbance returned. There was tenderness in the hepatic area, which was also swollen. There was some jaundice, but there was no redness of the skin. Later the scar of the exsection gaped; soon a membrane bulged, and on incising this pus squirted to the ceiling. A large quantity was discharged, the cavity was washed out as before, and the hydrogen peroxide injected.

From this time forth the child began to get better, and at the present time she is perfectly well. The digestion, nutrition, strength and endurance are up to the highest standard. The right side of the chest is flattened, and the right shoulder is depressed, but otherwise it is a perfect recovery. In this patient the hydrogen peroxide solution seemed to check the production of pus at once, consequently there did not appear to be any good reason why the aperture should be kept open.

In the *Medical Record*, October 30th, 1886, there appears a summary of an article by Lagrange, of Bordeaux, referring to the site of the incision in perforating the chest wall for the relief of empyema.

Lagrange reports a case when, after incising the left eighth intercostal space, the patient died the next day from peritonitis! *post mortem* examination showing that the diaphragm was pierced, letting the pus into the peritoneal cavity. According to this author many surgeons have met with a similar mishap in penetrating the chest wall by knife or trocar, or in exsection of bone. It appears, then, that as the diaphragm may be adherent to the chest wall, as high as the fifth rib, consequently the opening in the chest wall should not be made below the fourth space.

Curiously enough it would seem that there may be two sides even to this phase in the theory of the treatment of empyema. In my fifth case the surgeon excised the fifth rib, and completely evacuated the contents of the chest, the wound closing up in the meantime. After the lapse of two weeks another collection of pus presented itself and was evacuated through the same aperture. Of course the query will be suggested as to what would have been the effect if the incision had been made in one of the lower spaces of the chest in the first place. However, in view of the report of Lagrange there can be no question as to the wisdom of locating the opening above the fifth rib under all circumstances. Once inside of the chest, the propriety of making a section lower down can be considered.

Many operators have striven to exclude air from the pleural cavity after the pus has been evacuated. It has always seemed so difficult to do this and at the same time to keep the space free from pus, that I have never made the attempt, and in the light of my experience, it does not strike me as being either practicable or necessary. Donaldson, if I remember correctly, says it cannot be done.

In an article published in a former number of this journal, I have made reference to the danger of producing anæsthesia in empyema. In each of my cases ether was used, and I am convinced now that the individuals were in serious jeopardy from the anæsthesia produced. In the article referred to on anæsthesia, I advocated the use of the monoxide of nitrogen as being probably safer than any other agent known to me. I have not had an opportunity of trying it in an empyema, but I recently made use of the gas in aspirating the chest in an extensive serous accumulation, where, of course, the physical conditions were similar.

I will begin by stating that I am afraid of all anæsthetics; that I am never comfortable while any patient of mine is under the influence of any agent of this class ; that I never give chloroform, and finally, that I have never mixed these substances in any way.

In my case of serous effusion into the left pleura, upon introducing the needle of the aspirator my patient came so near to fainting outright that I was scared, and took out the needle before I had abstracted a sufficient quantity of the fluid to render the subsequent use of ether safe in my judgment. Inasmuch as I still felt that it was imperative upon me to remove more of the fluid from this patient's pleura, I was now placed in an awkward dilemma. The left side of the chest was so full that the apex impulse of the heart was not felt anywhere to the left of the notch below the ensiform. I did not dare to try aspiration without an anæsthetic again for fear that this dislocated heart would stop altogether, and for analogous reasons I was not willing to resort to the use of ether.   Everything indicated that this would be a good case wherein to test the action of the laughing gas.   And it was administered with the happiest of effects.   Under its influence the respiration became easier, deeper and slower, the pulse increased in volume, and there was less than usual of the cyanotic condition common to this form of intoxication.

Lest it shall be thought that I am fussy in the matter of my fears for this patient in case aspiration was repeated without an anæsthetic, I would refer the reader to the *Medical News* of January 1st, 1887, in which a case of sudden death, from aspiration, is reported by Reeve, of Ohio.

To summarize the foregoing :

I. Settle the diagnosis early by aspiration, removing enough fluid to render the subsequent use of anæsthesia safer.

II. Perform pleurotomy at once.

III. Use laughing gas for anæsthetic purposes, if attainable; if not, ether; but neglect no precautions.

IV. The site of the incision should be above the fifth rib.

V. Wash the pus out of the pleural cavity with warm water once.

VI. Inject the solution of hydrogen peroxide, diluted, to render the pus sweet and to check its production.

VII. Let the aperture close when pus ceases to be produced.

REMARKS ON INTERNAL URETHROTOMY, WITH CASES.*

By W. B. VAN LENNEP, M.D.,
Philadelphia.

EVERY originator of a new method of treatment or operation would seem to tend toward the extreme of too extensive application, would make the same a cure-all and an infallible one.   He is met, however, by a host of opponents, incited, some by personal motives, others by jealousy, but the majority by the above mentioned tendency on the part of the inventor.   These decry the same as useless, injurious, etc., in varying degrees, and it is only by the continued accumulation of testimony from disinterested observers that the procedure finds its real place.   With this end in view, I propose to relate my experience with internal urethrotomy as devised and taught by Otis, of New York.

· *Read before the Pennsylvania State Medical Society, September 23d, 1886.

I have practiced this operation for over two years, and have a series of nearly thirty cases observed for periods varying from the above down to a few weeks. They have been cut for the relief of gleety discharges, as a rule; for troublesome symptoms of the prostatic portion occasionally; and, jn two instances, for almost complete closure of the urethra. The number of strictures has varied from one to six; their location from one to four and a half inches down, the average depth of stricture following urethritis being, from my experience, between two and three or three and a half inches. Hence they have always been anterior to the triangular ligament, or in the superficial urethra, and readily reached by a straight instrument.

In two instances, there has been bleeding requiring attention subsequent to the operation, while but three have had more than the slight febrile reaction we might look for after any surgical interference. Cutting has been undertaken for hard, callous strictures, yielding only to a certain amount of dilatation, and then bleeding readily under manipulation; for elastic, recontracting or resilient strictures, which stretch six or eight sizes, perhaps, at one sitting, but are back again to the starting point at the next. With but one exception, sounds and local and constitutional medication have always been tried first.

I have operated without any anæsthetic, with cocaine, and with ether, and would give the preference, other things being equal, to the latter, on account of the complete relaxation produced, and because cocaine has, in several instances, disappointed me.

The after treatment has with some been *nil;* with others a course of sounding extending over a period of three weeks, during which the discharge of healing dries up. As a rule, the latter have done better. With this have been associated mild local applications of one form or another by means of injection, medicated bougie, or painting through the endoscope.

The majority of cases have been markedly benefited or cured of the troublesome symptoms; in a number, too, I have been able to find a "catch" with the bulbous sound at one or more points cut. In some the symptoms recur with the recontraction, in others they continue in its absence. In some, they disappear when this constriction is removed by a second operation, in others they do not. I ought to add, in justice to myself, that this recurrence or failure, if you please, has not been more frequent in my earlier than in my later operations. A certain number of failures are undoubtedly due to follicular disease which often seems almost impossible to cure, unless, perchance, it be kind enough to cure itself. A word concerning the technique of the operation may not be out of place.

The first step is to ascertain the full capacity of the urethra and accurately locate and measure the stricture or strictures. This is readily done with the urethrometer. The meatus and superficial constrictions are then cut to the full size with Otis' dilating urethrotome. I use this method almost entirely in enlarging the entrance to the urethra. The pressure seems to benumb the pain and the register enables one to be much more accurate than with the knife; the bleeding, too, is less troublesome.

The tightest stricture, usually the callous one, is then stretched and incised. My instrument registers one size too large, and in my later operations I have purposely overstretched and consequently over-incised the stricture. This is repeated if necessary until the urethrometer detects no "catch," and then the remaining constrictions, of which there are almost always one or more, situated anteriorly as a rule, are treated in a like manner.

It is hardly necessary to add a word in favor of cutting a tense stricture as compared with the older methods; Otis has argued the matter at length and in a convincing manner, to American surgeons at least.

.In incising a stricture I take pains to have the knife look upward as nearly as possible in the median line. As a result the consequent bleeding is, to my mind, very much less, and in the two cases when bleeding was at all troublesome I neglected to do this.

Another precaution, and by no means an unnecessary one with the instrument in question, is to have the knives *literally* sharp. I once tried to operate with a dull knife, and since that time have them ground immediately after use.

The operation done, a large Nélaton catheter is introduced to the bulb and a warm antiseptic solution freely injected. It runs out alongside the catheter, of course, and very soon flows clear, however free the hemorrhage. This is repeated if necessary after each urination for from twenty-four to forty-eight hours. Bleeding usually accompanies the flow of urine and erections, but has, in every instance, yielded as readily to the washing as at the time of operating. The penis is gently bandaged, a folded napkin laid over it as a pad, which is held in place by a towel or bandage fastened front and back to a waistband, thus allowing the patient to make considerable pressure by traction on the same.

The account of a few cases may be of interest.

I. Mr. A., clerk, between 30 and 35 years of age, came to me in the summer of 1884 with a chronic but free urethral discharge and a left sided epididymitis. On the subsidence of the latter, I found, on examination, a clean cut, short constriction, a trifle over three inches down. It admitted a No. 27 (French) sound, and, to make a long story short, was, with considerable difficulty, gradually dilated to No. 36. In the meanwhile he had topical applications and several remedies.

The urethral capacity was full No. 45, but beyond No. 36 the stricture would not stretch, each sounding, too, being followed by free bleeding. To complicate matters, the epididymitis relapsed, and he was induced to try urethrotomy.

I operated with the patient under ether, and by two stretchings and cuttings brought the stricture up to No. 46. No other constrictions were present, and he recovered without a bad symptom and without after treatment. The discharge ceased, and nearly a year afterward I was unable to find any sign of stricture. This is the largest urethra I ever met with.

II. Mr. S., mechanic, æt. 33 years, was sent to me on account of symptoms that caused a suspicion of stone. I examined him carefully and made out a decided prostatic catarrh with extreme hyperæsthesia. He positively denied having had a urethritis, and I began with five drop applications of a five per cent. solution of nitrate of silver to the prostatic urethra, together with pressure to the same by means of cylindrical sounds. When I reached No. 29 (French) it was arrested at three and three-quarter inches, and I found there a hard, resisting constriction that refused any dilatation. The urethral capacity was found to be No. 35, the stricture measuring No. 28, while anterior to it was another of larger calibre. They were both cut and a No. 35 sound readily introduced; the patient being etherized, the deep urethra and bladder were carefully examined. There was next to no bleeding, the annoying perineal pains and dysuria disappeared, and the urine cleared up. On the second day, however, patient had a severe chill followed by high temperature (104 degrees) and a sweat. He received *aconite*, but the chill recurred with a sweaty fever and symptoms indicating *gelsem.* Still the fever continued with occasional chills and sweating at irregular intervals until it assumed a typhoid character. *Baptisia* seemed to clear up everything and he is now in a fair way to recover.

III. Mr. J., merchant, æt. 31, came under my care in January, 1885. He had had several attacks of urethritis, and, for a long time, had never been free from a slight urethral discharge, which seemed constantly inclined to spring into full bloom on the slightest provocation. He had been the rounds and tried everything. I found a contracted meatus, a constriction behind the fossa navicularis, a stricture through which a No. 30 sound could, with difficulty, be squeezed just short of two inches down, and another admitting a No. 27 nearly two inches further. Both constrictions would only give two or three sizes, while the urethral capacity was No. 37.

Using a four per cent. solution of cocaine as an anæsthetic, I brought them up to full No. 37, and the other day, fifteen months later, a No. 37 bulb went through the urethra as smoothly as it did immediately after the operation. There has been no recurrence of the discharge. Patient had two smart hemorrhages on the second and eighth days, following erections.

IV. Mr. C., salesman, consulted me concerning a urethral discharge he had been troubled with for about fifteen years, every over-exertion or sexual indulgence bringing on a profuse flow. His urethra measured No. 43, and, besides a contraction at the orifice, there were three strictures, approximately at one, two and four inches. They could be stretched with considerable force to No. 40, or even No. 41, but would bleed quite freely and require, at the next sitting, a No. 33 or No. 34 to begin with, so rapidly did they contract.
Urethrotomy was performed without an anæsthetic, at his request. At the first sitting I cut the two anterior strictures, freely over-incising them. At a second sitting, number three was treated in like manner. Still the discharge continued, and three months later I again cut a "catch" I found at stricture number two.
There was no apparent change in the flow, which still resisted every topical application and internal medication imaginable. I gave him, among other things, *hydrast. sulph.* as an injection, and, to my surprise, for it had hitherto always disappointed me, the discharge was checked at once. It recurs, however, to this day from the same exciting causes; it is bland, milky and profuse, unaccompanied by pain or inflammatory symptoms and, from what I can learn, is non-infecting. About five months after the last cutting, I examined the urethra, but could find no sign of stricture.

V. Mr. M., sixty years old, contracted gonorrhœa when a young man, and used "very strong injections of nitrate of silver." He had noticed that, for some time, the stream of urine was getting smaller, and that he was obliged to use a good deal of force to expel the same.
I succeeded, with some difficulty, in getting the smallest filiform bougie into the urethra, and had to use considerable persuasion to make it advance. By degrees, a second was insinuated alongside, then a third, and so on until the urethrometer could be made to enter the canal. I found a capacious urethra measuring No. 35 or No. 36 up to within two and a quarter inches of the meatus; from that point on was a hard cicatricial tube. I cut up and down at several sittings, until I could readily pass a No. 35 sound. There was immediate improvement, which has continued, although the tendency to recontraction requires a stretching about once a month.

I would, in conclusion, heartily endorse internal urethrotomy in hard, callous strictures, which resist complete dilatation; in those which constantly contract, elastic or resilient ones. In tight stricture we must come to this procedure sooner or later in most cases. In giving a prognosis, however, we must remember follicular disease, and, in rare instances, an atonic condition of the mucous membrane. We can, I think, perform the operation with every promise of success in cases of prostatic disease, catarrhal or nervous, when such a stricture exists in the anterior urethra.

I am decidedly opposed to internal urethrotomy beyond the bulb ; hemorrhage is apt to be severe, and is hard to control, and reactions are frequent and dangerous. Further, the apparent constrictions in the triangular ligament, in many instances, certainly depend upon and disappear with the anterior strictures, while those of traumatic origin, so common in the membranous urethra, are best treated through a perineal incision.

SMALL-POX INOCULATION.

IN a lecture recently delivered at St. Mary's Hospital, Mr. Shirley Murphy adduced some evidence to show that there was a probability that the virus of small-pox obtained from the initial vesicle produced by inoculation of small-pox differed in its action from that obtained from the general eruption. The not infrequent death from inoculated small-pox led at first to much opposition to this method of protection against natural small-pox, but later it was found that inoculation could be performed without risk. In an account given by Sir George Baker of the extraordinary success attending the inoculations of Daniel Sutton, of Ingatestone, in Essex, who in three years inoculated some 20,000 persons without bad result, he attributed this success to the fact that Sutton allowed his patients to enjoy fresh air during their illness ; while Dr. Glass, of Glasgow, believed that Sutton's treatment in encouraging perspiration was responsible for their recovery. It is clear that Sutton professed to have a secret in his treatment, although this secret is only metioned in relation to the composition of certain medicines ; but Sir George Baker, curiously enough, observed that " What is extremely remarkable, he (Sutton) frequently inoculates people with the moisture taken from the arm before the eruption of small-pox " ;.and Dr. Chandler, who also witnessed Sutton's work, referred the chief benefit of his plan to the infecting humor being taken in a crude state " before it had been ultimately variolated by the succeeding fever." Baron Dimsdale, who took much interest in Sutton's proceedings, and subsequently himself practiced inoculation, closely imitated his method, and was very successful in his results. If, as Mr. Murphy pointed out, the virus of the initial vesicle differs in any respect from that of the general eruption, some difference may also be found in the ease with which the bovine animal is inoculated with the one and the other virus. Certainly this point deserves further investigation.—*London Lancet,* January 1st, 1887.

EDITORIAL DEPARTMENT.

EDITORS.

GEORGE M. DILLOW, M.D.,	Editor-in-Chief, Editorial and Book Reviews.
CLARENCE E. BEEBE, M.D.,	Original Papers in Medicine.
SIDNEY F. WILCOX, M.D.,	Original Papers in Surgery.
MALCOLM LEAL, M.D.,	Progress of Medicine.
EUGENE H. PORTER, M.D.,	Comments and News.
HENRY M. DEARBORN, M.D.,	Correspondence.
FRED S. FULTON, M.D.,	Reports of Societies and Hospitals.

GEORGE G. SHELTON, M.D., ... Business Manager.

The Editors individually assume full responsibility for and are to be credited with all connected with the collection and presentation of matter in their respective departments, but are not responsible for the opinions of contributors.

It is understood that manuscripts sent for consideration have not been previously published, and that after notice of acceptance has been given, will not appear elsewhere except in abstract and with credit to THE NORTH AMERICAN. All rejected manuscripts will be returned to writers. No anonymous or discourteous communications will be printed.

Contributors are respectfully requested to send manuscripts and communicate respecting them directly with the Editors, according to subject, as follows: *Concerning Medicine, 21 West 37th Street; concerning Surgery, 256 West 57th Street; concerning Societies and Hospitals, 131 East 70th Street; concerning News, Personals and Original Miscellany, 461 West 71st Street; concerning Correspondence, 152 West 57th Street.*

Communications to the Editor-in-Chief, *Exchanges* and *New Books* for notice should be addressed to *102 West 43d Street.*

CONCERT OF ACTION IN LEGISLATION.

DURING the past fifty years the legislatures of our States have been pestered with efforts of one party in medicine to suppress a section of the medical profession. After a prolonged struggle, the effort has signally failed. It is beginning to be realized that the tyranny of class or caste, of trade or profession, is incompatible with the spirit of American freedom and liberty—of fair play for all under the laws. Further, it is dawning upon the presuming old school party that, by irregular methods of procedure, it has degraded our law-makers' respect for the medical profession, and has thus barred the passage of good laws in relation to medical interests in general. Quacks have had the cover of the law because educated gentlemen, practicing a rival system of therapeutics, have been promiscuously classed with ignorant knaves of fraudulent intent. By endeavoring to put the ban of dishonesty upon conscientious men, by excluding them from professional privileges and respect to which they were justly entitled, and by setting them apart as a body to be deprived of legal rights through tricking of the State, the profession, as a whole, has been shorn of its power over public opinion, and has deservedly gained a reputation with legislators as too contentious and intolerant for more than trifling attention. The attention of the profession itself has been diverted from essential points, upon which all honest and public-spirited men ought to agree, by a boycotting spirit of hatred dominating their better feelings as good citizens, educated gentlemen, and members of a common calling, to which high honor would be granted if it were sought with that breadth of intelligence, feeling and purpose to which honor is due. The past has shown how fruitless and foolish it is to attempt to force or chicane American law with reference to medicine. Special privileges of one class over another class can never be erected. No section of the profession can ever control another section through the medium of the State. Fair play and an equal field for competition can never be defeated by any organization in medicine, however exclusive or wily. Constant recoil and repulse have taught their lesson, and medical legislation is approaching a more auspicious era.

In a recent letter to *The Medical Record* by Mr. W. A. Purrington, who has acted in behalf of old school societies before the legislature of this State, there is a practical confession that concerted action of the schools is essential to the enactment of laws regulating the practice of medicine. He makes clear, "First, why the bills to create a State Examining Board have failed to become law, while their discussion has made many legislators think it impossible to frame any bill on which practitioners of medicine will agree ; and, second, the points upon which agreement is possible, and legislation, therefore, attainable." He thinks "it a pity to sacrifice the bird in the hand to catch the bird in a particularly thorny bush." Agreement, therefore, is necessary to catch the bird of progressive legislation for the advancement of good law, and even Mr. Purrington's pachyderm will feel no joy in exploring the "bramble bush," which is spiked likewise with swords and ambuscaded with Gatling guns for the trampling rhinoceros. The birds of prey will be caged when pursuers unite, and the better educated physicians under the law will serve ignorance on toast when they will combine to cast the gridiron. There is no good reason why the legal medical bodies of the State should not act jointly in legislation through a common conference committee. Recognizing their powerlessness when acting independently, and ignoring the therapeutic tenets of each other, they can meet upon the higher plane of a just war against fraud upon the public health, and of deterring unfitted aspirants from the study and practice of medicine.

The programme for future legislation which is practicable would, therefore, appear to be joint respect between the schools for each others' equality under the law, joint overlooking of each others' therapeutic opinions, joint abnegation of efforts to hoodwink or override the other, and joint endeavor to combine practicable points of agreement, equitably applicable to all the schools. Mr. Purrington says: "It is safe to say that no reputable man will care to oppose vigorously a bill punishing offences, all of a fraudulent character." We feel sure in going further, and saying that, not only will homœopaths heartily forward such a bill, but other bills that fairly strike at the abuses within the profession itself. These are, essentially: defective preparation before matriculation, lax preceptors, too short a period of study. After these have been corrected, we can step up and forward to the question of State Examining Boards. The old school will find homœopathy fully abreast of it in laying the axe to the root of remediable abuses so soon as homœopathy ceases to be treated as the root, and is looked upon, in equity and courtesy, as a fellow pioneer before the law-making power.

ANTIPYRESIS AND FATALITY.

THE recent discussion before the Academy of Medicine upon the use of antipyretics in typhoid fever shows that this fascinating fashion of meeting a single symptom is palling upon its devotees. The theory that typhoid patients die from parenchymatous degeneration of the heart muscle, superinduced by long continued high temperature, and that, by reducing this same high temperature, heart failure is obviated and the patient necessarily tided over his period of danger, does not seem to square exactly with the facts as furnished. It is being questioned whether degeneration of the muscular fibres of the heart occur so frequently as German observers have reported; and the statistics of New York, from September 1st, 1886, to December 16th, 1886, furnish an appalling commentary upon present methods of treatment. During the time noted, out of a total of 527 cases of typhoid fever, 183 deaths have occurred, or a mortality rate of 34.68 per cent. After the paper of Dr. S. Baruch on "Do Antipyretics as at Present Employed Modify the Duration or Mortality of Typhoid Fever?" in which he presented the preceding authentic figures, and strangely enough argued from his impressions in practical contradiction of his statistics, the Chairman, Prof. A. L. Loomis, said : "He had brought this question before the section because it had seemed to him that the time had come for the profession in this city to stop and think as to what they were doing, as it had become the custom, or certainly was a practice too frequently indulged in, to attempt, at all hazards, to reduce a temperature of 102° or 103°—surely 104°F.—by the use of antipyretics ; and if one does not accomplish the end to resort to another. He had had the feeling for the last two years that we were doing harm by our heroic measure for the reduction of temperature in the treatment of dtsease." Dr. Kinnicutt said that the percentage of the relapses during the present outbreak had been largely in excess of that reported in previous outbreaks in this country. Dr. Wesley Carpenter used to have a mortality rate in the country of not over ten per cent. before the advent of the more modern antipyretic epoch. The general tone of the discussion certainly called halt to the treatment as at present employed, and nothing was presented save uncertain impressions upon the ultimate advantage of even moderate use of the antipyretic drugs. What was and what was not judicious use did not appear. Evidently the practice of making patients more quiet, tractable, and even more comfortable for the time being would seem to contribute to the more composed quiet and comfort of the grave. Antipyresis is apparently on its way to take its place by the side of blood-letting. Relapses, complications, sequelæ, and deaths, are now, as always, the tests of scientific treatment ; the thermometer measures final results with no more precision than the basin in the hands of an expert barber in the olden time. In the struggle between the antipyretists and expectants, homœopathic practitioners can wisely remain spectators, as they did in the conflict between the bleeders and anti-bleeders. By observing the consistency of their position as therapeutists, by treating patients with a view to all the symptoms, instead of making an onslaught upon one of many interconnected manifestations of a disordered organism, they can leave experimental empiricism to the long account which must be settled in the end. They will surely not be discouraged by their comparative results.

A QUESTION OF IDENTITY.

WHEN two editors of the same journal are on different sides of the fence, and each speaks with the editorial we, how is one to know which side of the fence is spoken from? When, for example, the *Medical Times* refers to the "school with which we are identified," which we is intended and what school is identified? Things are apparently mixed. It might be suggested to our contemporary, which has glossed itself anew with dual piety at the beginning of the year, that, for purposes of identification, it might be well to use one we with, and another we without, an asterisk. And if it would kindly indicate by some device, when it is speaking of the school with which it is identified by trusts, and when of the school with which it is identified in opposition to those trusts, how might the crooked be made to appear straight! Otherwise the eyes of its readers are likely to go asquint in watching its zig-zag straddle of the moralities, as well as of the schools. As the showman said of the anaconda boa constrictor: "It can swallow itself, crawl through itself, and come out again with facility; It can tie itself up in a double bow knot with its tail, and wink with the greatest agility."

COMMENTS.

REACHING ITS MAJORITY.—The *Hahnemannian Monthly* completed, with its December number, the twenty-first year of its existence and leaving the sponsors who have hitherto cared for it, announces that hereafter it will strike out for itself. In other words Dr. Pemberton Dudley and Dr. B. W. James, the present editor and business manager, become the owners of the magazine, the Hahnemann Club relinquishing all claim upon it. The magazine has an excellent record behind it and will doubtless steadily improve. We congratulate it upon the completion of its majority and wish its new proprietors all possible success.

ABLE AND EARNEST WORK.—The close of 1886 calls out an editorial in the *Homœopathic World* (Eng.), reviewing the work of the year and recounting the progress made. What has been done has been accomplished amid such difficulties and under such discouragements as to dismay the bravest. Nor is the outlook very inspiring for '87. The storm of bitter, ignorant opposition still rages and only here and there does a bit of blue sky appear. We, here in America, can form but a faint idea of the strength and fury of the current our friends in England have to stem. But neither in the *World* nor in the *Review* is to be found a word of weakness or of warning but an inflexible determination to continue the fight until success is attained. Both of these journals are very welcome visitors to our table. Fighting against odds, they yield no ground. A broad and refined scholarship leaves an impress on each number and every page. We are quite sure if our readers were better acquainted with our English friends they would wish them to become monthly visitors. They deserve a large subscription list on this side of the Atlantic.

THE PRESENT NEED OF HOMŒOPATHY.—There is a malady known as the dry rot which affects chiefly individuals and organizations lacking either brains or energy to undertake the honest work that lies before them. While its onset is insidious, its progress gradual, the result is not the less fatal. Its manifestations are marked. The symptoms cannot be mistaken and an organization so infected is doomed to a speedy dissolution unless prompt and radical measures be taken to afford relief. This disease is generally caused by dishonest indolence and once firmly seated the sluggish victim can scarcely be moved to action even by the sharp spur of self preservation. It is more than suspected that the homœopathic school of medicine is becoming infected with dry rot. It is true that in the last decade the new system of therapeutics has grown and flourished. Converts have been numerous, colleges and hospitals have increased in number, magazines have multiplied, an army of physicians now believe in and practice homœopathy. Yet the one thing that ought to have been done has been left undone. What work—original work,—has been done during the past ten years in our materia medica ? Of papers that have been compilations from other papers, of text book essays, of second hand and second grade work in every department, we have had enough and to spare. But of papers having the unmistakable impress of originality and painstaking research, there has been a most lamentable scarcity. And yet our materia medica is the corner stone—the bulwark of homœopathy. Strong as it is, much ought to be done—*must* be done if we would feel our position in medicine firmly assured. The great and crying need of homœopathy to-day is men who will devote some portion of their time to original and prolonged research. If we do not soon emerge from this slough of indolence into which we have fallen the whole superstructure, erected with so much care, will crumble to pieces before our eyes, and to mark the place it once occupied we may raise a slab bearing the words, "Perished of Dry Rot."

A SURVIVAL OF THE UNFITTEST.—The fruit of a complex civilization is sometimes bitter. The more intricate the machinery the greater the friction and the less satisfactory the results. Our civilization is as yet but a crust and it will not do to dig too deeply into it. However, it may be well to consider for a moment one of the results of our system of education, which is itself a product of our highly civilized condition. Nervous affections among children are becoming more and more common. The rate of mortality among the children of wealthy families is steadily increasing. Day after day the children go to the class-rooms and there breathe an atmosphere poisoned and vitiated by their own exhalations. This is well-known to be a most fruitful source of disease and produces a deleterious effect on the delicate organism of children by acting immediately upon the nervous system. Spinal troubles occurring in children are frequently due to faultily constructed seats together with the enforcement of rules that compel them to maintain unnatural positions for indefinite periods. The hours of study have been lengthened until they are much longer than they ought to be, especially in the lower grades. But the great trouble after all lies in the fact that educational systems do not recognize the great diversities of character and temperament that exist among children. The classification of children demands great care and superior judgment. From this defective system of grading comes also the complaint of over work in schools. On this point, Sir Spencer Wells, President of the Sanitary Congress, lately held at York, says: ''We have heard much of late about over pressure from work in schools. This is one of the novelties of our times. No doubt it exists, and yet, perhaps, it may in part be traced to some of our sanitary success. We have reduced the mortality of early infancy. Many children who would have formerly died off hand, are now saved and find their way into the schools. They are survivals of the least fitted. They live but they are not strong. They have to submit to the same routine and be forced up if possible to the same standard as the rest. But the effort is too much for them. Their frames are not hardy enough to resist the mental strain. The vice of the system is that it is indiscriminate. There is no revision of the recruits and the tasks are not apportioned to the feeble powers of the sanitary survivors.'' The remedy for these things undoubtedly lies in public agitation. It is the duty of the profession to speak out concerning these matters and in no uncertain terms.

BOOK REVIEWS.

''SYSTEM OF SURGERY,'' by DR. WM. TOD HELMUTH, Professor of Surgery in the N. Y. Hom. Med. Coll., etc. Fifth edition. F. E. Boericke, Phil., 1887. Pp., 1111. Illustrations, 718.

It is with pleasure that we welcome another edition of Dr. Helmuth's excellent surgery. The work is enlarged, revised, to a considerable degree rewritten, and with much new matter added. The print and typographical work is very much better than in previous editions. We also like the arrangement of the subject matter much

better. It is much more natural to place minor and preliminary surgery at the beginning than at the end, as it was in former editions.
Considerable new matter is to be found here, *e. g.*, cocaine anæsthesia,
various mixtures for local anæsthesia in small operations, numerous
new dressings, etc. The chapter on inflammation is rewritten and
gives much valuable matter, both as regards the essential nature of the
various states and stages, and also concerning the practical management of the different stages of the inflammatory process. The use of
topical applications is advocated as adjuvants to the homœopathic similimum. No doubt can be entertained of their usefulness, their condemnation being generally the result of a narrow experience. In the
chapter on tumors we notice much additional matter, both of classification and exposition, which is valuable. The author inveighs somewhat against the use of the microscope, claiming that it is of but little
practical value, but at the same time conforms to scientific demand by
classifying tumors according to their histological characteristics. The
structure of carcinomata is also placed as embryonal. It would be
well to modify this at least by explanation, as many of the best and
most recent authorities, *e. g.*, Agnew, Heitzmann, Billroth, Waldeyer,
Gross, etc., hold that the essential process which forms carcinomata
is an extensive and pathological proliferation of epithelial tissue
without any embryonal metamorphosis. The clinical exposition of
the different varieties of tumors is most excellent and furnishes a reliable guide, but the microscopical descriptions and illustrations seem
scarcely fair to the believers in practical microscopy. It would have
added greatly to the value of this chapter if reliable and natural illustrations of the histological appearance of the different varieties of
neoplasms could have been introduced, as those used could scarcely
be of much assistance in determining the classification of a growth
according to its histological elements. It is also nearly time that the
practical experience of surgeons should disassociate the term "semi-
malignant" from any connection with the sarcomata, as it is an
accepted fact that in point of malignancy there is but little preference
to be given to either division of these neoplasms. We know that such
is the author's experience, and in such matters classification should
always wait upon its results. The chapter as a whole is, however, a
great improvement over the ones in preceding editions. The chapter
on "A concise review of the present status of antiseptic surgery" is
new and forms a fair and impartial consideration of the vexed question of antiseptics. The result reached is that the antiseptic method,
as employed in the majority of hospitals, in which the cumbersome
details of Listerism are discarded, but in which wounds are treated
with perfect cleanliness and antisepsis, is the one which promises best
and yields the most satisfactory results. In the chapter on nerve
stretching we could wish that the author had entered a little more
freely into the details of the operations for particular nerves, and also
into the statistics of the results obtained. Various new methods of
treatment have been introduced in the article upon fractures which
add materially to its value. The treatment of hip disease is most excellent and all that could be desired ; it has been carefully rewritten,

antiquated methods discarded and the latest improvements introduced. We were much pleased, also, with the clear and explicit directions given for the reduction of dislocations of the femur by manipulation, and also with the article on hernia, which latter is particularly good. The latest statistics and methods of treatment are given, together with the author's favorite method of operating, which we have seen prove efficacious in many cases. The author's confidence and belief in the high operation for stone in the bladder is manifested in his article on this subject. It is one of the best in the book, and presents a most complete and definite picture of the advantages, dangers, and methods of performing the operation of supra-pubic lithotomy. The author has made an especial study of this question, being the first on this side of the Atlantic to advocate its performance in preference to subpubic or lateral lithotomy, and his views should be regarded as of great weight. Before any operator becomes prejudiced in favor of one or the other operation, he should at least attempt the high operation, according to the very clear and definite directions given in this chapter. For laceration of the perineum Emmet's new operation is advised. We are rather sorry to see the older operation discarded, as it has always yielded most excellent results. A new chapter on laceration of the cervix uteri, by Fred. S. Fulton, has also been added.

While much of the material is as in previous editions, new matter has been everywhere interspersed, bringing the work entirely up to date. It is written in a most pleasing and entertaining manner, entirely free from the heavy style of didactic writing. If there is any general criticism which is to be made it would be that methods of treatment are not given with sufficient detail, but in a work of this size such a course would be quite impossible. It is a work which every homœopath should have in his library, for in it its distinguished author has again demonstrated his rank among the foremost surgical writers and operators of the times.   F.

THE SURGERY OF THE PANCREAS, AS BASED UPON EXPERIMENTS AND CLINICAL RESEARCHES. By N. Senn, M.D., Milwaukee, Wis. Professor of the Principles and Practice of Surgery and of Clinical Surgery in the College of Physicians and Surgeons, etc., Chicago, Ill. · Wm. J. Dornan, Philadelphia, Printer.

It is with real pleasure that a reviewer meets with a work whose *raison d'être* lies in independent and scientific research. The volume is not large, but, thanks to the author's careful and systematic investigations, it has added materially to our rather meagre knowledge of the pathology, but particularly of the surgical procedures appropriate to the various diseased conditions incident to the pancreas.

The author first reviews the anatomy, development and physiology of this gland, after which he details a large number of experiments upon the pancreas of animals, mainly dogs and cats, the results of which are most instructive in determining the tolerance by the system of operative procedures upon the gland. The experiments were made to determine the effect produced upon the system and pancreas by section of the gland, laceration, comminution of a portion, complete and partial, extirpation, obliteration of the duct by elastic compression, and the formation of an external and internal pancreatic fistula. The different diseased conditions to which this gland is subject is next treated of, the diagnosis, pathology and treatment being given.

A few of the results reached were :

I. That restoration of the pancreatic duct does not take place after complete section of the pancreas.

II. Complete extirpation of the pancreas is invariably followed by death.

III. Partial excision of the pancreas for injury or disease is a feasible and justifiable surgical procedure.

IV. Limited detachment of the mesentery from the duodenum, as required in operations upon the pancreas, is not followed by gangrene of the bowel.

V. The formation of an external pancreatic fistula by abdominal section is indicated in the treatment of cysts, abscesses, gangrene, or hemorrhage of the pancreas due to local causes.

These conclusions may be accepted, as the author's experiments in each direction were upon a sufficient number of animals, and with results definite enough to warrant confidence. The whole is written in a clear, plain, scientific manner, which is in happy contrast with the florid and sententious style of many of the recent medical issues. Dr. Senn is evidently a man, who, by reliance upon independent work rather than upon the traditional theories culled by diligent clipping and copying from old authorities, is well calculated to advance any subject which may engage his attention. The operator who aspires to the performance of abdominal section should possess the monograph, as it throws much additional light upon the opening subject of intra-peritoneal surgery. F.

A LABORATORY GUIDE IN URINALYSIS AND TOXICOLOGY, by R. A. WITTHAUS, A.M., M.D. New York : Wliliam Wood & Co. 1886.

This is an excellent guide for those who have an instructor to aid them, or to those already somewhat familiar with the subjects, who desire to review the laboratory processes used in the examination of urine and poisons. The work is arranged in the form of a note-book, similar to " Draper's Laboratory Course in Medical Chemistry," and this form is undoubtedly most useful. Illustrations are introduced sufficiently to give clearness to the text.

After an introduction, giving the general rules for laboratory work and the use of the book, the qualitative and quantitative analysis of the urine is taken up. This part of the work is quite thorough, tests being given for paraglobulin, mucin and peptone substances, which are usually omitted in works of the kind. Following the directions for chemical analysis is a section, fairly well illustrated, devoted to the microscopic examination of the sediment, and then a section on qualitative analysis of urinary calculi.

The second part, in which the detection of poisons is considered, includes mention of the antidote to each, and is an excellent exposition of the methods of detection within reach of the general physician. Books like this have always a place in medical literature, and are of benefit to the practitioner as well as the student, by interesting him in more scientific methods of investigating disease, and so giving him an incentive to closer study.   L.

HAND BOOK OF PRACTICAL MEDICINE, by Dr. Hermann Eichorst. Vol. IV. Diseases of the Blood and Nutrition, and Infectious Diseases. Seventy-four wood engravings. New York : Wm. Wood & Co., 1886. Standard Library, Pp. 407.

The above work, as a whole, of which this is the concluding volume, is one of the best among recent publications in advanced information, brevity of statement and practical service in clinical observation. Its illustrations, especially reliable in clinical microscopy, mark it out among books of its class. The author is an eminent representative of the German school of physicians, or medical naturalists, and, using the didactic method of concisely compacting his matter, be has furnished a hand book suitable for authoritative teaching of students. For the practitioner the work has unusual value as a convenient summary of the latest German views in pathology and treatment. The present volume worthily sustains the high reputation of the author.

THE REVOLUTION IN MEDICINE, by John H. Clarke, M.D. London : Keene & Ashwell, 74 New Bond Street, W. New York : Boericke & Tafel.

The editor of the *Homœopathic World* has in this, the seventh Hahnemannian oration, delivered at the London Hom. Hospital, Oct. 5th, 1886, presented in enjoyable oratorical form a sketch of the birth, progress, results and present movement of homœopathy. Dr. Clarke is a working believer that "the same strenuous efforts, the same faith and fortitude, which enabled Hahnemann to accomplish all he did, are demanded of us, according to our measure, to maintain what he began." His own measure being large, his words fall with information, purpose and fervor. The address is therefore as stirring as it is instructive.

REPORTS OF SOCIETIES AND HOSPITALS.

NATIONAL HOMŒOPATHIC HOSPITAL OF WASHINGTON, D. C.*

THE appropriation of twenty thousand dollars, by the Congress of the United States, towards the establishment of a homœopathic hospital at the National Capital, may well be accepted as the final extinction, among intelligent men, of that blind prejudice which for more than sixty years has refused to recognize any virtue or merit in the teachings of Hahnemann.

The gift itself is significant, but the unanimity of the members of both houses who voted for it is even more so. It was given without reference to the medical preferences of senators or representatives, and indicates that the age of intolerance, so far as the United States is concerned, has passed, and that hereafter homœopathy is to be treated according to the rules of common sense, and is to stand or fall, as its merits or demerits are ascertained by practical experience and impartial investigation.

The most ardent advocate of homœopathy has never asked more than this, and its most bitter opponent should accord it no less. If its efficacy as a curative system cannot stand the most critical tests, honestly and impartially applied, it has no right to live. Thus far it has justified the confidence of its adherents. In its local and state institutions it has lowered the death rate and increased the percentage of cures, as compared with those under allopathic management. It has been steadily growing in public favor, and the most significant feature of this growth is, that it comes largely from the ranks of its opponents—from men and women, who, out of a bitter experience, have turned to it as a last resort, and found in it the healing virtues which they had sought for in vain elsewhere.

The friendly attitude of the United States towards homœopathy, as evidenced by the generous contribution toward the Washington Hospital, will be very gratifying to the friends of the system, not only in this country but throughout Europe. It will have a beneficial effect wherever known. It will strengthen the hands of those who seek aid from the several states for the support of like institutions. It will command for homœopathy not only the respectful attention of the states but of nations, and will ultimately lead to a more just and equitable distribution of the funds appropriated annually for the support of public charities.

As the history of the movement which led to this gratifying result must be regarded as part of the history of homœopathic progression, a brief outline of its inception and progress will be of interest. In the spring of 1881 a few ardent advocates of homœopathy met in the City of Washington for the purpose of organizing an association, having for its object the advancement of the system they believed in. In June of the same year they were incorporated under the title of "The National Homœopathic Hospital of Washington, D. C."

The distinctive objects of the Association were :

First.—To create, through intelligent discussion and the distribution of reliable data, a popular sentiment in favor of homœopathy at the seat of Government.

Second.—To establish a hospital in the City of Washington, so that the superior merits of the system might be brought into comparison with the hospitals under allopathic control, and wherein both pay and charity patients could find skillful treatment and comfortable accomodations.

Third.—To build up a sentiment, based on public necessity, which would eventually take the form of legislation, whereby some branch of the Government would be charged with the duty of collecting and tabulat-

---

* By Alonzo Bell, Ex-Assistant Secretary of the Interior.

ing the reports of all the hospitals throughout the country, showing, annually, the diseases treated, the results of the treatment, the school of medicine in charge of the patients, the percentage of deaths and recoveries, and such other statistics as would enable the non-professional to determine the relative merits of the two leading schools of medicine.

Fourth.—To break down, by the irresistible logic of facts, the Chinese wall of exclusion which has practically shut out the homœopathic practitioner from the Army and Navy of the United States.

The Hon. Montgomery Blair was elected President of the Association. and under his leadership the first earnest work was done. One of the early outgrowths of the Association was a Free Dispensary, and this did much towards popularizing homœopathy by carrying its benefits into the homes of the poor. A few noble hearted women gave both their time and money to support the dispensary, and from the hour when its doors were first opened it has steadily grown in public favor. Its hundreds of patients have grown into thousands, and to-day it may justly be ranked as among the beneficent institutions of Washington, quietly and most efficiently doing a good work in a field hitherto neglected.

The satisfactory work of the dispensary did much toward recruiting the ranks of the Association. It commanded the respect and substantial aid of the city authorities. It awakened a wide-spread interest in homœopathy among many who had been strangers to its virtues. It brought to the front earnest and influential men and women. It paved the way for the subsequent establishment of the homœopathic hospital.

In the early part of 1884 it was deemed advisable to open a hospital. The lack of funds was a serious obstacle in the way, and precluded the purchase or erection of a suitable building for the purpose. Therefore, a house was rented, fitted up in a modest manner, and the long wished for institution became a reality. What it lacked in size and accommodations it more than made up in the energy and faith of its managers. It soon became apparent that it was too small to properly accommodate the numbers applying for admission. Larger rooms, and more of them, became an absolute necessity. This was an easy conclusion to reach, but the more difficult problem to solve was, how to obtain the money to secure the change. Local subscriptions were inadequate, the good will of friends had already been sorely tested, and it became obvious that outside aid of some character must be invoked to provide funds for the proposed enlargement.

An appeal to Congress was decided upon. A committee of ladies was appointed to lay the appeal before that honorable body. The generous response of the 48th Congress, in the form of an appropriation of fifteen thousand dollars for the erection or purchase of a suitable building for a homœopathic hospital, is the best evidence that the duty entrusted to these ladies was faithfully performed.

Although the contribution was a small one, it was sufficiently large to emphasize a vital truth whose scope and influence will reach far into the future of homœopathy. A million dollars could not more effectually signalize the end of old time prejudices and the dawn of an era of toleration, wherein the supremacy of intelligence and reason is to be recognized by the representatives of the people.

After the appropriation became available, several months were consumed in the examination of proposed sites, buildings and plans. The aggregate of funds, public and private, in hand would not justify the purchase of such property as seemed to be needed for the new hospital. Some urged the buying of valuable lands and the erection of a suitable building thereon, and paying on it the cash in hand, securing the balance by deed of trust. Others insisted that the only safe plan was to purchase the best possible with the money available, and enter upon the enlarged field free of debt. Fortunately the voice of the prudent ones prevailed, and in due time a fine opportunity was offered to purchase a splendid site and a substantial building thereon, at a price within the means of the Association, and less than the original cost of the building. The transfer of title was soon effected, necessary alterations were made, toward which Congress appropriated an additional five thousand dollars, and on the first of February 1886, the Association took formal possession for hospital purposes.

The building is located at the corner of N. and Second Streets, N. W. The sight is a healthy one and free from all unpleasant surroundings. The view from the upper windows of the hospital is surpassed by few places in the City of Washington. The structure is of brick, the walls and foundation being of the most substantial character. It is four stories in height, the dimensions of the main building are 80x50 feet. A brick annex contains the kitchen, laundry, and heating apparatus. No sewer or waste pipe enters the walls of the main building. It is heated by steam radiators with proper openings in the walls for the admission of fresh air. The arrangement is such that the temperature of any part of the building can be easily regulated and controlled. The provisions for ventilation are simple and efficient. A system of lateral air conduits connect with two large vertical shafts, passing from the ground floor out of the roof. A current of hot air passing up through these shafts induces outward currents through the lateral conduits, and these being connected by registers at the top and bottom of the rooms, the vitiated air within is readily withdrawn. The management has given earnest attention to the proper sanitary conditions essential to successful hospital work, and it is believed that in this respect the National Homœopathic Hospital is equal to the best in the country. The building will accomodate about fifty patients, provision being made for their treatment in wards as well as in private rooms. An operating room, rooms for consultations, the necessary dining and reception rooms, complete the finish of a hospital building that any homœopath, whether a resident of Washington or elsewhere, might justly be proud of.

The organization consists of a President, a Vice-President for the District of Columbia, and one from each State and Territory, a Secretary and Treasurer, and a Board of Trustees. The management of the property and business affairs of the Association is in the hands of the Trustees. A Hospital Committee, appointed by them, consisting of three members of the Association and four members of the Ladies Aid Association, supervise the internal management of the hospital. A competent matron and a corps of nurses, under the general direction of the Hospital Committee, are in immediate charge. The Medical Staff is composed of thirteen physicians, members of the Homœopathic Medical Society of the District, and appointed by the Board of Trustees. Assignments are made from the Staff, by its President, to take charge of diseases of children, diseases of females, eye and ear, general and nervous diseases, obstetrics, respiratory organs and heart, surgery, venereal and skin diseases. A house physician is at all times within call. The rules and regulations in force are those which the most approved experience has found to be necessary. Quite as much freedom is allowed as is consistent with the proper care of the sick, the design of the management being to surround the sick room with something of the comforts and conveniences of home life. The present President of the Association is Hon. Morrison R. Waite, well-known as the Chief Justice of the United States. The Treasurer is Lewis Cliphane, of Washington, D. C.

Such in brief is an outline of the National Homœopathic Hospital, which enjoys the distinctive honor of being the first and only homœopathic institution in the land that owes its existence to moneys directly appropriated by the Congress of the United States. The maintenance of the hospital depends wholly upon private sources, and probably will so continue, until the fact is established beyond a reasonable doubt that the public funds, annually expended for purposes of charity, will go further and do more good in the hands of homœopaths, than in the hands of those who now expend them. It is confidently believed that the material already exists to establish this important truth, but it must be gathered together, collated by impartial hands, and, if possible, the conclusions reached should bear the stamp of government authority. Published to the world in this form, they would be accepted as reliable data, beyond the reach of partisan controversy, and would carry conviction wherever distributed and read.

To bring this about is part of the work of the Association yet to be performed, and every legitimate influence will be exerted until it is accomplished. While this work serves a local charity it is purely national in its scope. Its success will benefit every community in the land. The vindication of homœopathy, through a practical test conducted at the National Capital, and under the auspices of government patronage, will do more in a single year, to crystalize public sentiment in its favor, than could be accomplished by a century of partisan discussion.

The representatives of the people have given the friends of homœopathy a golden opportunity to make good their claims in a manner and at a place that will command the attention of the masses. It remains to be seen whether this opportunity is to be embraced by the advocates of the system, and an earnest effort made to build up a hospital at Washington, whose results can safely be accepted as a fair standard of the virtues of the system, or, whether the movement, as a national one, is to fail for lack of a hearty and generous support.

No more appropriate place for a representative homœopathic hospital could be found on the continent than the City of Washington. The location is central, the climate healthy. It is alike free from the rigors of winter and the extreme heat of summer. The city is, and always will be, an attractive centre for visitors from our own and other lands. As the seat of government, it will command the attention of all who seek to become acquainted with our institutions. Its population must continue to be more or less transient, as it is largely made up of persons connected in some capacity with the government service or of those directly or indirectly dependent on them. Thus the impressions formed at the Capital are likely to be widely disseminated throughout the land by the thousands of visitors and residents who are continually coming and going. How essential, then, to have the best practical exposition of the system we believe in at this important point.

In the movement so well begun there should be no possibility of failure. The homœopaths of Washington are active and willing, but the burden of the labor required should be shared by all who are in sympathy with their work. Every city, county and state should contribute to the success of the movement. Out of the aggregate of the small contributions, may come an institution that will prove not only a blessing to the capital of the nation but a vital blessing to the cause of humanity everywhere.

SOCIETY FOR MEDICO-SCIENTIFIC INVESTIGATION.

THE regular meeting of the Society for Medico-Scientific Investigation was held January 4th, 1887, at 201 East 23d Street, with President Cowl in the chair.

The President then read his opening address, after which Dr. R. N. Flagg presented a paper on " Bronchial Hemorrhage Resulting in Acute

Consumption," in which the Doctor held that a rapidly developing phthisis was the result of a rather profuse hæmoptisis.

Dr. Vehslage considered the case reported a rare one as to the sequence of morbid changes. Regarding the treatment of phthisis by nebulized fluids, he had not had sufficient experience as yet to enable him to speak of results.

Dr. Leal was inclined to believe that Dr. Flagg's case was tubercular in origin. If it were otherwise, it would partake of the character of catarrhal phthisis and would probably have run a longer course. He had used ergot with success, as far as the relief of the hæmoptisis was concerned, in several cases, and had seen no symptoms of ergotism follow its continued use.

Dr. W. Storm White then read a paper upon "Abnormalities in the Position of the Abdominal Visceræ."

Dr. Blackman stated that an examination of a number of cases had led him to believe that some of the usual statements as to the position of some of the abdominal visceræ were inaccurate. For example, the stomach is described as lying transversely, while, in most cases, it will be found to lie nearly perpendicularly, especially if empty. This is constantly true in infants. Often the distribution of the blood supply will decide whether the abnormality is congenital or acquired. If an organ be congenitally displaced its artery will be correspondingly dislocated in its origin. He has seen the kidney in the venter of the ilium and its artery given off from the abdominal aorta. The attachments of the peritoneum may also afford means for determining whether the abnormality is congenital or acquired. As in Dr. White's case where the liver was displaced to the right, the suspensory ligament was also displaced, thus showing this condition to be normal in origin. Anomalies of the muscular system are constantly encountered, and the presence or absence of certain muscles, as the *psoas parvus*, does not at all depend on the muscularity of the individual. Muscular anomalies occur in about eight per cent. of individuals. Dr. B. had found eight in 105 cases.

The vascular system is very often found to vary from the normal standard. He has seen the bifurcation of the axillary artery take the place of bifurcation of the brachial. Two kidneys have been found on one side. One kidney has had two and even three ureters. The spleen should be entirely above the last rib, and if recognized below it, even on inspiration, it is enlarged. The stomach varies more than any other organ. He had recently a case of typhoid fever with the tenderness and symptoms found in the ileo-cœcal region absent, but developed in the scrobiculus. Possibly the ileo-cœcal region was dislocated to that point.

Dr. Cowl had noted variations in the suspensory ligament of the liver. He had seen the transverse colon as low down as the pubes and the bowel held all on one side by adhesions. In a triangular aneurism of the abdominal aorta, at its bifurcation, the posterior wall of the sack became at last entirely absorbed and death resulted from hemorrhage into the abdominal cavity.

Dr. White stated that in his case the visceræ were held in the upper portion of the abdominal cavity, and the retracted abdominal walls filled the lower portion.

The Society then adjourned.

RECORD OF MEDICAL PROGRESS.

A NEW URETHRAL SOUND.—Dentue exhibited to the *Societe de Chirurgie*, the 6th of October, a sound devised by Bruch, of Algires; in which the terminal fifth only is rigid, the remainder being soft.— *Jour. des Soc. Scientifiques.*

PNEUMONIA IN UTERO.—Mr. Henry Strachan gives an account of a case of pneumonia in utero (see *British Medical Journal*, November 6th, 1886). A woman, eight months pregnant, suffering with left-sided pneumonia, four days after the onset of the disease was delivered of a female child. The infant died in less than twenty-four hours with symptoms of acute pneumonia. A *post mortem* examination showed acute pneumonic consolidation of the whole left lung.

AN INDICATION THAT UMBILICAL CORD IS AROUND THE NECK.—Mr. F. R. Humphreys writes to the *British Medical Journal*, November 6th, that in nearly all cases he has seen, where the umbilical cord was around the child's neck, the mother had cried out when the head was against the perinæum, much the same as in the early part of the first stage of labor, and had complained of sharp, acute pain. He says he has rarely noticed this cry when the cord was not around the neck of the child.

DURATION OF INFECTIOUSNESS IN SCARLATINA, SMALL-POX, MEASLES, MUMPS, AND DIPHTHERIA.—Dr. Pearse, in a paper on the above subject read before the British Medical Association, concludes as follows :—" My observations make the duration of infection in the several diseases as follows : Measles, from the second day, for exactly three weeks ; small-pox, from the first day, under one month, probably three weeks ; scarlet fever, at about the fourth day, for six or seven weeks ; mumps, under three weeks ; diphtheria, under three weeks."—*British Medical Journal*, November 20th, 1886.

CHALK OINTMENT AS AN APPLICATION IN ERYSIPELAS.—Sir Dyce Duckworth recommends equal proportions by weight of lard and *creta preparata*, the lard being melted before the chalk is added, as a cleanly, cooling, soothing and trustworthy ointment to be smeared thickly over the erysipelatous part. He considers it preferable to dusted flour and far superior to white paint, which is mischievous and cannot be removed. It is now the favorite application in St. Bartholomew's Hospital. The precipitated and prepared chalk act equally well.—*The Practitioner*, Jan., 1887.

TUBERCULAR INOCULATIONS IN A MAN.—Dr. Axel Holst mentions the case of an attendant on the phthisical patients at a hospital, who had suffered for a long time from atonic ulceration of the fingers, which had been treated with ointment, plaster, caustic, and scarification. No tubercle bacilli were to be observed with certainty in the sores. Later, the man was affected with a tuberculous glandular swelling of considerable size in the axilla, which contained a considerable number of Koch's bacilli ; and Dr. Axel Holst is of the opinion that it is highly probable the patient had received infection through the sores.—*London Lancet*, October 16th, 1886.

HEMORRHAGE FROM THE INNOMINATE AFTER TRACHEOTOMY.—Dr. Hutton, at the November meeting of the Manchester Medical Society, related the following :—A boy, aged eighteen months, with bronchitis and laryngitis (" diphtheritic ? ") of three weeks standing, suffered from urgent dyspnœa, and tracheotomy was performed. Great and unexpected improvement took place, and in twelve days the child was convalescent and able to do without the tube for four hours and a half. The same night violent hemorrhage occurred and caused immediate death. *Post mortem*, an ulcer was found in the anterior wall of the trachea, at the level of the lower end of the tracheotomy tube, implicating the innominate.— *British Medical Journal*, December 4th, 1886.

CATARACT PRODUCED DURING THE ADMINISTRATION OF NAPHTHA-LINE.—In June, 1886, Bouchard and Charrin presented to the *Académie de Médicine* of Paris, some results obtained by administration of naphthaline to rabbits. One of these results was the production of cataract. Last December they gave the results of more extended researches, pursued in the laboratory, for general pathology of the faculty of medicine. After the ingestion of the drug in doses of 1.50 gramme to 2 gramme *per diem*, mixed with glycerine, cataractous changes appear in the crystalline lens, more or less slowly, according to the case. It is rare, however, for the changes to fail to appear by the twentieth to the twenty-fifth day after the beginning of the experiment. Both eyes are usually affected at the same time. Exceptions however occur, the cataract appearing only in one. eye. Other substances have been administered, but with negative effect.

THE LIGATION OF LARGE ARTERIES IN THEIR CONTINUITY.—Messrs. Ballance and Edmunds give the following as the result of an extended series of experiments : The application of a ligature to a large artery in its continuity should be performed without damage to its wall. This is all the more important if the vessel be diseased, the non-irritating aseptic ligature so applied being a source of additional strength and making the occlusion of a diseased artery almost as successful as that of a healthy one. When the coats of an artery are uninjured by the ligature, the danger of ligation near a large collateral branch is wholly avoided, because (*a*) no danger can accrue from hemorrhage when the wall of the vessel is intact ; (*b*) the formation of clot, upon which the safety of the patient so much depends if the wall of the vessel be damaged, has really nothing to do with the adhesive changes which take place in a ligatured vessel ; (*c*) the plastic actions which proceed at the place of ligation are practically alike whether the tunics be ruptured or not. It is not necessary to use a flat ligature, but a non-irritating aseptic ligature such as kangaroo tendon or chromic catgut, which will remain for several weeks before being absorbed. The final conclusions are the advocation of—1. The employment of antiseptic precautions ; 2. The use of the small, round absorbable ligature ; 3. The maintenance of the integrity of the arterial wall.—*British Medical Journal*, October 20th, 1886, and *London Medical Record*, November, 1886.

OPTICAL TREATMENT OF STRABISMUS.—M. Javal presented, at the last meeting of the French Academy of Medicine, a paper in which he detailed his experiences in the treatment of strabismus without operative interference. In inveterate cases the surgical method alone is applicable ; and it is in recent cases, occurring in young subjects, that the optical method can be substituted. The first step in the method recommended by the author consists in making a practice of occluding the normal eye, and then training the deviated eye by means of the necessary ocular gymnastics. The strabismus, however, requires that the deviated eye concurs in binocular vision. That this may be accomplished, the author employs a stereoscope, so constructed that the angle of the lenses may be gradually changed from the normal. A scale attached to the instrument renders the variations apparent, and measures the progress made by the patient. A second instrument is used in those cases in which an oblique deviation is added to the lateral strabismus. Javal's methods are applicable to divergent strabismus, or to convergent strabismus, with or without myopia.— *Jour. des Soc. Scientifiques*, 13th October, 1886.

PHARYNGEAL AND LARYNGEAL NYSTAGMUS.—In our last issue we published some notes in the form of a letter on rapid rhythmic contractions of the pharyngeal and laryngeal muscles, associated with rapid rhythmic contractions of the ocular muscles, in a case of cerebellar tumor, in a girl aged twelve years. The importance of the nystagmus of the pharyngeal and laryngeal muscles lies partly in the interest attaching to the phenomenon, and partly in its suggestiveness. In the case in question great attention was paid to the state of the rest of the nerves of the body, but nothing in the same nature as nystagmus of any other muscle was observed, nor, so far as we know, was there any rhythmical recurrence of sensation in any sensory district. The rate of the rhythm in the pharynx and larynx was perfectly synchronous with the rate of action of the muscles of the eyeball. The ocular nystagmus was of a mixed, vertical and horizontal description. It is hardly likely that the symptom which Dr. H. R. Spencer discovered in this case of cerebellar tumor is of common occurrence either in tumors of the brain, or in any other disease of the central or peripheral nervous system, but its present recognition will doubtless stimulate observation, and may lead to still further extension of knowledge. The symptom is a genuine one, and evidently not dependent on a combination of conditions whose balance is easily upset, for the nystagmus has been in constant active operation for at least two months. The rate of the pharyngo-laryngeal contractions, like the synchronous nystagmus of the eyeball is 180 per minute. It is worth while remembering the circumstance that the muscles which are the seat of the rapid nystagmus in this case are sometimes employed volitionally, and at other times automatically or reflexly. Another feature of the case to which Dr. H. R. Spencer alludes is the rate of the pulse, which is unaccountably frequent, being 100 per minute. It may be that this is related in some way to the action of the pharyngo-laryngeal muscles, whose motor fibers in the vagus are divided, in part at least, from the spinal accessory muscles, which is also believed to preside over the rate of the action of the heart.—*London Lancet,* October 16th, 1886.

UNDEVELOPED SEXUAL ORGANS, ASSOCIATED WITH CONGENITAL DEFECT OF THE TONSILS.—At a meeting of the *Clinical Society of London,* held October 8th, 1886, Dr. A. Pearse Gould read a paper on the above topic. The case was that of a male, aged twenty-seven, over six feet high, slender, with fair, soft, smooth face, a boy's voice, and no hair on his face. The penis and both testicles were small, but the right epididymis was thickened, which Mr. Gould attributed to a blow on the part, when the boy was eleven years of age. The prostate could scarcely be felt through the rectum, and the seminal vesicles could not be felt. The man had no sexual desire ; the only sign of any sexual activity was occasional slight priapism. There was an oblique inguinal hernia on the right side. The pillars of the fauces were close together and only very small tonsils could be seen or felt between them. Mr. Gould said the case raised the question whether there was any intimate connection between the tonsils and the testicles. It was a popular notion that excision of the tonsils before purberty endangered virility, and Dr. Shorthouse, quoted by Dr. Ogle, was named as a writer who spoke of such an effect as a matter of common observation. The shrinking of enlarged tonsils and the cessation of repeated attacks of tonsilitis at puberty, were adduced in support of the influence of sexual maturity upon these organs. On the other hand, in Zanzibar, where all boys have their tonsils excised, the testicles are well developed and the operation now is so common that, were it liable to be followed by such a grave result as non-development of the sexual organs, abundant evidence of this fact would be forthcoming. The removal of an enlarged organ was different from its imperfect development and might be attended with different results. Mr. Gould had seen two women with absent or undeveloped ovaries, and in whom the tonsils were of full size, and Dr. Langdon Down, who had seen many cases of imperfect sexual development, had not observed any associated change in the tonsils. An interesting discussion followed the reading of the paper, and the concensus of opinion inclined strongly in the direction of the non-relationship between the tonsils and the sexual organs.—*London Lancet*, October 16th, 1886.

NEW TREATMENT OF RESPIRATORY AFFECTIONS AND BLOOD POISONING BY GASEOUS RECTAL INJECTION.—Dr. Bergeon, of Lyons, has recently presented to the *Académie des Sciences*, to the *Association Scientifique Français à Nancy*, and to the *Académie de Médicine*, the results obtained from the rectal administration of gaseous medicaments, G. Masson, Paris, publishes, in pamphlet form, an account of the experiments of Dr. Bergman and Dr. Morel, his assistant, an abstract of which will be found in the *Annales des Mal. de l'oreille, du larynx, etc.*, December, 1886. Dr. J. Henry Bennet, of Paris, has published his experiences with the process in the *British Medical Journal* for December 18th, 1886., where the apparatus used is illustrated. Dr. B. first tried the injection of large quantities of carbon dioxide in human beings, using even as much as four litres two or three times in twenty-four hours, without producing any toxic effect. The gas is expelled by the mouth in a few minutes without disturbance of respiration, nor pain. Carbon dioxide was found to have no medicinal action, but there is mixed with it sulphuretted hydrogen, which acts as a powerful germicide. The vapor of carbon disulphide appears also to have an antiseptic action. Sulphuretted hydrogen as ordinarily prepared does not, for some unaccountable reason, seem to have the same beneficial action as the same gas derived from some of the natural mineral waters, as the Eaux Bonnes. The process as applied in phthisical cases is, in brief, as follows : A rubber gas bag of proper size is filled with freshly prepared carbon dioxide, obtained by acting on bicarbonate of soda with dilute sulphuric acid. The tube leading from the gas bag is then connected with a bottle holding the sulphuretted water, in such a manner that the carbon dioxide must pass through the mineral water and become charged with the sulphuretted hydrogen, in its passage to the rectal tube, in which the apparatus terminates. The tube being introduced into the rectum of the patient, the gases are introduced slowly, twenty minutes being allowed for the injection of four litres. This gaseous enema must be given twice a day, beginning with one litre and gradually increasing the amount. The injections are given an hour before, or three hours after eating, Dr. Chantemesse reports nine cases of pulmonary tuberculosis which have been notably relieved. The increase of weight was rapid, a pound or more a day at first ; the strength improved ; the cough and expectoration and fever diminished; asthmatic and catarrhal cases were also improved. Spillman and Parisot have experimented with the process and note an additional effect.—See *Jour. des Soc. Scientifique*, 29th December, 1886. In a little over a month they administered the gaseous injections fifty times to nine patients, and give the following account of the results : About two or three hours after an injection, when the distention of the abdomen has almost entirely disappeared, the patient experiences an imperative impulse to sleep. The sleep appears to be natural and the patient awakens refreshed. This is a constant result and does not appear to be due to any general improvement in the patient, because, if the injection be omitted at night the conditions of sleep are as they would have been without the administration of any hypnotic. This action is due to the carbon dioxide and not to the sulphuretted hydrogen mixed with it ; and the single gas acts in the same manner.

NEWS.

THE Homœopathic Medical Society of the State of New York will meet at Albany, February 8th and 9th.

EDITORIAL CHANGE.—The St. Louis *Periscope* has had another change in editorship. Dr. Frank Kraft has resigned and Dr. J. Martine Kershaw has taken his place. We trust the new editor will find the editorial cushion a comfortable one.

SURGEON APPOINTED.—We learn from the *York Despatch*, that the Directors of the Harrisburg and Baltimore Railroad have appointed Dr. D. B. Grove, of Hanover, Pa., Surgeon of their road for the coming year. Dr. Grove, is a graduate of the N. Y. Hom. Medical College.

THE CHIRONIAN.—One of the handsomest of our exchanges is the *Chironian*, published by the students of the N. Y. Hom. Medical College. It is pleasant to look upon and affords entertaining reading. We advise all alumni of the college to subscribe for it. It is well worth the money.

RECEPTION.—On Friday Evening, December 17th, a reception was given Prof. Ludlam at Dr. George S. Norton's. "Everybody" was there and the rooms were well filled. An elegant collation was served during the evening. The occasion was a most pleasant one and was thoroughly enjoyed by those present.

THE LONDON HOSPITAL.—The London Homœopathic Hospital report for the past year is exceptionally small. Out of a total of six hundred and seventy-four cases treated, including both medical and surgical treatment the mortality was less than five per cent. The Homœopathic Hospital of Melbourne, Australia, reports a mortality of a trifle over five per cent. Such statistics as these annoy our old school brethren.

A SLIGHT MISTAKE.—A well-known dentist contributes the following: "A gentleman from the boundless West was calling at the 'parlors' for consultation and as the interview was about terminating, his eye chanced to fall upon the doctor's diploma, the leading lines of which, in very black text, ran thus: 'Academia Chirurgia Dentium' etc. As the Chirurgia struck him his face suddenly lighted up and extending his hand energetically he exclaimed! 'Why, doctor, I didn't know you were from Chicago, Shake.'"

A NEW ENTERPRISE.—The Good Samaritan Diakonissen is the name of an order recently established in this country but long known and tested on the continent. It differs from other charitable organizations, in that it provides trained nurses not only for the rich who may pay for their services but for the poor as well. A portion of the building at 201 West 38th Street, has been fitted up as an hospital and will be headquarters of the order for the coming year. The hospital was opened on the 14th of December.

A NEW SOCIETY.—The Homœopathic physicians of Hudson County, N. J. have decided to organize themselves into a society for mutual benefit and strength. On the evening of the 8th of December, '86, a meeting was held at Dr. Hoffman's office when the requisite steps were taken towards the formation of a society. The organization rejoices in the euphonious title of the "Hudson County Medico-Chirurgical Society." The officers for the ensuing year are :—President, Dr. L. J. Meyers; Vice-President, Dr. Pyle; Secretary and Treasurer, Dr. L. A. Opdyke. The Society meets on the first Wednesday of each month.

OBITUARY.—James A. Gwaltney, died at his home in Baltimore, Dec. 18th, 1886. At a special meeting of the Maryland State Institute of Homœopathy held December 20th, 1886, the following resolutions were passed: *Whereas*, under the dispensations of an all-wise Providence our *confrère*, James A. Gwaltney, M.D., has been removed from our midst; and *Whereas*, we, the members of the Md. State Institute of homœopathy, recognizing in Dr. Gwaltney a conscientious physician, an earnest member of the Institute and a devoted adherent to homœopathy, do appreciate the loss his death has occasioned. *Therefore, resolved*, that we tender to the bereaved family our sincere sympathy, and that a copy of these resolutions be sent to them and also published in the Medical Journals. V. EDW. JANNEY, *Secy*.

THE ADVANCE OF CHOLERA.—The epidemic of cholera which began at Brindisi last spring was carried up the western coast of the Adriatic to Hungary and prevailed in many Italian cities. A great stream of immigration from Italy has been pouring into the Argentine Republic, and it is known that the disease was carried to Buenos Ayres by these immigrants. From Buenos Ayres it was quickly conveyed to other cities on the Plata River and its tributaries and to points on the railways which have recently been built. Chili, the Argentine Republic and Uruguay are infected. It is probable, also, in spite of a most rigid quarantine that Brazil has not escaped. It is stated that at one time the mortality at Buenos Ayres became so great that the dead were burned in heaps in the outskirts of the city.

A TEST FOR IMPURE AIR.—The following method for determining the impurity of air is worthy of trial. If teachers and school officers were more careful concerning the quality of the atmosphere in class-rooms there would be less illness among the pupils. Dr. A. E. Burckhardt of Basle, warmly recommends a simple and small apparatus for determining the amount of carbonic acid in the air of schools, hospitals, etc., invented by Dr. Schaffer, of Berne. The apparatus is based on the fact that diluted lime water gives a violet red stain on phenolphtalein paper, which stain disappears in the air containing carbonic acid, and does so the more rapidly the larger the amount of acid present in the air. It is only necessary to mark the time which has been required for the disappearance of the stain and to consult an appended table which shows the amount of acid corresponding to the time.—*Ex.*

THE HELMUTH HOUSE.—The spacious edifice at 41 East 12th Street, long the residence of Dr. Willard Parker, has recently undergone a striking transformation. Some few months ago Dr. William Tod Helmuth obtained possession of the building and at once began the alterations and repairs necessary to fit it for a first-class private hospital. Entering the broad hallway a handsome reception room is found on the right. Opposite are the various offices and beyond a pleasant dining-room. Four entire floors are fitted up for the convenience and comfort of patients. Three operating rooms, furnished in most complete fashion, are at the disposal of the surgeons. The great charm of the house, however, is the home-like appearance of everything! Every room is cheery and comfortable and shows the exercise of much taste in selecting the furniture and pictures. Dr. S. H. Knight is the resident surgeon, and a corps of trained nurses is in constant attendance. The house is full of patients already, although it has been open but a month.

THE PERILS OF DAMP BEDS.—A respectable proportion of the deaths that occur during the winter season are either directly or indirectly due to sleeping in damp beds. As a matter of fact this peril is of the greatest and it is ever present with us. The experienced traveler rarely hazards the risk of sleeping between sheets which are nearly sure to be damp, until they have been aired under his personal supervision at a fire in his bed-room. If this be impracticable he wraps his cloak around him or pulls out the sheets and sleeps between the blankets—a disagreeable but often pru-dent expedient. The direst mischief may result from the contact of an imperfectly heated body with sheets which retain moisture. The body heat is not sufficient to raise the temperature of the sheets to a safe point, and the result must be disastrous in the extreme, if, as is sure to happen, the skin is cooled by contact with a surface colder than itself, and steadily abstracting heat all the night through. Country people in particular are specially culpable in this matter. A "spare" room is reserved for guests. For weeks it may remain unoccupied, unaired and unwarmed. A visitor arrives. Unconcious of the fate that awaits him he calmly passes the evening in social enjoyment. Later he is shown to the "spare" room for the night. The atmosphere of the apartment has the chill and damp of the tomb and the sheets of the bed are veritable winding sheets—shrouds, in fact. He is fortunate if he escapes with nothing more than a "cold." There is no excuse for the neglect of proper precaution to insure dry beds.

THE ALUMNI LECTURE.—The Second Annual Lecture before the Alumni Association of the N. Y. Homœopathic Medical College, was de-livered Thursday evening, December 16th, in the Concert Hall of the Metropolitan Opera House, by Prof. R. Ludlam, M.D., of Chicago. His subject was "Post-Graduate Education." A large and intelligent audience was present and listened with evident interest to the lecturer. Among other good things Dr. Ludlam said : "A practical professional education is a progressive affair. Much has been written on the higher education of medical students, but little or none on the higher education of physicians. The trouble with a large number of physicians is that all study and appli-cation stops on commencement day. My prescription will be :—I. A sys-tematic plan of reading and writing on medical topics. The doctor of our day is not so fond of his library. He has more books and periodicals, but is less familiar with their contents. For two reasons I apprehend that the medical publications of to-day are more satisfactory and helpful than ever before. First, because of the multiplication of encyclopedias, and second, because of the decrease of controversy in medical writing. II. Professional intercourse and correspondence. The scheme of a progressive medical training must include the *life* as well as the literature of our guild. With-out professional intercourse, men grow selfish, sectarian and short-sighted. Nothing so sterilizes our faculties as distance and separation. Our obser-vation is personal and individual, while our experience is general and many-sided. One is limited, the other continues the accumulated wealth and wisdom of the profession. We must pour our mental earnings into the common treasury of medical knowledge. III. The improvement of every possible opportunity to revisit the college for a review of studies. The mental faculties are like the metals—the most useful are the most prone to become rusty. That graduates do not more often return to college is not entirely due to pressure of daily duties, but something of it must be charged to the college. Perhaps the college does not offer an equivalent for a prolonged absence from practice. IV. Attendance upon Post-graduate schools and special courses of instruction." The doctor's prescription is an excellent one and it cannot be taken too often or in too large dozes.

VOL. XXXV.   *MARCH, 1887.*   (VOLUME II, Third Series.)   No. 3.

NORTH AMERICAN
JOURNAL OF HOMŒOPATHY.

ORIGINAL ARTICLES IN MEDICINE.

HICCOUGH AND TREATMENT.

By JAS. A. FREER, M.D.,
Washington, D. C.

I WAS called upon a short time since to treat a patient suffering from this distressing symptom, and not being thoroughly conversant with its nature, as to causes, course, etc., I sought to gain information from such text books on the practice of medicine, as were available, these being the productions of the leading authors of both schools, but, to my disappointment, all that I could find concerning it comprised only a few brief references, all of which gave only a very imperfect and unsatisfactory knowledge of this subject. Since then I have searched the literature of the subject as contained in the cases reported in the English language during the last century; having found these records to contain many items of interest, it is my object to embody them, as far as possible, in this paper, and to give the homœopathic treatment of the malady, together with such other treatment as has been found most successful.

Every one is familiar with this peculiar and often distressing spasmodic action of the diaphragm, called hiccough, which generally and frequently occurs as a symptom of some slight irritation of the stomach, arising from overheated or pungent articles of diet, or following the ingestion of substances difficult of digestion.

The treatment of these attacks, which may be called physiological, is also simple and well known to all : they either cease spontaneously in a few minutes, or are controlled by drinking a few swallows of cold water, the breath being held for a moment, or by allowing to dissolve in the mouth a lump of sugar saturated in cider vinegar; another simple remedy, which has often proved successful, is the taking of a full inspiration, and holding the inhaled air as long as possible in the lungs, this act keeping the diaphragm in a quiescent state for a moment; when the air is exhaled the spasm will, as a rule, be found to have

ceased. Occasionally cases arise where these simple remedies all fail
to effect relief, and the paroxysms may rise to such a pitch of intensity,
and last so long, and with such distressing characteristics, that they
deserve to be classed as pathological.

In such cases the spasms sometimes involve not only the diaphragm, but all of the other muscles of respiration, and occur in such
rapid succession, and with such violence, that the speech, deglutition,
and even respiration, are rendered almost impossible, and the diaphragmatic attachments become so sore from its spasmodic action,
that each contraction causes intense pain; in these cases the spasms
frequently continue during sleep; at such times the affection becomes
very grave, threatening the life of the patient. It is with these persistent and chronic cases that it is the object of this paper chiefly to
deal.

Etiology. The causes operating for the production of hiccough
may be classified under three heads.

I. Those that are centric in origin.

This class includes all those cases in which the origin can be
traced to lesions at the base of the brain or in the cervical portion of
the spinal cord. Numerous cases belonging under this division have
been observed and reported, and to this category belongs the case
which it was our province to examine, referred to above; the following
is a brief account of the case :   ·

CASE I, widow, æt. 69, Irish.—This patient was admitted into the
Ward's Island Homœopathic Hospital on June 30th, 1885, suffering
from chronic singultus. She presented a good family history and had
herself enjoyed excellent health until the commencement of the above
trouble, which dated from July 16th, 1884; it was inaugurated by a
spasmodic twitching of her facial muscles, this in a few hours being
followed by the spasmodic contractions of her diaphragm, characteristic of hiccough; from this sudden invasion it soon attained to a
degree of severity that was very distressing, and continued thus with
unabated vigor day and night. She stated that her life had several
times been despaired of on account of the dyspnœa caused by the
rapid succession of the spasms. At about the same time, with the occurrence of the above symptoms, she noticed tenderness of the cervical
portion of her spine, in which region she could sustain but slight
pressure, and from which proceeded, at intervals, severe lancinating
pains, which were greatly aggravated by motion. After about two
months of this suffering, during which she was under continuous
medical treatment, she decided to enter a hospital, and was accordingly admitted at St. Luke's in New York City, where she remained
until the time of her admission at the Homœopathic Hospital. While
there she came under the care of several physicians of eminence, from
whom she received careful treatment of every variety that it was

thought could benefit her, under all of which the only improvement was a slight amelioration of the severity of the spasms and a diminution of their frequency.

When she came under our care she was hiccoughing at the rate of about ten per minute, when in a quiescent state, but the frequency and severity of the spasms were increased by eating, and greatly so by emotions and exercise of the upper extremities. She was well nourished and enjoyed about her usual strength. Her bowels were slightly constipated, but aside from this her functions were normally performed. An opportunity was not afforded us for the exhibition of homœopathic treatment in her case, as she left the hospital in a few days to enjoy the hospitality of her friends.

The irritation in this case seems to be conveyed directly through the phrenic nerve, which has its origin from the third, fourth and fifth cervical nerves. These cases are exceedingly stubborn ones to treat, and it is with this class that the results of treatment have been most unsatisfactory. Hiccough has often been observed in protracted cases of anæmia ; here also its origin is supposed to be central, resulting from irritation of the nerve centers, set up either by an insufficient supply of nutrition, or by the circulation through them of blood rendered abnormal in quality, by the retention of impurities, these conditions arising from defective assimilation of nutritious principles, or from the non-elimination of the products of tissue metamorphosis. Similar phenomena are manifested in some of the exhausting fevers, especially in typhoid, where it is not an infrequent complication in the last stages of the more malignant types of that disease ; here practitioners have learned to regard it as an ominous symptom of dissolution, though it must not be regarded as the signal for the abandonment of hope, for the pathological processes may yet be stayed and health restored.

Here also must be classed the hiccough that occurs in the last stage of Bright's disease, when the blood becomes surcharged with urea ; in these cases it may be the first of the train of couuvulsive symptoms that terminate only with the life of the patient.

About twelve per cent. of all reported cases belong to this class.

II. This class comprises those cases which arise from irritation along the course of or at the peripheral extremity of the phrenic nerve; about thirty-one per cent. of all reported cases are of this variety; of these, slightly more than one-half occurred as epi-phenomena of pneumonia, with which it forms a very distressing complication, though it is not of such fatal issue as might be supposed, for in only one of the reported cases where it occurred did the complication terminate fatally, and in this case the brain was also seriously affected.

CASE II.—A good example of a case belonging to this class occurred in a man who suffered continuously from hiccough for about two months, when he died, apparently from inanition. The post mortem examination revealed an abscess located between the stomach and diaphragm; the irritation caused by this set up and perpetuated the spasms; the diaphragm was found considerably thickened by inflammatory deposits.

Pleuritis, of both the idiopathic and traumatic varieties, has been a fruitful source of the malady, especially when affecting the diaphragmatic portion of the pleura. Hepatitis has also acted as a cause, through secondary involvement of the diaphragm; in these cases the singultus subsides with the hepatitis.

CASE III.—Another case of somewhat unique nature occurred in a man forty-four years old. He had been in poor health for some months and had gradually lost flesh, when hiccough set in; he entered a hospital, where he obtained some relief, but the spasms were not entirely suppressed, and in a short time they returned with all of their former vigor, and were so distressing that in about three months the patient died from exhaustion. Post mortem examination revealed caseous deposits, three on the right side and two on the left at the roots of the lungs, where they exercised pressure on the phrenic nerves, the resulting irritation giving rise to the diaphragmatic spasm.

III. This division includes those cases which are reflex in their origin, arising from irritation in some remote part of the body.

About twenty-six per cent. of all recorded cases belong to this division; it presents a great variety of causes, some of which are of very remote nature.

CASE IV.—A man who was suffering from rheumatism affecting the ankle joint, which was very tender and much swollen; could not walk or scarcely move the joint at all without causing severe hiccough; subsequent to this attack of rheumatism his shoulder joint became affected in a similar manner, when he again experienced his old difficulty, hiccough resulting from the slightest motion of the affected joint, and continuing while motion lasted, and until the pain had subsided again; this condition continued until the rheumatism was cured when the spasm followed in its wake.

Another cause is masturbation, which has been known to operate in a few cases; of these a somewhat peculiar one was;

CASE V.—A young Irish girl, who indulged this vicious habit to the extent of producing four or five orgasms daily; she could by no means be persuaded to abandon her folly, and so her hiccough was perpetuated until she passed from observation.

One peculiarity of her case was that a species of spinal irritation was set up in the lumbar region, in relation to which she discovered some peculiar phenomena which she disclosed to her physician and allowed him to test to his satisfaction. By pressure over the lumbar portion of the spine the severity of the spasms was increased when they already existed, and when absent they were induced by the same means ; on the other hand, by exerting pressure over the upper portion of the vulva they were entirely suspended, thus, conditions of quiescence and of extreme exacerbation could be made to follow each other at will and in quick succession ; the whole therapeutic battery of the old school failed utterly in this case.

Another example, which shows how widely we are to search for causes in obscure cases, occurred in .

CASE VI.—A young lady of excellent reputation, and continued for almost five months, the most of the time under heroic treatment; as no cause had been discovered to account for her trouble it was thought to be advisable to make a vaginal examination, which was done, and an excoriation of the portio uteri discovered; this was cured by topical applications, and as it healed the singultus was gradually relieved.

A perineal abscess in another woman inaugurated an attack which subsided with the evacuation of the pus.

Other causes belonging to this category are fright, hemiplegia, constipation, and irritating substances in the stomach.

In about thirty per cent. of all cases no cause was discovered.

The predisposing influence of age and sex is not very marked ; childhood and youth are almost exempt from the graver forms, but beyond twenty the cases are about equally distributed over the different decades. As far as sex exercises any influence there is a little greater liability among males ; this is chiefly due to occupation, which in them predisposes to some of the diseases in which hiccough occurs most frequently, *i. e.*, pneumonia and typhoid fever.

Cause and duration : But little of value can be said in a general way under this head on account of the great variety of causes upon which they depend. The attacks usually commence by the manifestation of slight and infrequent spasms; these gradually gain in violence and frequency until the maximum is reached ; no limit can be fixed to this period of invasion as it is of very variable length. The degree of severity to which they attain also varies greatly in different cases, while in some cases only from five to ten convulsions occur in a minute ; in others they rise to such a pitch as to be a continuous succession of clonic spasms. A similar difference is also noticed in the severity of the spasms ; some are very slight, involving only the diaphragm, while others involve the diaphragm and with it all of the muscles of respiration, in convulsions so severe that the patient

and his bed are together violently shaken.   In the latter cases the
stomach is rendered entirely incapable of retaining food, all that is
swallowed being immediately pumped out by the spasmodic action.
In one case of a woman the paroxysms were so constant and so
noisy that her husband was unable to endure it, and so obtained a
divorce, after being disturbed by it for twenty years.

A word must be said on the periodicity of the spasms which
sometimes obtains; in some cases these occur at the same hour each
day, last a short time, and then are suspended until the following day;
other cases present a longer interval of rest, *i. e.*, a few days, and
sometimes they are extended to weeks and even months.

In all cases showing this periodicity the tendency is, unless treatment is successfully employed, for the intermissions to shorten and
the attacks to become more severe and of longer duration.   Sometimes
the periods of intermissions are very irregular in length, affording no
means of forestalling an attack.

This phenomenon of periodicity is assumed by almost all attacks
during convalescence.

The duration of attacks is exceedingly variable, being governed to
a great degree by the cause; when it is an epi-phenomenon of acute
diseases its course is generally not long; in pneumonia it usually
commences in the first stage of the disease, and in nearly all reported
cases it has shown a susceptibility to well directed treatment, and has
generally subsided in from a few hours to a few days.   Where the
cause is more obscure, treatment has been less successful, and the
spasms have lasted longer, often for months and even years, some
cases resisting all treatment, as the case mentioned above, which
lasted for twenty years and was then lost sight of.

It is surprising to note with what rapidity some attacks will exhaust
the energies and reduce the flesh of its victim, especially when the
spasms are continuous, as they so often are; the patient obtains no
peace by day nor by night.   A few days of such suffering will produce
a remarkable transformation ; the flesh becomes shrunken, the pulse
accelerated and weakened in force, the tongue gets dry, the countenance haggard, and death threatens, and, indeed, soon follows, unless
relief is obtained ; when relief is afforded convalescence is as rapid as
was the decline.

Prognosis : The prognosis of a symptom of such uncertain significance must, of course, be very uncertain, and can be rendered intelligently only upon a thorough understanding of the conditions which
give rise to it.

About eleven per cent. of all cases have terminated fatally; of these, one was complicated with pneumonia, two with Bright's disease, one with hemiplegia, one with spinal irritation, one with abscess between the stomach and diaphragm, and one with caseous deposits in the lungs, especially at the roots.

Treatment: The first requisite to the successful treatment of the affection is the discovery of its exact cause, if this is possible; the location and nature of this will then suggest the mode of treatment.

It is not within the scope of this paper to go minutely into the treatment, for if we recall the classification it will be seen that this would cover a broad field in medicine. The cases reported have almost all been under allopathic care, consequently the statistics are not rich in glory for homœopathy.

The treatment has been remarkably heroic in many cases and has partaken much of experiment, yet some excellent results have been achieved.

The following are a few remedies that have met with most marked success by the old school :

Chloral has been employed with very gratifying results in a large number of cases ; in those cases in which it has exercised a curative effect its action has been very prompt, cure following after the administration of a few doses. The dose varies in the hands of different practitioners, from five to forty grains. *Quinine* in large doses has cured several cases, as has *pilocarpine*, injected under the skin in doses large enough to produce free perspiration and salivation. Other remedies are *amyl nitrite, cannabis indica, strychnine, opium,* together with emetics, cathartics, and hot fomentations.

Electricity is recommended, though it has not been sufficiently tested to justify a high recommendation; there are two modes of applying it, both of which are about equally in favor; one is the passing of the current through from side to side in the region of the diaphragm ; the other the passing of it along the phrenic nerve ; this is accomplished by placing the anode over the clavicle and the cathode in the scrobiculum cordis. Compressing the chest also has a sphere of usefulness, and is highly recommended by some practitioners ; it is best accomplished by placing the tips of the fingers with the hands in a position of complete supination against the abdominal muscles at the lower and outer juncture of the epigastric with the hypochondriac region, and by then making firm and gradual pressure upwards and backwards against the diaphragm; this must be continued for some time after the spasms cease and then withdrawn gradually ; when judiciously employed this method will be found very efficient.

Homœopathic treatment :

Aconite. This remedy is especially indicated where there is intense arterial excitement, with evidence of local congestions of the brain, cord, or other organs—in fact, in nearly all cases where hiccough complicates acute congestive diseases. Its leading symptoms are great fearfulness and apprehension, dread of some accident happening, distraction of ideas, with great sensitiveness to all impressions. Great thirst. Hiccough comes on after eating or drinking. Long-lasting attack in the morning, accompanied by pain and restlessness.

Agaricus. Confusion and dull aching in the head. Tendency to spasmodic twitching of the muscles all over the body, especially in the face and upper extremities. Hiccough occurs in the afternoon. Several convulsions follow each other in rapid succession, first in the posterior portion of the chest, then in the epigastrium, afterwards in the hypogastrium, especially on the right side, attended with a sensation as if the body were shaken thoroughly, occurring in the evening and when standing. Inflammation of the upper part of the abdomen; abdomen distended.

Belladonna. This drug will sometimes be selected where the cerebral and circulatory phenomena characteristic of it are present. It has intense thirst for water, but when it is brought it is repelled. Aversion to all fluids. Inefficient inclination to eructate ; eructation half suppressed. Eructation and hiccough. Spasms, composed partly of eructation and partly of hiccough. Violent attacks of hiccough ; so violent that they jerk the patient up. Frequent spasmodic hiccough that goes on to suffocation. Hiccough and convulsions of the left arm and right leg alternating. Redness and heat of the head. Violent hiccough about midnight, accompanied by a profuse sweat. Nausea, with vomiting. Borborygmi, 'with feeling of heat in the abdomen. Violent cutting and pressure in the abdomen of erratic character. Violent pressure downwards as if everything would be pressed through the pelvis. Incessant moving of the body, especially of the arms. Single muscles contract continuously in different parts of the body.

Bryonia. Ill-humored, quarrelsome, fretful. Excessive thirst day and night ; must drink a great deal at once. Thirst for cold water. Frequent empty eructations, with confusion of the head ; eructations of tasteless gas. Hiccough after eructations without having eaten anything. Severe hiccough after eating, and with every spasm; pressure in the forehead as if the brain shook from behind forwards. Hiccough after vomiting. Hiccough, afterwards eructations lasting several minutes, aggravated by the slightest motion. Nausea and vomiting after eating and upon awakening in the morning. Stomach full and sensitive to pressure. Pressure in the stomach after eating, as from a stone.

Carbo vegetabilis. Violent and almost constant eructations. Eructations after eating and drinking. Eructations preceded by griping in the abdomen. Constant sensation of heartburn. Hiccough after a moderate dinner; after every motion; aggravated by slight causes.

Graphites. Constant eructations tasting of food. Ineffectual attempts to eructate. Water-brash at night in bed. Hiccough in the morning after rising and after dinner. Hiccough in the evening lasting for an hour or more, after every meal, whether hot or cold, with a dull, heavy head, or sleeplessness. Nausea and vomiting in the morning.

Hyoscyamus. Thirst, caused by sticking and dryness in the throat. Ineffectual effort to eructate. Bad-tasting eructations, with inclination to vomit. Frequent hiccough, with cramps and rumbling in the abdomen. Hiccough during abdominal inflammation. Violent hiccough at midnight, with involuntary micturition and frothing at the mouth. Violent hiccough, with constipation. Excessive long-continued hiccough after dinner. Heartburn.

Ignatia. The general characteristics of this drug, in its mental and nervous spheres, lead to its selection.

It has hiccough occurring in the evening and after drinking. Hiccough after eating or drinking. Hiccough from tobacco smoking in one accustomed to the use of tobacco. Aggravation from tobacco and coffee. Hiccough in children when they are restless and cry much at night.

Lycopodium. This drug may sometimes be thought of when the excessive flatulence characteristic of it is present; aside from this its indications are not characteristic.

Natrum muriaticum. Sometimes ravenous hunger, and again aversion to food, especially bread. Aversion to smoking, of which he has been fond. Excessive thirst. Heartburn and water-brash. Violent hiccough lasting for several days. Hiccough, with yawning and nausea, while in bed in the evening. Hiccough, alternating with yawning; at last yawning alone, lasting for a long time.

Nicotinum. Great thirst day and night. Bitter and sour eructations, with pressure in the stomach lasting for a half-hour or more. Violent hiccough for several evenings.

Frequent violent hiccough in the evening, renewed from time to time for several days; comes on nearly every evening after retiring, and lasts an hour or more. Nausea and sticking pain in the stomach.

Nux vomica. Hunger, though with aversion to food and drink, and to his customary tobacco. Excessive thirst, especially for beer, drinking followed by qualmishness. Eructations sour, bitter, rancid. Frequent hiccough, without apparent cause, coming on before dinner. Hiccough brought on by cold drinks. Heartburn, as from an overloaded stomach. Nausea after eating, aggravated by tobacco.

Sepia. Excessive appetite, never satisfied, hungry feeling in the stomach soon after meals. Desire for vinegar. Much thirst for cold water, drinks much and often, followed by thirstlessness. Hiccough after a meal lasting for a quarter of an hour or more. Hiccough during the habitual smoke, with contractions of the throat and a sensation as if a plug were in it, producing an excessive accumulation of water in the mouth. Hiccough after supper. Heartburn in the morning and afternoon. Nausea at intervals during the whole day, also after a meal, with an afflux of watery saliva; bitterish, sour taste in the mouth. Nausea in the morning, only passing off after eating something. Sensation of weakness and goneness in the stomach.

Staphis. Frequent hiccough, associated with nausea and stupefaction of head. Frequent hiccough while smoking tobacco, as usual. Severe hiccough, coming on half an hour after supper, always after eating.

Veratrum. Hiccough in the morning with customary smoke. Long-continued hiccough, with thirst for cold drinks; hot drinks bring on hiccough. Nausea, followed by violent and frequent vomiting.

Other remedies are: *Ant. crud., Amyl nit., Bismuth, Calc., Cham., Coccul., Crot. tig., Cupr., Gels., Lachesis, Ledum, Nux vom., Puls., Silic.,* and *Spong.*

Repertory.

TIME.

After eating: *Acont., Bry., Carbo. veg., Graph., Hyos., Ign., Ratan., Sep., Silic.,* and *Staph.*

Before eating: *Nux vom.*

Evening: *Graph., Ign., Nat. mur., Niccolum, Puls.,* and *Silic.*

Midnight: *Bell.* and *Hyos.*

Morning: *Acont., Graph.* and *Bry.*

INDUCED BY.

Cold drinks—*Nux vom.*

Cold fruit—*Ars.* and *Puls.*
Constipation—*Hyos.*
Diarrhœa—*Hyos.*
Drinking in general—*Ign.*
Motion—*Bry.* and *Hyos.*
Tobacco—*Ign., Sep., Staphis., Verat.* and *Nux vom.*
Warm food—*Graph.*
Warm drink—*Verat.*

ACCOMPANIED BY.

Confusion of head—*Acont., Agar., Graph.* and *Staph.*
Cramps in abdomen—*Hyos* and *Carbo. veg.*
Involuntary micturtion—*Hyos.*
Pain—*Acont., Cistus, Hyos., Verat., Verat. vir.* and *Stramon.*
Restlessness—*Acont., Ign.* and *Hyos.*
Thirst—*Bry., Hyos., Niccolum* and *Sepia.*

BACTERURIA.

By H. E. RICE, M.D.,
Springfield, Mass.

IT is not intended that this paper shall lay claim to scientific exactise, nor has it been published as a treatise on bacteria, but merely as a record of personal observations and ideas, which I have not found embodied in any work on microscopy, urinary analysis, or renal diseases. As such, it may excite comment and enable me to get the views of other observers, by that means leading to a more definite understanding of the relation this microbe may have to renal disease.

I can perhaps give no better idea of the conditions under which it is met, than by a report of two cases which have come under my observation during the past two years. The first patient, a man of forty-five, short, thick-set, previous history good, complains solely of a most atrocious odor arising from his urine as soon as past. He first noticed this some ten or twelve months previous, since which time it has been growing gradually worse, time of day urine is passed, or diet, having no apparent influence on the odor. His urine chemically showed a daily amount of 1,400 or 1,500 c. c., of extremely acid reaction. Specific gravity, $1.025°$—$1,030°$, urea 2%–2.4%, varying very little, a peculiarly disagreeable odor and a cloudiness which is charateristic, being persistent, even after twice or three times filtering, boiling, and the addition of acids or alkalies. This cloudiness gives the urine when agitated, a peculiar glistening appearance not unlike snow in the air. Neither albumin nor sugar was present, and when the specimen was left exposed in a conical glass, decomposition did not set in for several days—three usually. Under a power of 400 diameters, the freshly voided urine seemed to be crowded with micro-organisms, all in active motion, either single, or in pairs and occasionally forming chains of three, but never more than that number. They were much more active in urine freshly passed than in that which had stood for even a few hours. Keeping the specimen at a temperature of 95°, however, prolonged their activity. The bacillus, under a power of 2,000 diameters, appears to be about .006 m. m. in length, and .002 m. m. in thickness, possessed of one flagellum and sometimes two, and containing two spores. It multiplies by fission, becoming somewhat elongated (perhaps to .008 m.m.), and constricted in the middle. Division then takes place and each portion becomes a perfect individual, capable of locomotion.

I have never noticed colonies of these bacteria, but always find them existing as individuals.

Repeated examinations of this urine failed to reveal anything further, each day's accumulation being almost identical with that of the day before. Thinking this must be the same bacillus which inhabits alkaline urine occasionally, and whose migrations are confined to the bladder and urethra, I applied the cure for such conditions, and which had been successful in other cases ; washed out the bladder thoroughly with a solution of carbolic acid, 1–500, with the effect of materially sweetening the excretion for about twelve hours, at the end of which time it was as bad as ever again. A solution of mercury bi-chloride, 1–3,000, was then tried, with much the same result, except that it lighted up a cystitis which lasted several days, and taught me to be more careful in the use of the sublimate.

For eighteen months I watched this patient carefully, examining the urine from time to time, and searching for new developments.

They came about four months since, in the shape of a sub-acute croupous nephritis—with which is associated considerable cardiac irregularity, full carotids, some dizziness at times, headache in the occiput, dimness of vision, and general malaise.

In the meantime I was on the lookout for a similar case, examining every urine I could procure and finally found the microbe again, this time in the urine of a pale, anæmic, strumous girl of nine. In this case, as in the former one, the bad odor arising from the urine, even when freshly voided, being the cause of complaint. On examination it showed much the same characteristics as that of my other patient, being very acid; specific gravity, 1.025° or 1.030°; neither albumin nor sugar present. The cloudiness due to countless numbers of bacteria was present, and under the microscope it was recognized as the same one which I found in the other case.

There could be no possibility, in this case, of this bacillus being due to any septic condition, such as infection from impure catheter, for the girl had never been catheterized, nor had she even suffered from any cystitis or urethritis. After the bacteria had been present some fifteen months, I found, at my last examination three weeks ago, about $\frac{1}{75}$ of 1% of albumin, pus and fat corpuscles (a very limited number of the latter), and a few epithelial and hyaline casts from the straight and convoluted tubes.

Other cases in which the bacillus was present, have come under my observation, but occurred in urines handed me for examination by other physicians, and I have had no opportunities for following them up. They all presented the same characteristics as the two cases mentioned, however, the extreme acidity and the persistent cloudiness being the most noticeable. In the *Centralblatt fur Klinische Medicin, No. 37, 1886,* and copied in the *Medical Record* of December 18th, 1886, Drs. Schottelius and Reinhold report a case of "Bacteruria" and consider it a "most puzzling" one, as well as curious, but do not connect the presence of the bacillus with renal disease, or, in fact, with any disease. Their experiments with the bacillus are similar to my own, except that mine grew rapidly in hydrocele fluid as well as in bouillon, and like theirs, not at all in urine.

I am well aware that two cases are too few to afford a basis for a theory of disease, but as a result of my observations, I have come to three conclusions :

First.—That in some acid urines exists a bacillus not mentioned by observers.

Second.—That the *habitat* of this bacillus is the human kidney.

Third.—That it may be an element in the development of disease of that organ.

THERAPEUTICS OF SPINAL IRRITATION.

By FRANK F. LAIRD, M.D.,
Utica, N. Y.

(*Continued from page 81*).

Nux vomica—*Stiffness of neck, especially right side.* Drawing pain and a feeling as 'of a load on nape of neck, in morning. *Tearing pain by paroxysms in nape of neck in evening.* Bruised pain in nape of neck on stooping and on touch. *Pain as if the flesh were beaten loose from the last cervical vertebra ;* could hardly bear pressure of shirt against it. Cracking (painless) in the cervical vertebra on moving the head; *joints of cervical vertebræ are painful to touch.*

Drawing-tearing, *burning-tearing* and constrictive pains in back. *Constant-pain and bruised sensation in back and small of back.* Bruised pain in back, still more painful when touched and on pressure, as if congested with blood. Drawing in back extending down from nape of neck (while sitting), together with a violent pain in the pit of the stomach, like a crawling, obliging her to sit bent over (in afternoon). Pain between scapulæ and in nape of neck on motion. Pain as if beaten in the dorsal and abdominal muscles, even when not touched. Drawing, bruised, constrictive and burning-striking pain between scapulæ ; also *pressure as of a stone between the shoulder-blades.* Constrictive pain in small of back, extending into side. *Pain in small of back as if bruised or broken, worse 3 or 4 A. M. Pain in small of back at night, preventing turning over in bed ; must sit up to turn over.* Jerk-like, dull sticking in small of back and ischii, worse when coughing or sneezing. Small of back and loins seem tense and sore on touch. Pain in pelvic region as if dislocated, on slightest motion. *Pain across loins, passing to hips.* Pressive pain in loins extending toward spine, causing anxiety, with flatulency. Tearing and pulling in the lower portion of the back while walking and sitting, but not while lying.

Extreme irritability of temper. Over-sensitiveness, every harmless word offends, every little noise frightens ; cannot bear the least, even suitable, medicine. Great anxiety with inclination to commit suicide, but is afraid to die ; much lamentation and weeping. Cannot bear reading or conversation ; irritable and wants to be alone. *Over-sensitive to external impressions ; cannot tolerate noise, talking, music, strong odors or bright light ; the most trifling ailments are unbearable and effect him much. Hypochondriac mood worse after eating.* Time passes too slowly. *Dread of that kind of literary work requiring ratiocination ;* not averse to reading or committing to memory. *Inability for mental work ; unable to think correctly.* Easily makes mistakes while talking and writing, omits syllables and even whole words; in conversation, has great trouble to find the words and uses unsuitable expressions; slow flow of ideas ; can with difficulty collect his thoughts. Disinclination to bodily labor.

Vertigo, after dinner ; as if the brain were turning in a circle, with momentary loss of consciousness ; *with* obscuration of vision (while eating) and faintness ; as if bed were whirling around with her ; dizzy, reeling while walking, as if he would fall to one side or backward ; when sneezing, coughing or rising after stooping.

Intoxicated confusion in head ; intoxicated dizzy heaviness in the morning. Stupid feeling in head if he holds it erect ; when stooping, sensation as if something heavy fell into forehead.

Headache in the morning in bed ; in middle of brain, *felt before opening the eyes ; in forehead ;* in occiput ; as if the skull would burst ; *as if the head had been broken with an ax ; as if he had not slept ; makes him stupid, disappears after rising.* Pressive, boring pains in the head, commencing in the morning, *worse after eating, with nausea and sour vomiting* toward evening after lying down. Drawing, tearing, jerking, burning or pinching pains in head, especially in morning. Redness and heat of face with coldness of other parts of body (Arn). And after eating except, perhaps, hands (palms). *Heaviness and pressure in head after dinner, especially on moving the eyes.* Headache as if brain were bruised or beaten. Pressing pain as if a nail were being driven deeply into side of brain. *Tension in forehead* as if it were pressed in, at night and in the morning, worse on exposing the head to the cold air. Sensation as from a bruise in the back part of head. *Pressive and throbbing headache in vertex from fixed attention of the mind.* Pressing-downward drawing pain deep in the head in region of vertex. Pain in occiput as if brain were pressed forward or bruised. Headache externally ; pain in scalp, aggravated by touch ; especially on vertex ; pain in scalp as if beaten. *Aggravation—Head symptoms worse from mental exertion, exercising in open air, after eating* and *from wine* and *coffee.*

Amelioration—Better in a warm room and from sitting quietly or *lying down.*

Photophobia, worse in morning, wearing off as day advances. Painless injection of the white of the eyes. Vision cloudy. Blepharospasm. *Dilatation of pupils from irritation of the spine* (Vilas).

Ringing, hissing, roaring, or chirping as of locusts in the ears (at night).

Prosopalgia, of an intermittent or periodic type, worse from use of coffee, liquors or abuse of quinine. It comes on usually in the morning and is worse from standing and motion. The eye of the affected side is injected and watery and smarts as from salt ; redness, heat and numbness of cheek ; constipation. Is very irritable and wishes to be alone. Twitching and spasmodic distortion of facial muscles ; spasmus facialis *every time the patient gets angry.* Tension and drawing in face. Stiffness of jaws.

Dry cough with soreness in abdominal muscles. Oppressed breathing ; tightness of breathing from spasmodic constriction of lower part of thorax ; especially when walking and ascending. *Compression of chest as if drawn together, at night* in bed. Tension and pressure in external parts of chest at night as from a weight, and as if the sides were paralyzed ; *pain in chest as if it were compressed by a weight in open air.* Pressing-inward pain in sternum which is sensitive to touch as if beaten ; pain in side of chest below shoulder as if bruised, worse on touch and motion. Drawing beneath left breast, with anxiety, a kind of oppression of the heart, making respiration difficult. Pressing in the chest as from a heavy load.

Palpitation ; *on lying down after dinner ; after eating, from coffee ; from protracted study.*

"This remedy gives speedy relief after abuse of coffee, wine, tobacco, spices, etc. The palpitation does not last long and is attended with cerebral congestion or nausea."

Syncope—*Bad taste in mouth in morning, though food and drink taste natural ; taste sour ; bitter. Offensive odor from the mouth. Sticky, dry mouth without much thirst, in the morning, as if he had been on a spree. The taste of milk in the morning is disgusting, as if spoiled,* Speech difficult, tongue thick. *Constriction of pharynx with difficult swallowing.*

Hunger with aversion to food, especially bread, water, coffee and tobacco. Thirst ; *for milk* which often sours ; *and good relish for drink, but drinking is followed by nausea.* Want of appetite and *constant* nausea. *Bitter, sour eructations.* Spasm of œsophagus, preventing eructations. Hiccough. *Heartburn ; waterbrash ; after eating. Nausea ; in morning : after eating ; from tobacco ; with faintness. Vomiting ; of sour mucus ; of food* and drink ; of bile ; *retching as if to vomit while hawking mucus from fauces. Epigastrium sensitive to pressure ; could not allow the hand to lie on the stomach without causing nausea ; cannot bear clothing tight around the waist.*

Gastralgia—Clawing, cramping pains *increased by light but relieved by hard pressure*—hence *bending forward gives immediate relief ; feeling as if clothing were too tight* ; pain in back starting from posterior wall *of stomach* and spreading under short ribs of left side ; *feeling of weight, pressure and tension between scapulæ ; each paroxysm attended by a feeling as if the bowels would move ; better from hot drinks, worse from food. Tension* and *fullness in epigastrium ; pressure as from a stone, worse after eating. Fluttering,* sinking feeling at stomach *with palpitation. Scraped sensation in pit of stomach ;* or as if something were twisted about. *Pressure in stomach an hour or two after a meal with dulness of head and hypochondriacal mood.* Craving for *brandy, beer, fat food,* chalk.

The gastric symptoms appear an *hour* or *two* after *eating* (Puls, *immediately*) ; *general* aggravation *after dinner.*

Constrictive pain in hypochondria. Cramp-like pain in left side of abdomen with qualmishness. Bruised pain in side of abdomen 'and in loins when touched; also, drawing and stitches. *Loud rumbling and gurgling in abdomen in the morning. Flatulent distension of abdomen after eating.* Flatulent colic with pressure upward, causing dyspnœa and downward, *causing urging to stool and urination.* Periodical colic before breakfast or after meals. Pressure under short ribs as from incarcerated flatus. *Constrictive pain in abdomen. Pain in abdomen as if everything in it were sore, at every step. Jerking and twitching in the abdominal muscles (under the skin) which are painful as if bruised, on touch or motion of body. The band of the clothes above the hips always seems too tight. Sensation in abdomen as if everything in it would fall down, obliging careful walking;* also *sensation as of a weight.* Constriction, *forcing down toward genitals* and feeling as if puffed or swollen, in hypogastrium. *Pressive pain in the pubic region.*

Constipation with frequent and ineffectual desire for stool and sensation of constriction in rectum; after stool, sensation as if more remained but could not be evacuated. Frequent urging but passes only a little each time. Blind hemorrhoids. Alternate constipation and diarrhœa. *Proctalgia, worse after a meal and from mental exertion.* Paralysis of rectum (use strong tincture or strychnia).

Painful ineffectual urging to urinate, urine passes in drops with burning and tearing in urethra and neck of bladder. Retention of urine with above symptoms, where lower part of spine is affected; cystospasm, with twitching and jerking of muscles of extremities. *Incontinence of urine due to paresis of bladder* (strong tincture or strychnia).

"Spinal irritation due to sexual excesses suggests *nux vomica* when the pains are principally felt at night in the small of the back, aggravated by turning in bed; sore and bruised feeling in the lumbar region when pressed; dull pains in back when sitting; costiveness; more or less headache, sometimes with vertigo" (Hoyne).

Uterine and *ovarian neuralgia, the pains causing desire for stool* and *urination.*

Feeling of tension and stiffness in the extremities sometimes associated with jerking in the muscles. *Trembling of the limbs and jerking of the heart. The longer he lies in bed in the morning, the more pain he has in all the limbs especially in the joints, as if beaten and bruised; relieved after rising. Sensation of sudden loss of power of the arm or lower extremities, in the morning. Great weariness and relaxation in all the limbs, after taking the open air. Falling asleep of arms, hands* and *soles of feet.*

Shoulders pain as if bruised; paralytic heaviness in shoulders with weak arms.

Tottering and *unsteadiness of lower extremities. Paralytic drawing in muscles of thighs and calves, painful on walking. Painful bruised feeling in muscles of thighs* and *in knees. Stiffness and tension in hollows of knees, especially after standing ; sensation as if tendons were too short, on arising from a seat.* Numbness and deadness of the legs. Cramps in calves at night, also in soles, must stretch the foot.

Great debility with over-sensitiveness of all the senses. Stitches through the body in jerks, feels sore all over ; worse mornings. *Tremulous sensation over whole body, in morning. Greater weariness in the morning after rising than in the evening when going to bed.* Sensitiveness and aversion to open air.* Fainting fits after walking in the open air. Tendency to faint ; from odors ; in the morning ; after eating. Chilliness and shivering over whole body with blueness of the skin, *especially of the hands and nails. Heat with aversion to uncovering. Paralysis.*

Sleepiness early in evening ; on going to bed, falls asleep immediately ; awakens at 3 A. M. feeling well (Nux patient is always better after a short sleep if not aroused), lies awake for hours with a rush of thoughts, falls into a dreamy sleep at daybreak from which he is hard to arouse, and then feels tired, weak and averse to rising.

Sleeps mostly lying on the back, with one or both hands above or under the head. Loud snoring respiration during sleep. Much yawning and sleepiness during the day, especially *after eating.*

Drea ms with frightful visions, causing fear ; awakens in fright from the least noise.

Aggravation—From mental exertion (ratiocination) ; in the morning ; after eating, especially after dinner ; from motion; from slight touch ; in open air ; in dry weather.

The *Nux* patient is thin, irritable, choleric, with dark hair ; makes great mental exertion or leads a sedentary life. He is addicted to highly seasoned food, coffee, tobacco or alcohol ; or has dined upon drug mixtures, hot medicines and nostrums. Many of these patients have become slaves to the use of narcotics. The mental condition is *sui generis* and is one of the most marked characteristics of the drug, *viz.:* he can perform *automatic* brain-work, such as reading or memorizing, without difficulty ; but as soon as the attempt to *reflect, reason, think*, the head becomes "confusion worse confounded." In *nux* the faculty of *ratiocination suffers ;* in *lyc.* and *cocculus all* the mental powers are paralyzed.

PHOSPHORUS—*Stiffness*, soreness (right side), tearing and feeling as of a weight in nape of neck. The anterior cervical muscles are painfully sensitive to touch and motion. Twitching of cervical muscles.

Tension in all the muscles of the back with pressure. Back seems bruised, constantly obliging her to turn in bed. Violent pain in spinal column ; at insertion of last false ribs ; as if beaten, during menses ; on sitting a long time. *Dull sensation as from congestion in the whole spine* with, at times, a paralytic sensation in sacrum ; *heat in back, can't lie on it, it is so hot.* After mid-day nap, feels paralyzed in back and arms ; as if back were asleep or sprained.

The spinous processes of the dorsal vertebræ between scapulæ are exceedingly sensitive to pressure ; also muscles between spinous processes and left scapula ; much worse on left side ; sticking pains beginning at the bone near left scapula and extending forward through the chest or in reverse direction, at times also extending to upper arm, relieved by firm pressure upon the back, by rest and by warmth ; the pains are aggravated by lifting and by working ; worse during menses and *especially aggravated by unpleasant emotional excitement* and by vexation. Sensation as from a draft of cold air in muscles of right scapula and along posterior surface of upper arm to elbow, or feeling as if a raw wind were blowing on a moist surface. Sensation when lifting or carrying anything as if some one were tightly grasping scapula. Between shoulders ; *burning* or *dull pain ; throbbing in a small spot.* Tearing and stitches in scapulæ.

Great nervous sensitiveness, with weakness, especially in region of last lumbar vertebra and in sacrum ; every slight exertion causes pain along whole spine. *Pressure on spinous processes of two last lumbar vertebræ and neighboring parts causes a sensation of numbness and rigidity in both feet.* Paralyzed sensation in upper os sacrum and in lower lumbar vertebræ. *Transient pain extending from coccyx through spine to vertex drawing the head backward (during stool)*; coccyx painful to touch as from an ulcer. Pain in coccyx impeding every motion ; she can find no comfortable position ; followed by painful stiffness of neck.

Mental depression with excessive timidty is a great characteristic of *Phosphorus; constant apprehension of some impending misfortune. Anxiety and restlessness ; with much sweat on forehead and heat of head; when alone ; at twilight ; about the future ; during a thunder storm ;* with palpitation. *Anxiously solicitous as regards the termination of her illness. Great fear ; as if a horrible face were looking out from every corner;* anthropophobia (*lyc.*); An indescribable feeling of fear, fright and dread ; fears she will die, yet weary of life. Hysterical alternation of laughing and weeping. *Great sadness* alternating with indifference to everything, even her own children. Excitable, easily angered and vehement, from which she afterwards suffers. *Any lively impression is followed by heat as if immersed in hot water. Great indisposition to physical or mental activity, even to converse. Inability to think ; slow flow of ideas ; cannot keep* the *mind on any particular subject. An absent minded, dazed condition in which the patient seems unable to collect his senses or grasp any thought, is highly characteristic of the remedy. Stupid feeling with heaviness, dulness and confusion of the head.*

Vertigo ; staggers while walking ; *after rising from bed* or *from a seat ; like a heavy pressing downward of forepart of head* with faintish nausea and blackness before eyes when stooping ; on closing eyes ; *as though all the blood rushed to the head ; compelling recumbent posture;* with headache and exhaustion ; *worse morning and after meals.* Says Hoyne : "The following symptoms are relieved by this drug : vertigo as if the chair on which she was sitting were rising ; vertigo with op-pressive pains in the head ; vertigo with chills or with excessive secretion of saliva ; vertigo followed by diarrhœa with great heat and sweat ; vertigo as if she would fall." Great weakness of head, cannot endure sound of piano.   Dull headache ; as if he had not slept enough or as after night watching ; with dizziness, followed by red circular patch in middle of forehead.   Heavy headache extending to eyeballs as if head were drawn forward by a weight, face feels congested as after overstudy, at height accompanied by drawing in left side of occiput ; worse from mental application.   Pressive headache, mostly right side, relieved in open air.   Headache from slightest vexation. *Constrictive headache every other day.*   Violent numb and dizzy feeling with pressive pain in head, disinclination and inability to work, espec-ially mental labor, and sleepiness ; almost entirely relieved after lying quietly and partly sleeping, returning only after rising and moving about, with sore pain in various places in head when touched.   Vibra-tion in head when talking loudly, compelling her to converse in a low tone.

Dull pressive frontal headache extending to eyes and *root of nose ; feeling as if eyes would be pressed out ; worse from motion, better in open air.   Headache in forehead.   Sensation as if the skin of the forehead were too tight above eyes wakens her every morning,* with heat in head. Congestive pulsating burning in forehead.   Headache over left eye. Sick headache with pulsations and burning, mostly in forehead ; with nausea and vomiting from morning until noon ; worse from music, while masticating and in a warm room (Hering).   *Throbbing pain in temples.*   Shooting or sticking pains from one temple to the other. *Vertex; dull stupefying headache ;* spasmodic contractive pain ; *conges-tive pain ;* throbbing, also in left side of head especially occiput ; hot vertex after grief.

Coldness with pain in ear or cold, crampy pain on whole left side of head. Right sided headache from mental application. Drawing, tearing or throbbing in right side of head.

Sensation of coldness in cerebellum with sensation of stiffness in the brain. Pulsations, sticking and burning in the brain ; *the heat enters the brain from the spine*—hence in congestive headaches rising up from spine and spreading over head (*Silicea*). Headache increased by music and odors. The occiput or forehead is swollen ; touching the swollen part causes the most excruciating pain.

The headaches of *phosphorus* are congestive or neuralgic (hemicrania). Motion, stooping forward, mental exertion, warmth and noise, aggravate ; the reverse conditions relieve. They are generally the result of too close application to study or arise from sexual excesses. Vertigo, difficulty of application to intellectual labor, mental depression and a feeling of great fatigue, are common accompaniments.

Eyes give out while reading. *Distant objects appear to be covered by smoke or mist ; sees better in morning, in twilight* or *by shading the eyes with the hand.* Letters look red when reading. *Green halo around the candle. Sparks before the eyes* in the dark. *Black floating objects, points and spots before the eyes.* Paroxysms of nyctalopia ; or sensation as if things were covered with a gray veil.

Difficult hearing, especially of the human voice. Sounds re-echo in the ears, especially music. Roaring and ringing in the ears.

Over-sensitive smell, especially with headache. Tension in skin of face. Tearing, darting pains in bones of face, temples and jaws.

Nervous aphonia ; larynx sensitive to touch. Aphonia from prolonged loud talking. Spasmodic cough *with tightness across upper chest, worse in changing from warm to cold air.* Oppression and anxiety in chest, worse evening and morning. Nervous palpitation of the heart in tall, slender persons *with feeling of weakness in chest,* irritability, and aggravation *before a storm. Violent palpitation,* with anxiety, evenings and mornings in bed ; while lying on left side. Pressure in middle of sternum and about the heart. *Syncope.* Dryness of throat, day and night ; it fairly glistens. *Ravenous hunger at night. Great longing for acids* and *spicy things.* Great thirst ; longs for something refreshing. Loss of appetite alternating with bulimia. WANTS ALL FOOD AND DRINK COLD. *Regurgitation of food without nausea very soon after swallowing it ; also in mouthfuls.* Eructations ; empty ; sour ; *tasting of the food, even several hours after eating ;* ineffectual, with pressure in chest. *Much belching of wind after eating.* Hiccough. Constant nausea. AS SOON AS WATER BECOMES WARM IN THE STOMACH, IT IS THROWN UP. *Nausea disappears on drinking water.* Vomiting. Great fullness in stomach and painfulness to touch and pressure. *Pressure above pit of stomach ; as from a hard substance ; pressure at cardiac orifice, especially on swallowing bread, which remains seated there.* Pressure in stomach as from a heavy weight after eating. Oppression and burning in epigastrium ; drawing pain extending to chest; "goneness." Cardialgia ; gnawing, constricting, griping pains, worse after eating and from motion. Gross speaks highly of *phosphorus* in gastrodynia when there are paroxysms of pressing pain in stomach running into back, brought on or aggravated by eating, or relieved by yielding to a most ravenous appetite (Hempel and Arndt). Incarcerated flatus ; loud rumbling in abdomen ; *emission of much flatus.* SENSATION OF GREAT WEAKNESS AND EMPTINESS IN ABDOMEN ; also sensation of coldness. Enlargement of liver and spleen.

Burning or *needle-like stitches in the rectum. Constipation ; feces slender, long, dry, tough and hard, like a dog's ; voided with difficulty.* Painless diarrhœa.

Frequent micturition at night ; scanty discharge. Urine ; turbid and high-colored ; *brown, with red sandy sediment ;* deposits white, cloudy sediment ; variegated cuticle appears on the surface. Retention and incontinence of urine occasionally present. *Profuse watery urine.* Spinal irritation from sexual abuse ; *excessive sexual excitement both mental and local ;* frequent erections and emissions or *irresistible desire for coitus ;* full of lascivious dreams and thoughts ; *heat in and congestion of lower spine.* With palpitation of the heart worse from any emotion ; spine exceedingly sensitive to touch, with weakness in back and limbs ; trembles, stumbles and totters ; sleepless from excessive heat, must get up and walk ; tendency to cough or to painless diarrhœa. If impotent, he always gives a *previous history of hyperexcitement.*

Menstrual derangement. Amenorrhœa with blood spitting or hemorrhage from nose, anus or urethra.

Weakness in all the limbs as if paralyzed ; trembling from every exertion. Extremities, especially hands and feet, are as heavy as lead. Burning in hands and lower extremities. *The arms and legs easily fall asleep.* Cramps. *Numbness in limbs* is a prominent symptom. *Arms and hands become numb ; fingers, especially tips, feel numb and insensible.* Tensive, pressive sensation in deltoid and upper dorsal muscles, extending up the nape of neck. Tension, stiffness and heaviness of right shoulder, with pressure ; *great heaviness of the arm.* Heaviness and trembling of the hands while allowing them to hang down, with redness and distended veins, and a feeling as if blood was forced into them. *The fingers cramp.*

The nates are painful as if suppurating, on sitting a long time. Feet swollen in the evening or when walking. Ankles feel swollen and as if the skin were tense. Constant inclination to cramp in soles and toes. *Burning of the feet.*

. INABILITY TO LIE ON THE LEFT SIDE. *Small wounds bleed much. General nervous exhaustion ; inexpressible heaviness of the whole body so that every motion is unpleasant and difficult ; exhaustion of both mind and body, in the morning.* Sometimes this exhaustion seems to centre in the chest and the patient is so weak she can scarcely speak. Numbness of the whole body accompanied by pricking sensations. *Chilliness every evening, with shivering, without thirst. Cold extremities ;* COLDNESS IN KNEES CONSTANTLY *at night in bed. Perspiration on head and hands frequently alternating with coldness.* Sweat mostly on head, hands and feet, with increased urine, or only on forepart of body. Flushes all over, beginning in hands. Paralysis. *Great sleepiness ;* sleepy all day, restless all night. *Cannot sleep before midnight.* Frequent waking from heat or from hunger. Unrefreshed in the morning ; even quiet sleep does not rest her. When falling asleep, sees faces leering at him or imagines *he is in several pieces and cannot properly adjust the fragments.* FREQUENT ALTERNATION OF WAKING AND SLEEPING IS VERY CHARACTERISTIC. Dreams ; *of trouble and danger ; lascivious. Aggravation—Before midnight ; during a thunder storm ; when lying on left side* or back. *Pains are especially aggravated by unpleasant emotional excitement and by vexation. Amelioration—In the open air.*

Phosphorus finds its typical patient in the tall, slender, nervous woman who is startled by even the opening of a door ; and in the rapidly growing youth who has sacrificed his nervous energies to sexual indulgence or excessive brain-work. Like its analogue, *cocculus,* this drug produces such extreme prostration that the patient can scarcely stand upon his feet ; each presents the well known symptoms of cerebral exhaustion ; and in their entire pathogenesis we see a close similitude. But the resemblance is *apparent, not real. Cocculus owes its symptoms to anæmia ; phosphorus, to hyperæmia.* Bear this one fact in mind and the distinctive modalities are unerringly interpreted.

(*To be continued*).

HOW TO STUDY THE MATERIA MEDICA.*

By SAM'L LILIENTHAL, M.D.,
New York.

"Look here, upon this picture, and on this,—
The counterfeit presentment of two brothers."

Hamlet, Act III., Scene IV.

IN No. 20 of the *Allgemeine Hom. Zeitung,* Dr. Pfander, of Thun, and Dr. Hesse of Hamburg, publish some of their cases ; allow us to dissect them, so that we may learn therefrom how to study materia medica.

Dr. A. Pfander's first case reads as follows :

CASE 1.—C. K., 12 years old, took sick July 29th, suffering from hallucinations, appearing especially during sleep, but also when awake. *Stram.* 4.

July 30.—Slept well, head, free, right inguinal glands somwhat swollen and painful. Cold compresses.

September 3. Paroxysmal severe colicky pains in stomach and abdomen, shooting into the right leg, yesterday also vomiting.   During the forenoon the pain is continuous, the whole abdomen painful ; stool thin and black; temperature increased, pulse 100. *Aconite* 3 and *merc. cor.* 5, alternately.

September 4.—Pains the same, first sound of the mitralis not clear. Pulse 120, temp. 39.6 (103¼). *Bryon.* and *coloc.* in alternation.

September 6.—There was some improvement, but to-day pains return with dyspnœa. Murmurs of the heart clearer at the first sound of the pulmonalis ; the beat of the heart somewhat spread out ; temp. 39.2 (103), pulse 108. Same drugs.

September 9.—Colic somewhat easier ; heart the same ; painful swelling of the left knee, right knee was also painful. Temp. 38.5 ; pulse 116. *Natr. salicyl.* 4.0 (one drachm) to 200.0 water ; every two hours a tablespoonful. *Spigelia* 5.

September 11.—Swelling of knee gone, appetite good, no pains, pulse 88. *Natr. salicyl and spig.* are continued in rarer doses.

September 24.—Pains in heart and arm (stenocardia), left ventricle somewhat enlarged, a murmur takes the place of the first sound of the mitralis. *Kalmia* 2, cleared the case up.

In this case, Pfander says the colic was already of a rheumatic nature, showing itself more decidedly by the affection of the knees. *Colocynth* failed, *salicylate of soda* cured, though it showed no influence on the heart. It is questionable whether this drug has any influence in rheumatic affections of the heart, still its action in rheumatism is so prompt that the rheumatic trouble is removed before the heart can

---

*A paper read before the New York County Medical Society, December, 1886.

become affected. It perhaps was the epidemic remedy once, but its time may have passed.

CASE II.—Pauline J., 13 years old, suffered this year for the third time from articular rheumatism, which with two former cases was treated allopathically by *salicylate of soda.*

June 26.—The rheumatism attacked both articular ends of the left clavicle, which were red, swollen and very painful. *Vitium cordis,* insufficiency of the mitralis; pulse 120, fever moderate; urine full of phosphates. *Ferrum phosphoricum* 3.

June 27.—Less pain in the clavicula, but pains in both scapulæ, and small joints of left hand, which are swollen.

June 28.—The joints of right foot and left hand most painful. Pulse 104. *Ferr. phos.* 3.

July 1.—Discharged cured, and so far no relapse, whereas formerly she suffered pains for weeks; perhaps the quantities of the *salicylate* taken in former cases caused the relapse, for if this drug does not produce an amelioration in two days, it is of no use to continue it.

REMARKS :—It is easier to criticise than to make it better, still we cannot consider the doctor a strict homœopathic prescriber. Though *stramonium* removed the hallucinations, he forgets to tell us in what they consisted, for we have many drugs which produce hallucinations. It is only too true that a large majority of physicians claiming to be adherents to the law of similarity, are given to short alternation of two or three drugs ; but it cannot be denied that such alternation prevents a close study of our materia medica, and lands its adherents on the sand-banks of routinism. Alternation leads to pathological prescribing and to the neglect of these differential minute symptoms which are the pride of a student of homœopathic materia medica. On the third Pfander gives *aconite* and *mercur. corros.,* on the fourth, *bryonia* and *colocynth,* on the fifth *spigelia* and *natr. salicyl.,* and on the eleventh *kalmia.* He had to deal with an acute migrating rheumatism, finally settling in the heart and knees. Neither the doctor nor could we find any indication for a *mercurial,* for after twenty-four hours he changed to *bryonia* and *colocynthis.* Now we all know the great sensitiveness of the *bryonia* patient, who has to keep perfectly quiet to get some ease and mostly attended with constipation and relieved by a pasty stool. *Colocynth,* on the contrary, has violent colic with copious liquid stools ; colicky pains relieved for a time by a copious evacuation, but the sharp pains soon return until another discharge takes place. We deal here with a neuralgia of the bowels and not with an inflammatory state.

But, as the wandering rheumatism attacks now the knees and the heart, the doctor flies to *spigelia, kalmia* and the *salicylate af soda.*

We believe with the doctor that the *salicylate of soda* has been over-estimated by the old school in the treatment of rheumatism, and still it has its strict individuality as : Acute inflammatory articular rheumatism attacking one or more joints, especially elbows and knees, with great swelling and redness ; high fever and excessive sensitiveness to the least jar, motion impossible. It visits especially strong, robust persons with sanguineous temperaments. Notwithstanding the similarity of amelioration by rest we meet, under *bryonia,* rather a muscular than an articular rheumatism, and it may follow, when necessary, the *salicylic acid,* which, like *aconite,* is more indicated in the first stage, when it may prevent its spreading to the heart, where we find *bryonia* as often in-dicated as *kalmia* or *spigelia.* In fact under *kalmia* rheumatism we hardly ever meet fever or inflammation. It is a weariness and languor, with the wandering pains, which, in their migration, may also attack the heart and aggravate the valvular affection, whereas *spigelia* has high fever during the commencing valvular disease with purring feel-ing about heart, stitches about the heart, pulse strong, but slow. Often *kali carbonicum* is indicated when *spigelia* is prescribed.

Can any one from the recital of such a case, affirm which remedy cured or do we learn anything from such a report?

How much more instructive is the second case, which was rapidly cured by *ferrum phos.,* a drug proved by Prof. Morgan ten years ago. It is one of Schüssler's tissue remedies—I like the old name better, for our remedies cure by their dynamic action—and these twelve drugs, carefully studied and faithfully applied, one at a time, for alternation with them is an absurdity, will well repay the student and the practi-tioner for their clear-cut indications. Some fear their use would lead to routine work—be it so, it is preferable to know twelve drugs thoroughly, than to dabble hap-hazard among many. Alas, the laborers are few, the drones many. Articular rheumatism, shooting from one joint to another with loss of sleep and night-sweats not reliev-ing the pains with characteristic restlessness—he cannot lie down, must gently walk about to get relief; these are the indications of *ferrum phos.,* and with such symptoms we may expect a cure.

Let us look now at the other picture. My young friend, Dr. Hesse, of Hamburg, is a pupil of Kunkel, and no wonder he is strict in the use of drugs.

Case I.—A lady of thirty years, brunette and of good constitution, complains of a thousand and one things, but especially of no desire to work, headache, surging in ears, hammering in ear, head, in the whole body, palpitations and dyspnœa when ascending, pains in back, in stomach with eructations and flatus, sensation as if she ate too much, menses sparingly and regular. At every visit she had new symptoms, at her last visit she chiefly complained of all the former ones, of great desire for fruit, does not care for anything nor for anybody, sensation of emptiness. *Ignatia* 30, one dose daily, cleared up the whole state, so that she feels well again.

CASE II.—A strong, blonde lady of 36 years ; complaining already for several years, sought my advice after having refused treatment and operation by a noted gynæcologist. Her greatest troubles were pains in the right side of the abdomen, extending to the back of the right hip, at first only periodically, now continuous. The abdomen in the region of the right ovary is very sensitive to pressure, the bed-covering unbearable, her clothing must be kept loose. She can only lie on her back, never on the side affected. She lies awake at night for hours ; appetite variable ; stools only by the aid of purgatives, mostly very painful and with discharge of blood. Draughts and wet weather aggravate. Menses regularly every four weeks, lasting a week and followed by moderate leucorrhœa. During the first day of menstruation the pains are more severe and last more or less during the whole menstrual period, sometimes even up to the next one, so that she is obliged to keep her bed. Coitus also very painful. The gynæcologist diagnosed induration or tumor of the uterus and advised an operation.

She came under my treatment in December, 1885, and for four months I felt dissatisfied, though there was some improvement under *kali carb.* which regulated the stool, diminished the pains so that she only had to keep her bed during menstruation. April, 1886, she received several powders, *sulfur* 200, to take one powder a week. May 26th, she complains of an eruption over the whole body, similar to one she had four years ago and which was suppressed by salves. Otherwise she feels a great deal better. *Placebos.*—July 2d. Eruption gone, eats well and sleeps well ; menses nearly free from pain and can dress again fashionably. October 13th. Discharged, cured ; had no medicine during the last three months.

CASE III.—A women of 54 years complains for months; want of air, especially evening and night, has to sit up in bed and walk about to get relief. No appetite, thirst, stomach bloated, cannot bear anything tight about her, especially in the afternoon ; stool every third or fourth day, hard and after great exertion. Passes little urine and easily ; no sweat ; cold feet; the whole body feels cold; falls asleep late ; great anxiety ; much headache ; œdema pedum in the evening ; wants her head kept cool in a warm room. *Lycopodium* 30, a powder only.

A month later great amelioration ; breathing free, can sit or lie in bed ; good appetite and all other symptoms disappearing. *Lycopodium* 30, a powder every third day and then discharged cured.

Now look at this picture and at the other one. One physician alternates and guesses, the other studies and knows his materia medica and cures his cases with the single remedy and time.

There must be a cause for this difference and this leads us to the all absorbing question : how to study materia medica and how to prescribe according to the law of *similia similibus curantur.*

Every merchant is obliged to keep books of single or double entry in order to know how his personal standing is and how he stands with his customers. Therein lies the whole secret. Every physician ought to be well acquainted with the periodical literature of his own school as well as of the others, and journals ought to be read pen in hand. Take, for example, the last number of the *Hom. Physician,* and that sterling physician, C. C. Smith, gives us these hints for several remedies : You ought to have now a repertory volume of your own, wherein you enter these symptoms alphabetically : *e. g.* under R : *rhododendron :* Cannot get to sleep or remain asleep unless her legs are crossed.

A pathological repertory is another one. You read perhaps an article on tabes dorsalis which in its first stage was relieved by *baryta.* Now you put under T : Tabes dorsalis or locomotor ataxia—*baryta.;* No sensory paralysis yet, fulgurant pains; twitching in legs; genital excitation ; some disorder of vision.

You may also keep an inter-leaved edition of Hering, Lippe—materia medica or repertory—or Raue, Lilienthal, etc., and at your leisure you enter such symptoms in their respective places and by-and-by you will be astonished how much you profit thereby.

But the best lesson is one's own practice. In your ledger every case, trivial though it may appear, ought to be entered in full and carried from day to day, till your patient is cured, or otherwise. A post mortem study once and a while takes the pride out of a fellow and convinces us that we have yet much to learn. The case got well. Study your case anew to see whether your remedy set the ball in motion, and if so, enter it in your m. m. repertory. I am sure that Hesse put in his respective case under *ignatia, sulf. or lyc.* Our most successful practitioners do it and never say it is time lost or they have no time for it. Why, it does not take half an hour, after your day's labor is over to make these entries in your respective books ; and keeping your indices in order, you can find what you need, at a moment's notice. After a few years careful medical book-keeping you feel astonished at your own material, carefully gathered and garnered. You have your own repertory well indexed, it is. your own mine well worked out, and in similar cases we have only to refer to our own repertory in order to refresh our memory. We have our own experience founded on facts and we believe in it.

To be a successful homœopathic practitioner it is necessary to consider every case daily as if it were a new one, in order to detect the least change which might have taken place. It does not always mean that we must change the remedy or even the potency, but forewarned is forearmed and placebos might come in place in order to give the drug time to digest. We are all too much in a hurry and the study and application of our materia medica allow no hurry. One word more and I am done: it is better to be right with the few than to sail carelessly down the stream with a majority.

PRACTICAL HINTS FOR THE STUDY OF NEW GROWTHS.

By A. WILSON DODS, M.D.,
Fredonia, N. Y.

IT is not to be supposed that the writer of this paper expects to teach the members of the Society anything new in regard to the pathology or appearance—microscopical or otherwise—of new growths, but having found by experience that the ordinary works on Pathology and Pathological Anatomy leave the student utterly in the dark—or at best, give general directions which are almost as useless—as to those processes which have of necessity to be gone through with before a thorough microscopic examination can be made; he has thought that the brief detail of some of the methods he has found the most useful, might be of interest to the Society. It need scarcely be said that there is no claim of originality on the part of the writer in any of the methods here detailed, for all have been obtained in greater or less part from various authors, and with this general acknowledgment of indebtedness, the subject of credit will be dismissed.

In this paper, as little will be said of pathology and pathological anatomy as possible, as it is with the preparation for seeing and not what is seen that we have to do.

Broadly, then, the manner of examining any new growth may be considered under two divisions. First, the appearance presented by the tumor to the unaided eye as to shape, color, etc., and also on section through its mass. Second, its histological structure as shown by the microscope.

Of the first of these nothing need be said here, save that the naked eye appearance should always be noted and recorded as soon as possible after the removal of the tumor from the body. The main points to be noted are the color, shape, consistence and the appearance on section.

Before proceeding to the examination of the different methods of preserving, staining and mounting the tissues, it will be of advantage to consider what points in the structure of a new growth, we wish to determine by a microscopic examination, in order that an intelligent selection may be made of the means used in preparing the tissues, so that the structure to be demonstrated may be shown in the best possible manner.

Briefly the points to be made out, if possible, are these : the blood vessels and their relation to other parts; the lymphatics and nerves, if any, and in order, if possible, to determine the mode of growth, to be able to distinguish between the young and growing bioplasts, and the formed material ; these taken together will give a better idea of the true nature of the growth than any hunt for the so-called cancer cells.

There can be no doubt that the best and most certain modes of showing the blood vessels in any tissue is by injection ; for if this be well done, it places the differentiation of these vessels from the surrounding structures beyond question ; gives the best idea of their relationship to each other and to the adjacent tissues, and also allows the observer to form a more just conception of the amount of the blood supply to the part. The art of making injections is not very difficult of attainment for any one who is possessed of an ordinary amount of manipulative skill, plus patience and perseverance, although, no doubt, complete success will only be attained after repeated failures. Much more, however, can be learned from a partially injected specimen than from one which is not injected at all, and I cannot too strongly recommend that the attempt to inject new growths should be made at every opportunity.

When it is proposed to inject a tumor, the attempt should be made as soon after its removal as possible, and before it has lost its animal heat. When this is not practicable, the tumor should be immersed in warm water for some time before the process of injection is begun. Of the different injection masses which I have tried, the best by far is Beal's transparent Prussian blue. Its advantages are, that it does not have to be heated, that it is perfectly miscible with the blood ; its fluidity is so great that it permeates the finest capillaries with ease; it is perfectly insoluble, and therefore does not transude from the vessels and stain the surrounding tissues, and it is so transparent that not only the histological structure of the tissues, but even the elements of the vessels themselves can be perfectly demonstrated, provided the subsequent methods have been properly chosen.

The main point to be observed in all injecting, is not to use too much pressure and thereby rupture the vessels. Especial care needs to be observed in this when new formations are being injected, as the newly formed and young vessels are very delicate and easily torn.

It will, I think, be at once admitted that the demonstration of the exact relationship existing between the lymphatics and the new formations is of the first importance ; and I must ask the Society to bear with me, if I go more into detail on this subject than the limits of a paper of this character would seem to require ; but I wish, if possible, to make it plain, just what knowledge we possess of this important subject, and also why I am inclined to consider as not proven, what some authorities assert as a demonstrated fact.

Recognizing, then, that many of the different forms of new formations are in all *probability* supplied more or less abundantly with lymphatics ; and it is by supposing the presence of these vessels that many of the facts in this clinical history of the more malignant types can most readily be explained ; indeed, I admit it would seem as if their recurrence, and the proneness with which the lymphatic glands in the direction of the lymph current are affected, could hardly be explained in any other way ; still there is a great difference between what is probable, no matter how great the probability, and proven fact.

There is, so far as I can learn, only one class of tumors in which it is claimed the lymphatics have been demonstrated, *viz.:* the Carcinomata ; and it is because the authors whom I have been able to consult, do not agree among themselves, that I am in doubt as to whether these vessels have been actually seen. Of these authorities, only three—Green, Woodhead and Beal—mention the subject of lymphatics in connection with the new formations at all. Green and Woohead speak of them as one of the characteristics of carcinomatous growths. Dr. Green says : " In addition to the blood vessels, the cancers also possess *lymphatics.* These accompany the blood vessels, and, as has been shown by M. M. Cornil and Ranvier, communicate with the alveoli." Dr. Woodhead: "Imbedded in the fibrous stroma, and quite separated from the epithelial elements, run *well developed* blood vessels. If, further, it is stated that the alveoli are in direct communication with the lymphatics at the margin of the tumor, the essential features of the carcinoma are enumerated." It will be seen from the foregoing, that these two authors while agreeing as to the presence of lymphatics, are at variance as to their distribution. Beal, on the other hand, speaking of this system of vessels, says : "—— of the arrangement of which in morbid growths nothing is known." Add to this that neither Green nor Woodhead gives any drawing illustrating what they have seen, although they both do of the other histological structure of these tumors, and I think enough has been said to show that so far, at least, as the connection of the lymphatics with the tumor substance proper is concerned, our knowledge is, at best, extremely vague.

By this digression from what might be considered the original scope of the paper, I have endeavored to show that there are still very important facts even in the histology of the new formations for us to learn, and that an examination of one of these formations should never be undertaken without keeping this fact in view, that, we may, if possible, add to the general stock of knowledge on this subject.

As to the best methods to be used in attempting the demonstration of these vessels, I have nothing to offer further than that nitrate of silver staining is the one most commonly used. This is the method Klein used in his work on the lymphatics of the peritoneum and lung. If they could be injected, that would be the best evidence, but the injection of lymphatics, always difficult, would, in the case of new formations, be much more so, even if one could find a vessel large enough to admit a pipette. To thus show them would, however, repay the labor of many failures.

The next object to be attained is to, by some means, be able to distinguish between the living, growing parts of the tissue, and those which are formed or dead. This can be accomplished by staining the bioplasm with an alkaline solution of carmine. As soon as the injection process is completed, wash the tissues with a solution of glycerine and acetic acid; then cut pieces from the tumor about an eighth to one-quarter of an inch thick, taking care to include, if possible, a part of the healthy tissue, immerse them in the carmine fluid and leave them for four to six hours. After again washing them in the glycerine solution, put them away to harden in a solution of glycerine and chromic acid, or glycerine and bi-chromate of potash. I prefer the chromic acid, however, especially for tumors of rapid growth. After hardening, which will take from one to five or six weeks, according to which solution is used, place the pieces in strong Price's glycerine, with five drops of glacial acetic acid to the ounce, in which they will keep till it is convenient to examine them.

In cutting thin sections, the freezing method is much to be preferred to imbedding, as not only is it more rapid, but by it the tissues are kept continuously in *viscid media.* Before freezing, the pieces of tissue must be transferred to a U. S. solution of gum acacia, and left in it for from twelve to twenty-four hours, then freeze and cut sections. The sections as soon as they are cut must be placed in the solution of glycerine and acetic acid, to allow the gum to be displaced by the glycerine.

After the gum is thoroughly soaked out of them, they are ready for the next step, *viz. :* the staining of the formed material. This may be done either with hæmatoxyline, or with one of the analine stains.

If the foregoing methods have been followed, the nerve fibres will be well shown without any special staining. If, however, it is wished, they can be developed still further by the use of chloride of gold in a one to two per cent. solution.

The specimen is now ready for mounting, and this should be done in Price's strong glycerine—sp. gr. 1240—if the best results are desired. Three points only need be mentioned in this connection, *viz.* : be sure that the section is thoroughly impregnated with strong glycerine before mounting ; second, make a shallow cell on the slide with damar or asphalte, in which place the section ; and third, after it is covered, seal up at once with damar, asphalte or zinc white. I prefer damar or asphalte for glycerine mounts, as they are not so liable to run in as the zinc white, and are more easily removed if it is desired at any time to remount the specimen.

It will be noticed that glycerine plays an important part in the foregoing procedures, and I cannot too strongly recommend its use to any one who is working or intends to work in this field. It may be more difficult to keep specimens mounted in glycerine on account of its liability to leak, than if they were in balsam or damar ; but so much more structural detail can be seen, and better seen, that it is much to be preferred. This liability to leak is really the only objection to the use of glycerine, and with care it can be wholly or in large part overcome.

Much has been said and written against glycerine as a mounting medium, but I believe it has been by those who have never taken the time to do what is absolutely necessary to be done, in order to use glycerine successfully, *viz.* : To *thoroughly* impregnate the tissues with the strongest glycerine *before* mounting. The misconception which many good workers in the field of pathology have of this matter, is well shown by the following quotation from a recent work on Practical Pathology:—" Glycerine—is the most useful fluid for the preservation of thin sections, which are to be transferred at once from water to the slide. When pure glycerine alone is used, as for extremely delicate tissues, thin sections of lung or peritoneum, the section is placed on the slide, superfluous moisture drained away or removed with a soft cloth, and then a small drop of the fluid is dropped on the section with a glass rod."

No wonder that glycerine is condemned, if this is the method of using it. The thin sections of lung would—as I know to my cost—be just as likely to be torn to pieces as to be well mounted.

All I can say on this subject is, compare tissues mounted in balsam with those in glycerine, and I think, to any unbiased mind, the result will be in favor of glycerine. I have here a slide or two, mounted in different media, which I think will illustrate the advantage of glycerine as a medium for the preparation of animal tissues, which the members can examine at their convenience.

APPENDIX.

Injecting Fluid (Beal).

℞

Price's glycerine (1240)................ ....fl. ℨ ij.
Tr. Ferri perchlor.................................gtt. x.
Pot. ferrocyan....................................grs. iij.
Hydrochlor. Ac. fort........... ... .gtt. iij.
Aqua Dist...................... ....fl. ℨ j.

Mix the tincture of iron with one ounce of the glycerine, and the ferrocyanide, first dissolved in a little water, with the other ounce. Add the *iron solution* to that of the ferrocyanide *very slowly*, shaking *well* during the admixture. Lastly, add the water and hydrochloric acid.

Carmine for Staining Bioplasm (Beal).

℞

Carmine (*best*)................... ....grs. x.
Liquor Ammonia, fort....................... ....fl. ℨ ss.
Glycerine (*Price's*, 1240)................... ...fl. ℨ ij.
Aqua Dist............................... ... ..fl. ℨ ij.
Alcohol..fl. ℨ ss.

Dissolve the carmine in a test tube with the ammonia, by aid of heat and agitation. Boil the solution for a few seconds, and set aside to cool. After an hour, when much of the excess of ammonia will have passed off, then add the glycerine and water, and filter; then add the alcohol, and keep in well stoppered bottle. Should any of the carmine be deposited after a time from the escape of the ammonia, add one or two drops of liquor ammonia to four ounces of the solution.

Glycerine Solution for Washing.

℞

Price's Glycerine (1240)............... ....fl. ℨ ij.
Aqua Dist.................... ... .fl. ℨ j.
Acetic Acid, Glacial...............................gtt. xv.
Mix.

Hæmatoxyline Stain.

℞

    Alum.
    Price's Glycerine (1240).
    Aqua Dist.
Dissolve and mix.

Hæmatoxyline Crystals (Grüblers).

℞

    Abs. Alcohol.

Dissolve hæmatox. in test tube with abs. alcohol, and add slowly to solution of alum, stirring all the while with glass rod. Keep in glass stoppered bottle coated with asphalte, to keep off light. Dilute about one-half with water and glycerine before using.

Eosine Stain for Formed Material.

Make in watch glass a solution of equal parts strong glycerine and distilled water, and add thereto as much eosine in crystals as can be taken upon point of teasing needle.

Chromic Acid Solution.

Make a strong solution of chromic acid in water. Of this add to strong glycerine a sufficient quantity to make it of a pale straw color.

Bichromate of Potash Solution.

Make a saturated solution of the salt in distilled water, and add of this solution, twenty drops to the ounce, to strong glycerine.

Nitrate of Silver Staining (Woodhead).

Take a very thin section of the tissue, to be stained as soon as it is removed from the body, and wash well in distilled water to remove all chlorides. Expose to the action of a large quantity of a one-half per cent. solution of nitrate of silver for from five to ten minutes (until it becomes somewhat whitened) ; wash in water (not distilled), and expose to diffuse daylight until a delicate, brown tint makes its appearance. Care must be taken to protect the specimen from the direct action of the sun's rays, or the tissues become quite opaque. If specimens are not to be mounted at once, preserve in glycerine, two parts, and water one part, with five or ten drops of acetic acid to ounce of mixture.

Gold Chloride (Woodhead).

Soak the tissue as soon as removed from the body, in a one-half per cent. solution of chloride of gold, until it is of a lemon color ; then expose in one per cent. acetic acid solution to strong light, until it assumes a purplish tinge.

ORIGINAL ARTICLES IN SURGERY.

THE SARCOMATA.*

By FRED S. FULTON, A.M., M.D.,

New York.

WITH the advance of civilization and the constraints imposed upon humanity by an ever-increasing formality and binding custom, the ravages of malignant diseases have been steadily augmented.

They fasten themselves with a sort of pitiless irony upon those whom an abundant fortune most carefully guards, leaving those whom poverty and exposure have hardened to quit this life through the portal of a less hideous and loathsome calamity. The aged and decrepit do not furnish the large quota of its victims, but adolescence, maturity, and apparent health are laid under the heaviest tribute to satisfy its demands. The number who are yearly dying of malignant disease is greatly outrunning the increase in the population, as is shown by the statements of Mr. Dunn, taken from the report of the Registrar-General of England, which fact shows both the practical ignorance of the profession at large, and also of the specialists, regarding malignant developments, and also the need of greater efforts being made to augment our knowledge and to induce the profession generally to adopt what, at present, appears to be the course most promising of success.

Malignant neoplasms are divided into the sarcomata and carcinomata, the division being based upon both their origin and histological structure, which are essentially different. The best substantiated theory of the former is, that the sarcomata arise from fixed connective tissue cells, and have a distinct reversion to embryonic structure. Regarding their microscopic structure in general, the cells are the diagnostic features; with carcinoma it is different; the general topography of the growth, the *arrangement* of somewhat similar cellular elements, the quantitative predominance of one tissue over another, are the salient features in the diagnosis. In the sarcomata there is usually a great mixture of types, and also, very many times, a large amount of tissue, which is not embryonic, *[e. g.*, fibrous connective tissue, cartilage, bone, and sometimes muscular tissue. While these elements influence somewhat the malignancy, according to their greater or lesser quantity, they do not, in any manner, affect the par-

---

* Read before the Homœopathic Medical Society of the County of New York, November 11th, 1886.

ticular kind of sarcomata which it may chance to be, nor do they have any bearing upon the ultimate effect of the malignant growth. It is, to a certain extent, an adventitious product which, though present and characterizing the growth, does not hinder the legitimate action of the sarcomatous elements. The cellular elements, or, as Heitzmann calls them, the "sarcoma corpuscles," are the only features of real importance either as regards the malignancy, the ultimate prognosis, or the nomenclature of the growth. The terms fibro-sarcoma, osteo-sarcoma, chondro-sarcoma, etc., are wrong both in the real characterization of the neoplasm and in the ambiguity which it occasions in the practitioner's mind. For instance, some sarcomata, as those of the testicles, have a strong tendency to develop cartilage, which, in time, not infrequently ossifies in part. It might be called either a chondro-sarcoma or osteo-sarcoma. The usual idea, when a diagnosis is rendered, or a description given of a chondro- or osteo-sarcoma is, that such originate respectively from cartilage or bone in some part of the organism. In this case it would be radically false. And in this case this misleading nomenclature would both disguise the essential nature of the tumor, which is dependent upon its cellular constitution, and also mislead as to its origin and organizing or disorganizing tendency. To say that the term osteo-sarcoma or chondro-sarcoma is an appellation meant simply to classify the tumor according to its *tendency* to develop these various normal tissues, is to claim before the uniniatiated and ignorant what is utterly impossible, and what the microscopist knows is impossible to perform. These fine distinctions on tendencies are as reliable as the "baseless fabric of a vision," and would vary, not according to the pathological appearance under the microscope, but according to the vagaries which haunted the mind of the examiner.

In addition, the term osteo-sarcoma, etc., by one authority, is used to designate a sarcoma which originates and develops in bone; by another authority it designates a sarcoma wherever found or of whatever variety, in which osseous matter is deposited; while by another a tumor is classified as an osteo-sarcoma, in which, by some occult and psychic method, in which the use of material lenses are unnecessary, the *tendency* to such development is discovered. It forms a hopeless jangle of terms, for which the only excuse is the ignorance of early classification. What is wanted is to know whether the cells which characterize the neoplasm are round, spindle, net, giant, arranged in alveoli, or deeply pigmented ; for it is upon these features that the prognosis, malignancy, and characterization of the tumor essentially depend.

If, unfortunately, the tumor be a large, round-celled sarcoma, such as I will show you in a moment, the prognosis is bad ; if it be a small, round-celled sarcoma, it is the worst possible ; the spindle variety is less dangerous, and returns after a greater length of time ; while the giant-celled sarcoma is the least malignant of all, and offers, if thoroughly extirpated, a fair prospect of future immunity.   Moreover, if a surgeon removes a growth, which he feels confident is sarcomatous, from the bone or cartilage of the knee joint, what information is it if the microscopist returns a diagnosis either of chondro- or osteosarcoma ?   That is not what he desires to know, but rather to what particular species, with its respective malignancy or innocence, the neoplasm rightly belongs.   He was already confident that it was a sarcoma, and desires further knowledge as well as confirmation.   The peculiar site of a tumor also tends greatly to modify its structure. That is, if the tumor develops as a sub-periosteal or central bone sarcoma, while the cellular elements may be either round, spindle, giant, net, mixed, etc., there will be a greater or less amount of cartilage or bone in the growth.   If the neoplasm develops in the muscles or fibrous tissue, these normal structures will be more or less abundant.   These do not affect the prognosis or course of the growth, and should be slightly considered, except as manifesting a tendency towards organization or disorganization. · If a round-celled sarcoma present a chondrifying tendency, shown by the actual presence of cartilage, it is sufficient to classify it as such.   I have a specimen from which might be taken splendid examples of both fibro- and chondro-sarcoma.   It is a round-celled neoplasm, with a strong tendency towards disorganization, and should be classified as such. It is upon these grounds that I believe that the nomenclature, as adopted by many text-books and pathologists, is essentially wrong. We should exclude all such hybrid terms as fibro-sarcoma, chondro-sarcoma and osteo-sarcoma, as ambiguous and misleading.

`   The original classification of Virchow into

> Round-celled,
> Spindle-celled,
> Net-celled,
> Giant-celled,
> Melanotic sarcoma,

to which might be added the alveolar sarcoma of Bilroth, is a much truer and more scientific classification, beyond which it is both useless and misleading to go.

    The site occupied by the sarcomata is the same as that of carcinomata, with the exception that sarcomata affect primarily the bones and muscles, which is exceedingly rare, if it ever occurs, in carcinoma. Being developed from connective tissue corpuscles, their most common sites are the skin, subcutaneous tissue, bones, lymphatic glands, eye, upper jaw, testicle, breast, brain, kidney, and liver.

In one respect they differ markedly from cancers, appearing sometimes as congenital diseases, or developing in infancy or childhood. Macroscopically they have but little to differentiate them from cancers. Some rapidly growing sarcomata indeed present all the appearances of encephaloid disease. They may simulate every kind of benign or malignant growth. Their development, however, is generally slower, attended with but few evidences of inflammation; their form is usually oval; they are of unequal consistency, and rarely ulcerate; the cachexia is usually developed later than in cancer, and the lymphatic glands are not so frequently affected, owing entirely to the locality of the tumor. If, however, the site be favorable, as in sarcoma of certain portions of the thigh, the glands are affected with equal certainty and quite as early.

Regarding their microscopical appearances, I have prepared as illustrations the various kinds, drawings from slides, which I have prepared from tumors removed at the Hahnemann Hospital. They are quite accurate, being transfers from the slides by means of a reflecting mirror somewhat upon the principle of a camera lucida, which I attached to the microscope. I shall not pretend to show illustrations of all the varieties and hybrid varieties of sarcomata; only some of those which I have taken from my own specimens, as more interesting.*

The round-celled sarcoma has several sub-divisions :

I. The large round-celled sarcoma.

II. The small round-celled sarcoma.

III. Lympho-sarcoma, which is properly a sub-division of the latter; and

IV. The endothelial sarcoma, which is placed in this division, because its structure, and not similarity of origin, places it here. It is a species not recognized by Virchow, Heitzmann, Prudden and Delafield, or by most authorities. Agnew classifies it among the sarcomata, and we believe rightly.

These round-celled sarcomata approach most nearly to embryonic or granulation tissue, and are, consequently, the most malignant of this group of neoplasms. It appears true that the further the histological structure recedes from healthy adult tissue into the domain of the purely embryonic, the more deadly are its properties. The small,

---

* The paper was illustrated by large drawings of the different varieties of sarcoma.

round-celled sarcoma, which is of the most primitive type, is essentially the most malignant.

The great characteristic of this form of large round-celled sarcoma is the large cell, with its large and coarsely granular nucleus. These very closely resemble cartilage corpuscles, only in the latter the finely granular protoplasm which forms the body of the large round-celled corpuscle is absent, and you have merely a large cartilaginous ring, containing a coarsely granular nucleus, held in a structureless basement substance. The tumor, from which this specimen was taken, was removed from the knee joint by Dr. Wilcox; and exhibited in certain parts the degenerating cartilage, with its characteristic corpuscles. In this, as in most sarcoma, there is some connective tissue holding the cells together ; there is no definite arrangement of either these fibres or their contained cells. In some round-celled sarcomata, particularly the small round-celled, the fibrous material is very scanty; at times requiring a careful search to distinguish it. In such a case the cells simply lie in a structureless basement substance. In typical cases this would be the structure. The cells and their contained nucleus may vary greatly in size, as may also the relative size of the cells and their nuclei.

Many cells contain two or more nuclei, illustrating, no doubt, one method of the growth of the tumor by a constant segmentation and development of sarcoma corpuscles, as well as by the undoubted invasion and transmutation of healthy tissue into morbid structure.

The favorite site of these tumors is in the bone, skin, subcutaneous tissue, glands, and lymph nodes. There are no macroscopic appearances which serve to distinguish this form from others. In general, it has greater rapidity of growth, is more friable, often multiple, and invades the system correspondingly quickly. The above characteristics are true of all the group of round-celled sarcomata, and it is only by a microscopic examination that it is possible to determine its exact variety. The small, round-celled sarcoma and lympho-sarcoma are essentially the same variety, differing merely in the fact that the lympho-sarcoma, having invaded the tissues of some glandular body or lymph node, exhibits the characteristic epithelial structure of the ducts, as is seen in the central portion of the plate. There is but very little connective tissue in this variety. It is rather myxomatous tissue, having the characteristic enlargements at the junction of the diverging fibrillæ. In places slight and irregular bunches of connective tissue can be seen, with blood-vessels with which, in some localities, it is abundantly supplied. The large figure in the centre is a transverse section of a duct of a lymph node, lined with columnar epithelia and filled with lymph and blood corpuscles. The great mass of the tumor, and in cases of simple, small-celled sarcoma, the entire bulk, is composed of these small, round, multi-nuclear corpuscles, lying in a structureless basement substance, or held by small, fibrous fibrillæ, or, as in this case, myxomatous tissue. It is one of the most malignant neoplasms, and removal offers but small chance of long immunity from the disease. What was true of the large, round-celled sarcoma, regarding their site and clinical features, is also true of this. This specimen was taken from a tumor removed by Dr. Wilcox from the lower jaw of a colored man, whom many of you saw. As is the case with most of these, the removal has been too recent to warrant a prognosis or statement regarding their return, aside from that which the known characteristic of the morbid growth would warrant.

The growth from which the specimen of an endothelial sarcoma was obtained was a tumor of the jaw, removed by Dr. Helmuth, and was in a condition of ulceration at the time of its extirpation. It had already greatly invaded the system, and was in the latter stages of degeneration. This tumor develops, as is shown by different sections of the same growth, within the lymph spaces, crowding the fibrous tissue of the lymph walls and surrounding connective tissue aside to make room for the increasing and developing sarcoma corpuscles. It is not until the last stages of sarcomatous degeneration that the fibrous tissue is entirely supplanted by the malignant cellular elements. The characteristic structure, as you can see, consists of large, heavy cells, with large, coarsely granular nuclei, closely resembling the large, round-celled sarcoma corpuscles enclosed in a very scanty and degenerating fibrous net-work, forming large, partly broken down alveoli. In the lower portion of this large alveolus is a row of spindle cells, no doubt being an intermediate stage of degeneration of the fibrous connective tissue into sarcoma elements. There is a large amount of basement substance. The blood-vessels are in the bundles of connective tissue. If this sarcoma had been extirpated early, before it had so extensively invaded the tissue, while it was in its first stage, having a large predominance of normal structure, its return would have been much slower and the chances for lengthened life greatly improved. The large amount of sarcomatous tissue in the tumor exhibits its malignancy. It returned to its original site before the wound healed, and when last heard from, the patient was gradually sinking from exhaustion.

Of the spindle-celled sarcomata there are two recognized varieties. Properly, the net-celled sarcoma, as Professor Heitzmann has shown, by the form of its cells, should be classified as a sub-division of the spindle-celled sarcomata. The large and small-celled differ from each other merely in the size of their cells. In the large-celled variety the fibres are usually more abundant, and the corpuscles are less closely packed. Both have large, oval nuclei. In this specimen, which is from a tumor removed from the cervix by Dr. Helmuth, as is usual with this variety, the cells lie in perfect juxtaposition with no intervening fibres; simply a mass of small spindle cells, held together in a structure-less basement substance, without any intervening reticulum. The tumor in gross is very soft and friable, readily cleaving into sections or crumbling under touch. In some places, particularly in transitional stages, the corpuscles have no definite arrangement. In this illustration, which is taken from a tumor in a highly active and transitional state, you will see cartilage corpuscles in various parts undergoing degeneration ; and also that, except in two places, the symmetrical arrangement is greatly disturbed.

These varieties possess a great disposition to become organized into connective tissue, never, however, so as to destroy their malignancy. These tumors are often encapsulated and do not infiltrate the tissues. The infiltration of the surrounding tissues by sarcomata differs much from that of carcinomata. In the latter, the infiltrated tissue is hardened and changed both as to touch and sight, while in sarcomata the tissues may be extensively contaminated without manifesting any marked change of appearance or feeling. The favorite sites of the spindle-celled variety are in the bones, subcutaneous tissue, skin, periosteum, aponeurosis, fascia, testes, and breast.

It might be said of this, as of all sarcomata which affect the breast, that they do not involve the lymphatic glands of the axilla, which is in marked contrast to cancers of the same locality, and serves, when unfortunately present in the latter case, to diagnose between them. The spindle-celled sarcomata were classified by Paget as recurrent fibroids.

This illustration of the net-celled sarcoma is not from my own collection, but from a drawing which I made from one of Professor Heitzmann's specimens while studying with him. As you will see, it is in reality a spindle-celled sarcoma, the only difference being that the cells have long prolongations which reach to and unite with similar elongations of other cells, forming a large net-work, in the meshes of which lie granular protoplasmic bodies in a bed of finely granular basement substance. These cells, as others, have long, oval, granular nuclei. In its general structure and characteristics it resembles a myxo-sarcoma, or, more properly, a sarcoma, usually spindle-celled, containing an abundance of myxomatous tissue ; consequently it is

less malignant. Usually the spindle corpuscles from which the prolongations issue, are very large, greater in size even than the cells in
the large spindle-celled sarcoma.

Of the melanotic and alveolar varieties, time will not allow me to
speak. They are rare varieties, and not frequently met.

Excluding the hybrid or mixed varieties of sarcomata, such as
fibro-sarcoma, chondro-sarcoma, etc., as we shall do, the giant-celled
is the only one left. It consists merely in large multi-nuclear bodies,
much larger than those in any other growth, containing a mass of very
finely granular protoplasm, in which the nuclei can, with care, be
detected. These cells seem to be grafted upon the main body of the
tumor, and lie in a coarse net-work of fibrous tissue, or spindle cells.
The tumor exhibits a great tendency to organization, the large giant
cells being, according to Heitzmann, simply a fusion of the medullary elements under a strong tendency to form territories of cartilage
or bone. The malignancy of these tumors is the least of all the sar-
comàta, as would be expected from their microscopical elements.
Their favorite site is upon the periosteum, particularly of the jaw.
When in this locality, they are more familiarly known as "epulis."
Clinically, it is often impossible to distinguish the cancers from sarcomata. In general, it can be said that the latter do not tend to suppuration or ulceration, their form is often oval, they are often multiple,
not infrequently encapsulated, primarily affect the bones and muscles,
which primary cancers do not, and are not confined to maturity and
old age, but may attack infancy and adolescence, appearing at times
even as congenital defects.

The microscopist who expects to find decisive boundary lines
between the sarcomata will meet with disappointment. The types
merge and mingle. A round-celled sarcoma will have in places a
great abundance of spindle cells, and *vice versa ;* while fibrous connective tissue, cartilage and bone may help to form the same tumor.
Its classification must depend upon the predominant character of its
cellular constituents.

In all these cases the only chance of cure or lengthened days
depends upon early extirpation.

It is not safe to leave a tumor, regarding which there is the
slightest question of doubt, and even a benign tumor offers many
grounds for suspicion ; for microscopic, as well as clinical evidences,
show not only that an inherently sarcomatous growth degenerates
from a comparatively benign to a most malignant type, but also that
benign growths not infrequently, under favorable conditions, are
metamorphosed into either a sarcoma or carcinoma. Any benign

tumor which, by its position, is subject to irritation and disturbance, should raise in the physician's mind earnest considerations regarding its removal. We are aware that that is going further than is usual, but we believe that even present knowledge which the microscope and clinic have furnished us, had we time to detail them, will more than bear out the conclusion.

NEW METHOD FOR EXCISION OF KNEE JOINT.—Mr. Herbert Allingham proposes the following method, which he has repeatedly demonstrated on the cadaver, and twice on living subjects. He claims that the method is especially suited to those cases in which the synovial cartilage is chiefly involved, and that a movable joint will usually result. The method he describes as follows: (See *British Medical Journal*, January 15th, 1887, for full description and accounts of two cases.)

A vertical incision is made over the joint, extending from two or three inches above the patella to the tubercle of the tibia. Above the patella the knife splits the quadriceps tendon and passes into the synovial pouch. The soft tissues are divided down to the patella, the bone is sawn through, and the ligamentum patellæ is split down to the tubercle of the tibia. The halves of the split patella and ligaments are moved well to opposite sides of the joint, the head of the tibia and condyles of the femur being thereby exposed. The crucial ligaments, if not already destroyed, are divided, and, the leg being flexed, the condyles of the femur are pushed forward on the tibia and the necessary amount of bone removed. After completely flexing the leg on the thigh, the internal lateral ligament is carefully separated from the internal semilunar cartilage, the tibia is pushed forward on to the condyles of the femur, and, in order to avoid dividing the lateral ligaments, a thin slice is removed from the tibial articular surface with a strong knife or chisel. The synovial membrane had best be cleared from the joint as far as possible, and at this point in the operation drainage openings should be made at the postero-lateral aspects of the joint, on the outer side, between the ilio-tibial band and the tendon of the biceps, and on the inner side just above the inner hamstring tendons. If only a little of the cartilage of the patella is eroded, it is cut away with a knife. If, however, the bone is extensively diseased, it should be shelled out of the entire quadriceps tendon, without destroying the connection of the quadriceps muscle with the ligamentum patellæ. If the patella is to remain, the halves are sutured together by a strong catgut suture. If the bone has been removed, the halves of the extension of the quadriceps are brought together with catgut. Finally, the split ligamentum patellæ and quadriceps tendon are adjusted and stitched with fine catgut; the skin united with separate sutures, and the limb dressed antiseptically.

VESICAL PARALYSIS IN LEAD COLIC.—According to Jacob, the retention of urine sometimes observed in cases of saturnine intoxication, is due not to spasm of the neck of the bladder, but to a true paralysis.—*Deutsche Med. Woch.*, No. 32, 1886.

EDITORIAL DEPARTMENT.

EDITORS.

GEORGE M. DILLOW, M.D., ... Editor-in-Chief, Editorial and Book Reviews.
CLARENCE E. BEEBE, M.D., ... Original Papers in Medicine.
SIDNEY F. WILCOX, M.D., ... Original Papers in Surgery.
MALCOLM LEAL, M.D., ... Progress of Medicine.
EUGENE H. PORTER, M.D., ... Comments and News.
HENRY M. DEARBORN, M.D., ... Correspondence.
FRED S. FULTON, M.D., ... Reports of Societies and Hospitals.

GEORGE G. SHELTON, M.D., ... Business Manager.

The Editors individually assume full responsibility for and are to be credited with all connected with the collection and presentation of matter in their respective departments, but are not responsible for the opinions of contributors.

It is understood that manuscripts sent for consideration have not been previously published, and that after notice of acceptance has been given, will not appear elsewhere except in abstract and with credit to THE NORTH AMERICAN. All rejected manuscripts will be returned to writers. No anonymous or discourteous communications will be printed.

Contributors are respectfully requested to send manuscripts and communicate respecting them directly with the Editors, according to subject, as follows: *Concerning Medicine, 21 West 37th Street; concerning Surgery, 256 West 57th Street; concerning Societies and Hospitals, 121 East 70th Street; concerning News, Personals and Original Miscellany, 461 West 71st Street; concerning Correspondence, 152 West 57th Street.*

Communications to the Editor-in-Chief, *Exchanges* and *New Books* for notice should be addressed to *102 West 43d Street.*

HONEST SPECIALISM *VERSUS* TRADE.

" SINCE we have, therefore, but one principle to deal with in the living organism, and but one disturbance of that principle to prescribe for under the cognomen, disease, why should we have schools of medicine to teach specialisms in therapeutics? They should be taught, of course, in the colleges in the regular curriculum, but when they are not, the student should supplant the deficiency by forming classes for their special study, not, however, for the purpose of making separate, special or indiscriminate use of them, which can only result in error, but for the more perfect equipment of his armamentarium. Does not every method of treating disease (so called) belong to the science and art of medicine, each method, as well as each agent, having its particular adaptation in the treatment of particular cases of malady? How irrational it is, then, to establish schools for teaching specialisms in therapeutics, and for the avowed purpose of putting asunder that which in the nature of things are joined together and are one and inseparable? Is it not also a travesty on science as well as a scandal in the profession?

"So far as the propriety of perpetuating homœopathic schools of medicine and maintaining the titular distinction, homœopathic, by their graduates, are concerned, we are familiar with the reasons brought forward by their advocates in support of it. 'The system is not complete; their work not yet done,' say they. New drugs have to be proved and old drugs reproved, the materia medica revised and corrected, fallacies expunged, the truth placed in clearer light, etc.

We concede all this, and admit that no public work more important than the above can engage the attention of physicians. It is indispensable to the efficient application of the law of Hahnemann in any case of disease to which it is adapted. But it does not follow from this that it is necessary to establish a distinct and separate school of medicine, and make test of fellowship allegiance to the doctrine of *similia similibus curantur,* or *contraria contrariis curantur,* neither of which is of universal application, but each being true and applicable in its own sphere and special exigency. * *

We insist that homœopathy is *not* always 'a practical method of treating the sick.' While it is perfectly obvious to us that 'the great truths which it embodies are worth developing and improving to their furthest extent,' it will be admitted by every candid observer that they are not thus developed and improved at the present time, and that therefore they are not susceptible of certainty of application. Indeed, so great is the uncertainty of their application that in certain critical emergencies it would be highly culpable of a practitioner to trust the fate of his patient to them. But even were the truths of homœopathy fully developed and apprehended by the practitioner, we should still have to demur, * * on grounds the validity of which the vast majority of homœopathic practitioners must admit, since it were idle to dispute them, namely: *Its method is not a universal one;* that is to say, it is not adapted to all cases of sickness, but like other methods of therapeia has its special adaptation to particular cases and exigencies. It is, therefore, but a part—an important part—of medical science and art. And he who would not have the sphere of his professional activity narrowed to a single conception in therapeutics, and would square his professions by his practice, is in duty bound, therefore, to adjure the title, homœopathic, and adopt that of physician."

From its peculiar sophistry, our readers will have divined that the preceding extract is taken from *The New York Medical Times* (leading editorial, "Unity *versus* Specialism in Therapeutics," February, 1887). We quote as much as fairly represents the views of the editorial, the more inconsequential portions being omitted. In more succinct, logical form, the argument in our quotations (if argument it should be styled), runs about as follows : *First,* that because we have but one principle to deal with in the living organism, and but one disturbance of that principle to prescribe for under the cognomen, disease, therefore colleges for the purpose of teaching homœopathic therapeutics, which are now taught in no other colleges, are a travesty on science as well as a scandal in the profession. *Second*, that because there is no public work more important than proving new drugs, revising and correcting the homœopathic materia medica, expunging fallacies, placing homœopathic truth in clearer light, therefore the societies and institutions now organized for that special important public work should be denominalized, disorganized, and submerged in the regular organization of ignoring and suppressive empiricism, miscalled the science and art of medicine. *Third*, that because at the present time homœopathy is not developing and improving its great truths to their furthest extent, therefore homœopaths, some of whom are capable and some incapable of employing homœopathic methods in critical emergencies, (the emergencies being usually those of the pre-scribers ignorance and pocket-book), should commit those truths to oblivion by joining the ranks of those who catch at the fashions of palliative empiricism in lieu of an honest effort to master homœopathic resources to their furthest extent. *Fourth*, that because the homœopathic method is not universal outside of its own sphere, it is not universal within its own sphere, which is evidently not the sphere of knowledge of the editors of *The Times*, or one to which they have ever rendered any definite contribution, except by way of the scissors and the paste-pot. *Fifth*, that because homœopathy is an important part of medical science and art, it is, therefore, a therapeutic method of such narrow efficacy that, like the sentimental fly, it should buzz forthwith into the very mandibles of the beguiling spider. *Sixth*, that because the homœopathic practitioner exalts his conception of the rule of similars to the always paramount place, and, generally speaking, exclusive place, in his prescription of drugs, for the cure of disease, he should, therefore, square such conviction with the forswearing of the homœopathic name which designates him to the community among physicians as broadly and essentially different in his curative methods. Summed up in its shortest terms, the covert attitude under the sophistical sentiment of *The Times*, is this: Homœopaths and Homœopathy should commit suicide in disregard of principle, of righteous policy, and of honor before men, because it serves the selfish purposes of the editors of that journal to

fish for what will bite and what they can snare in both schools of
medicine. And the bait is sham science, and the snare not that of
pure philanthropy.

The above propositions not demanding amplification, it will be
seen that our logic leads to different conclusions from those of *The
Times*, and therefore is the "most peculiar of any ever observed outside
of Andover, or a lunatic asylum." We will confess that we were
not educated at Andover, and, so far, have managed to live outside of
a lunatic asylum. Yet, we even commend Andover for education in
the methods of logic and in the conduct of life, where a course might
be suggested as of probable benefit to the gentlemen so opposed to
"specialism." If they feel beyond the age when they can profit by
such instruction, we would direct them to the Middletown Insane
Asylum, of which the senior editor is a trustee, for a lesson of restraint
in critical emergencies. Without a dose of morphia, or other anodyne,
or hypnotic, or empirical makeshift of any kind, by the merciful
humanity which Hahnemann first adopted in the management of the
insane, by sound hygiene and proper food, by abstaining from that
harmful drugging which, under the name of science, palliates until it
cannot cure, and by unvarying adherence to the homœopathic method
of prescribing with the resources now known to our materia medica,
each year has shown a greater percentage of recoveries and a lessened percentage of deaths, as knowledge in using remedies homœopathically has grown with honest and longer study. In 1886 its percentage of recoveries swelled to 50.99 per cent., and its death rate
dwindled to 2.99 per cent., a record hitherto unknown in the history
of medicine, and impossible, if homœopathy were not now a distinctive and scientific school of medicine. Perhaps, after due treatment in such a homœopathic institution, one of its trustees would be
saner than to permit this utterance to go out under his responsibility:
"It is with profound regret, therefore, that we observe in certain
quarters the most strenuous efforts put forth to have it ('specialism' in
therapeutics) perpetuated and made eternal."

In conclusion, we would crave our readers indulgence for so much
attention to an unworthy topic. While it may seem too small in
interest, yet the principles involved in the dual position of profiting by

homœopathy and publicly betraying it extend wherever homœopathy exists. *The Times* and its editors, in themselves, may be of little significance ; but so long as that journal can speak of homœopathy as the school with which it is identified, and its editors can hold representative positions, which give them an implied authority of representative homœopathic voice, their endeavor to destroy the school whose trusts they have sought, and to which they have the shameless hardihood to cling, demands, we believe, the full candor of expressed opinion, which the interests of homœopathy demand. Moreover, the time has come when homœopathy should squarely deal with its empirical and commercial element, which, having lost moral grip upon the higher purpose through which homœopathy was founded and brought to great achievement, would trade away their sacred inheritance from the dead and the enlarged inheritance that they, in turn, owe to posterity for the expediency of an immediate mess of pottage. If persons need to be attacked, it is because that principles in this world take the concrete forms of men. The President and Secretary of the staff of the only great charity hospital in the world, which has been placed by municipal trust under homœopathic control, holders also of other trusts in homœopathy, cannot advocate such views as are presented in our opening quotations, without constituting a travesty on homœopathic honesty as well as a scandal in the profession.

A NAPPING SOCIETY.

THE recent meeting of our State Society gives evidence that our school is not in decadence. The number in attendance was smaller than usual, the number of interesting and valuable original papers fewer, the discussions tame, the politics more decided ; in fact, the whole proceedings showed a lack of interest that apparently argues very strongly in favor of the ancient remark, " homœopathy is dying out." But the argument is in reality in the opposite direction. In a nameless town there was a nameless deacon, who was noted as a regular sleeper in church, when his good pastor was in the pulpit; but if it ever chanced that his good pastor made an exchange, the nameless deacon was sure to be in 'his place, wide awake through the entire service. These things came to the ears of the preacher, and, feeling aggrieved, he unloaded his burdens to his parochial fellow-helper. "Why do you pay more attention to the stranger than to your own beloved pastor?" The deacon explained to this effect: "Now, Dominie, ye mustn't feel hurt! Ye see that when ye are to hum, I know we shall hear no unsartin sound from the pulpit, but when ye change with a stranger, I have to keep a look out for the doctrine."

Thus, for a number of years there has been a sleeping in our State Society. Easy success has served to lessen need for watchfulness in opposing hostile legislation. Our members are absorbed with work in private practice and local charities, and leave the central organization to run itself. And if one cares to look into the matter, he will find that those counties which have the largest, most active and interesting local societies, take least interest in the State organization, while the scattered members are usually in attendance and value the opportunity for fraternal intercourse. The excuses given for neglect of the central Society are uniformly the same : business, distance, local interests. Our legal status, our past success, our present prestige and future prospects are all recognized as in the keeping of the State Society, and yet these interests are left in the hands of a few who attend the annual meeting, the semi-annual being devoted to medical papers. If members grumble at rings, they have themselves to blame ; if the representatives of " liberal and rational homœopathy" elect their men, it is simply due to the fact that those who claim to represent a "pure homœopathy" do not care for their claims, or views, or convictions as much as their words would seem to imply. For, unlike the good deacon, whenever the strange preacher goes into the pulpit, they snore through all kinds of "unsartin sounds," and have no look out for the doctrine.

. Yet, these times demand alertness and activity. The homœopath of old could keep to his materia medica and his practice, and rely upon the allopath to spread homœopathy by his more conspicuous hatred and his more comparative ill-success. But the homœopath of to-day needs all the help from his fellows which can be gained by fraternity of purpose and interchange of knowledge. The student of the present time must join cause and cure, diagnosis and therapeutics, pure science and art, and compete with acute dissemblers, sharpened in wits by a livelier struggle for existence with each other and with rising homœopathy. Homœopathy, once despised, like a street urchin, in the gutters of practice, has grown to corpulent manhood, and lives in equal honor in brown stone fronts upon the fashionable thoroughfares. The "regular" of to-day envies his successful rival's possessions, and calculates upon the supposed existence of a fatty heart and degenerated moral fibre to one day make that brown stone front his own. But he miscalculates. Older homœopathy is but over-fed and under-exercised; lolls too much after its luxurious dinners; is lax in church attendance, and snoozes over points of doctrine. But the spur is coming, and the younger generation, under new conditions, will not only hold its own but demonstrate anew the old truth which has stood so well the test of time. While the deacons sleep, the young minds are awake and active, and their convictions are taking stronger hold upon the central core of truth. There is revival astir, as seen in the more active society interest in the larger centres of the State, and if we mistake not, the interest will soon extend to our State Society, which has been dozing on traditional methods between the passing of the old and the coming of the new. That it may be made adequate in efficiency and dignity with the needs of homœopathy in the great Empire State, should be the thoughtful purpose of the younger men who are merely reluctant to take hold lest they disturb the slumbers of the deacons.

COMMENTS.

ANOTHER STUMBLE.—The young person who comments on the news of the week for the *Record*, has again escaped from his apron strings and been eaves-dropping among the gossips. He says: "Homœopathy and Hypodermics. The dean of a homœopathic medical college in this city is reported to have bought another hypodermic syringe recently. This is not what Hahnemann taught; it is not homœopathic." This alleged purchase has evidently caused the youth much distress of mind. Evidently he fears for his neighbors' morals. Like many other zealots he is caring for the dean's morality at the great expense of his own. For on the very next page is found the following choice morsel : "*Pulsatilla* in Acute Orchitis. Dr. Gerard Smith writes in the following enthusiastic strain about *pulsatilla* : 'Having witnessed the striking curative action of *pulsatilla* in acute orchitis and epididymitis, I should like to persuade others to follow Dr. Brunton's advice, and give this drug in inflammatory states of the testicle, epididymus and spermatic cord. To have it in our power to subdue promptly the intense suffering of such cases is a great blessing, and the relief is so rapid that it is even unnecessary to employ morphine to subdue the pain, while the swelling and heat subside more rapidly than under any other drug.'" Clearly the fence around this young man's moral garden (if it ever had one) is in sore need of repair. As it is, most of his morality seems to have escaped. The dean may or may not have "purchased" a hypodermic. If he has one he came by it honestly. But the use of *pulsatilla* as described in the extract above was stolen bodily from homœopathic works and usages. The drug in question was introduced in medicine by the celebrated Baron Störck. He found it of service in affections of the eyes and secondary syphilis, but made no use of it in affections of the genital organs. Until within a year or two the drug had fallen into disuse by the allopaths, but was a prime remedy with the new school. *Pulsatilla* was proved by Hahnemann himself and its peculiar properties discovered. Two practitioners of the old school in England were honest enough to admit that they were indebted to homœopathic treatises for its use, but Brunton and others of his ilk prefer to steal. The *Record* will doubtless find it expedient to tie up its young man again.

INDECENCY IN MEDICAL LITERATURE.—Under the above caption, in the February number of the *New England Medical Gazette*, may be found an editorial so timely in appearance and so incisive in utterance as to entitle it to more than a passing notice. It is high time that indecent jokes and vulgar allusions be branded as they deserve, and the proprietors or editors of the journals in which they appear should be made clearly and definitely to understand that a clean and decent page is demanded by the profession. We cannot do better than quote the *Gazette :* "A religious journal which could give space to coarse jokes, conundrums and *double-entendres* at the expense of the names, beliefs, and observances which the church hold sacred, and yet could pass unrebuked of the clergy and be read and supported by them, would in the very fact of its continued existence be a serious reflection on the fitness of the clergy for their high office. The same should, to our mind, be true of any medical journal publishing indecent jokes whose point lies in allusion to those physiological functions of the human body, or those intimate relations of human life before which wise delicacy draws the veil that science or morality is at any time free to lift, but which should be held sacred from the prurient fingers of a bastard humor. * * * * *
The reading of them tends to foster in the minds of physicians, and especially of younger physicians, the idea which more than any other will be fatal to their growth in personal character and public usefulness—the idea that the ethical side of professional life is no very serious matter ; that the deep respect of a physician for the more in-

timate life of his patient has its place among appropriate phrases for commencement valedictories and for the preface to a work on gynæcology ; but that it is quite permissible for the physician, the doors once shut like the priests of old, to "wink behind the mask" if not to wholly cast the mask aside. Such paragraphs, sooner or later finding their way to the laity, serve as apt illustration for the theory which, to the crying shame of the masculine side of our profession, is so freely advanced to-day in private conversation, in essay and in fiction, that the diseases of women can and should be treated by women only, since among men the delicacy and dignity of mind, which should be brought to their treatment, are wholly lacking."

BOOK REVIEWS.

KEY-NOTES TO THE MATERIA MEDICA, by Henry N. Guernsey, M.D. Edited by Joseph C. Guernsey, A.M., M.D. Philadelphia: F. E. Boericke, 1887.

This little book of 267 pages, of which 178 pages are devoted to the characteristics of the more important drugs in use, offers no excuse for empiricism to those who constantly cry out against the bulk and confusion of our symptomatology. No man ever was more fitted to compile a work of this sort than the late Dr. Guernsey ; keen and critical in observing symptoms, enthusiastic in reporting the successful use of the remedy, he was ever on the alert to catch the genius of the drug and to find its similitude in the patient.

To our mind, this work serves a better purpose as a companion to the study of a complete symptomatology than as a work to prescribe by. It is just the book its name suggests, "Key-notes !"

We only wish that the symptoms were all reliable guides ; most of them are guides, but few are absolutely trustworthy. The addition of *selections from* Bœnninghausen's repertory is of the greatest value, as far as it goes ; we only regret that it is so fragmentary. Will not Dr. Guernsey give us a complete Bœnninghausen, with the additions made by Dunham and his father, the late Professor Guernsey? A few vulnerable points deserve notice and correction in future editions. *First*, as the book aims to give us key-notes, it should not attempt physiological theories of the action of a drug. *Second*, if it attempts to explain such action, it should do so correctly and fully. To give one example, under *Amylenum nitrosum* (should it not be *Amyl.,* which may be an undeclinable, neuter Latin noun?) we find "the heart and circulation soonest feel the influence of this remedy, thence the action passes through the nervous system." Under *Hyoscyamus*, "The general sphere of action of this remedy is found in spasmodic affections." The book is full of indefinite and incorrect statements of this sort, which detract from its value, and should be expunged. Would it not be well to give the section, "generalities," first? Such a group of "*key-notes*" is the best starting point in studying a drug and must first be learned and longest carried in mind. The repertory is a trifle difficult to use, from lack of headings ; one never knows whether the page is one of aggravations or ameliorations, and the index is not arranged alphabetically, as it should be. These defects make it annoying when one is hurried. Let us have next time a perfectly simple alphabetical index and good headings, and, if possible, a fuller list of remedies in the repertory.   *   *   *   *

REPORTS OF SOCIETIES AND HOSPITALS.

HOMŒOPATHIC MEDICAL SOCIETY OF THE STATE OF NEW YORK.

The thirty-sixth annual meeting of the Homœopathic Medical Society of the State of New York was held in the Common Council Chambers, City Hall, Albany, Tuesday and Wednesday, February 8th, and 9th. Between fifty and sixty members were in attendance.

President Henry C. Houghton, after the opening by prayer, delivered the annual address, in which he reviewed the progress of the Society, and the success and respect which had attended its members, collectively and individually; traced the gradual development of the fraternal feeling among different sects of medical belief, from the bitter animosity of fifty years ago, and showed the forces that had been working from without to render the old school more tolerant and respectful. He believed that we should hold fast our position of dignified adherence to our belief, allowing the truth of our doctrine and the increasing momentum of the old school towards our principles of practice, to carry the dominant school into fields of liberal thought and action. In conclusion, the Doctor recommended that the fraternal feeling which is the basis of the Society, should be perpetuated and guarded; that the Secretary's salary be abolished, and that physicians of the State be induced to join; that the transactions be issued semi-annually, promptly after each session, and that papers presented to the Society be exclusively its property, and not be published elsewhere.

The Treasurer, Dr. E. S. Coburn, presented his annual report, in which he called attention to the laxity of the county societies in paying the dues of delegates.

Dr. Moffat moved, that in the next transactions the names of delegates, whose dues are unpaid up to the current year, shall be omitted, and that the reason for such omission be stated. Motion was lost.

On motion of the Board of Censors the following were duly elected members of the Society:

Drs. G. T. Borden of Caledonia; F. S. Fulton, New York; J. D. Hineman, Buffalo; George Clinton Jeffrey, Brooklyn; George W. Lewis, Jr., Buffalo; Wm. E. Long, Buffalo; J. DeVello Moore, Utica; S. W. Skinner, LeRoy; J. H. Chamberlain, Belfast; Mark S. Purdy, Corning; Ferdinand Seeger, New York; C. E. Walker, West Henrietta.

Drs. Lewis, Watson and T. M. Strong were appointed a committee to select the chairmen of bureaus. Drs. Houghton and Bryan were appointed a committee on permanent and honorary members. Dr. H. M. Paine, chairman of the committee of legislation, then presented the report, which was accepted. In this he stated that the attempt on the part of the old school to establish a single State Board of Examiners had been frustrated, and that a joint bill, Senate Bill 485, had also failed to pass; that the old school had at present relinquished its attempt to establish a State Board, and were endeavoring to have the present laws codified and regulated; that the bill prepared by W. A. Purrrington, Esq., whose provisions are essentially the same as those of the previous Senate Bill 485, had been reported favorably by the Senate. This bill is Senate Bill 45, and should receive the support of all. The following resolutions were then offered:

Resolved: That in the opinion of this Society, it is desirable that the provisions of the law of 1872, whereby the different schools of medicine in the State are provided with separate Examining Boards, should be preserved and perpetuated,

Resolved: That whenever the provisions of this law are changed, they should be amended so as to confer upon the boards appointed thereunder, both examining and licensing powers.

Resolved: That we approve the enactment of the present bill, known as Senate Bill 45, the purposes of which are the codification of the present laws relating to medical practice, and to better regulation thereof.

Resolved: That the committee on medical legislation be instructed to endeavor to carry out and render effective the purposes and recommendations herein set forth.

All of which is respectfully submitted.

Dr. M. O. Terry, Chairman of Committee on Societies and Institutions, presented their report.

The Committee on the President's address presented their report, approving the recommendations of the President.

On motion it was resolved that no salary be attached to the office of Secretary at present; also, that the transactions be published semi-annually, and that the Society have exclusive right to the papers presented. Following this, the necrologist, A. W. Holden, reported the death of Dr. Pettit of Fort Plain, Dr. Lawrence of Port Jervis, Dr. Ormes of Jamestown and Dr. Liebold of New York.

The following were nominated for the respective offices:

For President, Dr. H. M. Paine, Dr. F. Park Lewis and Dr. T. L. Brown; 1st Vice-President, Dr. Moffat and Dr. Wm. Tod Helmuth; 2d Vice-President, Dr. J. M. Lee; 3d Vice-President, Dr. Geo. E. Gorham; Secretary, Dr. H. M. Dayfoot; Treasurer, Dr. E. S. Coburn.

The Committee on High Potencies reported that it was difficult to decide upon a suitable plan for work; that circulars had been addressed to the profession through the journals and the mails, asking for information and co-operation, but that the few answers so far received would be of little value unless accompanied by others. They recommended that Drs. H. W. Dods and W. C. Latimer be added to the committee.

AFTERNOON SESSION.

As Chairman of the Committee on Regent's Degree, Dr. F. Park Lewis reported that the Regent's Degree should be conferred only upon those who were eminent in medicine and surgery.

No report of the Bureau of Materia Medica was received, as the chairman was absent. Under the Bureau of Mental and Nervous Diseases, G. A. Gorton, of Brooklyn, presented a paper upon "The Home Treatment of Insanity," in which the Doctor stated that under the present method of treatment, it was doubtful if it was advisable to send lunatics to asylums. It was an error to herd together the insane, on account of the moral influences exerted over each other, each patient being the center of morbific causes which injuriously exerts itself against his fellows.

The patient should remain at home and enjoy liberty and the society of his family. Confinement in asylums will often make permanent lunatics of those who might have been cured. In certain cases home treatment is impossible for many reasons, but where feasible, it should be insisted upon. Incompetency in the treatment of mental diseases by home practitioners was reprehensible, and had originated the specialists in mental therapeutics, who were anomalies and should disappear. The unpardonable ignorance on this subject was largely due to the failure of medical colleges to furnish proper instructions in mental diseases and therapeutics. Following this, Dr. Chas. E. Walker read a paper on " The Diagnostic Points in Nervous Diseases."

Dr. Geo. E. Gorham, of Albany, said that in most cases, if careful search were instituted, some organic disease would be discovered as the cause of the subjective and functional symptoms, so called. For example, exhaustion of the sympathetic system was accountable for many cases of neurasthenia; while the rectum, prostatic urethra, prepuce, and uterus furnished the richest field for the development of secondary reflex neuroses of the most aggravated type. The operation for phymosis, and sounding the urethra had cured some ·of the worst cases of apparently functional disturbance.

Dr. Charles McDowell, New York, Chairman of the Bureau of Histology being absent, no report from this bureau was received.

Under miscellaneous business, Dr. L. B. Wells, of Utica, was placed upon the senior list. Drs. A. S. Ball, of New York and David H. Bullard, of Glen Falls were added to the senior members.

Dr. E. Hasbrouck, Chairman of the Bureau of Obstetrics, read a paper by Dr. J. N. Mitchell of Philadelphia, upon a "Case of Labor Obstructed by a Pelvic Tumor." When first seen, the patient had been in labor eight or nine hours,. the first symptom of approaching labor having been the discharge of a dark fluid. When the patient was seen, the pains were regular, and the discharge continued, but on examination, the vagina appeared to be a closed cul de sac much shorter than natural, and no cervix or os could be discovered. On bimanual examination, two tumors could be detected in the abdomen, one low down and to the right, the other higher and to the left. Forcing the tumor slightly upward, and crowding the hand between it and the symphysis, the cervix and os could be detected, with the breech presenting. The tumor was diagnosed as ovarian, and puncture of the sac, or lapero-clytrotomy was considered. Later, however, the hand was passed between the symphysis and the tumor, the breech grasped, drawn down, and the child delivered. No uterine contractions following, the placenta, which was adherent, was removed with the hand. The patient rallied well, but in the morning she became pulseless, restless and cyanotic, and died shortly after in collapse, with no external hemorrhage. Rupture of the uterus, and hemorrhage into the abdominal cavity were diagnosed. No autopsy was permitted.

The conclusions reached were that the greatest danger arose from the extensive bruising of the tissues. That in all cases where the tumor could not easily be pushed up, tapping or lapero-elytrotomy or Thomas's operation should be performed early.

Dr. Geo. E. Gorham, Albany, then related the case of a woman who, after a protracted labor, was delivered, when a tumor was discovered upon the posterior wall of the uterus. The placenta was delivered, and the patient did well for three days, when suddenly she went into collapse, and died. An autopsy disclosed a fibroma upon the posterior wall of the uterus.

Dr. Everitt Hasbrouck, Brooklyn, then read a paper upon " Obstetrical Memoranda and Experiences," in which he detailed the results of various methods of treatment practiced in 959 obstetrical cases which he had attended. Of these, the largest number in any month had been in the Julys, when 103 cases were attended. Twenty-four were still-born; prolapse of the funis occurred in seven; version was performed in seven; the forceps had been applied twenty-three times; the breach presented in eleven cases; there had been twelve twins; twelve mothers had died; one labor had been absolutely dry from beginning to end, and the child was the scrawniest he had ever seen. *Arnica* is usually given immediately after labor, followed by *bryonia* 12 or 30, until the breasts become normal, when *nux* 12 or 30 is given to relieve constipation if the bowels are dormant. Other remedies are given if necessary. The funis is invariably ligated in two places before pulsation ceases, and cut between the ligatures, after which it is wrapped in some piece of old cloth. In one case, two knots were found in the funis. The placenta is delivered by placing one hand over the uterus and the other upon the placenta, carrying the second hand within the cavity of the uterus if necessary. The bandage is not used, as it does not assist in the reduction of size. His method of supporting the perineum is by pressure upon the head of the child, to retard its passage over the perineum, at the same time to have the patient cease making expulsive efforts. Lubricants are also used, and if necessary the perineum is gently peeled down over the head of the child. In case of the death of the fœtus in utero, the patient is instructed to delay any active procedures for its removal until septic symptoms manifest themselves. In every case, the uterus has expelled its contents before such symptoms appeared. Cinnamon tincture is used in cases of post partum hemorrhage, or vinegar given internally, a wine glass at a time, if the former does not control it. Vaginal douches are not employed, unless the lochia becomes offensive. In case of threatened mastitis, rest and compression, together with the local application of Kierstead's ointment, are employed. If the breasts are very full and heavy, *bry.* and the breast pump once or twice in twenty-four hours is used. If milk is deficient, the mother is given *calc. carb.* 3 and ordered to drink milk freely. Dr. H. M. Dayfoot, Rochester, always gives *arn.* after delivery; the funis is not ligated until all pulsation has ceased. If the child is still-born, the funis is severed at once, and the child immersed alternately in hot and cold water, artificial respiration, assisted by blowing into the child's lungs, being kept up. In one case, seven knots were found tied in the cord. The vaginal douche is employed, and if the temperature runs up, intra-uterine irrigation is employed, which will reduce temperature and avert septacæmia. The perineum is not supported, but if labor is too rapid the head is retarded in its passage through the vaginal outlet. In mastitis, the breasts are supported, and *kali. iod.* given. He finds that the patients rest better when the abdominal bandage is employed. Dr. Geo. E. Gorham, Albany, uses maltine, a dessert spoonful three times a day, to increase the secretion of milk.

Dr. H. L. Waldo, West Troy, gave an analysis of 385 cases of labor attended by him. One prolapsed funis had been met; the forceps used fifty-five times, and he believes with no harm to the patient; he thinks that their more frequent application would be of benefit to the mother.

Used *arn.* for the first fifty cases, after which he discontinued it, and found that patients did quite as well without as with it. He resuscitates children by continuing artificial respiration, blowing into their lungs through a handkerchief, and rubs *amyl nitrite*, two drops, over the nose and lips of the child. Dr. John L. Moffat, Brooklyn, in one case, when the vulval orifice was very small, had incised the perineum, healing it afterwards by *calendula*. *Cham.* is sometimes used in place of *arn.*

Dr. T. L. Brown, Binghamton, urged the necessity of educating your patients to live hygienically, and to call their physician as early as the seventh or eighth month, that he may prepare them by proper hygienic measures and medicines for their labor. He is accustomed to use lard in place of oil for lubrication of the perineum. Dr. L. Faust, Schenectady, said that such a course, while beautiful theoretically, was not always practicable, as many patients did not inform the physician until parturition had begun.

Dr. Wm. C. Latimer, Brooklyn, cuts the funis without tying; uses small piece of absorbent cotton, in which to wrap the cord. Ninety per cent. of his patients engage him previous to labor. He uses simply a canton flannel slip, flannel bandage and the cotton for the cord in dressing the child. He has found no good in Kierstead's ointment. Forceps are rarely used.

At the evening session the discussion was continued.

Dr. Ed. S. Coburn, Troy, related a case in which death had resulted from giving a vaginal douche.

In another case, the water injected did not return, and the patient became weak, prostrated, with feeble pulse, and general symptoms of collapse. On inserting a pair of placental forceps within the os uteri, and opening them, the water gushed out, and the uterus contracted. The patient recovered. Since then, he has discontinued the douche. One woman under treatment has a constant flow of milk, which it seems impossible to stop.

Dr. Geo. E. Gorham, Albany, said that he never used injections, and that Dr. Fordyce Barker, in a late address, stated that he had now abandoned them, and since then the temperature approached nearer the normal. Dr. Fred. S. Fulton, New York, cited a case of violent hemorrhage from the uterus, caused by the extrusion of a mucus polypus, which was immediately controlled by injecting into the uterus and vagina, pure vinegar. The Doctor later removed the polypus, and the woman made a complete recovery. Another case of rigid os which had yielded to *gels.* was reinduced by *ergot*, fluid extract, given to hasten the pains. It again yielded to *bell.* The conclusion was that *ergot* in the first stage was a dangerous remedy.

Under the Bureau of Clinical Medicine, Dr. Titus L. Brown, Binghamton, detailed the history of a young girl who had brought on a persistent dyspepsia by excessive use of coffee. The intestinal disorder was entirely cured by stopping the coffee, and placing the patient upon a diet of eggs and milk beaten together. Dr. H. L. Waldo, West Troy, then read a paper on "Drinking Water as a Vehicle for Germs," in which he held that typhoid fever and cholera were often communicated by drinking water; that chemical and microscopical analysis of water to determine its purity, was not to be trusted, and that the only test for potable water was freedom from sewage contamination. The Doctor cited Albany as furnishing an example of a city furnished with impure water. The city derived its water supply from the Hudson, into which, and only a short distance above it, Cohoes, with its 20,000 inhabitants, Lansingburgh with 10,000, Waterford and Green Island with as many more, West Troy with 15,000, and Troy with 70,000 people, poured their entire sewage. The Doctor contended that the water must necessarily be impure, and originate many zymotic and infectious diseases. In reply, Dr. Geo. E. Gorham, Albany, claimed that there was but little typhoid fever in the city, and what did exist, was found in that section supplied by wells. Dr. N. Hunting, Albany, stated that we did not know how much typhoid fever there was in the city, but he was convinced that there was much more than was reported, and that it came from the impurities of the water.

Dr. D. B. Whittier presented a paper upon "Is Belladona a Prophylactic in Scarlet Fever?" The conclusions reached were that scarlet fever was a zymotic disease, with a definite course, and that it was uninfluenced by medicines; that *bell.* was prophylactic only in the Sydenham type of the disease, which at present is very rare; that the infection of scarlet fever has not been demonstrated to be a specific germ, and that the exfoliation of epidermis has nothing to do with its contagion. The real cause was at present unknown.

Dr. H. C. Houghton, New York, stated that the homœopaths appeared to be giving up theories just as the allopaths are accepting them. At the

Five Points House of Industry, it was formerly always their custom, on the outbreak of scarlet fever, to give *bell.* night and morning, to every child connected with the institution. They never had a second case under this method.

Dr. T. L. Brown uses lard during the fever, when the patient is restless.

Dr. W. C. Latimer said that the location of wells was often erroneous, and that it was of the utmost importance to·know the dip and direction of the water-shed which determined the course of the underground water.

Dr. H. L. Waldo then exhibited O'Dwyer's tubes, and explained their *modus operandi.*

Dr. L. A. Bull, Buffalo, stated that an improvement had been made in the tubes by placing a rubber instead of a metallic ring at the top. Feeding could then be carried on more easily.

Wednesday morning, Dr. F. Park Lewis, Buffalo, presented the report of the Bureau of Ophthalmology. The first paper was by Dr. Colvin, on "Foreign .Bodies in the Iris," in which was detailed a case of cystic tumor of the iris dependent upon a foreign body which had become lodged there. Iridectomy and subsequent puncture of the cyst gave promise of restored vision.

The second paper was " A Rare Case of Morbus Basedowii (exophthalmic goitre)." The patient, twenty-six years old, had been well until she became pregnant. At the time of examination, the heart was fluttering, the eye was protruding, and the seat of, at times, sharp darting, at others, dull heavy pains. There was general prostration, bad dreams, sharp uterine pains, but no abnormality could be discovered on examination ; nor could any organic heart lesion be detected. The protrusion was aggravated by anxiety or mental excitement, and was always preceded by epistaxis and congestion of the head. There was also severe pain in the head, beating in the ear, constipation, and increased hunger. There was no organic eye disease, the media being clear, and the retina normal. The history and apparent cause was domestic infelicity. The protrusion was unilateral, and there was no enlargement of the thyroid gland. *Nux mosch.* proved entirely curative, all symptoms and the protrusion of the eye disappearing under its use.

Dr. W. C. Latimer cited a case in which *ignatia* had relieved all the symptoms, excepting the protrusion of the eye.

Dr. Jno. L. Moffat detailed a case of cyst of the cornea, caused by a minute foreign body having lodged there, which was at once relieved of all pain and disease by rupturing the cyst, and allowing the foreign body to escape.

Dr. D. B. Hunt, New York, then read a paper upon "Kalmia Latifolia in Rheumatic Iritis," detailing several cases in which there had been intense, sharp pain, boring in the eye, with ciliary injection and tenderness of the eye, all occuring in rheumatic subjects. In every case, *kalmia* relieved at once, after the failure of *bry., spig., ac., rhus.,* etc.

Dr. L. Faust said that it had become almost a routine prescription for him to give *kalmia* in rheumatism of the shoulder, and neuralgias of the right side.

Dr. J. L. Moffat stated that *kalmia* had been of great service to him in rheumatic iritis, but that he had found *prunus* or *paris* were often indicated in pure neuralgias.

Dr. Selden H. Talcott, Middletown, then presented a paper on "The Practical Treatment of Insanity," in which he said that as long as a patient was not dangerous, and could be carefully attended, and the cause of his mental aberration did not lie in domestic unhappiness, or in business distractions, the patient had better remain at home ; but if a contrary state of affairs was present, the patient should be removed to an asylum. The first asylums were started by the monks of Jerusalem in the sixth century.

In the south of Europe, the monks established the first in the fourteenth century.   To the Quaker Christians of England is due the honor of transforming mad-houses into proper asylums.   The spread of Christianity and the rearing of asylums have been coincident.   A change of scene and climate, *e. g.*, from a low land or sea shore, to the mountains, and *vice versa*, is beneficial to the insane.   The buildings should have the best ventilation and drainage ; all sanitary conditions should be perfect ; the rooms heated with steam or hot water.   The proper treatment consists in gentle discipline, kindness, rest, exercise, proper diet, mental and moral hygiene, and medicines.   No form of punishment is suitable or justifiable, as the patient is always sick, and does not appreciate the end or reason for such.   If the patient is wasting in strength and flesh, he should have entire rest ; be put to bed until all mental excitement has subsided.   The diet is liquid, and should be given every three hours, milk and beef tea being used ; the former as a nutritive, and the latter as a mild stimulant. Later, toasted bread, rice, baked potatoes, etc., can be given ; then exercise can be resumed ; medical treatment being used constantly.   Up to September 30th, 1886, the percentage of cure had been 50.95%, the death ratio 2.99%, of all treated.   Homœopathic remedies are used exclusively, and with much better results than are shown from old school treatment. The main remedies used are *ac., ars., bell., hyos., stram., verat. alb.,* and *verat. vir. ;* a second group is formed of *bapt., bry., canth., cimcif., nat. mur., sulf., puls.*   Prescriptions are made on the totality of symptoms. The history of a lady patient was then detailed to show the results of treatment.   Admitted December 10th, 1886, at which time she had been under old school treatment for five years.   There was no hereditary predisposition.   Five years ago her menses were suppressed by cold.   At admission she weighed ninety-one pounds, temperature 100 1-5, respiration rapid, menses regular as to time, but very profuse.   The patient could not sleep, was excited and noisy on admission.

She was given *puls.,* hot milk and beef tea, and Mellin's food, and put to bed.   On the fifth of January she menstruated normally, and had no illusions or excitement.   On January 15th, sat up for the first time.   The pain in the ovaries had disappeared.   February 1st she weighed 114 pounds, sleeps well, and has no delusions.

The Bureau of Laryngology was then introduced by Dr. Geo. M. Dillow, New York, Chairman.   Dr. L. A. Bull, Buffalo, read a paper on " The Tissue Remedies in the Treatment of Diseases of the Air Passages."   For the past nine months he has used no others.   The main indications are as follows :

Calcarea phos.   In chronic catarrhal ear trouble, cough of chronic consumptives ; in scrofulous subjects with enlargement of the cervical glands.

Calcarea sulp.   Catarrhal condition bloody expectoration.

Calcarea fluor.   Hard, bony growths, osteo-sarcoma.   Secondary and tertiary syphilis, horrible odor.

Ferrum phos.   Takes the place of *aconite,* sore throats of singers ; pulmonary congestion.

Kali mur.   In throat trouble where formerly the mercurials were given, white-coated tongue and tonsils ; thick tenacious secretion.   Adherent crust forms in the roof of the pharnyx.

Kali phos.   Chronic pharyngitis ; bad odor from skin.

Kali sulph.   Stringy, thick secretion.

Mag. phos.   Chronic pharyngitis and cough which is spasmodic ; lungs are sore from coughing.   Gagging and choking on swallowing.

Natrum mur.   In catarrhs, aggravated on exertion and in the cold.   In one case it caused the reduction of a hydrocele.

Natrum phos.   Yellow coating at the base of tongue.

Natrum sulph.   Photophobia and scrofulous ophthalmia.

Silicea. Has had the best result from this remedy. Has cured cases of chronic pharyngitis, hay fever, tender feet. In one case caused entire relief in hay fever of long standing.

In all cases has used the fourth decimal.

Dr. Geo. M. Dillow, New York, has used the peroxide of hydrogen in syphilitic ulceration of the pharynx with remarkable results. The use of the tissue remedies he regarded as largely empirical, not being founded upon the provings of the drugs upon healthy subjects, but taken from the recommendations of Schüssler, which were founded very largely upon experience.

Dr. H. C. Houghton considered that these remedies offered a rich field for investigation.

The Censors reported for membership Drs. D. B. Hunt, H. D. Schenck, M. W. Vanderburg and D. G. Wilcox.

The following officers were elected for 1887–88 : President, H. M. Paine, Albany ; 1st Vice-President, Wm. Tod Helmuth, New York ; 2d Vice-President, J. M. Lee, Rochester ; 3d Vice-President, Geo. E. Gorham, Albany ; Secretary, H. M. Dayfoot, Rochester ; Treasurer, Ed. S. Coburn, Troy.

It was voted to hold the next meeting in New York, on September 20th and 21st, 1887.

The Bureau of Surgery then reported a paper on "The Treatment of the Sac in the Radical Operation for Hernia," by H. I. Ostrom, New York. It was read by title and referred. Dr. M. O. Terry, Utica, then read a paper on "An Old Author on the Symptoms Produced by Spinal Irritation ; Incidental Remarks," in which were detailed the symptoms ensuing from spinal anæmia, and cauterization, by the actual cautery, recommended as the most efficient remedy. Dr. J. M. Lee, Rochester, then read a paper on "The Diagnosis and Treatment of Wounds of the Femoral Artery," by L. L. Brainard, M.D., Little Falls, and another on "Ovariotomy," by himself. The author detailed the history and method of operating in five recent cases.• He does not employ antisepsis but pays great regard to cleanliness. The pedicle is tied with silk, cauterized, and returned within the abdomen. The parieties are closed with wire, silk or cat-gut. Calendula dressings are applied over the line of incision, which is as short as possible. One of his patients died. She was practically moribund before the operation, which was for cancer of the abdominal organs.

The following Chairmen of Bureaus were then appointed : Legislation, Dr. Geo. E. Gorham, Albany ; Medical Education, Dr. Chas. A. Bacon, New York ; Medical Societies, Dr. M. O. Terry, Utica ; Ophthalmology, Dr. A. B. Norton, New York ; Mental and Nervous System, Dr. Selden H. Talcott, Middletown ; Histology, Dr. Fred. S. Fulton, New York ; Obstetrics, Dr. Louis Faust, Schenectady ; Clinical Medicine, Dr. H. L. Waldo, West Troy ; Otology, Dr. E. J. Pratt ; Pædology, Dr. Wm. C. Latimer, Brooklyn ; Laryngology, Dr. L. A. Bull, Buffalo ; Surgery, Dr. J. M. Lee, Rochester ; Gynæcology, Dr. F. F. Laird, Utica ; Vital Statistics, Dr. A. R. Wright, Buffalo ; Climatology, Dr. C. E. Jones, Albany.

The following Censors were elected : Northern District, Drs. A. W. Holden, Jno. A. Pearsall, F. F. Laird. ; Southern District, Drs. F. E. Doughty, E. Hasbrouck. A. B. Norton ; Middle District, Drs. M. O. Terry, C. E. Jones, F. L. Vincent ; Western District, Drs. Asa S. Couch, N. Osborn, E. H. Walcott.

Drs. Henry C. Houghton and Wm. Tod Helmuth, of New York, were elected to the Regent's Degree.

A motion allowing members the privilege of printing their papers in the journals before their appearance in the transactions was lost by a vote of nine to seven, after which the Society adjourned to meet again in New York, September 20th and 21st, 1887.

RECORD OF MEDICAL PROGRESS.

OXMEL SCILLÆ IN PERTUSSIS.—Dr. Netter—*Arch de Pharmacie*, September 5th, 1886—states that whooping cough may be cured in a week or less, by the use of oxmel scillæ, 20-60 drops per diem.

SCOPOLINE, a new mydriatic, has been used instead of atropine, with success, by Mr. Dunn, in the treatment of corneal ulcers, keratitis and iritis.—*British Medical Journal*, January 8th, page 62. It is derived from the scopolia japonica, and was first recommended as a mydriatic by Dr. Pierd'houy. It is, so says Mr. Edgar A. Browne, rather more energetic than atropine, acts more quickly, and its effects pass off more slowly.

ANTIPYRIN RASH.—Dr. Daly writes to the *British Medical Journal*, January 15th, 1887, that antipyrin produces a rash resembling that of measles, but differing from the latter in the following particulars : 1. It did not make its appearance first on the forehead, and was most marked on the extremeties, though present on the trunk, and to a limited extent on the face. 2. Its color was rose-red, and it was not arranged in cresentic patches. 3. There was an absence of general symptoms. 4. Its duration was only from twenty-four to thirty-six hours, and it quickly subsided when the drug was left off.

MILK DIET AS A CAUSE OF DILATATION OF THE STOMACH.—Debove presented a patient at a recent meeting of the *Société Médicale des Hôpitaux*, who showed evidence of the harm sometimes resulting from an exclusive milk diet. Two years ago, while suffering from an alcoholic gastritis, with symptoms of ulceration, he was put on milk diet, finally taking as much as eight litres a day. After a certain time he grew weak and lost thirty-six pounds in weight. Debove then diagnosed gastric dilatation, and gave him one and a-half litres of milk, with a little meat, and the stomach was washed out by the usual method. The patient has since gained thirty pounds in weight, and is perfectly well.—Paris Letter to the *British Medical Journal*, January 15th, 1887.

NEWS.

PERSONAL.—Dr. E. C. M. Hall, formerly Instructor in Chemistry in N. Y. H. Medical College, was married to Miss Helen L. Rice, at Fair Haven, Conn., January 26th, 1877.

MISSOURI INSTITUTE OF HOMŒOPATHY.—The eleventh annual session of the Institute will be held at St. Louis, April 26-27, 1877. Joshua Thorne, M.D., is the President, and James T. Runnels, M.D., Secretary.

THE BURDEN OF LIFE.—Patient.—"But Doctor, it seems to me that your bill is rather steep. Ten years ago you would not have charged me half so much." Doctor.—"You forget that it costs twice as much to live as it did ten years ago." Patient.—"I do not know anything that has doubled in cost." Doctor.—"You forget your Doctor's bills."

SMALL POX.—The recent outbreak of variola in New York has thus far been kept within limits by the health authorities. The cases as reported to the health department have been as follows : Total number of cases from January 7th to February 5th were fifty-two ; deaths, eleven. There seems to be no reason to fear an epidemic of the disease at present.

A DANGEROUS GAS.—Some time ago the manufacture of water-fuel gas was begun at Troy, and its use proving satisfactory, the number of consumers largely increased. Its cheapness, (fifty cents a thousand) together with its great heating power, seemed destined to make its general introduction merely a question of time. But its deadly work in a Troy house where three corpses were found, shows that as at present manufactured, it is unfit for use. This gas is without odor, and may be as fatal to persons awake as ordinary illuminating gas is to those asleep. Besides it may enter buildings which are not connected with the mains, and kill the occupants almost without warning. Until this gas is made odorous so that its presence may be known by the sense of smell, it will be unsafe to use.

A LEGAL DECISION.—From August to December, 1886, Albert Eastman practiced as a physician and surgeon in Steuben County, Indiana. He was without a license, and upon an affidavit being filed against him was tried, convicted and fined. At the trial Eastman made a motion to quash the indictment on the ground that the law was unconstitutional and void, for the reason that the Legislature had no right to place restriction upon the liberty of a citizen in following any profession or vocation he might choose. The motion was overruled, and after the conviction Eastman appealed to the Supreme Court, where the decision of the lower court was recently affirmed. The opinion held that the case of admitting physicians to practice was the same as admitting of lawyers, and that the admittees should be thoroughly proficient in learning and skill, so as to protect the interests of the State. A physician was trusted with care of the health, life and limbs of the people of the State, and it was in order to protect such that the law of license was enacted.

FEES OF GREAT SURGEONS.—The fees of great surgeons and physicians have a general interest for the public as well as a special one for the recipients. Hunter never gained more than $30,000 a year, and for many years he gained less than $5,000. Sir Astley Cooper's profession brought him trifling sums for several years ; in the fifth year of his practice he only gained $500; but in time his income rose to $45,000 a year, and one year it reached $105,000. Sir Benjamin Brodie's receipts are stated to have far exceeded Cooper's. It was vulgarly reported of Dr. Chambers when his right hand was injured by blood poisoning, that his fingers had become crooked from the continual habit of taking fees. He was in great demand, yet his fees do not appear to have exceeded $45,000 per year. This is high remuneration, but if the fees of some distinguished American surgeons and physicians were known, it is quite possible they would equal or even exceed those given above. It may be judged from these figures that the medical profession is one of the most profitable. No doubt it is so to eminent doctors, just as the Bar is to eminent lawyers. Either profession is profitable to those at the top.

IPECACUANHA CULTIVATION IN INDIA.—The superintendent of the cinchona plantations of the Bengal government gives the following facts concerning the cultivation of ipecacuanha, taken from *The Living Age.* The facts are of considerable biological interest, as showing that amongst closely connected forms, which can scarcely be distinguished by palpable morphological distinctions, there may yet be unobvious constitutional differences which in the struggle for existence may determine the several and ultimate dominance of some one form in particular. "Our original stock of plants came from Kew and Edinburgh—the great majority from Edinburgh. The few plants from Kew differed a great deal in appearance from the Edinburgh lot, which again differed greatly from each other. After we were satisfied that we could make nothing out of ipecacuanha from a commercial point of view, we put all the plants out in the open air and let them take their chance. Very soon the Edinburgh sort began to disappear, until in the course of a year or two there was not a single plant of one of the Edinburgh varieties alive, while almost every plant of the Kew variety lived. Of it at the present moment we have a good stock. Probably our ipecacuanha experiments may prove another instance of the folly of giving up the cultivation of new crops as hopeless, until the most exhaustive experiments have been carried out." *The Living Age* is one of the best of our exchanges.

STRANGE BED-FELLOWS.—The prohibitionists by their recent action, seem to have put themselves in rather an unenviable position. Fanaticism and blind zeal are not the best guides to temperate and judicious action. An open alliance between the liquor dealers and prohibitionists would seem among the impossibilities. And yet that is exactly what the prohibitionists have done in their opposition to the High License bill. The liquor interest is energetically fighting the bill, for they know and do not hesitate to say, that it will burden the traffic so greatly as to crush out a great part of it. They are not afraid of prohibition, for they know that it will not, in this State, at least, prohibit. If it is said that the law cannot be enforced, and liquor will be sold without license, how much the more does that same argument apply to a prohibitory law. But the dealers know that a high license law can and will be enforced, and for that reason they are so determined in opposition. The Crosby Bill would undoubtedly put out of existence a great number of low groggeries and saloons, and while there would be still left by far too many dram-shops, yet it is an advance—a great advance—in the right direction. It is a move directly toward prohibition, and is the only way in which prohibition can really come. It is quite impossible to congratulate the prohibition party upon its new allies, but there is no inconsistency in the alliance. For years they have opposed practicable measures, looking towards the reduction of the liquor traffic, and the difficulty in securing any effectual legislation is largely of their making. That the High License bill ought to become a law is certain, and should it fail, the responsibility may be easily placed.

INSTITUTE AND HOSPITAL OF THE M. E. CHURCH.—There are in the City of New York some excellent schools for the training of nurses. But these nurses, so educated, go as a rule only where remuneration is given. The poor, therefore, who most sadly need their services, are neglected. This difficulty has hitherto been insurmountable, but recently some philanthropic ladies have associated themselves together and established the "Institute and Hospital of the Methodist Episcopal Church." The object and purpose of the Institute is to provide hospital accommodations and trained nurses for the poor, and others who require medical or surgical treatment, and to establish in connection with the hospital an institute or school for the training and education of women as nurses. These will be at the service of the poor as well as the rich. Not only will they give to the ignorant and indigent the care that illness requires, but they will also teach their patients how to live in health. Among the ladies interested in the Institute are Mrs. W. L. Harris, Mrs. W. F. Havemeyer, Mrs. J. D. Slayback, Mrs. W. H. Falconer, Mrs. W. B. Skidmore, Mrs. Richard Kelly, Mrs. Colgate, Mrs. I. P. Mesereau and many others. The Institute is located at 129 West Sixty-first Street. A resident physician will be needed, to whom will be given room and board, with privilege of moderate outside practice. The staff is as follows : Consulting Physicians, Dr. T. F. Allen, Dr. J. McE. Wetmore, Dr. J. G. Baldwin, Dr. Geo. Belcher. Consulting Surgeons, Dr. W. Tod Helmuth, Dr. F. E. Doughty. Attending Physicians, Dr. J. M. Schley, Dr. Wm. N. Guernsey, Dr. H. M. Dearborn, Dr. L. L. Danforth, Dr. E. V. Moffat, Dr. E. H. Porter, Dr. J. B. Garrison. Attending Surgeons, Dr. S. F. Wilcox, Dr. F. S. Fulton.

VOL. XXXV.   *APRIL, 1887.* $\binom{\text{VOLUME II,}}{\text{Third Series.}}$ No. 4.

NORTH AMERICAN
JOURNAL OF HOMŒOPATHY.

ORIGINAL ARTICLES IN MEDICINE.

SYMPTOMATIC vs. THEORETICAL INDICATIONS IN THERAPEUTICS.*

By J. T. O'CONNOR, M.D.,
New York.

IT must have been quite early in the period of the first drug provings by Hahnemann, when he recognized the duplication and reduplication of some symptoms of one drug in the pathogenetic records of other drugs, and we can easily imagine that it soon occurred to him to cast aside, as being of little value, those symptoms producible by the action of many different drugs. Hence it was an easy step to hold those symptoms as of the most value in a drug proving that were unusual, especially annoying or in any way peculiar. This is one of his fundamental principles in the application of the law of "*similia*" in the treatment of disease, and gives, in a certain sense, a short cut to the choice of a remedy, for he equally insists that the symptoms of the disease which are to guide us in our selection must be those not diagnostic of the disease, but special, peculiar or most annoying. Another step in the way of shortening the approach to a remedy was gained when he found that certain remedies were noticeably active in curing in certain bodily constitutions or at certain seasons of the year, and this apart from the usual conditions of aggravation and amelioration.

And just here appears to the philosophical observer a distinction between symptomatic indications and theoretical ones. For it must be admitted that his statement made in the *Organon* that a placid, mild-tempered person will not be helped by the employment of *bryonia* nor an irascible one by *pulsatilla* is not wholly deducible from an examination of the provings of these remedies, since contradictory emotional states exist in each. Other observers, following on the line

---

*Read before the Homœopathic Medical Society of the County of New York, February 10th, 1887.

laid down by Hahnemann, have collected, as a result of experience, many valuable indications for the use of certain drugs, indications which materially lessen the labor of selecting a remedy, and which are founded not upon the provings but upon experience with the provings. As instances of this may be mentioned, the use of *dulcamara* in conditions arising from exposure to damp cold, as in a cellar, or *rhus* for the effects of a wetting, etc. And these I have verified over and over again until they are as solidly established in my mind as is the knowledge that *spigelia* causes neuralgic pains of a certain character or that *ledum* produces pains having a characteristically definite direction.

The labor of simply reading over our enormous materia medica is one which we all recognize as requiring more time than the student can devote to one subject, and yet this subject is *the* one which the physician must master in some way if he hopes to be even fairly successful in practice. The existence of so-called laws has been invoked by different physicians to give a readier means of analysis of a drug proving, but so far all seem to be held by the mass of the homœopathic profession in slight esteem. Pathological change, too, consequent upon the lethal exhibition of certain drugs, has been brought into something like a relationship to the subjective symptoms as found in drug provings ; and such relationship has met with a more ready acceptance on the part of some homœopathic practitioners, while it has aroused the ire and secured the scorn of others. To say that because a drug, when given in large doses and to extremes, and thereby causing, it may be, pneumonia or peritonitis, is by that fact a homœopathic remedy for such disease, is to bring up a question which in this aspect it is not my purpose to discuss to night, but the question which I will endeavor to present is, whether there is any safe basis, pathological or otherwise, for the selection of the remedy apart from the symptoms as given in the materia medica, of provings, including, of course, the conditions of amelioration and aggravation.

The changes in pathological theories as to the cause of any disease are so constant in their recurrence as to remind us of the telegraphic reports from Europe concerning political affairs, wherein we find one day's paper to make positive assertion of a certain action by some high personage, only to deny this statement on the following day. Every new point reached in pathology seems to demolish some cherished theory of an earlier date, and yet there is always left a residue which the more recent findings do not overthrow. The results of pathological investigation in the dead house will remain true as far as the description of the "finds" goes, but theories based thereon are often ruthlessly overthrown by subsequent advancement in investigation under the microscope.

In illustration I may call attention to the very recent work done in establishing the entity, history, diagnosis, progress and outcome of multiple neuritis, a disease whose existence is as well established now as is that of typhoid fever, but which, very recently, too, was hidden under the mask of tabes, of anterior polio-myelitis, of neuralgia or of spinal cord affection due to the poison of diphtheria, typhoid fever and similar infectious diseases.

Let us consider a case of multiple neuritis which, say within a very recent period, might have been diagnosticated as one of anterior polio-myelitis. How would pathological views help us in prescribing under these circumstances when the pathological view of the case was, it is now admitted, at fault. Of the poisons, which, by their action on the human economy, produce inflammatory changes in the anterior grey horns of the spinal cord and disappearance of, or injury to the ganglion cells grouped there, the only one showing such result at an autopsy is *lead*. Now there is certainly no justification for the assumption that *lead* is the only poison capable of such action, but all that can be said is that it is the only poisonous substance which under present conditions enters largely into the daily life of certain classes of artisans, and hence the only one whose ultimate effects reach our notice. But *lead* also produces multiple neuritis, so that in the case cited for illustration, its employment might seem justified on the pathological basis of selecting a remedy, but the cure, if such resulted, would have been in spite of an erroneous diagnosis.

Again : an epidemic of poisoning by *ergot* occurred in Germany in 1879, and some twenty cases were taken to the hospital at Madgeburg. Of these, four came to the autopsy table, and all showed evidences of recently occurring sclerosis of the posterior columns of the cord. Now the employment of *secale* as a remedy in locomotor ataxia could be justified on the pathological basis of selection by the findings in these cases, and indeed the drug has been used for a considerable time by our allopathic brethren in this disease, but it is, I am sure, plain to any one who has a real appreciation of the homœopathic law that *secale* will never cure a case of tabes unless it is indicated by the symptoms. It is difficult to imagine that *secale* could act long enough and deep enough to cause the changes in the cord found in the cases noted, without, at the same time, giving rise to symptoms in plenty, known to be characteristic of the drug. But more than this. From recent investigations the theory has been advanced, based upon pathological observation, that there is a form of tabes in which the affection begins as a spinal meningitis, and consecutive inflammatory changes extend to the posterior columns so that even here a distinction must be made pathologically as to the special form of tabes produced by *ergot*, as well as the special form of each case of that disease under treatment. A report of this epidemic of *ergot* poisoning appeared in the *Archiv. f. Psychiatrie*, Vol. II., and in a recent issue of the same publication, allusion is made to the fact that in that very epidemic some of the cases under the poisonous influence of *ergot* had epileptiform convulsions. Are we then to prescribe *secale* in epilepsy because of this manifestation in some cases of *ergot* poisoning? My answer to this question will appear further on.

A relatively frequent manifestation of nervous disease, especially in dispensary practice in cities, was described by Putnam and Edes of Boston, in 1883, and has since been reported by other neurologists, especially Sinkler and Mills, Philadelphia, 1884. It consists of numbness and some loss of sensation in the fingers or hands, at times extending up the arms and it may affect the feet similarly. But it is usually confined to the distribution of one or more large nerve trunks and in the cases I have seen, now eight or ten in number, it is for the most part in the ulnar distribution. It is most noticeable after a hard day's washing—the disease most frequently occurring in women who do their own house work. The loss of sensation is great enough to render sewing or the finer manipulations with the hand well nigh impossible, and the tingling may amount to pain, so that there is at times some degree of suffering. From the disease appearing symmetrically in the two hands, the earlier observers thought that it must be of spinal origin, and now it must be plain enough to anyone that a prescription based upon such a view was necessarily a faulty one, even pathologically considered, since later researches bring the trouble under the head of multiple neuritis.

A neuritis is frequently set up by pressure in the region of one nerve trunk, as when a man sleeps with the head lying on one arm, or with the arm stretched out and resting on the sharp edge of the back of a chair. Here the patient wakes in the morning with the muscles supplied by that nerve paralyzed, and it may be weeks or even months before there is complete return of voluntary motion. Going one step farther, we find that Gowers says in his most recent work, "that this same form of trouble can and does occur when the arm is kept fixed for a long time in a bent position even without pressure." I saw one case some months since in which the extensor communis digitorum of one arm was paralyzed as a result of the patient's having carried a somewhat heavy article of furniture with its edge resting for a few minutes only upon the region of the extensor muscles of the affected arm. As the case came to me at a dispensary, and immediately as soon as the paralysis was discovered, I hoped to be able to use Hering's indication for *hypericum* which he thinks is specifically curative in injuries to the nerves, but the patient only came once more and I was unable to prescribe it. But I had already prescribed the remedy in ordinary cases of pressure paralysis without the slightest effect and the question now comes up is Dr. Hering's theory of the action of *hypericum* wrong or is the view that the trouble is due to pressure upon the nerve and injury to it from such pressure a correct one? From my own experience and from studying that of others, I am inclined to reject in great part the notion that such neuritides as those mentioned are due to injury to the nerve itself. I am inclined to look upon weakened or altered *tonus* of the arterioles as the immediate causal factor of these neuritides, and that the resulting mechanical congestion of the circulation in the channels of blood supply to the nerve branches themselves may be fairly considered as having a *preponderating* influence in impairing the function of the nerve and in the subsequent degeneration. Nervous elements are the highest development in the animal organism, and the extraordinary rapidity with which the nerve structures decompose outside the body may, I think, find some parallel within the body when the blood current, in any degree, stagnates. It is hard to believe that pressure over the trunk of a nerve buried as deeply in the tissues as is the musculo-spiral can have any effect on the trunk itself, even though it lies next the bone, and a distinct form of neuritis is known to occur after pressure upon a popliteal aneurism, as a result of which there may be a cure of the aneurism, but paralysis of the nervous supply below it.* Such are the cases of what is known as ischæmic paralysis, and the œdema and marked vaso-motor changes also present are, I think, to be accounted for in the sudden and complete stoppage of the whole circulation in a vessel supplying so much of a limb as does the popliteal artery.

Is there anything in the clinical history of the cases of so-called numbness of the fingers, or in those of pressure paralysis and allied types of neuritis to justify this view? I think there is. In the first place, in the cases of so-called numbness of the fingers, there is usually a history of hard work, of faulty nutrition and almost always the use

---

*Based on the clinical observation of one case, the explanation resting upon a reading at second hand of Leser's experiments. Leser's monograph (*Untersuchungen über ischæmische Muskellähmungen und Muskelcontracturen*, Volkmann's Sammlung, No. 249, 1884,) shows that ischæmic paralysis is purely muscular, the nerves giving no evidence of degeneration or even impaired conduction.

of some form of alcoholic stimulus, with impaired appetite and possibly insufficient and improper food. The woman who does a hard day's work takes a pint of beer at one or more meals daily, and the effect of the constantly repeated dose of alcohol must have, and does have its paralyzing influence on the vascular *tonus*, and it is notorious that the cases of pressure paralysis commonly seen, occur after the patient has gone to sleep in a condition of more or less advanced intoxication. When a patient comes showing drop wrist and giving a story of having slept with the head lying on the arm, the physician, who is acquainted with such cases, invariably says, "well, you had been drinking, hadn't you?" and the answer is almost always in the affirmative.   The predisposing cause here being the loss of vascular *tonus*, it only requires an added exciting cause, such as a venous stasis by pressure on the return flow of the blood, to determine in a few hours the loss of nerve function and impairment of nerve nutrition, or in cases where the primary cause goes on, this loss of function and impaired nutrition will increase, and affecting the peripheral divisions of the limbs, there will be in time a well marked multiple neuritis.   This view does not in the least do away with the accepted one concerning the trophic influence of the ganglion cells in the anterior grey horns upon the principal nerves.

In the old days of the Cæsars it was the proud boast that all roads lead to Rome, but can it be said now that all pathological roads lead to truth? If so they only do it after many devious windings, much retracing of steps already gone over, much tearing down of guide-posts leading to error.   In this view a pathological basis for prescribing cannot be supported scientifically.   The pathological findings of to-day may to-morrow be interpreted entirely differently from or contrary to views at present accepted, and hence to rely on changes of structure produced in lethal provings of a remedy as indications for the selections of that remedy in some disease characterized theoretically by such changes, is, to say the least, unsafe.   Hering's dictum that *hypericum* is indicated where nerves are injured may be correct, but it is inapplicable, as I think I have already shown, where it cannot be fairly considered that the nerve itself has been *primarily* injured; indeed from his qualifying observation, "injury to parts rich in sentient nerves" it is possibly applicable rather to affections from injury to the terminal or end organs of the *sensory* nerves.

It has been already stated that epileptiform convulsions have been seen in cases of *ergot* poisoning, but to assume that *secale* is a remedy in epilepsy cannot, I think, be justified in the absence of well known *secale* symptoms.   Indeed to select any remedy for epilepsy because it has caused epileptiform convulsions is to be deprecated, and I am strongly of the opinion that convulsive symptoms are the least valuable of all in our materia medica as indications for the selection of the remedy for this disease, and I am not sure but that the infrequency of our cures in this affection is due to our tendency to limit our choice of drugs to those which have caused convulsions ; in this regard I am sorry to have to admit that I have been as great a sinner as anyone.

Are, then, pathological changes, either in cases of disease or in fatal cases of poisoning, of no value? By no means. The value to the studious physician is enormous in the first instance, since we have every reason to believe that pathological findings will finally lead to a more accurate knowledge of what is of the greatest importance, *i. e.*, the knowledge of the beginnings of disease and also of its successive stages of development. As to the second instance, it is of value as giving him some positive knowledge of the final possibilities in drug proving, for we may be misled into rejecting a remedy in a given case because there has been no evidence of its power to cause similar changes.

From the foregoing considerations I would conclude that the neuritides to which such prominence has been given in this paper and with them many, perhaps most, of the system diseases of the cord, begin in the vaso-motor system of nerves which we may consider to act as both the outposts and quartermaster's department of an army. They give warning of noxious influences and through their governing action all parts of the organism are supplied with nutrient material. Strike them down and the warnings are not forthcoming ; impair their efficiency and the supplies needful for nutrition of parts are not delivered or are delivered in unmanageable quantity. So that, the symptoms at this early stage are the best guides in selecting the remedy and doubly so when we consider, as we must, that most of the symptoms in our provings find their starting point also in the vaso-motor system. I must say what many a better and abler writer has said before me, that I believe that under fairly good homœopathic treatment in the beginning such diseases as are recognized in the later stages by well-known pathological changes do not fully develop ; they are cured, as it were, before they are well under way. At the same time we do see cases, from time to time, in well advanced stages of disorders of this class, and to these cases we must give our best endeavors, and I believe we will do far more towards their cure by ignoring as a factor in the problem of selecting a drug, the pathological condition, real or supposititious, rather than by relying upon it as a guiding indication for the choice of the remedy.

It has been already stated that we are in possession of indications for the use of certain drugs in diseases, which indications are not really symptomatic or directly from the provings, but are the outcome of experience in using remedies according to the symptoms. Such indications are in that sense theoretical, and, in my experience, are of the highest therapeutic value. This rank was given to them years ago by Jahr in his *Clinical Guide*, wherein he says : ''The symptoms of a case if arranged as to their value will fall into three classes : First and most important, the cause of the disease ; second in value, the aggravations and ameliorations ; third and lowest in value, the symptoms proper, *i. e.*, character, location, direction of pains, etc.''

Unfortunately in many cases the cause of the trouble cannot be determined, but where it can be ascertained with any large degree of probability, half our work is done. At the same time it must be confessed that the number of remedies which can be administered according to causal indications is somewhat small, but where such application is possible the remedial influence makes itself manifest, as a rule, very soon. I have seen so often and with such marked rapidity, curative effects from the administration, following the causal indication, of such remedies as *arnica, conium, belladonna, arsenic, staphysagria, rhus, dulcamara, ranunculus,* and many others, that I am glad indeed when I can find a causal indication in a case, and I am sure that many other physicians have had similar experiences. A collection of such causal indications would, if contributed by the active workers in our ranks, be of the highest importance, and if this suggestion can arouse any number of my hearers to concerted action looking to this end, it will, I am sure, be of great profit to all. Why the cause of a disease should keep up the initial impulse which started into activity the disease process is a question that I am not able to answer ; that it does so is, I think, amply proven by the remarkable success following a prescription based upon such causal indication. It is difficult to get the early symptoms of a case which has lasted for months or years, but the causal factor is often known to the patient. To prescribe accordingly is not symptomatic prescribing, but such theoretical prescribing is to be commended and urged.

DR. S. G. SHARTEY, reports a case of infantile paralysis which remained through life—the patient, a man, dying at the age of sixty years from epithelioma.— *Jour. des Soc. Sci.*

AMMONIUM CARBONICUM.

By HENRY M. DEARBORN, M.D.,
New York.

THIS drug is a union of the atoms of hydrogen, oxygen, nitrogen and carbon, and its molecular formula is $2 N H_4 O, 3 CO_2$. Its composition is stated to be one equivalent of bicarbonate of ammonia, one equivalent of mono-carbonate, and the same of water—making, if pure, a sesqui-carbonate.

According to another theory, which supposes the existence of the quasi metal, ammonium—the equivalents of water disappear and the salt becomes a sesqui-carbonate of oxide of ammonium. In this theory also there is a strong analogy to the salts of the alkali metals in molecular formation, as well as chemical properties.

Ammonium carb. has been obtained from various sources; it is said to have originally been prepared from decomposed urine; in recent times it has been manufactured by subliming the muriate or sulphate of ammonia with carbonate of lime, the former having first been produced from coal gas liquor and bone spirit.

Freshly prepared *ammonium carbonicum* is fibrous and crystaline in appearance, in white, hard and translucent masses of pungent ammoniacal taste and smell.

It has an alkaline reaction and changes turmeric paper held over it, brown, by the escaping mono-carbonate; if this continue, it gradually passes into the bicarbonate, becomes opaque and falls into powder and loses its power to change turmeric paper, even when evaporated by heat.

It is completely soluble in both *cold* water and alcohol, but is decomposed in hot water or spirit with escape of carbonic acid; it is also decomposed or changed by acids, acid and earthy salts, lime water, etc.

Carbonate of ammonia is the chief ingredient of common smelling salts; it has been used for medicinal purposes in the form of ointments and plasters externally, and internally in doses up to thirty grains, in pill form, or more often in mixture with mucilage. Homœopathic preparations are triturations and percussion potencies, beginning with the fifth centesimal and aqueous solutions, commencing with the first, and carried up to the 1,000, if not higher. In what trituration or dilution the drug disappears or becomes incorporated in milk sugar or alcohol so closely as not to be detected, I am unable to state.

Applied to the skin, carbonate of ammonia first stimulates, and later, if continued, irritates, and is absorbed probably in small quantity. Placed at the nose, the mono-carbonate escapes, stimulating the mucous membrane of the air passages, especially the nose, with increased secretion, at the same time the heart action becomes stronger, and sensations from increased circulation follow.

Introduced into the stomach in sufficient quantity, it neutralizes the gastric juice and excites the action of the mucous lining; the process of digestion is retarded by its alkaline effects, unless an excess of acid is present, when it may be a temporary aid to digestion. In twenty to thirty-grain doses it acts as an emetic. It probably passes into the circulation in union with the acid of the stomach; but in excess it may pass by osmosis into the blood without molecular change, there to break up into its primary elements, or form other compounds. The blood plasma normally contains all the simple elements of *ammonium carbonicum*, either free or combined in proximate principles; and, to some extent, they are present as gases. The changes which it undergoes in the blood are little understood. Ammonia exists in the blood in small amount in health and is constantly eliminated; this elimination is increased when carbonate of ammonia is taken into the body, but whether direct or indirect through tissue waste, is uncertain; as an alkaline element in the blood, it helps to maintain its fluidity, although the escape of it does not cause coagulation, as once supposed. The carbonate has been said to be the noxious principle in the circulation, in cases of uræmic poisoning, but this is not supported by proof, unless the large exhalation of ammónia from the lungs in that condition can be regarded as such.

Whatever the chemical or vital transformations are in the blood, the result is increased heart action and blood pressure of short duration, followed by lower than normal blood pressure, unless the dose is repeated; increased circulation is accompanied with more color in the skin and a general sensation of warmth, beginning at the pit of the stomach, also with feelings of greater physical strength. These results are more decided if the *ammonium carbonicum* is injected directly into the venous circulation, showing its action is somewhat modified by the changes it probably undergoes in the stomach or mechanism of absorption. Its effects on the nervous system are explained by augmented circulation, irritation of sensory nerves and reflex action.

The continued use of carbonate of ammonia interferes with digestion and causes irritation of mucous membranes of stomach, bowels and respiratory tract. Like the fixed alkalies, it causes waste of tissue; in sufficient amount in the blood it injures the red globules and retards nutrition, which, together with disturbance of digestion and increased waste is manifested by emaciation, loss of color and feebleness.

This drug is said by Bartholow to be a physiological antagonist to hydrocyanic acid.

The high rate of diffusion and volatility of *ammonium carbonicum* are named as reasons for its rapid elimination; it is thrown out in the sweat in small quantity, and has been classed with diaphoretics.

A larger proportion passes off by the lungs, stimulating secretion, and by its alkaline properties helps to render liquid the products of inflammation, if present, or is claimed to do as a so-called expectorant. The largest elimination is through the kidneys, with increased action of these organs, and, in sufficient doses, renders the urine alkaline.

The physiological action of *ammonium carbonicum*, as understood at the present time, may be summed up briefly as an excitant and irritant locally to the skin and mucous membranes, with antacid or alkaline effects, local and general; in the blood it stimulates the heart, increasing circulation with subjective nervous phenomena, irritative and reflex, and is eliminated by kidneys (chiefly), lungs and skin, with usually increased action of these parts, and is characterized by rapid and brief effects; long used, it causes great depression, disorganization of the blood and tissue changes.

In toxicological doses the action resembles the other alkalies, except in being more rapid and accompanied with more marked dyspnœa, but with better chances of recovery after the first stage is past; death may take place quickly from collapse, or later from disorganization of mucous membrane of stomach and bowels.

PROVINGS.—It is not purposed here to give any list of symptoms which may be found systematically arranged in works on materia medica. Allen, in his work, collected 1,010 symptoms, nearly 800 of which were recorded by Hahnemann and his fellow observers. The number of symptoms is surprisingly large for a drug whose obvious action is so rapid and brief; beginning with chemical changes of varying degree, it passes quickly into the blood and has barely time to leave its impress upon the tissues of the body before it is expelled with the excretions. When an agent like *ammonium carbonicum* has credited to its pathogenesis a large number of distinct symptoms, it is a logical inference that they represent not only the largely varying differences of a few individual provers, but also a great variance in defining the same phenomena.

Most of the symptoms have their origin: first, from effects of *stimulation;* second, from *irritation;* and third, from *disorganisation* of blood and tissues, either with or without consecutive inflammation.

These effects of the drug may follow each other with comparative slowness, or in large or toxic doses, with marvelous rapidity. The stimulant action comes with increased blood pressure and corresponding functional activity, notably of mucous surfaces. The mental sphere does not, however, share in the general augmented activity, but remains unaffected or depressed, with a varying headache of a full, bursting character. In the stage of irritation functional activity is diminished and secretions changed in character, and both sensory and reflex nervous symptoms appear, of greater or less intensity. With the disorganizing effects on the blood and blood corpuscles, impairment of nutrition is manifest in general exhaustion, hemorrhages, local tissue change, or low grade inflammation—such as infiltration and induration of glands, serous effusions, boils, pustular eruptions, redness of the skin, resembling scarlatina or erysipelas, etc.

Therapeutical uses.—It might seem, from a superficial consideration of *ammonium carb.*, that from its chemical properties and rapid course of physiological action, it was better adapted to antipathic rather than homœopathic application in the treatment of disease; in fact it holds a more fixed and prominent place in the therapeutics of the old school than in those of the new school; but no one who carefully examines the records of cases of poisoning and of the effects produced on animals by this drug, and then notes the conditions existing when it is most successfully used in free doses, can fail to detect its homœopathic relation to disease, even in the ordinary doses prescribed by practitioners of the old school. The size of the curative dose does not impair its homœopathicity.

The *headache* caused by use of *ammonium carb.* in health is of two kinds. First, a primary headache due to blood pressure, most severe in the temples, and aggravated by closing teeth hard (Guernsey). Similar headaches are relieved by small doses of this drug. In this class of headaches, however, more often the indications point to other remedies—*aconite, bell., bry.*, etc. The second variety of headache is reflex, with a dull, confused feeling in the head, and associated with general physical and mental depression. It subsides with the local disturbances which gave rise to it.

Nasal catarrhs, beginning with acrid, watery discharge and lachrymation, followed by dry sensations in the nose, obstruction and forced mouth breathing, worse at night, and in *long lasting* colds in the head, especially of children, *am. carb.* is a very useful drug. In some of these cases it may be used with advantage by olfaction. I have seen obstinate coryzas greatly benefited by the drug administered in the latter way, or by the mouth, other remedies having failed to give relief.

In *pharyngitis* and *tonsillitis*, when there are burning and rough-
ness of throat, or in low inflammatory states of the throat of the
putrid, ulcerative or gangrenous forms, *am. carb.* may share the
honors, with *baptisia, mer.* and *mur. ac.*

Chronic laryngitis, with much dryness and hoarseness, worse from
speaking, *am. carb.* has benefited.

It is useful in *gastritis* and *gastro-enteritis*, when the parts are sensitive to pressure, with oppressed feelings after eating and from contact of clothing, empty sensations, eructations and vomiting of all
food.

In *dysmenorrhœa, metrorrhagia* and *leucorrhœa*, not dependent on
local conditions alone, but having systemic depression, poor quality
of blood favoring hemorrhages, menses premature and too free, sometimes with bleeding from the rectum, cholera-like colic before, and
with the flow and whitish leucorrhœa between the menses, *ammonium
carb.* is one of the best remedies.

In cases of *bronchitis* or *broncho-pneumonia* (later stages) when the
respiratory symptoms are proportionately more severe than the local
state of bronchi or lungs, indicating irritation of respiratory tract in
medulla (probably from vitiated blood) and hence very frequent
respirations, oppression of breathing, violent asthmatic or loose cough,
contractions of the chest, bloody and difficult expectoration, stitches
and burning sensations, symptoms aggravated by moving and generally present depression of mind and body, *am. carb.* is a superior
remedy.

In severe *scarlatina*, when the zymotic poison early and profoundly
affects the blood, as evidenced by hard, glandular swelling of the neck
and gangrenous ulceration of the throat, *am. carb.* has often proved of
service. It is also serviceable in *erysipelas* of old people of low
vitality, listless and dejected mind, and showing a tendency to gangrenous destruction of the skin.

Dr. Thomas Nichol *names it as a remedy in *small-pox* with
hemorrhagic and gangrenous tendencies, putrid sore throat and
extreme prostration.

This summary does not include all the pathological states in which
am. carb. might be a valuable curative remedy, and in the diseases
named more often other remedies are indicated; but its pathogenetic
relation to morbid conditions have been traced enough to show that it
does not deserve the neglected place it now holds in homœopathic
therapeutics.

---

* N. E. Med. Gazette, vol. xxi., p. 522.

Three things are essential, I believe, to the best use of *ammonium carbonicum.* First, it should be used in *dilution freshly prepared;* second, it should be dispensed from *stoppered bottles,* and not from open glasses; and third, it should be given *low.*

The first two essentials are self-evident by reason of the unstable chemical nature of the drug, and experience has proved that the lower dilutions (first, second and third decimals) act best in most instances where it is indicated, while in the severer types of disease which simulate the poisonous or prolonged effects, the administration of 1, 2 or 3 grains at a time becomes a proper homœopathic dose, and the writer does not hesitate to assert acts with the greater promptness the closer the existing similarity.

INSPECTION AS AN AID TO DIAGNOSIS IN DISEASES OF THE CIRCULATORY AND RESPIRATORY ORGANS.*

By J. W. DOWLING, M.D.,
New York.

IT is customary for the diagnostician, in making an examination in any given case, to first make a careful inspection of the body, noting all that is abnormal—and by abnormal in this connection is understood any physical sign which under any circumstances could be the result of disease process in any portion of the body—and at such times, that a proper comparison may be made, always endeavoring to carry in his mind's eye the form and appearance of the perfectly modeled and healthy man or woman.

The artist studies models of health and beauty, till he becomes an expert in matters relating to the form of the human body, even in its minutiæ. You will hear him expatiate on what constitutes the beautiful, the perfect mouth, nose, eye, forehead, ear and how these should be combined to form the perfect face, till you wonder and are actually alarmed at your lack of knowledge of the human form and face divine. Losing sight of the beautiful and perfect, the expert diagnostician will detect and point out imperfections, many of them apparently so trifling as to escape the eye of the ordinary observer, but insignificant as they are, indicating most positive pathological changes in organs vital to life, conditions which have been progressing for years and of which the patient is totally unaware; one glance

---

* Read before the Homœopathic Medical Society of the County of New York, March 10th, 1887.

will sometimes tell him of indiscretions of the past, of the present; will tell him of the future of the individual as regards health, the probabilities as to life, and in many instances the probable mode of death.

To the enthusiast in this line of research every form and face is a study ; he notices the spinal curves, the manner in which the head is carried, whether the shoulders be on a level, whether they be thrown forward, the shape of the thorax and abdomen, the gait, the position assumed in lying or sitting, the color of the skin, a diminution from the normal as regards the amount of adipose tissue, or a superabundance of the same.

He notices pathological changes in the superficial blood vessels, the course of the temporal arteries, the pulsations of these vessels, as well as those of the vessels of the neck.

He notices the appearance of the eye—its expression, and whether the pupil be unusually large or contracted ; whether the cornea has undergone degenerative changes, and notes if there be unnatural puffs on the cheek-bones, premature lining of the face and œdematous swellings beneath the eyes. Frequently before he has advanced to palpation, mensuration, percussion or auscultation, he has formed an opinion as to the condition of the various organs of the body, which is confirmed by his subsequent thorough and complete examination.

It will be impossible in the time allotted to me this evening to dwell at length on the visible physical signs of diseases of the respiratory and circulatory organs. I shall therefore content myself with an enumeration of them and dwell briefly on the significance of some often overlooked, but which are really of grave importance in the diagnosis of disease.

Changes in the color of the skin, the most common of which is blanching, are rarely overlooked and are so common to various forms of disease, that as a rule they are thoroughly understood, and the cause is generally investigated. Except in cases of pigmentation, the color of the skin is dependent on the quantity of blood circulating in the superficial vessels, and on the quality of this fluid. Unusual redness is an evidence of dilatation of the blood vessels on the surface, and this dilatation may be temporary, arising from vaso-motor paralysis, or it may be permanent, and under such circumstances would lead us to suspect hypertrophy of the walls of the left ventricle, possibly with insufficiency of the aortic valve.

Cyanosis is always of serious import, and whether diffused or appearing only at the points where it first shows itself and is always the most marked—namely, in the lips, on the point of the nose, on the eyelids, nails, tips of the elbows and the front of the knees—is positive evidence that the blood is not properly arterialized. This excess of carbonic acid in the blood may be, and generally is, evidence of grave disease either of the respiratory organs or of the heart.

Blanching of the skin is common to all debilitating diseases and often arises from vaso-motor irritation which prevents a proper filling of the capillaries of the skin ; under such circumstances it is but temporary, when persistent it is conclusive evidence that either the quantity of blood in the vessels is less than normal, or that it is pathologically changed in quality by a deficiency in the number of blood discs, or by a diminished amount of hæmoglobine, the number of red globules being normal or nearly so.

Where this blanching exists our attention would naturally be called to the heart or lungs, for it is from diseases of these organs that it is often most pronounced.

The so-called "phthisical habit" is familiar to every student of medicine, and is generally an evidence of phthisis or a predisposition to it. That great pathologist, Niemeyer, said : "This term is used to signify that peculiar build of the body indicative of a want of proper nutrition and development, and which is found in persons who have been subjected to debilitating influence capable of stunting the healthy growth of the system before their bodies have become fully developed. The bones of such persons are slender, their skin is thin, their cheeks have a delicate redness, the sclerotica is bluish, the subcutaneous connective tissue contains but little fat, the muscles are ill developed ; those of the neck allow the thorax to sink, causing the neck to seem too long. The intercostal muscles permit the ribs to spread apart, making the intercostal spaces broader ; the angle at which the ribs are attached to the sternum is more acute ; the entire chest is flatter, narrower and longer than in robust, muscular persons. The shoulders also are apt to sink forward and the inner edges of the scapulæ are tipped up like wings." He adds : "Many persons possessing such a conformation do live exempt from phthisis and attain a good old age. But such a circumstance does not in the least conflict with the belief that the phthisical habit is a valuable index of feebleness and delicacy of constitution, hence of a tendency to consumption."

There is greater danger that a catarrh at the apex of the lung will invade the air vesicles in a patient of this kind than in a muscular and robust man. Add to this picture of the phthisical habit, superficial breathing, with but little movement of the ribs in inspiration, a depression in one or both supraclavicular regions with perhaps a fossa beneath the clavicle of one or both sides, and the characteristic hectic flush, and you can, without advancing beyond inspection in your physical examination, diagnose almost to a certainty advancing destruction of the lung, or pulmonary consumption.

But it is not to these grosser signs of pulmonary and heart disease—signs familiar to all—that I wish to call attention to-night, but to signs which are too often overlooked and which, when they exist, are evidences of pathological changes which often endanger life and which require on the part of the individual bearing them the greatest care to avoid sudden serious illness, or even sudden death.

Many of these are visible on inspection of the face alone.

Probably the most important of these signs of danger are the full and tortuous temporal arteries. The temporal artery in the perfectly healthy man or woman is scarcely perceptible to inspection, but in those who have undermined their constitutions by reckless living, whether it be in matters relating to food or drink, heavy and prolonged mental strain, or excessive physical strain, the temporal artery enlarges and becomes lengthened, and to accommodate this increase in its length it becomes tortuous and is sometimes entirely misplaced from its normal position. While the nutrition is good it is full and bounding and its pulsations are visible to the eye; later, while the end is gradually approaching, the pulsations cease to be visible, the artery is compressible and the vessel is lost to ordinary inspection. Accompanying this state of the temporal artery there are frequently visible twigs of dilated vessels upon the cheek bones, on the alæ of the nose and on the ears; these twigs are atheromatous vessels and are, as a rule, indicative of a like change going on in vessels permeating vital organs—the brain, the heart, the kidneys. What is their significance? The condition mentioned of these vessels of the forehead and face is evidence of hypertrophy of the walls of the left ventricle of the heart, which in itself is not a disease, but compensatory and calculated to overcome the obstruction to the blood current in these vessels, for here the disease process has commenced; but this very compensating enlargement of the walls of the heart becomes dangerous to life, for an extra effort, mental or physical, involving, as it does, increased heart force, is liable to rupture one of these atheromatous vessels at its weakest point, and that is often in the brain, and apoplexy results from the cerebral hæmorrhage. Small capillary aneurisms are very common in the brains of such subjects, and a trifling effort often ruptures their walls; sometimes the flow of blood is so small that the effect is trifling, a slight paresis of one side of the face, a little thickening of the speech, a shuffling gate, passing off in a few days; at other times the flow is so great as to produce serious, often fatal, results.

This occurs often in the midst of health and vigor, while the temporal artery is full and bounding and the heart strong.

If this is escaped and the period is reached when the temporal loses its prominence, another significant physical sign often makes its appearance to inspection of the face; I refer to the so-called *arcus senilis*, not the white, calcareous *arcus* which so frequently involves the entire circumference of the cornea and encircles the pupil like a ring, and which is often seen in the apparent vigor of health in lithæmic subjects, but the yellowish arc, the fatty arc—for it is in reality a fatty degeneration of the cornea and appears on its upper border—it is an evidence of fatty degeneration of the heart; not that there is any direct relationship between the heart and the cornea, but as atheromatous vessels in the face are evidence of an atheromatous process in the vessels of other portions of the body, so fatty degeneration of the cornea is evidence of fatty disease, of fatty degeneration in other portions of the body; and experience tells us that this fatty *arcus senilis* is a frequent accompaniment of fatty degeneration of the walls of the heart, where an autopsy has done away with the possibility of a mistake in diagnosis.

Fatty degeneration of the heart is the ultimate result in the cases I have been describing, if the patient be unfortunate enough not to be stricken with fatal apoplexy, or to die of some accidental disease or injury. I say *unfortunate* enough, for I can imagine no greater blessing in such a condition, than to be stricken down, as was the lamented Beecher, in the midst of apparent health, vigor and usefulness.

Visible pulsations of the carotid arteries are always significant signs. Ordinarily these arteries, or rather their pulsations, are not visible to inspection; when they are, it is an indication of a plethoric condition of the system with a powerful, perhaps hypertrophied, hard working heart. This condition of the vessels of the neck arises also from aortic insufficiency with compensatory hypertrophy of the walls of the left ventricle. Where this lesion of the aortic valve exists, if the nutrition be good, and it occurs before the heart walls begin to fail, if the patient live long enough, the pulsations in all of the arteries is more pronounced than is normal, and the arteries finally become dilated. I have seen cases of aortic insufficiency where the arterial first sound could be heard distinctly through the stethoscope placed over the wrist. Frequently the *arteria innominata* is dilated to such an extent that it can be seen to pulsate in the supra-sternal notch.

There is another pulsation in the neck, a physical sign of grave omen. I refer to the pulsation of the jugular veins. This is always an evidence of approaching left-sided heart failure or of obstruction to the proper emptying of the right ventricle, as in croupous pneumonia involving a large area, or in pulmonary vesicular emphysema.

In mitral or aortic disease, when the walls of the left heart become weakened and the contents of the left ventricle are not freely sent into the aorta, there is, of course, great pulmonary engorgement, and the right ventricle fails in its efforts to expel its contents, and consequently dilates, sometimes to such an extent as to render the tricuspid valve insufficient to close the auriculo-ventricular orifice ; under such circumstances there is imperfect emptying of the auricle above, and the veins emptying into it. With every contraction an impulse is conveyed to the column of blood in the auricle, and thence to that in the descending *vena cava*, and thence to that in the jugular veins. If in doubt whether a pulsation in the neck be in the carotid artery or in the jugular vein the doubt can be dismissed by simple pressure with the finger ; it will be difficult to compress the carotid to such an extent as to obliterate the pulsation above the point of pressure, and even then the pulsation will be more pronounced below that point; but if the pulsation be in the jugular vein pressure will readily obliterate it. Slight pressure under such circumstances will prevent the return current of blood and that which is in the vein below the point of pressure will flow onward into the *vena cava descendens*, and there will be no column of blood in the vein below that point to receive the impression from that in the vena cava. As was said, this sign is of grave omen, and is rarely found in cases of valvular disease till great heart weakness is fully established.

In this connection, to leave the face, a pulsation is sometimes visible over the hepatic region from a like cause, and nearly always in the epigastrium from concussion of the dilated, often hypertrophied, right heart, against the left lobe of the liver.

A very pretty physical sign of weak heart is prominence of the veins of the arms, when the arms are permttted to hang down; always disappearing if the hands are elevated above the head ; often the location of the valves of the veins can be made out by the prominence of the vessels at these points.

All of these signs are visible on inspection of the patient before he has bared the chest or abdomen.

There are many, on inspection of the thorax, the shape of the chest, the extent of præcordial pulsation, the location of the apex beat, pulsations in unusual localities, the latter evidences of aortic aneurisms, or of a misplaced heart, from congenital transposition or traction from a cicatrised lung, or from the pressure of a pleuritic exudation with the traction of the lung of the opposite side.

Frequently is seen on the chests of phthisical cases a blue net-work of vessels. This is an evidence of adhesion of the two layers of the pleura at that point. Niemeyer explained this. He said: "Many branches of the pulmonary artery becoming destroyed in phthisis, those of the bronchial dilate, and conduct arterial blood to the lungs. Many newly-formed vessels, springing from the intercostal arteries, also advance through pleuritic exudations into the lung."

Thus the phthisical lung receives more arterial blood than the sound lung; part of it passes into the pulmonary veins, a part into the bronchial veins, and a third portion passes through the pleuritic adhesions into the intercostal veins, as the discharge of blood from the cutaneous veins into the over-loaded intercostal veins is thus impeded they, too, are apt to become over-filled and distended, and *a blue network of veins appears on the skin of the thorax.*

Oedema and dropsy show themselves on inspection—that in the face generally in the loose cellular tissue beneath the eye; if appearing here first always being an evidence of an hydræmic condition of the blood from loss of albumen, owing to Bright's disease, or arising from profuse hæmorrhage; that appearing first in the feet being an evidence of heart disease; and when appearing first in the peritoneal cavity being an evidence of portal obstruction, probably due to cirrhosis of the liver, but sometimes this latter form of dropsy is due to disease of the peritoneum itself.

In a case of general dropsy, with evidence of cardiac, liver, and kidney disease, if in doubt as to which of these organs was first affected, the question (properly answered), 'When did the dropsy first appear?' will set aside all doubts.*

SALICYLATE OF SODIUM POISONING.—A woman, æt. 55, took 120 grains salicylate of sodium in 30 grain doses, four hours apart. On admission to St. Mary's Hospital, London, where she applied for relief, she complained of a buzzing noise in the ears, some headache, and great deafness; she was naturally slightly deaf. The pupils were extremely contracted. The urine contained a large quantity of salicylic acid and albumen. The albuminuria persisted after the acid had disappeared from the urine. Three days afterward the symptoms, including the albuminuria, had disappeared.—*Brit. Med. Jour.*, February 5th, 1887.

---

* The different points in physical examination, dwelt upon in the paper, were demonstrated upon the chests of a large number of patients brought before the Society by the author.—ED.

BAPTISIA IN TYPHOID FEVER.*

By B. G. CLARK, M.D.,
New York.

THERE has been much written in regard to the virtues of this remedy in typhoid fever. Among the most noteworthy was a paper read before the British Homœopathic Congress of 1872, by Dr. Richard Hughes. In his *Pharmacodynamics*, third edition, he thus refers to this paper : "It is on this point that the interest of *baptisia* is centred. I have collected, in this paper referred to, fifty-three recorded cases of continued fever, in all of which, the effect of the medicine was either to induce a speedy crisis or materially to abate and curtail the disease."

In the discussion which followed its reading at the Congress, speaker after speaker rose up to confirm from his own experience this estimate of its value, and there was not a dissentient voice. Two of those who spoke were from the United States, and it was from this source that we first heard of its virtues and reputation.

Among the reports, examined in the paper, is one on the treatment of the "colonial fever" of Melbourne, and Dr. Kitching has just given us his experience with the corresponding disorder at the Cape, where he has found *baptisia* as potent as Dr. Madden found it in Victoria. So, from four continents the fame of the medicine comes borne to us ; and we cannot but give it a full consideration and trial. * * * *

"My own observations and inquiries dispose me to think that, excluding febricula, there is but one non-epidemic species of low fever, and that is the enteric. The typhus and relapsing forms are seen only in large towns, or under peculiar circumstances. Typhoid is constant everywhere in greater or less degree, having every now and then, from local causes, a special outbreak. It is the epidemic fever of all countries, having many names and many varieties of manifestation, but characterized everywhere by the specific process it sets up in the Peyerian and solitary glands of the intestines. If this be so, then it is for typhoid, that we have in *baptisia* a remedy so strongly accredited. I need hardly point out the claim set up for it.

"Typhoid is a disease of such frequent occurrence and such ghastly mortality ; it invades such high quarters, and threatens, if it does not actually destroy, such valuable lives ; it has, even when not fatal, so lengthened a process, so tedious a convalescence, such frequent sequelæ

---

* Read before the Homœopathic Medical Society, County of New York, February 10th, 1887.

of even direr import than itself, that any professing addition to our power of controlling it, cannot but be welcomed. Especially is it so, when the promise held out is of more than mitigation of severity only, more than sustainment of the patient ; when it is of actual abortion and breaking up of the disease, we shall, without controversy, have gained a priceless remedy."

Dr. Hughes then speaks of the pathogenetic action of *baptisia* and reasons that it is homœopathic to the first stages of typhoid fever, that is, " to the period antecedent to the full development of the intestinal affection."

He then says in closing the article, "I have gone fully into this matter, on account of its great practical importance. I hope that the facts alleged may induce some of those who hear me, to test the remedy in their own sphere of work, and to report the results.

" It need not be given in infinitesimal quantities. Drop-doses of the mother tincture, or small portions of an infusion were administered in most of the published cases. Such doses, moreover, will probably insure a wider range for the medicine.

"The tendency in America just now is to restrict its action in typhoid, to cases in which its minutest symptomatology is reproduced—as soreness in lying, a sense of being all to pieces, etc. But it will be observed that those who write thus, use the higher dilutions exclusively. For more substantial doses, it seems only necessary that the patient shall be within the first ten days of the fever, or, at any rate, shall not have passed from the 'gastric' into the 'typhoid' condition (I use the terms phenomenally), to ensure excellent effects from the drug."

I have quoted thus at length from Dr. Hughes, that I may not be accused of doing him an injustice. It was from the writings of Dr. Hughes, published as " Letters to a Friend," that I became a believer in the law of "*similia similibus curantur*," and, as a repentant sinner is thankful for the glorious truths of the gospel, so is he grateful to those who have prepared him to receive its blessings. In like manner I wish to record my gratitude to Dr. Hughes for the grand truths his writings first unfolded to me, and although my early obedience to his teachings, I believe, led me to prescribe *baptisia* when it was not the true similimum, the fear that others may do likewise, makes me feel it my duty to offer my feeble protest against this great teacher's advice on this subject. With that confidence borne only in theory, I welcomed my first case of typhoid fever, with feelings of no little assurance that I would soon abort it with *baptisia*. I gave the 3x potency and I had a case of nearly six weeks to attend. I thought I had given it too high, so my next case received three drop-doses of the tincture every three hours.

The second week showed as typical a case of typhoid as one seldom sees. My next case received the 1x, still the case went on regardless of *baptisia*. About this time I met one of the old school physicians, a neighbor of mine, and I asked him how one of his typhoid cases was getting along. He said, "pretty well, but the girl's brother is coming down also, but I expect to break it up." Now that interested me immensely, and I said, "you do? what are you giving him?" "*Baptisia*, fifteen drop-doses of the tincture, four times a day—it's a new remedy." "Is that so," said I, "try it faithfully and we will compare notes. I have used it some." About three weeks, or more, after the above conversation, he said to me, "that case turned out the worst one I ever had."

By this time I came to the conclusion that the cases collected and reported by Dr. Hughes were, to say the least, of a different type from those we had in Vermont. I betook myself to Jahr's Forty Year's Practice, Raue's Pathology and my Materia Medica, for the true similimum, in my next cases, and had much less trouble with them and a much more rapid convalescence. It seems to me that *baptisia* is more often indicated in the later stages when we have the dry, brown streak in the center of the tongue, the patient answers disconnectedly, he cannot get his thoughts together, and he even feels scattered about himself, is very drowsy, with fetid excoriating diarrhœa ; with these indications *baptisia* has done for me good service.

Dr. H. I. Elsner, of Syracuse, N. Y., read a paper before a branch of the N. Y. State Medical Association, June 9th, 1886, on "Typhoid Fever, as we see it in Central New York," in which he makes an observation which seems to me to be correct. He says, "the accurate, skilled and careful observer will be cautious how he makes a diagnosis of any fever during the first week, and yet some of our friends would have us believe that they have cured their patients before *we* have had time to make a diagnosis." Now, if we cannot make a correct diagnosis of typhoid fever before the eighth day, how can we say we had a case of typhoid and aborted it with *baptisia* on the fifth day? It is my opinion that the abortion of typhoid fever on the fifth (or any other day) with *baptisia*, or any other remedy, is a mistake and the abortion is one of diagnosis only. I would like to add here a few words from Dr. Raue's Special Pathology (second edition). "The right remedy cures a disease without a crisis ; and thus we have an indisputable proof that the selected remedy was THE remedy.

"When, after the administration of a homœopathic remedy, a crisis takes place notwithstanding, we may be sure that we did not 'hit' the case, and that the patient got well without our aid." It seems to me that the only way for a disease to terminate if our prescriptions have been correct is by lysis and it should be the aim of every physician to have his cases terminate in that way.

If I have not in your judgment rightly tested *baptisia*, or you have any experience with it that would lead you to different conclusions, I shall be glad to learn of them.

ON THE NECESSITY OF DIFFERENTIATION BETWEEN FALSE AND TRUE CROUP.*

By MALCOLM LEAL, M.D.,
New York.

I HAVE chosen to use the term false croup because it—being a symptomatic designation—is applicable to several pathological conditions. By it I mean any acute, non-membranous affection of the larynx, characterized by dyspnœa, proceeding from laryngeal obstruction.

By true croup I mean any acute *membranous* affection of the larynx, and although not believing in the pathological identity of diphtheria and croup, I shall include both in the above term.

Among the cases of false croup, there is one class in which the diagnosis from symptoms may be quite positive. In this class of cases there occur sharp attacks of suffocation, which are soon over, ending in partial asphyxiation, and unconsciousness, from which the patient rallies and is for a time free from dyspnœa. Or an attack may progress more gradually but still rapidly to an almost complete stenosis, but it readily yields to remedies and recovery quickly ensues. Such attacks are usually purely spasmodic.

The cases to which I wish to call your attention particularly are those in which the severity of the symptoms of laryngeal obstruction gradually increases, without intermission, for a period of several days, when the dyspnœa becomes alarming.

This condition suggests several pathological states, the prognosis and treatment of which differ very decidedly.

CASE I.—On the 11th of January I was called to see a little girl, five years old, who, two weeks after an attack of measles, had had a cold with slight hoarseness, and croupy night-cough. As she had

---

*Read before the Homœopathic Medical Society of the County of New York, March 10th, 1887.

been subject to attacks of *laryngitis catarrhalis*, her mother had not given her any special attention ; but when, after several days, the child complained of sore throat, I was sent for. I found my patient to be a well-built, rosy cheeked blonde, nervous and spoiled.

She complained of painful deglutition. The cervical glands, especially on the right side, were enlarged and tender. The tongue was coated with a thin, white fur, through which, at the lip, projected enlarged and reddened papillæ. The temperature was not taken, but there was little if any fever. The pulse was full, regular and quickened by excitement. A few discreet spots of exudation could be seen on each tonsil, more numerous on the left. Hoarseness was quite marked, but the larynx could not be examined as the child would not permit it, and the mother was not strong enough to hold her.

The next day, January 12th, the hoarseness was more marked, but the exudative spots on the tonsils were less numerous and thinner.

On the 13th my case record reads : "Exudation has disappeared from tonsils ; but on both sides of posterior wall of pharynx near tonsils are thick patches, membranous in character, each about 3 *m.m.* in diameter, and surrounded with a narrow areola of redness. Hoarseness more marked, and breathing slightly stridulous. Larynx cannot be examined. Patient bright and playing around room. Pulse good ; face flushed and plump (as is natural)."

In spite of the good condition of the circulation, a guarded diagnosis of diphtheria was given.

January 14th, at 2 p.m. The laryngeal stridor was marked ; with retraction of epigastrium ; aphonic cough with tenacious sputum, free from shreds of membrane.

No examination was made, the child becoming too much excited at mention of it to expect any result.

At 6 p.m., she was reported as being worse, and I prepared to intubate the larynx, making an appointment with Drs. Beebe and A. W. Palmer, to meet me in consultation with that end in view.

At nine o'clock in the evening we saw her, and found her much worse. No pulmonary sounds could be heard. Respiration was shallow and all accessory muscles were brought into use.

The child was perspiring ; the face flushed, and without that drawn appearance of the mouth so common in diphtheria. We decided to force an examination of the larynx before resorting to intubation ; so she was held firmly while Dr. Beebe introduced the mirror.

The examination showed that the pharyngeal exudation had entirely disappeared ; and, to our utter surprise, not a trace of membrane was to be seen in the larynx.

The anterior two-thirds of the cords were rigidly approximated, both in inspiration and expiration, while posteriorily the triangular inter-artyenoid opening was left. There was intense congestion, but no swelling whatever. Intubation was postponed and remedies relied upon. At the same time Dr. Palmer remained during the night, having O'Dwyer's tubes and tracheotomy instruments ready for use in case of need.

January 15th, at 8 a.m., the condition was much the same but gradually grew worse until towards evening, when patient became more quiet, and by midnight, loose bronchial rales were heard through-out the chest.

January 16th. No change, except that stridor was not quite as constant. Epigastric retraction, and motion of alæ nasi still the same. In the afternoon respiration was easier, 30–36 ; bronchial rales were more sibilant ; cough looser.

January 17th, 8 a.m. Case record reads : "Pulse full and strong—about 120 ; respiration, 28–30 and easier; cough more aphonic and dry." Pulmonary sounds obscure though respiration is deeper. At mid-night I was sent for, as patient was reported as very restless, starting from sleep and clutching at throat. I found her sleeping, breathing more quietly than in the morning. Sibilant rales were heard over both lungs posteriorily. Laryngeal obstruction moderate.

Without continuing the daily history of the case, I may say that by the 20th the laryngeal stridor had disappeared, leaving the child com-pletely aphonic ; that by February 1st the aphonia gave way to hoarse-ness, which has now, March 10th, almost entirely disappeared.

Without the aid of the laryngoscope, this case would undoubtedly have been diagnosed as membranous laryngitis, and had intubation or tracheotomy been performed, an unnecessary operation would have gained the credit of the cure. It is a question now as to the correct diagnosis, whether the stenosis were due in part to diphtheritic paralysis of the abductors of the larynx, or to spasm of all the adductors except the inter-arytenoid muscles. I do not know, though I am in-clined to consider the former condition as being largely instrumental in producing the symptoms.

Case II.—Dr. T. C. Williams kindly permits me to refer to a case of his, in which I was called with the idea of performing tracheotomy, the night of December 19th, 1885. The child had suffered from a progressively increasing dyspnœa, and when seen, the laryngeal stridor was very severe and constant. Examination revealed absence of membrane ; moderate œdema of epiglottis with spasm of adduction of the glottis. The use of steam and anti-spasmodic remedies saved the child from tracheotomy, to which otherwise might have been given the credit of a cure of membranous croup.

Case III.—Boy, æt. 6.—On the twenty-ninth October '84' developed a peculiar tonsillitis, which in six days gave place to croupy cough with stridor which had increased to an alarming extent on the seventh of November. Examination showed an œdematous laryngitis, which gradually yielded to treatment and terminated in recovery.

Case IV.—In November last was called by Dr. B. G. Carleton to see a woman æt. thirty-five, who had had gradually increasing suffo-cative attacks, with remissions, but no intermissions, for some hours. The case was supposed to be one of œdema, and tracheotomy was prepared for. Examination revealed tonic spasm which steam and other remedies relieved in a few hours.

Many other cases might be recounted illustrative of the same point but they would be merely repetitions of those already referred to.

Two of the forms of false croup, namely, œdematous laryngitis, and paralysis of the abductors of the glottis, must be watched carefully, for operative interference *may* become necessary at any time. The result of tracheotomy in such cases is usually good, the dangers arising from the operation itself being the only ones to fear. In cases of spasm, however, I cannot but believe that relief may always be secured by other means.

• There are cases, as I have said, where there is little if any doubt as to the cause of the trouble, but it is impossible from the symptoms alone to differentiate between :—tonic spasm of the adductors, paresis of the abductors, œdema glottidis, and some cases of membranous laryngitis. A laryngoscopic examination is necessary to enable us to determine which condition exists. True, a digital examination may enable us to recognize œdema ; but even that is uncertain, for it by no means follows that, because the epiglottis is œdematous, the glottic margins are in the same condition.

Such examination as is necessary need not be referred to a specialist. The conditions are well marked and easily recognized. The difficulties attending the examination of a child are the same to all.

Furthermore, the treatment of a paralysis of one set of muscles is probably directly opposed to the treatment of a spasm of the opposite set, and I am not prepared at present to believe that the treatment of an œdematous laryngitis, a spasmodic laryngitis, and a membranous laryngitis is the same, even though the external symptoms are the same.

But suppose, if you please, that the treatment *does* depend on the external symptoms alone, the question of prognosis is an important one. There are few of us who have not at some time felt the need of a correct diagnosis to aid us when asked, "will the patient get well?" With what a feeling of relief the physician can go home and to sleep when he knows that the suffocative attacks are purely spasmodic, no one knows but those who have experienced it.

The important question then, is one of diagnosis.

Is the obstruction spasmodic, paralytic, œdematous or membranous? and the answer is to be found by following a very simple rule, "look and see."

A PLEA FOR PURE HOMŒOPATHY IN OUR COLLEGES.*

By S. LILIENTHAL, M.D.,
New York.

WHERE there is so much smoke there must be a fire; and even if it arise only from burning out the chimney, it may be advisable off and on to follow the careful attention of the good housewife and see to it that everything in our household is in order.

In the February number of the *Homœopathic Physician*, my old and, venerable friend, Dr. P. P. Wells, of Brooklyn, opens fire against all homœopathic colleges, and accuses them of many sins of omission and commission:

1. Doctors speak of the necessity of a better medical education and the members of our college faculties *talk*, but never tell us how the want is to be supplied. They never have a thought that this better education can only come from better teaching. Even some changes made must be put on the wrong side, for a little more than a year ago one of our colleges made it the duty of one of their professors to teach the manner of preparation and the *use* of pukes, purges and poultices.

2. The *Organon* is hardly ever taught in any homœopathic college. In one, three attempts were made to *talk* of the *Organon* and were miserable failures.

3. Adjuvantia are openly advocated without exhausting the mental effort to find out the similimum to a given case; for this similimum is the *grand good thing* in homœopathy.

4. A homœopathic medical education consists of a thorough knowledge of homœopathic law and its corollaries, together with a knowledge of how to apply the science of therapeutics, founded on these, for the cure of the sick.

5. Why is it that such a homœopathic medical education is neglected in our colleges? and if an exceptional teacher tries to do his duty to the pupils, he is made to feel that he labors in a fighting opposition to his colleagues, and that in so doing he exposes himself to the danger of losing his place. And when he asks where is a homœopathic medical education to be gained, echo answers—ALMOST NOWHERE.

These are grave charges; and though we are convinced that Doctor Wells, in his blind zeal, may have gone too far, still it cannot be denied that there is much truth in his article; and when I asked

*Read before the Homœopathic Medical Society County of New York, February 10th, 1887.

myself, have such college matters anything to do with the Bureau of Materia Medica of the Homœopathic County Society, my conscience approved of the choice of this essay, for from the ranks of our younger members the future professors must be chosen ; and it is the duty of every college that its pupils know how to teach and how to apply homœopathic drugs :

1. In relation to the three P's of Dr. Wells, we must confess that our worthy foe takes a very narrow view of the subject of medical education. We reply to the accusation that it is the duty of every homœopathic medical college to teach everything which *is taught in any medical college, fully aud thoroughly*, PLUS HOMŒOPATHY. The latter is only the science of therapeutics, as far as homœopathic drug action is concerned, and even a puke or a purge may be necessary in cases of poisoning, to remove rapidly the poison out of the body; and when collapse threatens, woe to the physician who does not know when and how to apply electricity. How often has a warm, or even a cold bath or sponging quieted the raving maniac? Sleep followed, and allowed the physician time to get at the similimum of the case. The homœopathic healer must be the peer of his allopathic colleagues; he must know how to handle the whole medical and surgical armamentarium, and he must feel an honest pride that in most cases *homœopathy alone* suffices to restore that equilibrium which some known or unknown potency had disturbed.

2. There is some dense smoke for the second charge; for even the President of the American Institute of Homœopathy raises this charge and makes the teaching of the *Organon* obligatory upon the colleges. It ought, certainly, be the introductory part to any course of lectures on materia medica ; and it can be exhaustively treated in eight or nine lectures.

3. Let the *Organon* be the foundation on which our materia medica palace is reared. We acknowledge, with sorrow, that too many of so-called homœopathic physicians and *homœopathic patients* thirst and hunger after the fleshpots of Egypt, and to please the latter, the former are too apt to nurse the prejudices of bygone ages. One false step leads to another, and by and by many leave our ranks, or might as well leave them, to join the other side. The use of mere dietetic adjuvantia need not lead us to the constant use of M., N., O., P., morphine, narcotics, opium, and purges, and the safety of the patient is certainly far better secured by studying faithfully for the simile and applying it according to the precepts laid down in the *Organon*. Teach the application of our materia medica in every branch of medical art and science, be it surgery, gynæcology, obstetrics, or any other

specialty, and the hydra-headed bacillus will lose its terrors; keep your patient aseptic and you will have very little use of antiseptics.

4. As we all agree on that point, let us hope that our teachers may take it to heart, so that their pupils may become true homœopathic healers.

5. We come finally to the severest condemnation of our colleges, when Dr. Wells boldly asserts that almost nowhere a homœopathic medical education can be gained, and we may well propound the question, whether there is any truth in this assertion. We feel grateful for the "*almost*," and still it cannot be gainsaid that there is some smoke ! In some colleges some of their truest teachers were ostracised on account of their strict adherence to the principles of homœopathy; and I feel proud that such a thing never could happen in the New York Homœopathic Medical College. Let liberty rule, but let license be rebuked. If bigotry sometimes raises its head in the camp of the International Homœopathic Association—and here it may be excusable, for its members are intrenched behind the walls of the most strict application of homœopathic principles—the same bigotry raises its false beacon lights in our national and in our state societies, where chemistry, miscroscopy, spectrum-analysis try to confine our powers within narrow limits. Who are the members of these societies? The homœopathic physicians all through the land—and they are also the preceptors who send their students to the different colleges. Let this fountain-head be pure and clear, and you may rest assured that the colleges must follow suit, so that even a Wells has to change his dictum, and he may have to acknowledge that *a thorough homœopathic medical education can be gained* ALMOST ANYWHERE.

How careful we ought to be not only in our teachings of unalloyed homœopathy, but also in the practice of it. Let me cite a short article from the last number of the New York *Medical Record*, February 5th, 1887, page 145—"Homœopathy and Hypodermics." "The dean of a homœopathic medical college in this city is reported to have bought another hypodermic syringe recently. This is not what Hahnemann taught ; it is not homœopathic."

Although the fact of our good friend, the dean, buying a hypodermic syringe may be true, the conclusions based thereon are all false, for the dean may inject a high potency hypodermically, just as Hahnemann advised us to give sometimes our remedies by olfaction ; the very fact of buying another one shows that he keeps a separate syringe for each drug. In fact, I consider hypodermic injections of the similimum mighty useful, for it is well known that its action is more rapid, and alternation is thus more frequently obviated.

The animus of this short paragraph shows how we are watched by the enemies of our school on one side, and by the members of the International Homœopathic Association on the other side, and it is well that it is so.   If vigilance is the eternal price of liberty (but not of license), it behooves us in our teachings and in our practice to follow out the precepts of the father of homœopathy.

The Bureau of Materia Medica is the Bureau of Homœopathy, *par excellence,* and clinical facts in all the different branches of medical art and science only attest the truth of our Shibboleth—*similia similibus curantur.*   Let it be our aim that our pupils are fully up to the mark in every branch pertaining to a thorough medical education; but let it be our chief aim that they are thoroughly imbued with the principles of our school.   Homœopathic colleges must send out homœopathic physicians, so that success will be the rule in their practice and failures the exceptions.

The last lay of a minstrel !   This is probably the last time that I will have the honor and the pleasure to address the members of this County Society.   My beloved children wish that I should pass with them the winter of my life.   As they reside on the Pacific coast, it will bring me out of the jurisdiction of this State.   Relinquishing active practice, it will give me more time to devote myself to literary pursuits, and I hope to teach the *Organon* in the Pacific medical college.   With malice toward none, with charity and love for all, I tried to do my duty to my colleagues in and out of the college; and whenever a New York physician visits that far off coast, he may be sure of a hearty welcome, for California hospitality is no idle dream.

ORIGINAL ARTICLES IN SURGERY.

ROTARY LATERAL CURVATURE OF THE SPINE.*

By SIDNEY F. WILCOX, M.D.,

New York.

TO THE orthopædist it is curious to note the diversity of opinion on this subject, and this diversity exists in discussing every point from etiology to treatment.   In this short article I shall, of course, not attempt to discuss the various theories, but only to present those which seem to me the most satisfactory.   By rotary lateral curvature of the spine, we mean that condition of the spinal column in which a

---

*Read before the Homœopathic Medical Society of the County of New York November, 1886.

lateral inclination of the column is accompanied by horizontal rotation
of the bodies of the vertebræ upon each other.

In the generality of cases there are two curves—one the primary,
and the other the secondary, or compensatory curve.   This is not
always the condition, however, for sometimes there is only one long
curve.   This lateral deviation and rotation are not due to any actual
diseased condition of the vertebræ themselves, or of the intervertebral
substance, but are the results of conditions external to the spinal
column, and the changes which take place in the vertebræ and the
intervertebral substance result from unequal pressure.   The anatomical change consequent on rotary lateral curvature of the spine is a
sort of spiral twisting of the column upon itself, so that the anterior
portion of the column, consisting of the bodies of the vertebræ, swings
around to the convexity of the curve.   This causes a change in the
planes of the articular surfaces, and also in the relation of the ribs to
the spinal column.   The ribs on the side of the dorsal convexity are
thrown backward and separated, while on the side of the concavity
the opposite condition ensues.   One marked change is that in the
shape of the vertebral bodies, and the intervertebral substance, which
becomes wedge-shaped, with the base of the wedge towards the convexity of the curve, and the apices pointing towards the concavity.

In speaking of the etiology of rotary lateral curvature, I like the
remarks of Mr. Wm. Adams (Quain's Dictionary of Medicine, p. 1505),
in which he says : " The causes of lateral curvature are both local
and constitutional, and as one or other of these causes may predominate, so the cases admit of being arranged in three classes—

"CLASS 1.—Cases in which the constitutional largely predominate
over the local causes.

"CLASS 2.—Cases depending upon constitutional and local causes
in about equal degrees.

"CLASS 3.—Cases essentially depending upon local causes acting
mechanically, so as to disturb the equilibrium of the spinal column."

In the first class the cases occur mostly under twelve years of age,
some even being congenital.   Most of the cases occur between seven
and ten years of age, and sometimes it seems to be hereditary.

The second class he divides into two sub-classes—"(*a*) *cases depending upon induced constitutional or general debility, combined with
local causes acting mechanically ; and (b) those clearly of a rickety character.*"

The first sub-class includes cases induced by bad positions, which
tend to incline the column from the perpendicular, and the second

sub-class those cases clearly of a rickety character, accompanied by indications of rachitis in other parts of the body.

The third general class comprises those cases in which the curvature is not accompanied by any constitutional symptoms, but is induced by unsymmetrical muscular development, or from any condition which may cause a deviation of the axis of the spine from the perpendicular, as when one leg is shorter than the other.

My belief is that these causes act first, and that then the column, becoming bent, loses its power of vertical support.

The cases with which I have come in contact in private practice have been mostly of the mixed variety. Generally there has been a condition of constitutional weakness from some cause or another, and this has usually shown itself in the form of weakened ligaments or muscles—especially of the lower extremities—this condition being generally much more pronounced on one side than the other. As a result of the unequal muscular or ligamentous development, the conditions of knock-knee, or flat foot, or both, have been induced.

Now, it is plain to see, that, if the knee on one side, or the arch of one foot gives way, the leg on that side becomes practically shorter than the other, and the plane of the pelvis, taken from one acetabulum to the other, and which in a normal condition should be perfectly level, becomes tilted and drops down on the side of the practically shortened limb. Then the spine, which is supported by and firmly fastened to the pelvis, at a perpendicular with this plane, must make a curve toward the opposite side, or the equilibrium of the trunk will be lost. This, if allowed to run on, with the superincumbent weight still unsupported, induces a permanent curvature. But, if early in the case, the leg is straightened, or the arch of the foot raised, and the plane of the pelvis once more restored to the horizontal, the column will show a decided tendency to right itself.

All of the cases of this class of which I am now speaking, have been children of the sort generally denominated by the mothers as "weakly;" they are very likely to be poor feeders or desiring kinds of food not the best for them ; "finicky" is an expression which describes them.

This condition often follows contagious diseases, such as scarlet fever, measles, whooping cough, etc., and in one case, now under treatment, there is paralysis of some of the muscles of the leg following cerebro-spinal meningitis.

Of course anything which would make one leg practically shorter than the other would produce a similar effect, as bow legs, or in-knee.

Sometimes the pelvis is not tilted, as in two cases of girls, aged respectively fifteen and sixteen, both of whom were unusually large and well developed, and both with curvature, one with decided rotation. And yet their limbs were straight and the arches of the feet unusually high. I could imagine no cause for the curvature unless induced by faulty positions in sitting or standing. Both were languid and easily tired out.

Dr. Shaffer believes that in many cases the cause of the curvature is a paralysis of the intrinsic muscles on one side of the spine and a consequent contraction of the corresponding muscles on the other side, while Sayre and others believe that it is the long muscles which are thus effected.

It is probable that all of these causes enter in, more or less, as factors in the production of the simple curvature, and thus *its* occurrence seems to be easily explained. But it is not so with rotation, the cause of which is still an unsolved problem.

It is true that reasons almost without number have been brought forward to explain its occurrence, but only the one given by Dr. A. B. Judson seems to me to be tenable. I quote his own words (*Med. Record*, vol. XXII., p. 372):

"The distinguishing feature of rotation here proposed is the recognition of the fact . . . . . . that the posterior portion of the vertebral column, being a part of dorsal parietes of the chest and abdomen, is confined to the median line of the trunk, while the anterior portion of the column, projecting into the thoracic and abdominal cavities and devoid of lateral attachments, is at liberty to and physiologically does move to the right and left of the median line.

"When the median line curves to the right or the left under vertical pressure, which is the direct cause of lateral curvature, their freedom from control allows the bodies of the vertebræ to fall away from the median plane to the right or the left, while the posterior portions of the column are held in the median line by their muscular and fibrous attachments. This deportment of the two components of a vertebra, its anterior and posterior portions, is rotation in the vertebræ as a whole."

While this does not explain all the conditions present, it is, to my mind, the most reasonable explanation offered.

Among the earliest symptoms noticed in a case of rotary lateral curvature is the fact that one shoulder is a little lower than the other, or that one hip projects more than the other, or that one scapula seems unduly prominent. Any of these symptoms may be noticed by the mother or nurse, or, if the patient is a girl, the dressmaker may be the first to call attention to the lack of symmetry.

If the disease progresses, a decided deviation of the posterior spinous processes from the median line will follow, but it must be remembered that the bodies of the vertebræ swinging farther toward the convexity than the apices of the spinous processes, which are held nearer the median line by the muscular and ligamentous attachments, the curve, as seen externally, is apparently less than is really the case.

The shape of the thorax becomes changed by the forcing backward of the ribs on the side of convexity of the dorsal curve, and flattening of the anterior portion of the corresponding side of the chest. On the side of the concavity the opposite condition ensues. The ribs on the side of the convexity become separated, and on the side of the concavity they are crowded together, the sternum becomes very oblique, and, as the disease continues, the organs are more or less pressed upon and their functions interfered with.

Spinal muscular pains vary much in intensity, from a dull aching to violent lancinating pain, which is often excited by the slightest touch in the dorsal region. (Lateral Curvature of the Spine, Tivy — p. 35).

If the curvature arises from, or in connection with, knock-knee or flat foot, the child's gait will be awkward, the knees knock together, and the foot "splays," or turns out badly while walking.

Sometimes the projection of the ribs on one side and the consequent projection of the angle of the scapula, indicating that rotation has already set in, is one of the first symptoms, even while the line of the spinous processes seems almost straight.

Speaking of the Prognosis, Tivy (Lateral Curvature of Spine, p. 27) says : "The prognosis must in all cases be cautious, as sometimes cases which seem at first sight likely to increase rapidly, become spontaneously cured with slight deformity.

"This, however, is exceptional ; the natural tendency of all cases of lateral curvature is to produce increasing deformity.

"The rate and extent of increase depend, however, on various circumstances. Those cases which occur in infancy, in which there is, in all probability, great weakness of the spinal muscles, are likely to develop considerable deformity unless carefully treated, as are also those that depend upon rickets and cases in which the chief deformity is in the lumbar region.

"In all these cases a favorable prognosis must be given with great caution. Cases occurring between the ages of twelve and sixteen, when the health is fairly good, and the curves neither very large nor very unequal in size, will, in all probability, prove more amenable to treatment, and are less likely to result in serious deformity than those that occur at an earlier age. Should the curve be situated in the lower dorsal region, a part to which better support can be given by instruments, we may speak favorably as regards the prospects of a good cure.

"There are, however, exceptions to the rule that the occurrence of lateral curvature at a very early age is always unfavorable. One, at least, of my best cases, occurred at the age of six and was perfectly cured at nine, no deformity remaining, by wearing an instrument.

"Certainly I must allow that in this case, the patient was healthy and the muscles less weak than they usually are in such early cases."

Of course the prognosis is greatly influenced by the condition of the patient at the time he is first seen. A great mistake is often made by physicians who make light of a slight deformity and say that it will come all right of itself. Thus often the case becomes incurable by the time it is brought to the surgeon.

TREATMENT.—The treatment consists first of all in the correction of the constitutional and local predisposing causes.

If the child is thin and weak, with a tendency to knock-knee and flat foot, and, as is often the case, has some predisposing tendency, either inherited or otherwise, to tuberculosis or rachitis, then the diet must be carefully looked after. Since Mr. J. Milner Frothergill's "Manual of Dietetics" has come out I have read it assiduously, and have gained a knowledge of the subject which has been most helpful in the treatment of these cases.

My experience has been that either through a misguided appetite, or, what is about as bad, the urging of misguided parents, the children have eaten altogether too much meat, especially lean beef. This should not be so.

Without entering upon any further discussion of the subject, I will say, that instead of meat they want first, fat and plenty of it, either in the form of butter, animal fat, or even cod-liver oil. Then the grains and fruits come in, and oftentimes, if well digested, sugar and sweet things are not bad. The next thing is to get a proper remedy, and these are generally of the class known as "nutrition remedies," in which *ferrum* and *calcarea* and their salts largely enter. *Calcarea hypophos.* has been especially useful.

Then come those methods especially calculated to restore the tone of the weakened muscles. Under this head comes first, electricity *properly applied;* and second, friction. In speaking of electricity I use the words properly applied with emphasis, because my belief is hat when improperly applied it is worse than useless, while if applied properly it is a powerful instrument for good.

Take, for instance, those cases where certain muscles or groups of muscles are affected. Each muscle or group must be treated separately, by exciting its contractility from the motor points.

To differentiate between the forms requiring the galvanic or faradic current, I shall leave to the gentlemen who are at work in this branch to bring out in the discussion.

With regard to rubbing, I have my patients rubbed with the hand from one to three times daily, according to the case and the length of time. The rubbing extends over the back and the affected muscles.

As for exercise, I usually recommend only that which especially tends to straighten the spine.

Two horizontal bars, one of them about two inches above the other, by which the patient draws himself upward, taking hold of the upper bar with the hand on the side of the lower shoulder, furnish a simple apparatus for straightening the spine.

Sayre's suspensory apparatus, in which the patient draws himself up two or three times daily, is excellent. Another measure is to have the patient lean the convexity of the curve on some object, and attempt to straighten it. There are some other exercises, each adapted to special cases, which time will not permit me to mention here.

Lastly comes the apparatus. Some cases are cured spontaneously, and some by the afore-mentioned means, but by the time the case is sent to the specialist it generally requires some form of apparatus. In the use of apparatus we must first begin at the base of things. As I have already said, bow-leg, knock-knee, or flat foot often exist with the curvature, and either produce or aggravate it, so the arch of the foot must be raised first, or the knee brought to the proper position, before any good can be expected from treatment of the spine.

The method of treatment which I employ usually includes some form of corset, either of plaster-of-paris, or felt, or an unusually strong and well-fitting corset, which is made to order, and supplemented by a Y piece going over the shoulders. I do not believe in steel braces, unless the pelvic band is fastened to leg braces which run to the feet. Unless this is done I have never seen one which does not tilt and slide up on the projecting hip. Another objection to steel braces is their weight; a third is the difficulty of keeping them in order; and a fourth the difficulty in fitting them.

Dr. Shaffer's brace comes the nearest to the ideal of any I have seen. It is light and acts upon physiological principles, but in one case where I tried it the patient could not endure the pressure.

The plaster jacket makes a good support if judiciously employed. For lateral curvature it should be made so that it can be removed at night, and in order to obviate the cracking of the plaster by its removal, I have a leather hinge at the back. But a plaster jacket is neither so durable nor so light as one made of felt, and for that reason I prefer the latter.

Although I had seen and read more or less concerning the felt jacket I did not become particularly interested in it until I read a little book by William James Tivy, of London, on lateral curvature, in which the use of the felt jacket was strongly urged. Having had some experience with it since then, I prefer it, in a general way, to any of the other forms of apparatus. My reasons for preferring it are :

1st.—It is light and has no machinery to get out of order,

2d.—It is not easily broken, and if the shape changes under the influence of very warm weather, it can be easily restored and the felt stiffened,

3d.—The shape of the jacket can be readily changed as the patient improves ; and

4th.—It is easily put on and off, and, when on, its presence is no more apparent than any other form of corset.

For the felt corset the heavy "Russian felt" is probably the best. It can be softened by steam and fitted to the patient's body, and this is the method most generally employed and the one used by me at first. But I found that it was disagreeable to the patient on account of the heat, and it is difficult to stretch the felt sufficiently in order to bring it into shape on the patient, as a good deal of force is required to do so. Therefore, I now first make a cast of the patient's body in plaster-of-paris, and using this as a block, find it much more convenient both for patient and operator. The mould is made while the patient is suspended by the Sayre's apparatus, as this straightens the column as much as possible. Some surgeons apply the jacket with the patient lying down, but I prefer suspension. The advantage of having the plaster cast is that it can, from time to time, be straightened, as the patient can bear increased pressure on the convexity of the curve and the case improves. This straightening process consists simply of chiseling away the plaster from the convex side of the curve and adding to the concave side. This is, of course, done a little at a time, the cast gradually becoming more and more symmetrical in shape. The jacket is remoulded to the cast each time it is changed, which is about once in two weeks. The patient is thus gradually *forced* into shape, and I have been greatly pleased with the success attained by its use.

The jacket should be worn all the time when the patient is in the upright position, the patient being always suspended for its application.

The jacket should be removed for one or two hours in the middle of the day, during which time the patient remains in the recumbent position.

The patient should be seen by the surgeon as often as once in two weeks and, if possible, the shape of the jacket improved as frequently. As the patient improves it will be observed that the shoulders assume equal height, the projecting hip becomes less prominent, and the thoracic deformity less marked, until, if it is a curable case, it disappears altogether.

But such results are not always to be attained and the surgeon must be wary of promising a cure, for in some cases all that can be done is to keep the deformity from growing worse. Also persistent and patient co-operation on the part of both patient and parents must be insisted upon, and they must understand from the beginning the seriousness of the case and the difficulty of obtaining a cure.

INDURATIVE ŒDEMA.—Sigmund has described under this title a syphilitic affection, appearing as a gradual, painless and feverless thickening of the mucous membrane of the labia majora and minora and clitoris, as well as the skin of the prepuce, penis and scrotum. The affection may extend to the mons veneris and occurs either as an independent affection or as a complication or other syphilitic manifestions. It remains stationary for a time, (in one case five to six months), and then gradually disappears, leaving behind, as a rule, some thickening of the skin ; anti-syphilitic treatment is followed by prompt results.

Finger, of Vienna, had the opportunity of finding a series of interesting changes in a case of this disease which succumbed to an intercurrent erysipelas and pneumonia. The details of his findings are too long for our pages but consist in the main of small-celled infiltration and connective tissue, hyperplasia and alteration in the walls of the vessels. The combination of acute and chronic changes is considered noteworthy ; the latter is chargeable to syphilis, the former to the presence of numerous streptotococci. The relation of this organism to erysipelas cannot be well established and Finger holds that it must have existed previously. The existence of syphilis, together with the presence of this organism, produced the peculiar special features of œdema indurativum and thus is explained the exceptional location of this process. *Berlin, Klin. Woch., No. 46, 1886.*

EDITORIAL DEPARTMENT.

EDITORS.

GEORGE M. DILLOW, M.D., ... Editor-in-Chief, Editorial and Book Reviews.
CLARENCE E. BEEBE, M.D., ... Original Papers in Medicine.
SIDNEY F. WILCOX, M.D., ... Original Papers in Surgery.
MALCOLM LEAL, M.D., ... Progress of Medicine.
EUGENE H. PORTER, M.D., ... Comments and News.
HENRY M. DEARBORN, M.D., ... Correspondence.
FRED S. FULTON, M.D., ... Reports of Societies and Hospitals.

GEORGE G. SHELTON, M.D., ... Business Manager.

The Editors individually assume full responsibility for and are to be credited with all connected with the collection and presentation of matter in their respective departments, but are not responsible for the opinions of contributors.

It is understood that manuscripts sent for consideration have not been previously published, and that after notice of acceptance has been given, will not appear elsewhere except in abstract and with credit to THE NORTH AMERICAN. All rejected manuscripts will be returned to writers. No anonymous or discourteous communications will be printed.

Contributors are respectfully requested to send manuscripts and communicate respecting them directly with the Editors, according to subject, as follows : *Concerning Medicine, 21 West 37th Street ; concerning Surgery, 256 West 57th Street ; concerning Societies and Hospitals, 121 East 70th Street ; concerning News, Personals and Original Miscellany, 461 West 71st Street ; concerning Correspondence, 152 West 57th Street.*

Communications to the Editor-in-Chief, *Exchanges* and *New Books* for notice should be addressed to *102 West 43d Street.*

A DANGER IN MAGAZINE READING.

A SHORT time ago the Board of Directors of the New York Ophthalmic Hospital called the attention of its surgeons to the injurious effect upon the eyes resulting from the use of too highly calendered paper in many of our popular periodicals. And it is a subject which really requires agitation, not only by the medical press, but also by the daily secular papers, in order that it may more fully be brought before the public mind. For there is no doubt but that temporary, and even permanent injury to the vision, has been brought on from this cause.

Let one blessed with perfectly healthy eyes take up one of our monthly magazines, printed upon this highly glazed paper, and attempt to read it in the evening, by ordinary gaslight, and he will soon find that he is turning the page from side to side to enable him to see the print and avoid the dazzling reflection. After repeated ineffectual efforts to accomplish this object, if he does not lay the book down in disgust, he will experience a feeling of heat and dryness in the eyes, or a tired sensation, with a desire to close the lids, which must at last be yielded to or a headache will be the result. Now, if this is the effect produced upon the normal healthy eye, how much more serious must be the results when the organ of vision has been weakened by disease or overuse. Then we find the retina more sensitive to light especially to variations in intensity, and the muscular apparatus less ready to adapt itself to the changing angles and distances. As a sequence, existing asthenopic symptoms are aggravated and diseases induced which, sooner or later, cause permanent weakness or impairment of the sight. By the light of day the evil is mitigated, but by the evening light, when one naturally turns to his favorite magazine for recreation, he finds no rest or amusement from the perusal of its pages, only a feeling of fatigue and weariness to both mind and eye. That this is no overdrawn picture, colored by a vivid imagination, can be attested by thousands of readers of the current literature of our enlightened age.

The question may now be asked, "Why is high-calendered paper used in the printing of this class of books, if it is so injurious to the eyes ?" The answer which at once comes from the publishers of these journals, and it is, no doubt, the correct one, is, that the public demands it, by requiring the highest degree of artistic excellence in the appearance of the journal it patronizes. It is well known that a clearer impression and finer work can be brought out upon a smooth, glossy paper, than upon a duller, coarser surface ; especially is this true in relation to engravings.

Most publishers realize the danger to the vision which follows the use of highly-glazed paper, and some of the most prominent endeavor to lessen the evil as much as they dare and still successfully compete with their rivals, by using different grades of finish in the paper of the same journal, retaining the highest calender for engravings, and employing a lower finish for the text.

It is always less difficult to find a fault than to correct it, as it is easier to give advice than to follow it. So here, we may succeed in pointing out the injury which results from the employment of too highly finished paper, but it is more difficult to suggest a remedy which will prove acceptable and satisfactory to the public in general. The time, however, will come when the growing importance of this subject will demand more and more attention, and public opinion will require that greater efforts be made towards the solution of the problem of how to avoid the injurious effects of this method of printing and yet not materially impair the artistic beauty of our journals. As the constant drop, drop of water will wear away the stone, so the medical profession and the press, by continually directing attention to the danger to vision which lies hidden in much of our literature, will be the means of awakening the public mind to insist upon its correction in terms so forcible that publishers must, of necessity, heed the warning and follow its demands.

QUININE IN PNEUMONIA.

OUR readers are aware to how great an extent quinine has been administered by the theoretico-empirical school of therapeutics as an antipyretic in pneumonia; almost a universal fashion for a number of years past. But now, submitted to the scrutiny of more scientific analysis, it is being doubted whether it has the effect which it has so long been believed to possess. In a paper read by Dr. John Ripley, before the New York Academy of Medicine, experiments exactly carried out and recorded in forty-eight cases showed meagre results. Dr. Ripley is an acute observer, and, unlike many who appeal to what is called "experience" for the authority of his opinions, understands with clearness what constitutes genuine experience; that is, experiment undertaken under scientific conditions. His experiments can therefore be relied upon. In general deductive summary he states: "Practically, then, so far as can be judged from these experiments, the most that can be expected from twenty to forty grains of quinine, administered daily to patients in the active stage of acute lobar pneumonia, is, that it will reduce the temperature between 1° and 2° F. in about half the cases, while in the other half the reduction will amount to less than 1°. When we add to this statement the fact that the lowest points reached are not even approximately held with certainty more than two to four hours, the results appear even less striking. It is not improbable, also, that in a number of instances the effect of the drug was apparent only, as such recessions of temperature occur, during the course of pneumonias, in the absence of all medical treatment. That quinine is a feeble and uncertain antipyretic in pneumonia is the conclusion arrived at from an analysis of the foregoing experiments. But this is not the only argument against its use. Contrasted with its inefficacy as an antifebrile are some marked deleterious effects on the digestion, circulatory and nervous systems. When given by the stomach, even in moderate dose, if frequently repeated, it soon produces anorexia and nausea. In larger doses it not infrequently excites violent retching and vomiting, and prolonged intolerance of food and stimulants. Marked cardiac weakness, lasting several hours, and sometimes associated with dicrotic pulse, generally followed the maximum doses in these cases. Profuse, often cold perspiration was another effect taking place in from one to two hours after giving the quinine. Epistaxis occurred in about twelve per cent. of the cases. Profound nervous depression, somnolence, muscular twitchings and tremblings, dilated pupils, and in two instances opisthotonos, were some of the results on the nervous system. In three instances the urine was examined both chemically and microscopically, before and after the ingestion of the larger dose of quinine. Chemically, albumen was much increased in quantity after the quinine in one case, and there also appeared in this specimen renal mucus and hyaline casts not present before." The author further remarks "that portions of the affected lung hitherto unaffected, as also opposite parts of the sound lung, have become inflamed while the patient was under the influence of it." In the discussion which followed the drift of opinion was substantially with Dr. Ripley.

So is passing another fashion in therapeutics. But who can compute the miseries, small and great, which humanity has paid? Quinine by the mouth, quinine forced into struggling children, quinine in ejecting stomachs, quinine by the rectum, quinine under the skin, quinine administered by every device which scientific ingenuity can command, quinine to produce an active diastole of the heart, quinine to arrest cell migration, quinine to reduce temperature, quinine irrationally conceived to cure pneumonia by meeting a single symptom in disregard of a protesting and complexly deranged organism, such is one of the phases of fanciful therapeutics, called the science of medicine. One fashion follows another, and after being sanctioned by experience is abandoned by experience. Amid the changing fancies of the treatment of pneumonia, one method alone is stable. The so-called irrational, unscientific, irregular, homœo-pathic method in therapeutics treats patients with pneumonia as it did forty and even sixty years ago. With a scientific principle for the discovery of its remedies, the same remedies remain now as always a firm reliance. With law, experience has fixed them in their place where they stand forever; but, without law, experience has drifted from one catch to another, and has tied certainly to none.

A GAIN FOR CALIFORNIA.

IN removing to San Francisco, Cal., Dr. Samuel Lilienthal retires from active responsibilities to enjoy the closing decades of a singularly well spent and useful life in the companionship of his children and to secure the leisure in which to labor on, undisturbed by the cares of practice, for his beloved homœopathy. As scholar, teacher, editor and author, he has made a home for himself wherever he may choose to select his abiding place. New York regrets the loss of his presence, but, so long as he can use the pen, there is the satisfaction that he will continue among his friends wherever homœopathic litera-ture is read. Few have led a life of more unflagging work, and none have labored in greater kindliness of heart.

Now that he is on the Pacific slope, he has the warmest wishes from the East for the full measure of happiness. He left no enemies, and he will find none but friends who will welcome his unfailing geniality of nature, and learn of him how youth is carried into old age—the youth that always learns and freely gives. Our Board of Editors would especially tender to him their kindest hopes for his welfare, and express their appreciation of the example he has set for them in the performance of their work.

THAT "FLAMELESS LAMP."

THE *Medical Era* has pinioned the *Medical Times* for setting forth as editorial one of its selections from the *British Medical Journal* without a quotation mark. "A Flameless Lamp" appears identically in the editorial columns of the February (1887) number of the *Times* as it was published in the *Era* of September, 1886, a few closing sentences only being omitted. By throwing in a parenthetical, "says the *British Medical Journal*," the impression is distinctly conveyed that the composition, though not the information, was the product of editorial brains. *Suppressio veri, suggestio falsi*, being the peculiar ear marks by which the *Times* can be identified, it seems really cruel for the *Era* to so vilify, traduce and insult our New York contemporary, regardless of professional decency. Why should not the *Times* trick itself out with shams unexposed? It is hard pressed for original matter, and how could it honestly indicate that it scissored an editorial outright? In other issues there appear editorials which the *Era* might enjoy tracing to their source.

The query naturally arises, how much of the *Times* would remain if all matter where quotation marks rightly belong were subtracted from its columns? Evidently "something is rotten in the state of Denmark," and about ready to drop to pieces. At any rate, "it smells to heaven."

DR. BRUNTON'S PREDICAMENT.

THE growing use by the anti-homœopathic school of remedies in small doses, according to indications long followed in the homœopathic school, is becoming a knock-out reply to the charge that there is no efficacy in the homœopathic method, *per se.* Hence the dishonest desire to conceal the sources from which information is derived becomes the greater as the appropriation of homœopathic remedies proceeds. The most conspicuous sinner up to date has been Dr. Brunton, whose conveyances from homœopathy have been so numerous that, high priest as he is of modern batrachian therapeutics, he can no longer cover his neighbor's possessions in the voluminous folds of his garments. Dr. Dudgeon has been crowding him for more than a year past for explanation, until it would appear that he will stand before the assembled congregation and, decked out with his thefts, proclaim his opinion of the party from whom he stole his adornments. This he has announced his intention to do in the third edition of his book. Whether he can successfully clear himself of conviction at the bar of public opinion will be gathered from a letter of Dr. Dudgeon's in the *Lancet* of February 12th. Dr. Dudgeon writes: "Dr. Brunton gives in his book a bibliographical index, with lavish references about the remedies used in your school, but not a single reference about the medicines which homœopathy has introduced into medical practice. Why is this? Did Dr. Brunton rediscover all these remedies and their indications for himself? I know that Dr. Brunton is a very clever man, who has made many experiments with drugs on many frogs; but if his researches in this field had taught him the above uses of these drugs, he would certainly have told us. So we are driven to the conclusion that Dr. Brunton has borrowed extensively from homœopathy, but has studiously withheld from his readers the source of these borrowings; and, for anything that appears to the contrary in his book, he assumes to himself all the credit of all these remedies and all their indication, so strange to the practice of your school. Is this the right thing for a medical author to do? We may be a contemptible sect in the eyes of an orthodox author, but it is surely carrying cynical contempt for the rival school a little too far to convey a large number of their chief remedies into his book and to conceal carefully the source whence he has taken them. Does not Dr. Brunton owe the profession some explanation of his extraordinary conduct?" In the resolute push which is being made in England to make the public see homœopathy as it is, attention cannot be directed too pointedly towards Dr. Brunton's uncomfortable situation. The hook appears to be too well caught for him to dive from sight beneath the scum upon his frog pond. We trust that he may dangle becomingly at the end of Dr. Dudgeon's pole, as his dimensions have waxed large on homœopathic tidbits.

COMMENTS.

SYSTEMATIC RELIEF. — The Charity Organization Society, in its circular recently distributed, states one of the objects of the society to be as follows : To investigate thoroughly, and without charge, the cases of all applicants for relief which are referred to the society for inquiry, and to send the persons having a legitimate interest in such cases full reports of the results of investigation. There is another object that the society might have stated in its circular, not less important than any of those given—to suppress dispensary begging and dispensary charity—falsely so called. Although this object is not directly stated, yet the society will accomplish it if it be allowed to do so. Any dispensary may avail itself of the resources of this organization in investigating those cases which present for treatment. There is absolutely no excuse for indiscriminate and blind medical charity. The officers and physicians of every large dispensary know that a large proportion of patients who apply for relief are amply able to pay for it. But nothing is done, for every patient counts one, either in the clinic or on the hospital roll at the end of the year. "Professional beggars are encouraged and charity abused by gifts to those of whose real wants nothing is positively known." This is as applicable to medical charity as to any other sort. A small outlay will secure positive and valuable results. Those dispensaries which refuse to make use of this method of investigation, must be termed hereafter not charitable institutions, but, rather, advertising agencies.

BOOK REVIEWS.

"DISEASES OF THE LUNGS AND PLEURÆ." By R. Douglas Powell, M.D. Wm. Wood & Co. New York : 1886.

This work adds one more volume to the valuable books on diseases of the lungs and, as such, it is a pleasure to heartily commend it. It treats of the anatomy and functions of the lungs, the physical examination of the chest and the diseases to which its various structures, including the heart, are subject.

The normal and diseased sounds to be heard on physical exploration are treated of at length with a clearness and definiteness which cannot fail to instruct an old examiner and furnishes the most complete and practical guide for the novitiate which we have yet seen. The tabulated sounds with their definitions, synonyms, and clinical significance give, in a condensed form, all the desired information and furnish a most useful epitome for ready consultation.

The chapter on pleurisy and empyema is most able. The treatment is rational, little dependence being placed upon tremendous doses, but chiefly upon rational and common sense methods. Evacuation is recommended at an early date. The surgical aspect of pleuritic effusions receives a fairer consideration than is usual at the hands of a purely medical author. If more reliance were placed upon such interference and the author's recommendations for early evacuation followed instead of trusting to the efficacy of medicinal action, much suffering and not a few lives might be saved. Throughout the entire work, one can but feel that a large amount of well utilized clinical experience furnishes the foundation for deductions and treatment. The detailed symptoms are graphically accurate, and present the disease as an entity which would be readily recognized a second time. The clinical rather than the ideally-typical signs, both subjective and physical, are given.

The learned clinician rather than the fanciful theorist stands out prominently throughout the entire work. The author always gives the results of his experience in an honest, straightforward fashion, not as endeavoring to establish any given pet theory or idea, but holding himself always as an impartial observer, to whom facts appear in their right relation and not through the distorted method of an un-scientific craze. The work is free from the lurid prognoses, and uniform fatality in description which blind the eyes of readers and cause dismal prognoses to their patients, nor is it too hopeful. It simply looks on disease, particularly phthisis, as one which has been often met and many times subdued. The subject of hemorrhages is treated of rationally, the difference between true and false hæmoptyses plainly insisted upon, and the relation between hemorrhages whether single or repeated, and immediate danger or later developed phthisis shown to be less intimate than is often supposed. The whole ten-dency of the work is to place diseases of the lungs and pleuræ upon a more rational and correct basis, and to free them from the close asso-ciation with that secret dread and hopelessness with which most patients and many practitioners have come to regard even the slightest hæmop-tysis or the first evidences of impaired pulmonic function.

The consideration of the climatic treatment of phthisis, viewed from a European standpoint, is most complete but of comparatively little value to American practitioners. A similar, thorough, definite, dis-cription of the climate and climatic effects of the various health resorts of the United States would be exceedingly valuable. We regard the book as an important addition to our fund of knowledge of pulmonary diseases.   F.

AMERICAN MEDICINAL PLANTS, by MILLSPAUGH. Fascicle V.

This fascicle contains illustrations and descriptions, botanical, chemical and pharmacological, of the following : Aesculus glabra; Absinth., Ambrosia Anagallis, Argemone, Artemisia, Arum draco., Chenopod. anthel., Cistus, Collinsonia, Convolvulus, Euphorbia hyper., Euphorbia lath., Helonias, Humulus, Hydrophyllum, Hypericum, Lachnanthes, Lactuca, Leptandra, Lilium superb., Lycopus, Pen-thorum, Phaseolus, Polygonum acre, Ptelea, Ranunculus scel., Salix purp., Sinapis alb., Solanum nigrum.

The illustrations are for the most part good. Aesculus glabra gives one no idea of the spike of flowers of the tree, which would have to be reduced to come within the limits of the page, but the leaf and the single flower are good.

Absinthium is hardly an American plant, but it is cultivated some-times, as most European medicinal herbs are.

Some of the plates, such as Lachnanthes, are particularly good. The text maintains the high standard of the previous numbers, and renders the work of the greatest value to all medical men.   * * *

THE PRESCRIBER. A Dictionary of the New Therapeutics. By JOHN H. CLARKE, M. D., Edin., Physician to the London Hom. Hospital. Editor of the *Hom. World*. Second Edition, carefully revised, with numerous additions, including a glossary of medical terms. London : Keene & Ashewell. New York : Bœricke & Tafel, 1886.

This little volume, almost of pocket size, is not fully a dictionary, although such it might be styled on account of its alphabetical arrangement for rapid reference. It is designed for rendering prescription easy to the beginner who, having made out his diagnosis, would prescribe accordingly on dogmatic authority. The lines of distinction between remedies are mainly of the broad empirical order. Its tendency is to routine prescription. Yet it has the value of offering a ready catch at many clues which one may not know or have forgotten. As one physician on meeting another may say, "What do you give for such and such a disease?" so one may inquire here. It is not a skeleton key to successful practice, but rather a bunch of keys, which the beginner will do well to try first upon his materia medica. In other words, it is too meagre in indications for an authoritative prescriber or a dictionary of homœopathic therapeutics, but it is a salient epitome of the author's siftings, carefully indexed, from his own experience and study. Not being of the hackneyed order, it will be welcome to practitioners.

TRANSACTIONS OF THE THIRTY-NINTH SESSION OF THE AMERICAN INSTITUTE OF HOMŒOPATHY, held at Saratoga Springs, N. Y., June 28–July 2, 1886. Edited by the General Secretary, J. C. BURGHER, M. D.

TRANSACTIONS OF THE HOMŒOPATHIC MEDICAL SOCIETY OF THE STATE OF NEW YORK, for 1886. Vol. XXI.

HOMŒOPATHIC MEDICAL SOCIETY, STATE OF OHIO. Twenty-second Annual Proceedings, 1886.

If we judge the thirty-ninth Institute of Homœopathy by the bulky volume of transactions it left behind it, it may at least be,said that the days spent at Saratoga were not all days of idleness. A volume of 938 pages may be reasonably expected to contain valuable additions to homœopathic literature. Three subjects which are of special interest to the homœopath, and which relate directly to the new system of therapeutics, may be looked for, in the expectation that extended consideration, the result of prolonged investigation, will be given them. It may be supposed that the greater part of the transactions would be given up to papers on topics which embody and exemplify the central truths of homœopathy; that the major part of the work done at Saratoga would be done in the way of strengthening the weak points of homœopathy—and especially would we look for original work in the vast field afforded by the materia medica. But many things are looked for in this world that are not found. Seven pages and a half are devoted to the report on drug proving; and the papers of worth on materia medica occupy but small space. The volume contains nearly seventy essays on various subjects. Some of these are both interesting and instructive. Others are mere compilations prepared for the occasion. A few of the articles are so markedly distinguished by the absence of anything homœopathic, that the bewildered reader involuntarily turns to the title page to reassure himself that he is reading the transactions of a homœopathic body. But the book, as a whole, is valuable, and does credit to the

Institute. The binding is excellent, but typographical errors are too many.

The Transactions of the New York Homœopathic Medical Society make a good sized volume, well printed and bound. There is no report on drug proving to be found in the book, but the Bureau of Materia Medica presents quite a number of papers. The Ohio Society gives a proving of nitrate of sanguinaria. In all the reports there is too much "paper" and too little discussion. The theoretical crowds out the practical. Routine reports, business reports, statistics, etc., take up a great deal of room in all. The amount of specially homœopathic study to the square inch is small. Without neglecting the business that must necessarily come before the societies, or slighting routine work that must be done, it seems as if a little more attention might be given to the materia medica and therapeutics. The Proceedings of the Ohio State Homœopathic Society are neatly bound in paper, and contain papers of great interest. Greater promptness in issuing these reports would enhance their value.   P.

CORRESPONDENCE.

HOMŒOPATHY IN NEW ENGLAND.

To the Editor of the NORTH AMERICAN JOURNAL OF HOMŒOPATHY :

Last year I wrote of the activity of homœopathy in this vicinity, and to-day I can make an equally encouraging report. The latest topic of interest among us is the approaching semi-centennial of the introduction of homœopathy into New England, which we propose to celebrate with appropriate exercises. It is now fifty years since Dr. Samuel Gregg became a convert to homœopathy and introduced its practice into New England, twelve years after it was brought from Europe to your city. Plans for this celebration are being made by committees, and the following outline of what is proposed may be interesting: On Monday, April 11th, Hahnemann's birthday, there will be an excursion to the new State Homœopathic Insane Hospital, at Westboro, where the building and grounds will be inspected and appropriate addresses delivered in commemoration of the day. On Tuesday, April 12th, a large evening reception will be held in our most spacious hall, under the auspices of the Boston University School of Medicine. On Wednesday, the State Society will hold its annual meeting. We expect to make this a particularly interesting occasion, and hope many of our New York friends will give us their assistance. Our genial friend Talcott, of Middletown, N. Y., has already promised to come.

In my former letter I spoke of our success in obtaining admission into the City Hospital as only a matter of time. I must acknowledge that that time has been further postponed. By our petitions and work, however, we certainly accomplished something ; we stirred up our opponents pretty thoroughly, and gave the trustees a great deal of work to satisfactorily reply why part of our petition should not be granted—that referring to the admission of homœopathic physicians to practice in the City Hospital.

We are assured by the laity on all sides, by those favorable to our school of practice and by others that our claim was a just one and ought to be granted, and that it was the place of the trustees to formulate some plan for complying with our demand, but the result has proved unfavorable, and the trustees report "inadmissible." We asked for the introduction of homœopathic treatment for a portion of the patients. This can be done, they say, only by a change in the administration of the hospital in one of the following ways :

I.—By introducing another and independent body of physicians and surgeons, side by side with the present staff; or

II.—By setting apart separate existing wards for a separate staff; or,

III.—By building new wards for the homœopathic treatment.

Their objection to the first plan was that the introduction of another staff into the same ward, having the same assistants, would be attended by so many difficulties that it was dismissed as impracticable. Second, the idea of setting apart for homœopathic treatment some of the existing wards was thought inadmissible as it would interfere with the harmonious administration of details and, by preventing a proper classification of cases, add to the expense of running the hospital. The third plan, which would be most acceptable to us and easiest for the trustees to carry out, they consider beyond their province and say that the city government and not the trustees of the City Hospital are the body proper to determine how and when the city shall provide homœopathic treatment to such citizens as desire it. You may hear of this subject again, therefore, when we make another attempt to secure justice from the city. The only result really accomplished by the petition was to open to women all the privileges of the hospital instruction which our male students have for some time enjoyed.

The work of our homœopathic hospital has increased during the past year, and the results have been eminently satisfactory. 425 patients were treated, of which 165 were medical and 260 surgical. The mortality has been only a little over four per cent. although there have been many grave cases under care. Ten ovariotomies, sixteen amputations, and twelve cases of typhoid fever without a death, give evidence of the success of our treatment. $35,500, have been added by bequests and donations to the permanent fund of the hospital during the past year, which now gives us an invested capital of $107,650. The total expense of maintainance for the year was $24,810. The training school for nurses connected with the hospital has now been in operation a year, and all connected with it are thoroughly satisfied with the result. The nursing has been better done because there was less for each to do and the moral effect of the presence of healthy, conscientious and devoted women has been inestimable. During the year, after much stirring effort on the part of the Ladies' Aid Association, a nurse's home has been provided and equipped. A house about a quarter of a mile from the hospital has been secured and accommodations provided for eighteen nurses. This takes them away from the hospital air when off duty, gives them an attractive home, and necessitates daily a certain amount of out-door exercise, a thing which too often is neglected. A glance at the nurses connected with our hospital would assure one of their good health and morals, for it would be difficult to find a better collection of women as nurses in any hospital. There are now three head and thirteen assistant nurses.

The work of the Boston Homœopathic Dispensary shows a slight falling off from last year. 15,000 patients were treated and 40,000 prescriptions were dispensed. Since the foundation of the dispensary in 1857, there have heen 170,786 patients and 462,043 prescriptions.

Recently a new homœopathic dispensary has been established in the part of Boston called Roxbury, where the poor until now have been almost entirely without medical assistance, and obliged to go long distances to the old established dispensaries. It is a well-known fact that there is a large number of people who abuse medical charity at all of our dispensaries, patients applying for and receiving treatment who are able to and should patronize some physician in their neighborhood. The question is often asked how can this form of imposition be stopped? and I never have heard any satisfactory method suggested except the one which is put into practice in this new institution. Each patient on first presenting himself to the receiving physician is obliged to sign a book having blanks as follows :

No..... Name,.......... Address,.......... Reference,.......... Date,..........	No..... Date,....................188....
	My circumstances at present compel me to seek medical charity.
	Name,...........................
	Address,........................
	Reference,......................

These blanks are arranged so that they can be torn from a book, and a stub containing a duplicate of the first form remains. The slip is given to our associated charities, a most valuable organization, and the case looked up and reported back to us. Should the person prove an impostor, he will not be allowed to again receive treatment. Of course all this system would be comparatively useless without the aid of a thoroughly organized charitable society, which is able to investigate each case or has information upon the status of the people in its district. By means of following up this system we hope to prevent improper distribution of charity and the physicians in the neighborhood from suffering loss of fees. A charge of five cents is made to cover the cost of medicine, but even this small sum is remitted when we know that the patients cannot afford to pay it. How often these persons are able to spare that amount for beer, tobacco or patent medicines, only those who visit the poor really know.

This dispensary has been duly incorporated and its twenty-five trustees are among the best known and most influential people in that part of the city. In working up the interest in this institution much enthusiasm was met with, which indicates that the success of the undertaking will be permanent. The experience in organizing and establishing this dispensary and the assistance rendered by prominent citizens show how easy it would be to establish a homœopathic dispensary in each of our principal cities and towns.

The annual meeting of the Boston Homœopathic Society held at the Parker House, on January 20th, was as much of a success as that of last year. The society now has a membership of 157. Several good speeches were made, but a few extracts must suffice. President Boothby in his address spoke of the wonderful progress homœopathy has been making during the past year, and estimated that in that time all over the country over $1,000,000 had gone into our hospitals. He urged a continuance of the work by each member of the society, and showed by computation how much might be accomplished in the year should each member devote even fifteen minutes daily to the work of improving our materia medica. As special guests of the evening we were honored by the presence of Mr. J. A. Dewson and Mrs. I. T. Talbot, the building committee of the Westboro Homœopathic Insane Hospital. Mr. Dewson gave some account of the two years' work which the committee had done and spoke glowingly of the results. Taking under their charge at the outset the old buildings of the State Reform School for boys, which were more suitable for a prison than a hospital, they had transformed them into one of the most perfect insane hospitals in the country. The development of the congregate dining-room plan has been watched with interest by similar institutions. The first attempt made in this country to bring insane men and women into the same dining-room, it has proved, as Mr. Dewson said, a "perfect success," the patients who were most excited when by themselves calming down and behaving in the most decorous manner if told that any misdemeanor would exclude them from the room. Mr. Dewson closed with a warm expression of the appreciation in which the superintendent, Dr. N. E. Paine, is held by the trustees and all who have been brought into relations with him ; and said "The efficient work we are doing in our asylum is chiefly due to the faithful services of the superintendent." Dr. I. T. Talbot answered for the Boston University School of Medicine. In a sketch of the history of homœopathy, he compared its growth and activity in this country with that in the land where it originated. Although in Europe the number of homœopathic practitioners hardly holds its own, the practice has spread considerably among the people, many families having their box and book and depending upon themselves. There, as we know, all medical students have to follow the same prescribed course and few have the courage to hold to their convictions. How many students prejudiced in favor of homœopathy pursue their studies in the old schools of medicine, and, knowing nothing of the truths of homœopathy are turned from us by the ridicule of their professors. In the course of the past sixty-two years since the arrival of the first homœopath in America, we have grown into a powerful body of over 10,000 physicians. This wonderful development is due to the freedom of this country which allows the establishment of schools in which our principles are properly taught. This is the first satisfactory explanation I have ever heard of the difference between the growth of homœopathy abroad and in this country, and it ought to impress this upon our minds : If we have students whom we desire to make homœopaths, better would it be for them to be grounded in the principles of homœopathy than to have the most perfect theoretical knowledge which the old school can give.

Fraternally yours,

BOSTON, February, 1887.   WILLIAM L. JACKSON.

REPORTS OF SOCIETIES AND HOSPITALS.

HOMŒOPATHIC MEDICAL SOCIETY, COUNTY OF NEW YORK.

THE regular monthly meeting of the Homœopathic Medical Society of the County of New York was held in the reception room of the New York Ophthalmic Hospital, on Thursday evening, February 10th, at eight o'clock.

President Beebe in the chair. There were present eighty-three members.

Dr. S. Lilienthal read the first paper of the evening on " A Plea for Pure Homœopathy in our Colleges."

Dr. T. F. Allen :—I think the article of Dr. Wells referred to in Dr. Lilienthal's paper is open to just criticism, as not presenting the facts of the case. The truth is Hahnemann's *Organon* and homœopathy—good homœopathy—is taught in our medical colleges, with scarcely an exception. Our students are in no danger of losing sight of homœopathy, although their has been a general onslaught on the medical colleges by some who, I think, are apt to lose sight of true homœopathy, being blinded by prejudices in regard to high potencies.

As regards the hypodermic syringe which has been spoken of here to-night, I will say that I have not bought one for many years. I think it is probable that I have used a hypodermic injection of morphia on an average of once a year. We are through and through physicians and homœopathic only in therapeutics.

Dr. L. P. Jones, of Greenwich :—I have not much to say about the paper that has been read. There may be cases in which the remedies will not control the patients, and have been obliged to use the hypodermic syringe several times myself. I had a case of hydrophobia yesterday, in which I tried a hypodermic injection of morphia, but it was a failure, then thirty grains of chloral per rectum every two hours, but I lost my patient this morning. I do not know any remedy that has cured a case of hydrophobia or that has produced all the symptoms. If we had a direct method of teaching the materia medica from the more positive symptoms, I think it would be a great advantage.

Dr. S. Lilienthal :—We have no remedy for hydrophobia, nor has the other school. Pasteur claims to cure it, but I have no confidence in his treatment.

Some of us sometimes use morphine unnecessarily, for we have remedies which allay pains more satisfactorily as, *pulsatilla* or *antimonium tartaricum* for euthanasia. There is much truth in the remark of Prof. Hale, that for primary symptoms of the disease we ought to give the higher potencies, and for the secondary symptoms the lower ones. The application of our drugs needs yet careful study. Homœopathy is only one hundred years old and we are yet only babies therein.

A paper by Dr. T. F. Allen on "Colchicum in Acute and Chronic Nephritis," was then read, in which the doctor said : There are many forms of acute affections of the kidneys to be most speedily cured by attention to symptoms directly due to the diseased condition of the organ. Among the drugs suitable for this later condition we may instance *colchicum*. So far as present knowledge goes it produces no profound or lasting tissue changes within the body, and is rather a remedy for acute than chronic disorders. So, in some forms of chronic nephritis it is a temporary expedient and relieves only some of the acute manifestations while the general dyscrasia goes on unchecked.

My attention was first called to *colchicum* in the case of a pregnant woman suffering from albuminuria, who complained of *coldness in her stomach*. Colchicum was prescribed, and it not only relieved that symptom but also the necessity to lie with her legs bent up to avoid the distress in the stomach caused by straightening them ; it also stopped annoying attacks of vomiting from which she had suffered, diminished the amount of albumen in the urine, and enabled her to pass the full term and be delivered without any complications.

Later, a man suffering from chronic nephritis complained that he could not lie at night with his legs out straight on account of *the hurt in his kidneys*. This symptom always came on as an acute aggravation of his chronic trouble. If he had been worried by his business or exposed to wet and had taken cold, he was in the habit of complaining of this *soreness in the kidneys, aggravated by straightening his legs*, or *distressing pulsation through the sides of the occiput, aggravated by lying down, with a weak, heavy head*. Whenever he suffered from this headache one or two doses of *picric acid* would promptly relieve, but it readily changed to the soreness in the kidneys on straightening out the legs. I then prescribed *colchicum*, because it had relieved cases of *gastric troubles aggravated by straightening the legs*, and it was now found to relieve completely the last patient of this distressing symptom, and in relieving it did not bring on the headache. This symptom has served well as a keynote for the use of *colchicum* in acute nephritis or in acute aggravations of chronic nephritis. The association of *colchicum* symptoms now and then met with in such cases or during pregnancy, I have found to be as follows :

Urine scanty, dark, bloody.

Feeling of soreness in the region of the kidneys, aggravated by straightening out the legs.

Violent pinching in the region of the loins and urinary passages, with constant desire to urinate.

Feeling of tension in the region of the kidneys.

He is obliged to bend himself double and lie still the whole day without the slightest movement to avoid most violent attacks of vomiting.

Feeling of icy coldness in the stomach with constant nausea.

Dr. S. Lilienthal :—In the January number of *l'Art Medical*, Dr. Piedvache coincides with the remarks of Prof. Allen, that in treating Bright's disease, or any other one, we must not only attend to the present symptoms, but go back in the history of the patient to get at the origin of the disease. An antipsoric may be the similimum, just as Allen cured a case of morbus bri htii with *sulphur*.

acute albuminaria during pregnancy. I lost a case about a month ago. Patient had been unusually well; no œdema of extremities; heart seemed all right; urine abundant, and two months previous to this time there was no trouble with the kidneys. I found her in convulsions; had had one before I saw her, and more followed. I found she was having regular contraction of the uterus and that labor had begun. During the day she was delivered. She died that night. I had no remedy.

Dr. Allen :—In treating the various forms of kidney lesions, we must make a distinction in estimating the value of symptoms. In acute nephritis we must look chiefly to the symptoms directly caused by the lesion in the kidney, but in searching for the remedy for the chronic lesion, I am more and more persuaded that to be successful we must eliminate in a great measure the symptoms directly dependent upon the function of the kidney, and therefore, in prescribing, I ignore these acute symptoms as far as possible and search back in the history of the patient for other indications, a method of prescribing which I think we have to follow more or less in all chronic cases. I think fully seventy-five per cent. of the cases of chronic Bright's may be cured readily in the earlier stages or may be so modified that the patient can enjoy fair health. As Dr. Jones has said, some of the patients will die in spite of us, just as they do in phthisis pulmonalis, cancer and the like. I think a physician rarely loses a woman who has albuminuria during pregnancy.

Dr. J. T. O'Connor's paper on "Symptomatic *vs.* Theoretical Indications in Therapeutics," was then read.

Dr. Deschere :—I am positive, from my own experience, that in order to be successful we must prescribe according to the symptoms present, but in regard to the *value* of the symptoms, I think there has not been sufficient reliable material gathered to justify us to prescribe according to the causes *only.* Another reason why I don't wish to have too much stress laid upon that point is, that in cases of disease the indications of remedies according to causes are rather a matter of experience, which has frequently led to the selection of the drug, but has as often misled. We certainly do not give *rhus toxicodendron* because its symptoms coincide with cases that have been caused by getting wet. We have symptoms in *rhus tox.* that are very similar to rheumatic conditions among others, caused by getting wet; but this alone would not justify us to conclude that *rhus tox.* would necessarily cure that special case before us. We may erroneously suppose a case caused by certain circumstances, and I therefore think that the causes of a disease should not be the *first point* of value in the selection of the remedy. The accompanying symptoms, as to circumstances, etc., the aggravations, ameliorations, etc., are those that should be considered first, and then the others should follow. The cause is certainly a good point that can be taken into consideration with the rest.

Dr. O'Connor :—I am afraid Dr. Deschere has misunderstood what I tried to say, which was that theoretical prescriptions on pathological grounds, as against symptomatic prescription, had not been successful, but in my experience I had had some remarkable results in prescribing theoretically in other ways, and I was supported in that by the authority of Hahnemann, Bœnninghausen and others. I was led to the consideration of this subject by noticing the frequent occurrence of cases of colds and so-called muscular rheumatism, from changes of clothing. I have seen favorable effects follow the use of mercury of different kinds, so that I am inclined to prescribe that when such cause can be shown to exist. Among the cases I had in mind, I have seen what would be diagnosed now as paraplegia of spinal origin, cured by *dulcamara,* prescribed simply on the causal indication. The case was one which Dr. Wood sent me of incipient ocomotor ataxia, having the lightning pains, and in some degree Romberg's symptoms. The patient had been exposed repeatedly to wettings, and had been sent to New York for treatment. I gave him *rhus*, and he got well, and he is well now.

Dr. B. G. Clark read the last paper of the evening, on "Baptisia in Typhoid Fever."

Dr. Schley:—I have used *baptisia* with success in typhoid fever, also in pneumonia with marked typhoid symptoms. As to the statements of Dr. Raue in his work cited by Dr. Clark, that medicines have a decided effect upon the limitation of disease, I must state that I think Dr. Raue is in error. We all know that pneumonia (croupous) is a disease the crisis of which is *not* reached ordinarily until the fifth, sixth or seventh day, and it matters little whether the patient is treated on the expectant plan or not; the sharp turn will occur. It is the same in typhus and typhoid fevers. The so-called typhoid fevers that were aborted *within a week* were not such cases, in my opinion. It takes twenty-one days in the large majority of cases to reach a crisis. We must consider the different stages of the malady during that time: first the congestion and inflammation of Peyer's glands, then ulceration, then the retrograde changes and cicatrisation. In a certain measure these medicines do allay many symptoms, but they have no decided effect upon the duration of the disease. Dr. O'Connor puts the diagnosis of the case cited by him as that of tabe dorsails, and claims a cure. It would give me great satisfaction to know if this was a *bona fide* case of locomotor ataxia. I have seen five well-marked cases of this trouble in my private practice, three of these being of syphilitic origin, and in none of them did medicines seem to have any effect. They (3) had been receiving the best homœopathic treatment before they came to me. They all terminated fatally. Locomotor ataxia is a disease upon which medicines seem to have had very little effect. In its *incipient* stages we may diagnose and perhaps cure it, but it must be before any destructive changes in the cord have occurred.

Dr. S. Lilienthal:—The indications for *baptisia* are perfectly clear. The tincture in repeated doses can only be useful in the later stages of typhoids, where sepsis prevails, and the blood of the patient is thoroughly poisoned. To give such strong doses in the first stage damages the whole case, and it is a blessing if the patient does not die; whereas, the middle and higher (30 to 200) dilutions are suitable at the beginning of the disease. The tincture finds its place during the acme of the fever. I have seen many cases of typhoid fever.

Dr. Clark:—As regards the crisis, I would like to say that I do not consider it at all necessary to have a crisis. I understand by a crisis to mean that time when there is a sudden falling of the temperature. The fever has broken suddenly. I have treated some sixty cases of typhoid fever, and have had only one case that terminated by a crisis, and I hope I shall never have another in my practice, for I shall feel that I have not done as much good as I ought by my prescription.

The President:—You will permit me, in this connection, to refer briefly to the closing portion of Dr. Lilienthal's paper. I am positive that I but voice the feelings of the entire Society in giving expression to our respect and sincere affection for our departing colleague, and to our regret that removal from this city necessitates the sundering of the pleasant relations which have always existed between him and the members of the County Society. It would be impossible for any one of our number to leave behind him a greater void; and I am sure that, should circumstances permit him to visit us in the future, every one will delight in the privilege of extending the right hand of fellowship to Dr. Lilienthal, with the most cordial affection. We wish him long life, and the happiness he deserves amid his new surroundings.

CORRECTION.—Dr. E. Hasbrouck, Brooklyn, writes that in the report of the proceedings of the State Society, in our March issue, he was credited with the disposal of several more mothers than is his due. In 959 obstetrical cases only seven mothers died instead of twelve.

RECORD OF MEDICAL PROGRESS.

ABSENCE OF HYDROCHLORIC ACID IN CANCEROUS STOMACHS.—Lépine holds, contrary to the opinion of Debove, that hydrochloric acid is not formed in the gastric juice of a cancerous stomach.—*Jour. des Soc. Scientifiques*, February 9th.

FRACTURED CERVICAL SPINE.—Mr. G. H. Hawes, reports a case of fracture of the spine in the upper cervical region, probably the atlas. The treatment consisted in rest, sand bags being used at first to maintain the head in proper position and to insure its stability ; later these were substituted by a rubber air collar. Perfect recovery ensued in ten weeks. *Brit. Med. Jour.*, February 5th, 1887.

FRECKLES.—Halkins believes that in carbolic acid we possess a certain cure for freckles. The skin, first washed and dried, is stretched with two fingers of the left hand, and each freckle is carefully touched with a drop of pure carbolic acid (ninety-eight per cent.?), which is allowed to dry on the skin. In from eight to ten days, the cauterised scale falls off and the spot, at first red, soon assumes its natural color.—*Edinb. Med. Jour.*, February, 1887.

HYSTERICAL HYPERTHERMIA.—Debove reported to the Société Médicale des Hôpitaux of Paris the case of a young woman who had, a year and a half before, fever attacks coming on every eight days, with temperature in the axilla of 39° to 39.5° C. During the whole month of December, 1885, Debove found the temperature to be 41°, and during the whole of January, 1886, 41° and 41.3°. This fever showed no evening exacerbation, and finally disappeared quite suddenly.—*Neurolog. Centralb.*, No. 2, 1887.

PAROXYSMAL HÆMOGLOBINURIA.—Bamberger reports a case of paroxysmal hæmoglobinuria in which the patient, a cab-driver aged 45, whenever exposed to cold had a chill, immediately followed by the secretion of blood-colored urine. After some hours the urine became normal. Bamberger made the experiment of having the man dip his hands in ice-cold water, and then sending him, lightly clad, into the open air. The attack quickly followed in the above-mentioned way. The urine contained hæmoglobin in solution, but hardly a single blood corpuscle.—*Internat. Klin. Rundschau*, No. 1.

PLUGGING THE POSTERIOR NARES.—Dr. James Brydon suggests the following (see *British Medical Journal*, January 8th, 1887, page 61) : "Take a piece of twine of sufficient length and fasten to the end of it a pledget of lint, rag, or a small globular button. Form a ring a quarter of an inch in diameter, on the end of a probe or wire, and bend it down. Run the twine through the ring till the pledget or button is close against it. Pass the wire along the floor of the nose to the posterior nares ; tell the patient to hawk and spit out, and the pledget with twine attached, is ejected through the mouth." The usual method is then followed.

CUTANEOUS HÆMORRHAGES BY AUTO-SUGGESTION.—Mabille and Ramadier have described cutaneous hæmorrhages on the places of the so-called stigmata. Further observations in auto-hypnotism show the occurrence of self-suggested cutaneous hæmorrhages at a specified time, and upon a selected locality: a letter A upon the forehead, the four letters of his name upon the left thigh, etc. The right side was anæsthetic, the left hyperæsthetic ; as through suggestion this circumstance was reversed it was impossible for the patient to cause the stigmata to appear on the left, they now appeared on the right.—*Neurolog. Centralb.*, No. 2, 1887.

SENSIBILITY OF THE DRUM MEMBRANE A FACTOR IN RECOGNITION OF THE DIRECTION OF SOUND. — Gellé has positively determined in several cases, in Charcot's clinic, that in cases of complete cutaneous anæsthesia, where the skin of the auditory meatus, and *the membrana tympani also,* was anæsthetic, the patient, who could in other respects hear perfectly, could not tell with the eyes closed from which direction, either right or left, the sound of a ticking watch came. Gellé believes it may thus be assumed that the sensibility of the drum membrane is necessary to the recognition of the direction whence a sound comes.—*Neurolog. Centralb.,* No. 3, 1887.

PUERPERAL PHLEBITIS.—Lancereaux, in the *Gaz. Méd. de Paris,* February 19th, 1887, reports in full a case of puerperal phlebitis in which there were involved in succession the utero-ovarian and renal veins, the vena cava, the hypogastric and femoral veins, from which the trouble extended to the renal arteries, then to the aorta, iliac and femoral arteries. The last two named were obstructed, and gangrene of both limbs resulted. The autopsy which established the diagnosis also served to show the propagation of the inflammation from the veins to the arteries, and the author questions whether the gangrene in phlebitis is not oftener due to such propagation than to the formation of thrombi or emboli.

EFFECTS OF TOBACCO ON THE MENTAL POWERS.—Rouillard in *L'encephalie No. 3, 1886,* is of the opinion that the use of tobacco is in a slight degree stimulant to brain function like alcohol; but much more, it exercises a dulling, stupefying influence which can only be tolerated through becoming accustomed to it, and that the deleterious influence of chronic nocotism is particularly exhibited in the memory. The statistics of insane asylums offer no positive testimony as to the injuriousness of tobacco, but on the other hand it is known that among children of women-workers in large tobacco factories there exists a much higher percentage of brain and nervous affections. *Neurol. Centralb. No. 1, 1887.*

CONSANGUINITY AND OFFSPRING.—M. G. Lagneau read, at the February meeting of the Société d'Anthropologie de Paris, a note relative to the influence on children of consanguinity in the parents. Lagneau quotes statistics furnished to him by Aubert, to show that the offspring of consanguineous marriages are healthy provided no morbid inheritance exists. In a manuscript addressed to the Académie de Médecine, Aubert states that the canton of Croisie with 2,783 inhabitants, of which 890 have the same name, finds itself in first range of forty-five cantons of the department in military aptitude. This canton counts only six exempts, while those of Ancenis and Loroux are 142 and 145 per 1,000.

STROPHANTHUS HISPIDUS.—A correspondent of the *Brit. Med. Jour.* writes: * * * "I had occasion to order a small quantity of the tincture (of strophanthus hispidus) from one of our principle chemists, and was surprised to hear that the gentleman engaged in preparing it was suddenly affected with a severe headache about the junction of the skin and hairy scalp, which gradually spread to the temples; this was accompanied by double vision, succeeded by impaired sight of left eye, nausea, but no actual vomiting, coldness of extremities and faintness. It was several hours before the effects passed off. The manager of the compounding department was similarly affected, but in a less degree." * * *

HYSTERIA AMONG SOLDIERS.—Duponchel reports a number of cases of severe hysteria among soldiers, thus supporting anew the opinion that this disease is by no means confined to females. He holds that the diagnosis can frequently be made outside the time of the hysterical attacks, if the examination be done with sufficient care. As specially important diag-

nostic signs he gives : hemianæsthesia, or single circumscribed anæsthetic zones, narrowing of the visual field and irregularity of the same for
single colors, loss of reflex irritability of the pharyngeal mucous membrane, anomalies of muscular sense. In severe cases the other well-known
phenomena, paralysis, contractures, etc., naturally appear.— *Neurolog.
Centralb.,* No. 2, 1887.

OBSERVATIONS ON THE PROGENY OF ALCOHOLICS.—Dursout gives sixteen clinical histories in a series of observations on the degeneration of
posterity from alcoholism. The material was from the department of
Finisterre, where drunkenness in men and women has become a scourge
to the country. Experience in these cases shows that dipsomania descends
as an inheritance from ancestors to their progeny ; that in the parent it is
the basis of mental weakness and idiocy in the offspring ; that the children
of such parents fall into vice and crime ; that alcoholism in the parents is
followed by epilepsy in their children ; that it is the cause of hydroceph-
alus, and that the families of dipsomaniacs rapidly die out.— *Neurolog.
Centralb.,* No. 2, 1887.

CANE-SUGAR SOLUTION FOR TRANSFUSION.—Dr. Lewin gives high praise
to the addition of cane sugar in three per cent. solution to the already employed solution of salt for injection into the blood vessels in place of transfusion of blood. Among other advantages which this method offers, not
the slightest is that the system receives a nutritive material. The mixture
acted well in animals that had been bled, and also on one man. The
former, after having lost six-sevenths of the normal blood-quantity, after
the infusion of this solution not only survived, but recovered very rapidly.
In a man 400 CC were infused. In chronic anæmia, in poisoning, especially by substances that alter the blood itself, such as *carbon mon-oxide,
nitro-bensol,* etc., this procedure is to be recommended.

INFLUENCE OF NICOTIN AND TOBACCO SMOKING UPON THE NERVOUS
CENTERS.—Schtscherbak reported to the St. Petersburg Psychiatric Society,
in December, 1886, his experiments upon animals with tobacco smoke and
nicotin. He deducts from them the following conclusions : the influence
of tobacco smoke upon the brain (increase of irritability) is to be ascribed
to the nicotin taken up in the organism. Apart from these experiments,
it is shown by cases of excessive smoking, of accidental swallowing of
tobacco leaf, enveloping the surface of the body with tobacco, that tobacco
intoxication is due to nicotin. In two subjects the author, investigating
the nervous system after acute tobacco poisoning, found loss of cutaneous
sensibility, lessened sensibility of hearing, limitation of the visual field
(especially for green), and weakened tendon reflexes.—*Neurolog. Centralb.,*
No. 3, 1887.

PENETRATING WOUND OF BRAIN—RECOVERY.—Brigade Surgeon Wilson,
of Perth, sends the following remarkable record to the *Brit. M. Jour.,* 1887,
p. 278. He was called on January 28th, '86, to see a child who had fallen,
while standing in a chair, onto the point of an upright paper-file of copper.
The weight of the child and the force of the fall had caused the wire to
penetrate the right side of the occipital bone near its junction with the
petious portion of the temporal bone, a little below the level of the external
auditory meatus. When withdrawn, it was found that the file had penetrated more than three inches into the brain, in a direction somewhat upwards and forwards. The child when seen shortly after the accident was
in a state of profound collapse, but the breathing was stertorous ; the
pupils reacted to light ; the child had vomited. The treatment consisted
in absolute quiet. The comatose condition relaxed by the second day, and
by the twelfth day the child was apparently perfectly well.

PREVENTION OF IRRITATION OF THE AUDITORY MEATUS.—Dr. Duncan J. Mackenzie, of Glossop, writes to the *Brit. Med. Jour.*, January 8th, 1887, that the irritation at the external auditory meatus, caused by the mixture of discharge and boracic acid, after the application of the latter for suppurative otitis may be, in part, prevented by drying the meatus thoroughly with cotton, so as to prevent the adherence of the powder on moist spots and to allow its free passage towards the membrane. After applying the acid in the way described, a small piece of absorbent cotton is rolled tightly around the end of the probe, which is then introduced into the meatus and carried around its circumference so as to remove all the adherent particles. The probe is then removed and another piece of cotton applied, as before, with the exception that it is first dipped into an ointment of eucalyptus one part, and vaseline seven parts. The ear is then closed in the usual way with cotton. Dr. Mackenzie finds that this method not only prevents but cures the irritation.

ACTION OF POTASSIUM NITRATE.—Mairet and Combemale presented to the Société de Biologie, January 29th, the first part of their results on the action of nitrate of potash, and at the meeting of the fifth of February, their results with large doses. In small quantity, the action of the nitrate is to increase the water of the urine. The twenty-four hours' urine is augmented by from ten to sixteen fluid ounces, rarely more; while the urea and uric acid are not increased: The authors set themselves the task of explaining this action, and conclude that the nitre produces the diuresis by a direct action on the blood corpuscles, from which the water is in part extracted. The action of large doses of the drug is to provoke a gastro-enteritis, as manifested by the following symptoms: Vomiting, diarrhœa, depression of temperature and strength, weakness of heart's action and pulse, with increased frequency and diminished number of respirations. Depression is its marked characteristic.— *Jour. des Soc. Scientifiques*, February 9th and 16th, 1887. Nos. 6 and 7.

TO ASCERTAIN WHETHER GANGRENE IS LIKELY TO FOLLOW SEVERE INJURY.—Dr. W. Scott Lang contributes to the *Edinburgh Medical Journal*, January, 1887, page 597, an article on the above subject. He says that, to obtain an accurate idea of the probability of circulation being restored to an injured limb: "Gently raise the limb and keep it raised for two or three minutes, in order, to some extent, to empty it of blood, then apply a tourniquet or piece of elastic webbing on the proximal side of the injury and keep it applied for about a minute; lower the limb, remove the compression, and if sufficient circulation remains, the part beyond the seat of injury will blush rosy red, and will show in an unmistakable manner the condition of the blood-vessels." The procedure is especially recommended in those cases where a part is almost severed, in cases of frost-bite and embolism. It will promptly show the extent of approaching gangrene, and amputation may probably be performed without waiting for the appearance of the line of demarcation.

NEW FORM OF EXOPHTHALMUS.—Hack, *Deutsche Med. Woch.*, No. 25, 1886, describes a case of a girl, seventeen years old, who had double exophthalmus since early childhood. In May, 1885, she complained of pains and cardiac palpitation. Soon there appeared signs of cardiac hypertrophy. At the same time the exophthalmus was aggravated, and tumefaction of the left lobe of the thyroid gland increased. She had had obstruction of the nasal fossæ, which then increased to such a degree that operation was deemed advisable. Cauterization was, therefore, resorted to in the right nostril, with the surprising result of decreasing the exophthalmus at that side nearly to disappearance. The left side remained as before. Some days after, the left side of the nose was operated on in the same way, and on that side the exophthalmus diminished, but more slowly and less completely than on the right. After several months the nearly absolute cure of the exophthalmus was maintained, the palpitation disappeared, and the heart regained its normal volume. The enlargement of the thyroid diminished, but did not disappear.—*Edinb. Med. Jour.*, January, 1887.

HYSTERICAL MONOPLEGIA, WITH CONTRACTURE OF THE RIGHT ARM, LASTING FOR SIX MONTHS, CURED IN HALF AN HOUR BY HYPNOTIC SUGGESTION.—Dr. A. Voisin, while on a journey, found himself in a small station in southern France, and had to wait before a train would start. There was brought to him a woman, aged 40, who for two years had had different kinds of hysterical attacks, and for six months had suffered from a paralysis, with contracture of the right arm. The nails of the fingers had dug deeply into the tissues of the palm, and the ulceration gave out a horrible smell. Besides, there were obstinate constipation and retention of urine, necessitating the use of the catheter. Voisin hypnotised the patient deeply, commanded her to extend the fingers one after the other, to move the hand, to extend and to flex the fore-arm and the arm. Then he ordered her to go away and wash the hand and have the nails cut. The paralysis and contracture were permanently relieved, as he afterward heard. Unfortunately he had not time to remove the constipation and retention of urine by suggestion, so that the patient still suffers from these.—*Neurolog. Centralb.*, No. 3, 1887.

NEWS.

IT is said that coffee is one of the best antidotes for the effects of tobacco.

AMERICAN INSTITUTE OF HOMŒOPATHY.—The annual meeting of the American Institute of Homœopathy will be held at Saratoga, June 27th–July 1st, 1887.

TRAINING SCHOOL.—The Trustees of fhe Buffalo Homœopathic Hospital have completed arrangements for the establishment of a training school for nurses.

COMMENCEMENT EXERCISES.—The New York Homœopathic Medical College will hold its annual commencement exercises at Chickering Hall, April 14th, 1887, at 4 P.M.

HON. JOHN S. NEWBERRY, of Detroit, who recently gave $100,000 toward the establishment of a free homœopathic hospital in Detroit, died January 2d, 1887. The hospital he so liberally endowed will be his most enduring monument.

OBITUARY.—Mrs. Lucy M. Arndt died at Ann Arbor, Mich., on December 14th, 1886. She was the wife of Dr. H. R. Arndt, editor of the *Medical Counsellor*. Dr. Arndt has the sincere sympathy of his friends in his great bereavement.

PERSONAL NOTE.—The late Henry Ward Beecher was attended during his illness by Dr. W. S. Searle. Dr. Searle graduated with honor from Hamilton College in 1855, and from the University of Pennsylvania in 1859. He is one of the prominent homœopathic physicians of Brooklyn.

ALBANY SOCIETY.--At the twenty-seventh annual meeting of the Albany County Homœopathic Medical Society, Dr. H. M. Paine was elected President, and Dr. R. B. Sullivan Vice-President. Dr. Schwartz was elected a delegate to the State Society in place of Dr. Wright. The annual report showed the society to be in excellent condition.

MAY SOCIETY MEETINGS.—The thirty-second annual meeting of the Illinois Homœopathic Medical Association will be held at Joliet, Ill., May 17th, 18th and 19th. Dr. C. M. Beebe, Secretary, Chicago. The Indiana Institute of Homœopathy meets in Indianapolis in May. The Ohio Homœopathic Medical Society will meet at Cleveland, May 10th and 11th.

LEAGUE WORK.—The Homœopathic League is extending its work. While pushing the publication and distribution of its excellent tracts, it has also opened another branch of its work in the way of giving lectures in the principal towns. Dr. Pope delivered the first of the series at Leicester recently, upon an invitation extended by the Leicester Literary and Philosophical Society.

STAFF APPOINTMENTS.—The following changes in the Surgical Staff of the New York Ophthalmic Hospital have been made during the past year: C. C. Boyle, M.D., O.et A.Chir., has been appointed surgeon in the Ophthalmic and Aural Department; Geo. M. Dillow, M.D., and Malcolm Leal, M.D., surgeons in the Department of Laryngology; and C. E. Teets, M.D., and A. W. Palmer, M.D., assistant surgeons in the same department.

A NEW TREATMENT OF GONORRHŒA.—The treatment is based on the view that gonorrhœal urethritis is a parasitic disease; that the microbe can only live in an acid medium. Injections of bi-carbonate of sodium are commenced as soon as the discharge appears, or the patient comes under observation—three or four injections being made daily of a one per cent. solution. The urethral secretion is tested every day with litmus paper, and the injection is kept up until the discharge becomes alkaline or neutral.

A MATCHED PAIR.—"Moxie's Nerve Food" was recently shown, by careful analysis, to be innocent of any properties that would enable it to affect the nervous system in any way, being simply a mild and harmless drink, and now the much advertised "Kaskine," "The New Quinine," has been analyzed and found to be granular sugar, with a minute trace of quinine—one one-thousandth of a grain to a pellet. These are but samples of scores of similar remedies widely advertised in the daily and religious press, and still Simple Simon buys and swallows.

BOSTON UNIVERSITY SCHOOL.—The friends of the Boston University School of Medicine are possessed of a commendable zeal. A circular issued by a committee of citizens states the origin and aims of the school, its work in the past, its ambition for the future, its wants and necessities, and appeals to those who may be interested to contribute toward raising a mortgage of $35,000 now resting on the property of the school, and also toward a proposed endowment fund of $200,000. The Boston School has an excellent record, and is worthy of a good endowment fund. We wish our Boston friends good speed in their work.

WESTERN SOCIETY.—The meeting of the Western New York Homœopathic Medical Society held at Buffalo recently, was of special value to those in attendance. It is reported that the papers presented are rapidly diminishing in length, and that the discussions following are growing in interest and fulness. It would not be amiss if some larger and more pretentious organizations, emulating the good example of this Western Society, should summarily abbreviate the time now given up to ponderous and musty compilations called essays by courtesy, and so afford more opportunity and encouragement for the discussions which may be made the most valuable part of every meeting.

LIBERTY OF OPINION.—The Margaret Street Infirmary of London is an institution of some years' standing. Recently it became the scene of a contest between the adherents of allopathy and the friends of homœopathy. The result was a complete victory for the new school. In great disgust at this unexpected ending of the dispute, the allopathic members of the staff have tendered their resignations. This partisan attempt to check all liberty of opinion in therapeutics became a most dangerous boomerang for those who originated the attack. The places of those who resigned will be promptly filled by men of wider views and more liberal education, and the infirmary will do better work than ever before.

ALUMNI BANQUET.—The Alumni Association of the New York Homœopathic Medical College will give its yearly dinner at Delmonico's, April 14th, 1887. The business meeting of the association is called at 7 P.M. Nearly 200 alumni and invited guests attended the dinner last year, and the indications are that the attendance this year will surpass that number. It is believed that this will be the most successful dinner ever given by the association, and the committee desire particularly to invite those who have not heretofore attended. The toast-master of the evening will be Selden H. Talcott, M.D., and an enjoyable literary programme may be anticipated. Tickets for the dinner may be procured in advance from the Secretary of the Executive Committee, or from the Treasurer, the night of the dinner.

ALVAN E. SMALL, M.D.—On the last day of 1886 Dr. Alvan E. Small suddenly died at his residence in Chicago. For nearly half a century he was a prominent figure in the profession, always found in the van of progress. Dr. Small graduated from the University of Pennsylvania in 1841. Shortly after beginning practice he became convinced of the truth of homœopathy, and ever since that time labored earnestly for the advancement of the school to which he belonged. From 1849 to 1856 he was connected with the Homœopathic Medical College of Philadelphia as Professor of Pathology. In 1856 he resigned his chair and removed to Chicago, where he resided during the rest of his life. When the Hahnemann Medical College was organized in 1859, Dr. Small was elected Dean, and until the time of his death was connected with it in some capacity, as Professor or Trustee. He was the author of a large work on "Domestic Practice," and just before his death had completed a work on "Practice for the Use of the Profession." His genial and kindly nature had endeared him to his friends and his memory will long be cherished.

TEST FOR ARSENIC.—A simple and easily applied test for arsenic in wall-paper has been devised by Mr. F. F. Grenstted. No apparatus is needed beyond an ordinary gas jet which is turned down to quite a fine point, until the flame is wholly blue; when this has been done a slip of the paper suspected to contain arsenic is cut one-sixteenth of an inch wide and an inch or so long. Directly the edge of this paper is brought into contact with the outer edge of the gas flame a gray coloration, due to arsenic, will be seen in the flame (test No. 1). The paper is burned a little and the fumes that are given off will be found to have a strong, garlic-like odor, due to the vapor of arsenic acid (test No. 2). Take the paper away from the flame and look at the charred end; the carbon will be colored a bronze-red; this is copper reduced by the carbon (test No. 3). Being now away from the flame, in a fine state of division, the copper is slightly oxydized by the air, and on placing the charred end a second time not too far into the flame, the flame will now be colored green by copper (test No. 4). By this simple means it is possible to form an opinion as to whether any wall-paper contains arsenic, for copper arseniate is commonly used in preparing wall-paper. Tests 1 and 2 would be yielded by any paper containing arsenic in considerable quantity.

Vol. XXXV.   *MAY, 1887.*   (Volume II, Third Series.)   No. 5.

North American
Journal of Homœopathy.

ORIGINAL ARTICLES IN MEDICINE.

HOMŒOPATHIC MEDICAL SOCIETY, COUNTY OF NEW YORK.
QUERY: HAVE THE CAUSES WHICH LED TO ITS ORGANIZATION CEASED TO BE ACTIVE?*

By HENRY C. HOUGHTON, M.D.,
New York.

MR. PRESIDENT, LADIES AND GENTLEMEN.—The recently enacted changes in our Constitution require of your presiding officer that he give an address upon retiring from his duties, as well as upon his inauguration; so I can follow the example of Ahab, King of Israel, and say, "Let not him that girdeth on his harness boast himself as he that putteth it off." My duty is a review of the past year; I can safely trust the future to my esteemed colleague, whom you have honored by your suffrages, and whom you will support by your coöperation.

My theme is the Homœopathic Medical Society of the County of New York. Have the causes which led to its organization ceased to act? Should the Society be abandoned?

In order to answer this question, it will be necessary to look briefly at the status of the medical profession in New York City previous to 1857, the date at which this Society was organized, under the laws of this State. The inheritance of the ages had come down in an accumulating flood of empirical knowledge, till it struck a snag in the shape of Hahnemann's completed work on materia medica, issued in 1821. Soon after, in 1825, Dr. Gram, of Copenhagen, son of a cultivated Dane, nephew of the physician to the Swedish king, a com-

---

* Address before the Homœopathic Medical Society, County of New York, by the retiring President, January 13th, 1887.

petent and successful physician, had, at forty years of age, attained
such financial status as to be above want ; this gentleman had become
a convert to Hahnemann's views, after his return to Copenhagen from
America, on account of his father's death in New York.

During 1823, '24 and '25, he tested the truth.   In 1826 he returned
to America and located in this city.   He was introduced to the late
Dr. John F. Gray, by a patient of the same ; this led to an investigation of what Dr. Gray calls " an entirely novel mode of practice."
This was in 1827.   Dr. Gray acquired a knowledge of German in
order to master the materia medica, and a year later became, as
he says, "a competent prescriber of and a full convert to Homœopathy."

Dr. A. D. Wilson was the second convert ; then came Drs. A.
Gerald Hull, J. T. Curtis, Wm. Channing, and later, Drs. Freeman,
Joslin, Bayard, Ball, Bowers, Barlow, Hallock and others.   The only
organization for fraternal intercourse in the city, of which I can learn,
was the New York Homœopathic Physicians' Society, of which Dr.
Joslin was president, in 1843.   The evolution of homœopathic practice
was a process of personal, individual instruction, in many cases, after
a way like that followed by Nicodemus.   My revered friend, Dr. A.
S. Ball, recently gave, in a social interview, some idea of the experience through which the pioneers of our school were compelled to
pass.   He had removed to this city from the central part of the State,
and practiced according to his old school training.   Becoming
acquainted with Dr. Curtis, he was led to investigate the effects of
medicine prepared and exhibited according to the new method ; his
study was Nicodemus-like, going to the doctor's office at night ; there
he detailed cases and went out to give the medicine, as advised.   In
some cases he placed the patient in Dr. Curtis' care.   When he was
ready to treat his patients independently, and it became known that
he was using the "little doses," he was not only dropped from all
fraternal relations, but his former associates, to whom he brought
letters of introduction, ignored him entirely, passing him with averted
faces when they met upon the street.   Everyone who was known to
be even tolerant to homœopathists, although they did not fraternize
with them, were under suspicion and their apostacy anticipated by
invidious remarks.

From 1826 to 1856 all efforts to obtain any fraternal organization
as a representative body failed, because of the opposition of the
"regular school"—so called.   A glimpse of the nature of this opposition may be had from the following sentence quoted from a letter to
Hon. Wm. Kelly by Dr. J. Vanderburgh, written upon the occasion of

the passage of the Senate Bill, March 1st, 1856, authorizing the formation of homœopathic societies : "What shall we render to you for such service? You have abolished the sentence of outlawry, confirmed by the approval of three generations, against us; you have legalized a profession that has borne the finger of scorn for fifty years, and have given us the consolation of knowing that when the pilgrimage of this life is ended, we may be buried in consecrated ground."

The younger members of this society can have little idea of the bar put upon those who adopted homœopathic practice. It must be a sad case that called for such words as the following, from the lips of the late Carroll Dunham, M.D. : "The most bitter aspersions upon Hahnemann's personal character"—"abounding in the most concentrated contempt and scorn of the system which Hahnemann had unfolded !" . . . "And from that day to the present, all the utterances of the old school, whether from the press, the council, the professors' chair, or in the forum of the academy, have been bitter, personal denunciations of the character and motives of Hahnemann, and of all who have adopted, or have even shown a disposition to investigate his method."

A few weeks will complete a term of thirty years since the homœopathic school of the practice of medicine was made "regular" by State legislation, as regular as any other practitioners; a term of sixty years since Dr. Gram found his first American student, Dr. Gray. What a change ! The homœopathic idea dominates the medical practice of to-day ; the seed sown of Hahnemann's thought now waves like autumnal fields ; protected by legislation, our practitioners become public teachers, in State and County Societies, in public journals and medical schools, so that the progressive minds of the old school have had ample opportunity to read and digest the literature of the new. What is the result of this dissemination of new ideas ?

The last reports to the American Institute of Homœopathy give two national societies, five special societies, twenty-eight state societies, ninety-four local and county societies, nineteen medical clubs, six medical associations (miscellaneous), twenty-five general and twenty-nine special hospitals, forty-eight dispensaries, thirteen medical colleges, two special schools, twenty-one medical journals, forty-five new books and pamphlets and fourteen reports and transactions of societies. These figures give some slight idea of the influence exerted by the homœopathic wing of the profession. Many books and tracts have been issued for the purpose of popularizing the new practice, with remarkable results ; such, that the laity have been in advance of the profession, in adopting this simple, pleasant, effective mode of medication ; indeed the lay demand has compelled attention on the part of many physicians, who would otherwise have been ignorant of homœopathy.   It is to the intelligent, progressive layman that the profession is indebted for the liberal spirit that has controlled legislation, specially in this, the Empire State.   Our friends of the opposite side have come to recognize the fact, that no important medical legislation can hope to succeed that does not recognize the claim of the homœopathists to, at least, a respectful hearing.   We have and hold a large percentage of the wealth, the culture of the great cities of America, and the public sentiment to support our practice.

Perhaps the most remarkable result to be noted as following the teaching and practice of the new doctrine has been the effect upon the methods of the dominant school.   Dr. Pemberton Dudley thus gives a retrospect in an address entitled "The Test at the Bedside."   The medical practice of fifty years ago bears a not very close semblance to that of to-day.   The orthodox old doctors of those days, could they look in upon the sick chambers of our time, would be amazed, perhaps horrified, at the transformation of things since they fell asleep.   The click of the trigger lancet is heard no more, the blood bowl has vanished, the slimy leech has disappeared, the cup is broken, the seton is unheard of, the actual cautery is consigned—covered with merited anathemas—to the lowest depths of oblivion; the blister only rarely obtrudes its unwelcome presence ; the patient, exhausted by disease, is not still further exhausted by the rude and crude and violent methods of fifty years ago, nor of twenty-five years ago.   The disease is no longer regarded as a monster of hideous mien; to be vomited out, and purged out, and sweat out, and salivated out, and blistered out, and suppurated out, and burnt out.   The physician's visits are no longer dreaded, the sick room is no more a chamber of horrors, where once there were noisome odors and nauseating drugs, and the pangs of "treatment" worse than the pains of disease, and thirst unassuaged, and loathing and dread unutterable ; to-day there is a clean bed, the clean room, the clean atmosphere, the clean and quiet surroundings, the confident expression, the bodily needs satisfied, the pains alleviated, the strength carefully husbanded, the convalescence shortened.

"What has brought about the change ?   How has this rapid transformation been accomplished ?   Why does it come about that medical men have abandoned as not only useless, but positively harmful, those heroic measures that only a few short years ago were considered absolutely essential to the safety of the sick ?   Ask the allopathic professor and you will be told : 'We were compelled to discontinue our heroic treatment. Public sentiment and the demands of our patients forced us into milder measures.' Ask the people what brought the change in public sentiment, and they will tell you that it was the fact that homœopathy could cure its patients without a resort to those violent and dangerous methods. And so this is the first decided test of the efficacy and power of homœopathy. It has revolutionized the practice of the opposing school, and has changed the whole appearance and condition and circumstances of the chamber of sickness, where-ever an enlightened medical art carries its ministrations."

Coincident with the abandonment of the items mentioned by Dr. Dudley, we see an adoption of Hahnemann's discoveries under the guise of "physiological medicine." Following the lead of Ringer and Barthelow, the students of the new therapeutics have become the most audacious plagiarists ; unless it be true that on account of the degen-eration of the race, the brain has come to exercise unconscious cere-bration to an extraordinary degree, and in the special line of medical literature, selecting for the greatest functional activity, the department of materia medica and therapeutics.

In keeping with the adoption of " physiological medicine " we see a change in pharmaceutical methods. The old bolus and draught have retired, to give place to the sugar-coated pill, the granule, the parvule, the tablet triturate, " according to the method of Dr. Robert Fuller," *i. e.*, a Fuller genesis of the Hahnemannian idea. There is one farther evolution to be devoutly desired : a practice of the old injunction, "honor to whom honor is due."

It is just twenty years since I became a member of this society, and my retrospect is not calculated to discourage. On graduating from the medical department of the University of New York, the Hospital of the Five Points House of Industry was the only public institution in which homœopathy was officially recognized and prac-ticed ; two other institutions for children had medical care by homœo-pathists. The N. Y. Ophthalmic Hospital was placed in our hands the next year, and rapidly in succession during a score of years have we come to our present status. The record of the society for the past year is in some respects its best. As reported by the secretary, the membership is larger than ever ; this is in a measure due to efforts made to induce physicians practicing homœopathy in this city to join the society. When in Albany last February, with the Committee on Legislation of the State Society, the features of the law compelling membership in some county medical society were brought out, and on my return I urged the presentation of this fact to our colleagues. A fraternal circular was sent to such, and a gratifying response, leading to increased numbers, has been the result.

Every physician practicing homœopathy in this city should be a member of this county society, not merely for the sake of numbers. The matter is mutual ; every member receives as well as gives, but the obligation is greater on the part of the society so far as the introduction to membership is concerned. Those who come to the city ought to join the society for their own benefit, but we may well engage in a little winsome wooing. With the exception of a few persons who may be lapsing in fraternal spirit, every one practicing according to our methods may be induced to co-operate with us. It might be well to have a standing committee on initiations whose duty it should be to aid the secretary in this matter.

In view of the work that has been done by this society in thirty years, what reply shall be made to those who ask us to abandon our distinctive organization ? The " new code " departure of the allopathic wing of the profession is the result of a demand, voiced in public sentiment, rather than professional conversion. The spirit that has resisted the new school idea is not dead ; it is repressed, but similar in nature, and is manifested whenever it is warmed into temporary activity ; if you doubt it go and study medical legislation at Albany. The old school society of this city is not ready to reconsider the action which compelled our veteran members to organize this society, that they might have an opportunity to confer with each other, without being subjected to ridicule. The standing rule of the old school society is a menace to free expression of our views. He who enters there must abandon all hope, at least of being listened to with respect, if he advances any statement of therapeutics based upon the truth as held by the members of this society.

Well did Dunham say, in 1863, ''Now, as in the days of Hahnemann, there is an *antagonism* between the homœopathists and the old school. The former hold out to the latter what they believe to be that method which has ever been a *desideratum* in medicine. The latter refuse even to examine it, and expel the homœopathists from all associations over which they hold control. We cannot unite with them in any associated labors without ignoring and disavowing what we believe to be the true theory and practice of the all-important part of medical science—the science of therapeutics. *They will not unite* with us in associated labors for the development of this science."

Some one may suggest that physicians who were members of this society have withdrawn and have been cordially received by the old school society. The fact I admit; but the terms ! ! ! A virtual admis-

sion that they have no belief to guide them in the practice of the healing art ; possibly some were not strained by that admission ; but we
know that others did practice—do now practice—as we do, guided by a
law, a principle ; yes, a dogma, if one is dogmatic. As to the matter
of cordiality, if one can judge from the reports of Dame Rumor, it is
like in kind with that manifested in a Modoc council, where the pipe
of peace is held out with the right hand, while the tomahawk is
grasped under the blanket with the left, and negotiations for peace are
mingled with plans for a future massacre.

I am reminded of the cartoons issued during Greeley's historic campaign, in which Brown always appeared in diminutive contrast, labelled,
" Me, too." We respectfully decline any " *Me, too,*" relation. A
stranger may be invited to a friendly game of cards in a miner's cabin,
but if the tenderfoot insists upon his views of.methods, there come a
lively time and the possibilities of an autopsy. We respectfully decline.
I sympathize with the views of the most liberal men on both sides
who desire a union of the profession. No one likes to be under a ban.
Principle may interfere with progress of a certain sort for a time ; but
good, and only good, can come from faithful adherence to truth. In
the meantime, we may rest assured that the transformation will go on.
We invite the practitioners of medicine to.be students of physiological
medicine, to read the books of our best authors, to put our remedies to
the test at the bedside, and they will find what thousands of old school
men have found, that the new methods of practice are true, sure,
safe !

What of the outlook? I am not a prophet, although a seventh son.
I cannot say when the two schools will unite ; they may be two
lines separated by a radicle, always approaching, yet never to meet ;
at least organically. I can see a possible outlook. When *similia* is
admitted to be *a* law of practice, *a* truth which any medical man can
hold without being subject to contempt; when it is taught in all
medical schools, leaving the option with the student ; when the public
hospitals are open for service without discrimination against us ; when
remedies prepared according to the " *Fuller* " method are furnished in
the hospitals and can be dispensed, with the guarantee that the test of
results shall be clear and untrammelled ; when service in the army
and navy is open to us, then we will abandon our separate organizations, into which our fathers were forced, and we can then do so without fear, because the truth will demonstrate itself.

I can find no more fitting words with which to close than those of
Hahnemann, used by Dr. Dunham on a similar occasion. His pro-
phecy has already been partially fulfilled:

"Our art needs no political lever; no worldly badges of honor in order to become something. Amid all the rank and unsightly weeds that flourish round about it, it grows gradually from a small acorn to a slender tree; already its lofty summit overtops the rank vegetation around it. Only have patience! It strikes the more certainly, and in due time it will grow up to a lofty, God's oak, stretching its great arms, that no longer bend to the storm, far away into all the regions of the earth; and mankind, who have hitherto been tormented, will be refreshed under its beneficent shadows"—(*Dudgeon Lectures—Introduction.*)

COLCHICUM AND CAULOPHYLLUM.*

By JOHN L. MOFFAT, M.D.,
Brooklyn, N. Y.

HAVING occasion the other day to prescribe for an old lady with painful swollen finger joints, *colchicum* and *caulophyllum* at once came to mind; the question was, which shall it be? These drugs, while having a marked similarity in symptoms when presented in the Hahnemannian *schema*, are so diverse in their physiological spheres of action that, viewed from that standpoint, one would hardly think of comparing them.

COLCHICUM.	CAULOPHYLLUM.
Head.	*Head.*
Pressive heaviness deep in cerebellum on mental exertion. Boring headache over eyes. Very painful drawing tearing, eyeball to occiput, left side. (*Spig.*)	Headache, pressure behind eye; dim sight; from uterine trouble. Severe pain in temples, as if they would be crushed together.
Eyes.	*Eyes.*
Drawing, digging pains, deep in orbit. Pressure and biting in canthi, with moderate lachrymation.	Pressure behind eyes; profuse flow of tears.
Face.	*Face.*
Sickly expression; yellow spotted.	"Moth spots" on forehead (with leucorrhœa).
Teeth.	*Teeth.*
Sensitive on pressing them together; feel too long.	Teeth all feel sore, elongated.
Tongue.	*Tongue.*
Coated white, or bright red; *heavy, stiff, numb.*	Tongue coated white.
Mouth.	*Mouth.*
Heat in mouth, with thirst.	Mouth feels hot and dry.

* Read before the Kings County Homœopathic Medical Society.

COLCHICUM.

Throat.

Inflammation of tonsils, palate and fauces ; swallowing difficult.

Stomach, etc.

Great thirst, but no appetite.

Loathes the *smell* or sight of food.

Frequent eructations of tasteless gas; eructations with burning in stomach. Violent burning in epigastrium. *Stomach icy cold*, with great pain and debility.

Violent vomiting and retching motion. (*Tabac.*)

Nausea, with great restlessness.

Abdomen.

Griping pains in the abdomen. Colic, after flatulent food.

Colic, with great distension of abdomen, until diarrhœa sets in. Distension as if he had eaten too much. Flatulent distension of abdomen, with less frequent and less copious stools.

Pain in right hypochondrium, as from incarcerated flatus.

Stool.

Dysentery.

Copious, frequent, watery, or bilious —often without pain, sometimes with cutting colic.

Transparent, gelatinous, membranous.

Urine.

Copious, watery, frequent, but generally *scanty, dark, turbid*, with burning and tenesmus.

Male Sexuals.

Every few minutes sharp, stinging pain in the glans penis.

Female Sexuals.

Menses too soon.

Feverish restlessness in the last months of pregnancy.

Larynx.

Voice hoarse, or deeper than usual.

Breathing quick and audible, or slow ; irregular. Oppression or tension of the chest. Night cough, with involuntary spurting of urine.

Lacerating pains in chest; violent, cutting ; dull stitches *during expiration.*

CAULOPHYLLUM.

Throat.

"Distress" in the fauces, causing frequent inclination to swallow.

Stomach, etc.

Great thirst.

Canine hunger, with white coated tongue.

Empty eructations. Heat in the stomach ; fullness.

Spasmodic vomiting, cardialgia, excessive nausea ; (from uterine irritation.)

Abdomen.

Spasmodic and flatulent colic.

Spasms in the intestines from motor irritation, or from rheumatism. Distension of abdomen, with tenderness. Rumbling in the bowels.

Distress in stomach and bowels, with drawing in right hypochondrium.

Stool.

Constipation.

Watery stools ; great quantity but no pain.

Soft stool, very white.

Urine.

Copious, pale or straw colored.

Male Sexuals.

Tearing in glans and left spermatic cord.

Female Sexuals.

Menses too early.

Threatening abortion; vascular excitement ; tremulous weakness.

Larynx.

Loss of voice (reflex from uterus.)

Spasmodic affections of chest and larynx.

Spasmodic intermittent pains in chest.

COLCHICUM.

Neck and Back.

Stitches and tension between the scapulæ.

Tearing and drawing pains in neck, back and shoulders, preventing motion of the head.

Sudden tearing and shooting in loins.

Limbs.

Tearing pains in the muscles and joints; more marked action in the small joints.

Tearing, tensive pains, quickly changing location.

Arms.

Laming or paralytic pains in arms, so violent he cannot hold anything firmly. Rheumatic pains in arms, extending into ligaments of finger joints.

Oedematous swelling; numbness and pricking of hands. Inflamed finger joints.

Legs.

Tearing pains. Numbness and pricking.

Oedematous swelling of legs and feet, with coldness. With the pains, weariness, heaviness and inability to move.

Toes tingle, as after being frosted. (*Agar.*)

Generalities.

Sudden and extreme prostration.

Trembling weakness. Paralytic feeling with the pains. Very sensitive to slightest touch.

Paralysis after sudden suppression of sweat, specially of the feet; after getting wet.

Sleep.

Sleep disturbed or prevented by pains; starting, jerking in sleep; waked by frightful dreams.

Drowsy during the day.

CAULOPHYLLUM.

Neck and Back.

Pains shift to nape with spasmodic rigidity; high fever, nervous excitement. Rheumatic stiffness in nape.

Severe drawing · pains in sterno-cleido-mastoid muscle, drawing head to left.

Dull pain in lumbar region.

Limbs.

Rheumatism of the small joints. Drawing pains in the joints.

Constant flying pains in arms and legs; remain only a few minutes in any one place.

Arms.

Cutting in joints when closing hands; fingers very stiff.

Severe drawing in wrists and fingers, with swelling.

Legs.

Drawing pains.

All joints crack when walking or turning.

Drawing pains in toes, worse at night.

Generalities.

General debility; emaciation, anæmia.

Partial loss of sensation. Pains are intermittent.

Paraplegia, with retroversion and congestion of uterus after childbirth.

Sleep.

Sleepless, restless, nervous.

COLCHICUM.	CAULOPHYLLUM.
Fever.	*Fever.*
Cold stage predominates; febrile symptoms few and moderate. Frequent localized chilliness or shudderings. Sweat suppressed, or copious and sour.	High fever, nervous excitement.
Aggravation.	*Aggravation.*
Better in open air. Worse night; mental exertion; motion.	Worse in open air; better in room.
Often indicated for old people.	Especially suited for females.

Colchicum, the autumn crocus, or meadow saffron, was well known to the ancients, being named from the island Colchos. Dunham classes it with *ledum, rhododendron, kalmia* and *spigelia.*

I condense from his lecture the most lucid exposition of the remedy within my reach.

It acts mainly on the periosteum, synovial membranes of the joints, digestive organs, and the nerves of voluntary motion. That is, about equally upon the vital force and tissues, yet not, to any degree, upon the mind, which in fatal cases of poisoning is clear to the last. Most of the mental symptoms encountered are secondary to the general depression of the system.

Large doses cause muscular *prostration*, slow breathing, slow and feeble pulse. Death comes by paralysis of the heart.

There is an intense action upon the digestive tract, resulting in a picture of *Asiatic cholera* to collapse, or in an attack of *gastro-enteritis*, or of *dysentery*.

Tympanites, nausea and loathing of food are emphatic symptoms, but not necessarily associated.

The pains are *tearing*, and drawing or tensive; they frequently change their location and come in small spots, or they consist of tearing shocks, involving half the body at a time.

"The most distressing pains are the sticking shocks or jerks, which are felt deep in the soft parts and, as it were, upon the periosteum."

We also find creeping, shuddering, numbness and prickling sensations, "accompanied by a symptom which is characteristic of *colchicum*, viz., a feeling of muscular weakness or paralysis, worse in the arms and legs." There is a sensation of trembling all over the body, the weakness is so great. The whole body is sore and sensitive.

There are sticking pains in the joints, which are painful and inflamed, but do not suppurate. Pains in the bones, the shoulder and hip joints, but especially in the small joints.

Colchicum cures gout by its specific action, not by affecting the elimination of urea or uric acid, or by any hydragogue properties. Dunham observed that it relieved gout most effectively when means were taken to prevent its action on the bowels.

Old school authorities have for years been united in cautioning its administration in gout as a dangerous remedy, only to be given to strong, vigorous patients, who are able to withstand its depressing effect.

Its pathogenesis shows clearly that it is especially homœopathic to the asthenic form of this disease, and of rheumatism also. Dunham, in cautioning against too large doses, says we should strive to obtain the specific without the physiological effects, and thinks it not safe to give a larger dose than the fifteenth potency in a well-marked *colchicum* case.

The study of this drug has been too much neglected in cholera and typhoid fever. Many of us associate it in our minds solely with disgust for the smell of food and with autumnal dysentery, but if we prescribe it according to its pathogenesis its usefulness will not be so restricted.

Asthma has been cured by it, and palpitation. A peculiar chest symptom is the "dull stitches *during expiration.*" In many cases of poisoning, cataracts have formed before death occurred. Hoppe greatly benefited three cases of soft cataract, but did not cure them.

Colchicum may prove of value in spinal irritation ; beside the tearing, tensive, stitching pains in the back and neck, there is a spot on the sacrum, as large as the hand, which feels sore as if ulcerated, and is very sensitive to touch.

Caulophyllum thalictroides, "blue cohosh," or "squaw root," was known to the Indians, and noted for its effect upon the uterus.

Hughes seems inclined to classify it with *cimicifuga, pulsatilla, sabina, secale.*

Cowperthwaite with *cimicifuga, actæa spicata, pulsatilla, sabadilla, secale.*

Hale with *cimicifuga, viburnum, cannabis indica, asarum, ruta, pulsatilla, senecio, uva ursi, secale.*

Caulophyllum acts upon the *small joints* and short muscles, but principally upon the muscular tissue of the female generative organs, causing *intermittent contractions of the uterus.*

It covers *spasmodic pains in the hypogastric region; spasmodic dysmenorrhœa; after-pains; menstrual colic; irritable uterus;* feeling of fullness, as if the uterus were congested ; vaginismus, irritable vagina,

intense spasmodic pains; aphthous vaginitis; profuse mucous leucorrhœa; acrid, weakening, with heaviness of the upper eyelids.

It is not certain whether this drug acts directly upon the muscular
tissue or on the motor nerves. We certainly find an irritable condition of the system : nervous sleeplessness, high fever, with nervous
excitement, amounting even to delirium, chorea, hysterical and epileptiform spasms, with various other reflex disturbances dependent upon
uterine irritation, as paraplegia, headache, vertigo, "moth spots," nausea, vomiting and cardialgia.

Then for the reverse picture we have atony of the uterus, weak,
inefficient pains, general languor and weakness.

Its claim as an uterine tonic seems well substantiated, a course of
this drug for two or three weeks predisposing to a quick and easy
labor.

At the Brooklyn Maternity some years since *caulophyllin* was given
three times a day to every woman about to become a mother, for periods ranging from one to, if I remember correctly, nine weeks. The
experiment, covering several months and several dozen women, satisfied us that when administered for a long enough time—over two
weeks—the labor was certainly easier, and usually quicker.

The symptoms of the fauces, and probably to a certain extent those
of the stomach and stool, are due to some acrid principle in the tincture, aside from the *caulophyllin.*

Caulophyllum is frequently curative in articular rheumatism of the
small joints, and also when the arm, back and neck are involved. The
pains are *"drawing"* and severe, sometimes sharp, occasionally a dull
ache or stiffness.

Shifting pains are very marked, especially in the arms and legs.

While of value in chronic cases, *caulophyllum* earns its laurels in
acute articular rheumatism, and especially in acute hypogastric pains.
So far as we now can say, it is of no service in gout.

Unfortunately our knowledge of this remedy is principally clinical. Its literature, aside from clinical cases, is but a repetition of what
Hale wrote.

It is a blot upon our reputation that the homœopathic school should
have possessed such a valuable remedy for so many years without
proving it systematically.

THE RELATION OF THE PHYSICIAN AND THE SANITARIAN TO HEREDITY, WITH STATISTICS AS TO IT.*

By LABAN DENNIS, M.D.,

Newark, N. J.

IN the following article no claim is made to original discovery of the truths presented. Many of them have long been the common possession of the medical profession. The interested perusal of some of the writings of Francis Galton, F.R.S., followed by Ribot, Greg, Elam, Brooks, and others, suggested the thought that if the facts which they present could be laid before physicians and sanitarians, even though imperfectly, they would, perhaps, be aroused to study the subject more thoroughly, to read its accumulating literature, and thus to make practical application of these truths for the benefit of mankind.

While it has been in preparation, an article on "Heredity," by Dr. Maudsley, has appeared in the *Fortnightly Review ;* an address on the "Relation of Heredity to Health and Longevity" was delivered in June last by Dr. Carpenter, of Baltimore, before the Pennsylvania State Sanitary Association, and published in the *Annals of Hygiene ;* Dr. Preston has published an article in the *Popular Science Monthly* for September, 1886, on "Hereditary Diseases and Race Culture ;" at a recent meeting of the British Scientific Association, Sir George Campbell, President of the section of Anthropology, took for his theme "Man Culture" and considered its relations to heredity. A reply to this by Grant Allen has appeared in the *Fortnightly*. These facts suffice to show that the minds of scientists and physicians are being aroused to the importance of our subject.

Some one has said, "Give me the first five years of a child's life and I care not who has charge of him afterward." Solomon said several thousand years ago, "Train up a child in the way he should go and when he is old he will not depart from it." On the other hand, Carlyle in *Sartor Resartus* says : "It is maintained by Helvetius and his set, that an infant of genius is quite the same as any other infant, only that certain surprisingly favorable influences accompany him through life, especially through childhood, and expand him, while others lie close folded and continue dunces. * * * 'With which opinion,' cries Teufelsdröckh, 'I should as soon agree as with this other, that an acorn might, by favorable or unfavorable influences of soil and climate, be nursed into a cabbage or the cabbage seed into an oak. Nevertheless,' continues he, 'I, too, acknowledge the all but omnipo-

---

*Read before the N. Y. Medico-Chirurgical Society.

tence of early culture and nurture. Hereby we have either a doddered dwarf bush, or a high-towering, wide-shadowing tree ; either a sick yellow cabbage or an edible, luxuriant green one. Of a truth, it is the duty of all men, especially of all philosophers, to note down with accuracy the characteristic circumstances of their education, what furthered, what hindered, what in any way modified it.'" *   *   * Thus are stated briefly the opposing views which have been held as to the two great factors in human development, nature and nurture. •

By *nature* we mean the product of those influences which for ages in the past have modified the human race, controlling, directing, stimulating or repressing ; and so, presenting us the man inheriting all the vices and virtues of his progenitors. In this view we may say with Emerson, "Every man is a bundle of his ancestors." By *nurture* we mean the sum total of the agencies which may be brought to bear upon individuals after birth, whether by himself or his fellow-beings, for the direction and development of this nature.

Let us consider for a few minutes the relative importance of these two, and the physician's duty with reference to them. Heretofore the medical profession have been working on the side of nurture almost exclusively. But have we not duties yet unrecognized and consequently undone in the direction of nature? M. de Candolle, of the French Academy of Sciences, in a recent work on the laws of heredity, after an analysis of the lives and characters of two hundred scientific men of the last two centuries, arrives at the following general conclusions as stated in *Science* :

1. Heredity is a general law which admits but few exceptions.

2. The interruption of heredity through one or more generations (atavism) is rare, perhaps five or ten times in a hundred.

3. The more remarkable a person is for good or ill, the more numerous and pronounced are his characteristics.

4. Women show fewer distinctive characteristics than men.

5. All groups of characteristics are more likely to be transmitted by fathers than by mothers.

6. It is difficult to determine whether characteristics which have been acquired by education and other external circumstances are transmitted by heredity.

7. The most marked characteristics in an individual are generally those received from both parents, especially those received both from parents and other progenitors.

Mr. Galton, after carefully studying the lives of 180 distinguished scientific men of England, sets forth certain facts in a prominent light, which, for the purpose of understanding more clearly some of the laws that seem to govern heredity, we will analyze briefly.

Taking into consideration the antecedents of 107 of these men, we find descended from the upper and middle classes 104, from the lower, three. Hence, he says, "It is by no means the case that those who have raised themselves by their abilities are found to be abler than their contemporaries who began their careers with advantages of fortune and social position. They are not more distinguished as original investigators, neither are they more discerning in those numerous questions, not strictly scientific, which happen to be brought before the councils of scientific societies. There can be no doubt but that the upper classes of a nation like our own, which are largely and continually recruited by selections from below, are by far the most productive of natural ability." Thus he indicates the hereditary value of education extending through several generations.

As to the value of primogeniture, in a total of ninety-nine recorded cases, sixty-one belonged to the elder half of the family.

He concludes, therefore, "that the elder sons have, on the whole, decided advantages of nurture over the younger."

Under the head of fertility he finds the families to which scientific men belonged usually large. Thus, in about one hundred cases, the total number of brothers and sisters of these men averages 6.30, while of those who attained thirty years of age the average is 4.80. Comparing with these figures the number of the children of the scientific men themselves, he finds the number of *their* living children (say of ages between five and thirty) to be 4.70. "This implies," he says, "a diminution of fertility as compared with that of their own parents, and confirms the common belief in the tendency to an extinction of the families of men who work hard with the brain. "On the other hand, I shall show," he says, "that the health and energy of the scientific men are remarkably high; it therefore seems strange that there should be a falling off in their offspring." He finds the only characteristics common to those scientific men whose families were the smallest to have been that they possessed a relative deficiency of health and energy in respect to that of their own parents. "Their absolute health and energy may be high, far exceeding those of people generally, but I speak of a noticeable falling off from the yet more robust condition of the previous generation. It is this which appears to be dangerous to the continuance of the race."

Speaking of the qualities possessed by these men, he says, "It will be seen that the leading scientific men are generally endowed with great energy; many of the most successful among them have labored as earnest amateurs in extra professional hours, working far into the night." Of those who reported definitely as to the energy of their parents, by far the greater number derived this quality hereditarily from one or both.

As to their health, he says, "The excellence of the health of the men in my list is remarkable, considering that the majority are of middle and many of advanced ages. One quarter of them state that they have excellent or very good health, a second quarter have good or fair, a third have good health since they attained manhood, and only one-quarter make complaints or reservations.

"It is positively startling to observe in these returns the strongly hereditary character of good and indifferent constitutions. * * * All statistical data concur in proving that healthy persons are far more likely than others to have healthy progeny ; and this truth cannot be too often illustrated until it has taken such hold of the popular mind, that considerations of health and energy shall be of recognized import-ance in questions of marriage, as much so as the probabilities of rank and fortune."

Perseverance he finds to be a third quality upon which great stress is laid, and which is uniformly possessed by these men, and almost universally derived from their parents.

Practical business habits are generally prevalent, and fully one-half of those endowed with them in a decided degree accredit one or both of their parents with the same faculty.

Memory he finds an important ingredient in that aggregate of facul-ties which form general scientific abilities. That is shown by the fact that about one-quarter of the men on his list possessed it in a high degree ; but it is not an essential one, because it is defective in about one case in fourteen. Its hereditary character is abundantly illustrated by the histories of his subjects.

Independence of character, as among the qualities of especial ser-vice to scientific men, he finds marked in excess in fifty of his corre-spondents. In only two was it below par. Its hereditary character is shown by the fact that the home atmosphere which these men breathed in their youth was generally saturated with it. In confirma-tion of this he refers to the strange variety of small and unfashionable religious sects to which they or their parents belonged. Thus some were Quakers, Faraday was a Sandemanian, others were Moravians, Bible Christians ; and Unitarians were numerous.

As showing the influence of hereditary causes in the production of the taste for science, his correspondents' replies show a larger propor-tion due to innate taste than any other cause.

Mr. Galton declares, "When nature and nurture compete for supremacy on equal terms, in the sense to be explained, the former proves the stronger. It is needless to insist that neither is self-sufficient; the highest natural endowments may be starved by defective nurture, while no carefulness of nurture can overcome the evil tendencies of an intrinsically bad physique, weak brain, or brutal disposition. Differences of nurture stamp unmistakable marks on the disposition of the soldier, clergyman, or scholar, but are wholly insufficient to efface the deeper marks of individual character. In the competition between nature and nurture, when the differences in either case do not exceed those which distinguish individuals of the same race living in the same country under no very exceptional conditions, nature certainly proves the stronger of the two."

This opinion strikingly corresponds with that of the physiologist Burdach, who says, "Heritage has in reality more power over our constitution and character than all the influences from without, whether moral or physical."

In two previous works, most interesting and instructive, "The Origin and Development of Human Faculty," and "Hereditary Genius," Mr. Galton shows how markedly those intellectual and physical powers which give stamina and distinction to families run through generations. He points out how early marriages give rapidly increasing advantages in point of numbers to those stocks indulging in them., "Hence if the races best fitted to occupy the land are encouraged to marry early, they will breed down the others in a very few generations."

This brief summary will suffice to indicate Mr. Galton's estimate of the value of heredity in producing men of distinguished abilities.

Dr. Elam, in "A Physician's Problems," arrives at the following general conclusions : "In procreation, as in creation, we everywhere trace the operation of two principles, similarity and diversity. In obedience to the law of similarity, 'like produces like,' equally in species and in families. In obedience to the law of diversity, children differ from their parents and from each other. In accordance also with this law, there is the power of returning to the specific type, whatever may have been the modifications produced accidentally, or by the influences of circumstances, upon the race ; even as, according to Dr. Darwin, the different varieties of pigeon evince a tendency to return to the 'Blue Rock' type. The diversity is produced by the very potency of operation of the law of similarity, whereby temporary and accidental conditions are propagated. Every formation of body, nternal or external, every deformity or deficiency, from disease or accident, every habit and every aptitude—all these things are liable to be, or may be, transmitted to the offspring.   In the case of accidental defects and modifications of the specific type, the off-spring usually do not inherit them but return to the normal type.   Intellectual endowments and aptitudes are liable to transmission, and according to the mental cultivation or neglect of the parents will 'be, as a general rule, the capacity and facility of learning of the children.   This will be more evident in proportion to the number of generations through which such cultivation or neglect has been practiced.   All moral qualities are transmissible from parent to child, with this important addition, that in the case of vicious tendencies or habits, the simple practice of the parent becomes the passion, the mania, the all but irresistible impulse of the child.   Even when the very identical vice is not inherited, a morbid organization is the result, which shows itself in some allied morbid tendency or some serious physical lesion. All chronic diseases appear to be transmissible, either in the original form or in a transformation of the morbid tendency.   These inheritances, normal or abnormal, are not always immediate from the parent, or even in a direct line, but they miss one or more generations, and sometimes have only appeared in collateral branches, as an uncle or grand-uncle.   This may be due to the fact that some of the inherited qualities may lie dormant in one member of a family and be active in others.   Of all morbid heritages, unsoundness of mind, in its numerous forms, seems to be the most certain and constant, and the results form a considerable proportion of our criminal population. But whilst by the law of similarity children become subject to the imperfections of their parents, by the law of diversity they are enabled to escape from them.   These evils are not necessarily entailed, and a proper comprehension of the principles upon which these diversities depend enables us to take such measures as will facilitate this escape. The offspring of that large portion of our population given up to intemperance and other forms of vice, inherit from their parents strong impulses and feeble wills, so as to become more or less irresponsible, and bear a peculiar relation to the law, such as needs special investigation.   Matrimonial alliances should be so regulated as to avoid the most glaring evils mentioned above."

In support of these propositions, he adduces numerous facts which we can but briefly hint at.   Thus he shows that the direct transmission of the qualities of the parent to the child is exhibited in external resemblance, in similarity of internal organization, in habit and gesture, in temperament, in instinctive impulses, and in moral and intellectual tendencies and aptitudes.   Also accidental defects and diseases are occasionally transmitted; certain vicious habits in parents and violations of hygienic law give rise to transformations and degenerations of both physical and moral nature, which may be said to foredoom the offspring to an unfortunate and miserable existence.

Resemblances of person, feature, etc., are illustrated by the Jews, gypsies, the aquiline nose of the Bourbons, the thick lip of the reigning house of Austria, which is said to be due to the marriage of the Emperor Maximilian with Mary of Burgundy over 300 years ago. The gigantic figures of the men and women of Potsdam are said to be due to the guards of Frederick William of Prussia having been quartered upon the town for fifty years.   Breeders of cattle can modify at will a race by lengthening or shortening the limbs, increasing or diminishing the fat or muscle, or placing them in particular localities, as illustrated by the race-horse and dray-horse. Modes of walking, talking, peculiar gestures, left-handedness, fecundity, susceptibility to the action of certain drugs, longevity, albinism and melanism, superfluity of parts, as six toes and fingers, peculiar tastes and dislikes for certain foods and drinks, are all transmissible.   Education has power to modify the capacity of the offspring, as shown by pointers and St. Bernard dogs.   The same is true of men ; for example, the children of savages are less amenable to instruction than those of civilized people.   Mathematical and linguistic aptitudes run in families.

Elam says: "I cannot see any reason for acknowledging that bodily habits and faculties are hereditary, and denying it in regard to those of the mind."   In this matter, he says, "there is not that kind and amount of regularity which bespeaks law."

Genius in its highest forms seems not to be transmitted; but, as Mr. Galton has shown, talent, ability and superior powers are.

Elam shows that the moral faculties are subject to the same law. Propensities and tendencies to virtue and vice are hereditary, *not the acts themselves*.   Man's freedom is not obliterated, but he is destined to a life of more or less strife and temptation, according as his inherited dispositions are active and vicious, or the contrary.   Lecky says: "There are men whose whole lives are spent in willing one thing and desiring the opposite."

All the passions appear to be distinctly hereditary, as anger, fear, envy, jealousy, libertinage, gluttony, drunkenness.

Of the latter, a writer in the *Psychological Journal* says: "The most startling problem connected with intemperance is, that not only does it affect the health, morals and intelligence of its votaries, but they also inherit the fatal tendencies, and feel a craving for the very beverages which have acted as poisons on their system from the commencement of their being."

M. Morel says : "I have never seen the patient cured of his propensity whose tendencies to drink were derived from the hereditary predisposition given to him by his parents."

Special forms of crime are also hereditary. Lucas believes that in the formation of the criminal classes, hereditary influence is more powerful than education or example, adding "that as the latter would fail to make a musician, orator, or mathematician, in default of inherited capacity, so they would fail to make a thief."

Theft has been known to run through at least three generations ; so beating of parents, suicide, cruelty, vindictiveness and insolence are hereditary.

Not only are the permanent and established characteristics of parents transmitted to children, but often also temporary, transitory, accidental and morbid modifications of structure. Thus youth, maturity, age and precocity may be reproduced in the offspring with qualities belonging to each.

From fifty to eighty-four per cent. of the cases of insanity are estimated to be due to hereditary influences. Maudsley calls attention to the immense importance of hereditary taint as a cause of insanity, and says that two considerations are to be borne in mind : first, the taint is of varying intensity, and may be developed only under certain favorable conditions. Second, not only may insanity in the parents predispose to insanity in the children, but any nervous disease, epilepsy, hysteria, or neuralgia, may do the same; so, conversely, insanity may predispose to other forms of nervous disease.

Thus, by combinations of nervous disorders and physical and moral sins in the parents, there are developed in the offspring morbid temperaments, special deformities and anomalies, intellectual and moral aberrations, impulsive natures, proneness to yield to certain temptations, imbecile judgments, enfeebled will and torpid conscience. In all such, moral liberty is weakened, and these are the parents of the "dangerous classes."

The evils attendant upon consanguineous marriages should likewise be considered in this connection. They have been pointed out very frequently to be idiocy, scrofula, deafness, blindness and insanity. Even the union of persons unrelated, but of temperaments nearly alike, is not unattended by corresponding dangers.

(*To be concluded.*)

THERAPEUTICS OF SPINAL IRRITATION.

By F. F. LAIRD, M.D.,

Utica, N. Y.

(*Continued from page* 151.)

PHOSPHORIC ACID.—"*Phosphoric acid* is very efficacious in spinal anæmia *when due to long continued sexual excesses.* Emaciation, palpitation of heart, impotence, weakness of memory, spasms in chest, *headache on top of head,* numbness of hands and feet and *extreme languor* are the prominent indications." (Hoyne).

Great weakness and prostration, especially in the morning. Passing large quantities of clear, colorless or milky urine. In females *pain in liver during menstruation.*

In *phosphoric acid* cases, *the skin of the* face often *feels tense, as if white of egg had dried on it.*

The spinal irritation is *the result of long continued grief* or of *vital losses.*

Spinal irritation due to venereal excesses or resulting from protracted grief. Emaciation, palpitation of heart, weakness of memory, spasms in chest, *headache on top of head,* numbness of hands and feet, extreme languor, *frequent emission of pale watery urine* or *urine looking like milk and even coagulating.*

PHYSOSTIGMA.—Dr. Moffat extols this drug in the asthenopia of spinal irritation. (Transactions of Hom. Med. Society of State of New York, 1885).

PIPER METHYSTICUM.—Vessels of neck and base of brain full, as if circulation had been cut off with a cord; whole back of head, neck and cerebellum feel congested, sore inside and tender to outside pressure; these parts feel as if double or treble their natural size. After business anxieties, pain in middle of forehead, extending around sides to occiput; all the cerebellum and medulla feel compressed, especially from before backward, causing great restlessness; feeling as though he must move, or head and neck would be compressed to death. This constriction also extending to chest and stomach. *Pains in head relieved temporarily by turning the mind to another topic.* Soreness in back about second dorsal vertebra. *Right arm especially affected.* Trembling sensation in bowels and lower extremities. *Better in open air and when moving.*

Pain in back of head and spine, and relief from all sufferings temporarily by change (mental or physical), slight excitement or diversion of the mind to some other topic. (Raue).

PLUMBUM.—Paresis and paralysis of cervical muscles. Tension and stiffness in nape of neck, more on the right side, extending into the ear, on turning the head sideways. *Pressure in neighborhood of last cervical and first dorsal vertebræ causes pain.* Pains in neck, walls of chest, back and loins.

Weakness and neuralgic pains in back. "Spinal irritation." Pains in back, hips and down spine extending occasionally up the neck to back part of head.

Dorsal region of spine tender on pressure. Tearing, burning, sticking pains in scapulæ, especially *right.*

Lancinations and cramps in lumbar region of spine, worse by paroxysms ; relieved by pressure but aggravated by motion. *Painfulness of loins, nates, posterior portion of thigh, knee, sole of foot and toes. The pain, which is equally severe on both sides, is felt somewhat on the inner surface of lower limb ; it usually consists of prickings or lancinations, together with occasional attacks of cramp, dragging,* aching, drawing, tearing, pains in lumbar region, sometimes very violent. *Sticking in small of back, which is sensitive on leaning against the chair, disappearing by rubbing it* (*relief of pain from friction is quite a marked symptom of plumbum*).

Slow perception ; apathetic. *Loss of memory ; unable to find the proper word while talking.* Quiet and melancholic mood. Impairment of memory is a *late* result of lead poisoning ; hence we shall find the above symptoms *only* in long-standing cases.

Vertigo ; especially on stooping, or when looking upward. "It meets frequent attacks of vertigo with trembling of the head. The paroxysms are of short duration and are less liable to occur in the open air." (Hoyne).

Heaviness in head and dulness of mind. The patient *rubs his forehead* as if to clear the brain. Severe headache involving whole head. Tearing and contraction in forehead. Throbbing of temporal arteries ; temples feel as if compressed in a vice, with lancinating pains. Sensation of increased weight in occiput. Dull pains in back of head, with pressure, from spine upwards, sometimes extending forward to forehead. "Cephalalgia, when chronic, often yields to this remedy. The pain frequently commences in the occiput, while asleep, extends to the ears and temples and is somewhat relieved by getting up and moving about ; much frontal headache, worse by paroxysms ; the hair becomes fatty ; obstinate constipation." (Hoyne).

Yellowness of conjunctivæ.—Diplopia, hemiopia, amblyopia amaurotica. Everything seems yellow. Paresis and paralysis of upper eyelids.

Complexion, sallow, pale, like a corpse. Lips often have a *bluish* tint.

Distinct blue line along margin of gums.

Voice weak; aphonia from paralysis of laryngeal muscles. Constriction of larynx, constriction of chest, with oppressed breathing; short breath on motion, especially on going up stairs; sighing respiration. Severe pressive pain in lower part of left side of chest, apparently in the intercostal muscles. Pulse apt to be small and retarded.

Margins of tongue red; centre, *white, brown* or yellow. *Taste sweetish,* less often bitter or metallic. Constriction of throat; or paralytic condition with difficult swallowing. Globus hystericus. Sensation as if something in the throat moved suddenly up to the base of the skull and thence to left orbital region where it becomes a sticking. *Loss of appetite with great thirst. Fetid breath.* Eructations *sweetish,* sour, offensive, empty. *Nausea. Incessant vomiting. Hiccough. Pressure, distress and tightness about stomach.*

Cardialgia; violent pressure in stomach and pain in back, sometimes relieved by bending backward, and at other times by bending forward; *hard external pressure always relieves,* but frequently causes the pain to shift its location; the pains radiate into chest *all over abdomen* and *even into legs,* often with the *sensation as if abdomen or bowels were being drawn toward the spine; hot or cold drinks increase the pain; tepid drink agrees best; rubbing frequently relieves.*

Violent colic with hard retracted abdomen, as if drawn toward the spine by a string; the pains starting from the umbilicus as a centre, radiate to distant parts and even all over the body; *better from hard pressure and by rubbing.* Sensitiveness in hepatic and splenic regions.

Constipation; stools scanty, hard, in lumps or balls like sheep's dung, generally of a *black* or green color; *passed with difficulty; the arms are constricted and drawn up as if by a string; stool only once in eight or ten days, of scanty, blackish feces, whose expulsion causes acute suffering; colic, loss of appetite, sweet taste, dryness of the excretion* and *muscular atony* are the two prominent features in the constipation of *plumbum.*

Strangury, urine dark colored and *scanty, passed guttatim;* cannot pass urine, apparently from want of sensation to do so or from paralytic atony of bladder. Incontinence, the urine high colored and fetid.

Violent pains in the limbs, especially in muscular part of thighs, worse evening and night. Twitching and jerking in limbs with paralytic weakness. *Tendency to "wrist drop."* Coldness of hands and feet, *with fetid sweat of the feet. Sharp neuralgic pains in lower limbs, mostly from hips to knees, occurring in paroxyms.*

Numbness of arms and legs. Tonic spasm of muscles. THE PAINS IN THE LIMBS ARE WORSE AT NIGHT AND ARE RELIEVED BY RUBBING. *The extensor muscles are weakened more than the flexors.*

Emaciation, anæmia, anæsthesia or *hyperæsthesia. General prostration; lassitude; faintness.*

Arthralgic and neuralgic pains in trunk and limbs. Sensation of constriction with pain and spasm in the internal organs.

Entire absence of perspiration, except during the paroxysms of colic.

Skin dry, yellow or livid blue.

The ailments develop themselves slowly and intermit for a time; intermission every third day.

Paralysis with atrophy. Epilepsy, *the attack being followed by long lasting, stupid feeling in head.* Sleeplessness at night; sleepy during the day.

Aggravation—At night; while lying in bed.

*Amelioration—*FROM RUBBING.

Plumbum is not a remedy often called for; yet occasionally cases present themselves with the obstinate constipation, colic and gastric symptoms so characteristic of the drug. *Violent neuralgic pains in the extremities, worse at night,* should always lead to a careful study of *plumbum.* The victims of confirmed epilepsy, after years of suffering, frequently exhibit the spinal irritation and mental condition so well portrayed in the pathogenesis; and in these cases, the steady administration of this remedy will often render the most signal aid.

PULSATILLA NIG.—Painless cracking in first cervical vertebra on moving head. *Stiffness and pressive pain in left side of cervical muscles. Rheumatic pain in nape of neck with weariness of the feet; the pain is drawing tensive. Drawing, fine sticking pain in nape, between scapulæ and in back. Pain in neck as if he had lain in an uncomfortable position at night.* BACK IS PAINFULLY STIFF LIKE A BOARD. Drawing in back during stool, rarely at any other time. *Sticking pain in back and across chest.* Sensation in back-bone as if it would come out. Feeling as of cold water being poured down the back. Stitches in the back while coughing. Cracking in scapula on slightest motion, in the morning.

Between scapulæ; *pain increased by inspiration ;* pain as from a heaviness (*nux*)*;* sticking pain on motion impeding respiration. Stitches in scapulæ at night. *Stiffness and pain in small of back while lying, as if suppurating or as if tightly bandaged.* In small of back; *pain as if sprained on motion, can scarcely rise after sitting; labor-like, constrictive pain taking away her breath (especially in the morning).* Pressive pain in fourth lumbar vertebra, especially after walking.

Drawing pain extending from loins to pit of stomach where it becomes a sticking on inspiration. *Drawing tensive pain in loins. Pressive, tired pain in sacrum in evening.*

Mild, gentle, timid, yielding disposition with inclination to weep, cries when telling her symptoms. Tremulous anxiety.

Vertigo; *worse from looking upward; sitting; stooping; in morning on rising—always associated with chilliness.*

Headache; *mostly frontal above eyes, pressive or constrictive, often aggravated by raising the eyes; better from external pressure and in open air, worse during rest, (especially sitting)* and *toward evening; associated with chilliness, pale face, palpitation of the heart and chilliness.* Headache when the pains, occurring in paroxysms, increase to an intense point of severity and then decrease to a complete cessation (Dr. Gallupy).

Profuse lachrymation in the wind or open air. Desire to rub the eyes. Dimness of vision like a fog or veil before the eyes. Styes.

Sensation as if ears were stopped with roaring. Prosopalgia, pain twitching, tearing; worse in a warm room and toward evening.

Aphonia; *voice comes and goes without apparent reason.* Dr. Katka gives the following case: "Lady aged 32. Loss of voice for six years. Talks in a whisper and, if long continuing it, it causes a dry, straining cough, with a feeling of compression in the chest; constant dryness and burning in the last cervical vertebra which is sore to the touch; mucous membrane of fauces dry and red; menses scanty; sleep disturbed by frightful dreams, with crying and moaning; tearful disposition; easily irritated to anger. *Bell.* 2 relieved her nervousness, *Puls.* 2 brought her voice back in fourteen days." (Hoyne's Clinical Therapeutics).

Shortness of breath, anxiety and palpitation when lying on left side. Dry cough at night or in evening after lying down, disappears on sitting up in bed, returns on lying down; causes dryness of throat and prevents sleep. *Pain in chest as if ulcerated.*

Catching pain in region of heart subdued for the time by pressure of the hand. The pulse beat is felt in the pit of the stomach.

Mouth and tongue feel very dry but in fact are moist. Repulsive taste with white or yellowish-white tongue in the morning; at other times *a bitter, bilious taste* (even to the food), worse after eating ; or *taste of food diminished.* Eructations ; *tasting and smelling of the food ; bitter, bilious, rancid, sour ; like putrid meat.* Nausea, and vomiting of food and bilious or sour material or *of food eaten long before* (kreos). *Sensation of a lump at mid-sternum ;* of weight at epigastrium an hour after eating, relieved by eating again. *Thirstlessness ; cold water disagrees. Aversion to fat food which cannot be digested.* Much flatulence which moves about, causing pinching pains and rumbling; worse on awaking or just after supper (Farrington). *Gnawing distress in stomach as from ravenous hunger. Hiccough after cold food.*

Tendency to attacks of diarrhœa *at night* with *changeable stools;* or constipation with difficult evacuation, painful pressure and pain in back.

Tenesmus vesicæ. *Involuntary micturition while coughing or passing flatus; at night in bed.* Urine increased, watery, colorless; or scanty, red-brown.

Menses; too late and scanty, with thick leucorrhœa like cream or milk: suppressed after getting feet wet. Menstrual colic. Amenorrhœa. Chlorosis.

"Spinal irritation due to sexual excesses or masturbation requires *pulsatilla* when there is weariness and stiffness of the back, seminal emissions with excited sexual desire" (Hoyne).

Drawing, tearing pains in the extremities. Hip-joint painful as if dislocated. Boring pain in heels, toward evening. Soles of feet painful as if beaten. *(Retarded venous circulation in the extremities, varicose veins often being present).*

Violent trembling of whole body. *Longing for fresh air, cannot tolerate a warm room. Feeling of discomfort over the whole body, in morning after rising, disappearing on moving about. Pains; drawing tearing* or as *of subcutaneous ulceration* SHIFTING RAPIDLY FROM PART TO PART *; always accompanied by great* CHILLINESS *which increases pari passu with the pains; decrease and disappear when lying upon the back,* but when lying upon either side they increase or recur. Come suddenly, disappear gradually. *Symptoms ever changing;* especially violent every other evening. *Thirstlessness with all complaints.*

Late in getting to sleep and late in awaking; the longer he lies in the morning the weaker he becomes and the more he wants to sleep.

Dreams confused with crying, talking and moaning; *lies upon back with hands above head.*

Aggravation—In the evening; every other evening; at night; from warmth of bed; while lying down, *especially upon left side; in a warm room;* after eating; *especially after fat food, pork, ice cream, fruit, pastry.*

*Amelioration —*IN OPEN AIR *; in a cool place; when lying upon the back; when slowly moving about.*

Sandy hair, blue eyes, pale face, inclined to silent (*ignatia, demonstrative*) grief and submissiveness—this is the *pulsatilla* patient who is generally a woman or a girl at or near puberty. Her spinal irritation is commonly the result of ovarian or uterine troubles. Frequently she is the chlorotic victim, carrying a heavy load of iron and quinine and tears. *Melancholy, thirstlessness, chilliness with intolerance of a warm room, wandering pains, characteristic menstrual and gastric symptoms*—this is the combination almost invariably present.

RHUS TOX.—*Rheumatoid stiffness of nape of neck*, sometimes with pain as if a heavy weight were lying upon it. *Pain in the cervical muscles, as if the parts were asleep and as if one had been lying for a long time in an uncomfortable position, towards evening.* Drawing pains in the back. *Sticking in back while stooping, in evening.*

A constrictive pain in dorsal muscles, while sitting, relieved by bending back, aggravated on bending forward. Violent rheumatic pain between scapulæ, neither relieved or aggravated by motion or rest, only relieved by warmth, aggravated by cold. Lumbar region; *stiffness and aching ; bruised pains in small of back when sitting still or when lying; better from motion, or when lying upon something hard (natr. mur.); burning feeling in the loins.*

Sad, apprehensive, especially in evening and *at night; anxiety, with great restlessness.* Fear and dread of death, yet tired of life. Forgetful; difficult comprehension. THE MENTAL SYMPTOMS ARE WORSE IN THE HOUSE, RELIEVED BY WALKING IN THE OPEN AIR, and are accompanied by UNCONQUERABLE RESTLESSNESS.

Vertigo, *as if intoxicated, when rising from bed.* Headache, characterized by aching pains in the occiput, the pain extending to the ears and malar bones, and aggravated by exercise in the open air, or by damp, cloudy weather, are speedily relieved by the poison oak" (Hoyne). *Fullness and heaviness of the head, with pressing downward, as from a weight in the forehead.* Sensation as if brain were loose when stooping or shaking the head. *Headache in occiput that disappears on bending the head backward. Head as painful to touch as a boil (Sulph.)* Headache seeming to be external, as if skin were contracted, or as if she were pulled by the hair, yet scalp is not painful to touch. *Heaviness and stiffness of eyelids, as if paralysed.* Eye-ball sore when turning the eye, or pressing upon it. Obscured vision, as if a veil were before the eyes.

Cramp-like pain in the articulation of the lower jaw, close to the ear, during rest and motion of the part, relieved by hard pressure upon the joint and by warmth (Compare *caust.*) Prosopalgia *every time the patient gets a wetting.*

Hoarseness, even aphonia from overstraining the voice; or hoarseness *better from continued talking. Spasmodic cough, often with taste of blood in the mouth*, although no blood is present.

Violent palpitation of heart better from walking about. A sensation of *weakness and trembling of the heart.* "A tongue with the red tip in the shape of a triangle; a soft tongue with imprints of the teeth; a dry, red tongue, cracked at the tip; and a tongue coated white on one side only, are all indications for *rhus*" (Hoyne). *Sore sensation of tongue with red tip.   Great thirst for cold water or* COLD MILK. Incomplete eructations.   Nausea after eating and drinking.   After eating fullness and heaviness in stomach, as from a stone (*bry., nux., puls.*)   Flatulency.   *Colic pains and contractions in abdomen force him to walk bent.* Cutting, griping and jerking pains in abdomen, especially after eating; better after stool (*coloc.*)   *Soreness, as if beaten, in hypochondriac region, and still more of the abdomen; worse on the side on which he lies; worse when turning and when beginning to move* (Hawkes).   Sense of constriction in rectum, as though one side had grown up.   Diarrhœa, with *tearing pains down thighs during stool.*

"Incontinence of urine during rest, with urinary tenesmus, and afterward profuse discharge of urine, is a condition readily controlled by this medicine" (Hoyne).   Frequent urging day and night, with profuse emission.   Urine, *hot, high-colored, scanty ; dark, soon becoming turbid ;* colorless like water, with a snow-white sediment.   *Retention of urine ; backache, restless, cannot keep quiet.* Urine voided slowly, spine affected (*from getting wet*).   Involuntary urination at night and *while at rest.*

"Spinal irritation, the result of onanism, sexual excess, etc., is well met by *rhus*, when the pain in the back is of a tearing or contusive character, worse during rest; the sexual desire is increased and nightly pollutions are quite frequent.   Also when the result of getting wet" (Hoyne).   Uterine and ovarian troubles giving rise to spinal irritation, especially if *caused by straining, lifting, or becoming wet.*

Drawing, tearing pains, with stiffness and feeling as if sprained in arms; *better from motion.*   In tips of fingers, *when grasping anything, feeling as if pins were pricking tips and palmar surfaces of first phalanges of fingers; crawling as if asleep.   When lying upon the side the hips hurt, and when lying upon the back the small of the back hurts.* GREAT AND PAINFUL SENSITIVENESS TO TOUCH IN THE ANTERIOR MUSCLES OF THE THIGHS, *especially left.   The legs seem heavy and weary, as after long walking.*   Cramp-like, tensive pains in muscles.   *Painless swelling of feet in evening* (*bry.*)   *Feel painful as if sprained or wrenched in the morning on rising.*   In heels, *pain as if stepping on pins* on first standing in morning ; *sharp pain like running nails under the skin ; stitches* when walking.   *Drawing, tearing (rheumatoid) pains in lower extremities,* WORSE WHEN AT REST and IN COLD, WET WEATHER.

Great weakness paralytic debility and soreness, especially when sitting or at rest.

GREAT RESTLESSNESS AND UNEASINESS, *must constantly change position, especially at night.*

Very sensitive to cold air, which sometimes causes pain in the skin.

Paralysis—PAINS AS IF SPRAINED. Ailments, from spraining, straining, lifting, particularly from stretching arms high up to reach things (Hawkes); FROM GETTING WET, TAKING A COLD BATH, etc., *especially when over-heated; after drinking cold water. Tendency to rheumatism, erysipelas, or eczema.*

Sleeplessness, with restless tossing about. Dreams: *of his business* (Comp. *bry.*); OF GREAT EXERTION, AS ROWING, SWIMMING, ETC.

Sweats from warm drinks.

Aggravation—WHILE AT REST; *after midnight; before storms; on rising from a seat or bed;* on *beginning* to move; FROM GETTING WET; *in wet weather;* from north-easterly winds; *from cold in general.*

Amelioration—FROM CONTINUOUS MOTION; *in warm, dry weather; from warmth in general.*

Rhus is one of our foremost remedies in spinal irritation, and its use in old-standing cases is often attended with the most surprisingly brilliant results. Its leading indications are the CAUSATION BY STRAIN (LIFTING, ETC.), or BECOMING WET, GREAT RESTLESSNESS, WITH RELIEF FROM CONTINUED MOTION and INTOLERANCE OF COLD. Such patients generally give a rheumatic history and frequently complain that "*their legs are one mass of pains,*" a symptom which should always direct your attention to *rhus,* than which no drug in the materia medica presents a greater array of painful sensations in the lower extremities.

SANTONINE.—"Spinal irritation is not unfrequently due to the irritation caused by worms. Nervous, irritable cough, general and frequent twitching of the body; chorea, enuresis, tenesmus vesicæ; dreadful, disturbed sleep, picking at the nose, etc., are indications for *santonine.* In nervous failure of sight *santonine* has proved useful. Sometimes *cina* acts better than *santonine,* and should therefore be used in its stead" (Kershaw).

(To be continued.)

ORIGINAL ARTICLES IN SURGERY.

BLOODLESS AMPUTATION OF THE TONGUE.*

By WILLIAM H. KING, M.D.,
New York.

I AM well aware that many articles have appeared on the above subject ; but believing the operation which I am about to describe is more entitled to be called bloodless than any other, is the only excuse I have for presenting it to this society.

Mr. Bryant, of England, has for many years been the most prominent authority on galvano-cautery operations on the tongue. In a lecture published in the *Lancet* of February 28th, 1874, after giving the primary details of the operation, he says : "It (the wire) should not be heated beyond a red heat, and the redness ought to be of a dull kind. Above all, the process of tightening should be very slowly performed, the wire of the écraseur being screwed home only as it becomes loose by cutting through the tissues." The lecture from which the above is taken is quoted either in part or whole in nearly every text-book on electro-surgery, and in a great many works on general surgery; consequently it has become the most popular method of operating on the tongue. It is to the last sentence of the paragraph given above that I wish to direct attention, for I believe it is this sentence which causes Mr. Bryant's operation, in all other respects so perfect, to be a failure, so far as the bloodless operation is concerned.

Professor Helmuth once said to me that he had seen seven amputations of the tongue with the galvano-cautery, all of which were more bloody than those he had seen amputated with the ordinary écraseur. Some of these operations I knew were performed by Mr. Bryant's method, and it is but fair to suppose that all were, inasmuch as the operator was a strong advocate of it. I might also call as witnesses members of this society, some of whom I know have seen the operation performed after the Bryant method, and have expressed wonder that the operation should be called bloodless. It would be only a repetition for me to give all the details of the operation. They can be found in any work on surgery; I only wish to refer to that part of it in which I would differ from Mr. Bryant.

I use a large string of platinum wire, twenty-two, Brown and Sharp's gauge. This is important, for I knew a smaller one to break, and thus delay an operation. The handle I use is composed of two

---

* Read before the New York Society for Medico-Scientific Investigation.

strips of hard rubber tubing, placed parallel, separated from each other about one-half an inch, and held in position by two blocks of hard rubber at each end.

Running through the rubber tubing are two large copper wires, one of which is cut with a connecter, so placed that the operator can open or close the circuit with the thumb of the hand in which he holds the instrument. Between the hard rubber tubes is a screw running the whole length of them and which is held in position by the hard rubber blocks.

This screw has a large milled wheel, which gives the operator a powerful traction. Sliding in the screw is a hard rubber block with strong pegs for fastening the loop of the écraseur. This block is first screwed down to the end of instrument nearest the loop. The wire is placed in position and fastened to the pegs on the movable block. The screw is then turned until the wire is imbedded in the tissues of the tongue. When this is done, the wire is allowed to heat just enough to cut its way with constant traction on the loop. To do this it need never come to a perceptible redness. The operator should keep constant and strong traction on the loop. In fact use it as you would an ordinary cold écraseur, except that the traction used is just short of enough to cut the tissues, but requires a very small degree of heat to complete its work. It is this one point, the constant and strong traction, that I would change in Mr. Bryant's operation. First, I believe that it is on this one point that the success of the operation, so far as its bloodless character is concerned, depends.

The advantages derived from this method of operating over that of Mr. Bryant's are :

First—The tissues are rendered so tense by the traction that much less heat will sever them than when the wire is left loose.

Second—You will be able to maintain a much steadier heat, as the wire is continually imbedded in the tissues; while with the Bryant operation the wire cuts itself loose, the heat rises rapidly, and if the operator is not continually on his guard, it will rise to a white heat before he is aware of it.

Third—You get all the combined advantages of the cold écraseur and the cautery. The walls of the blood-vessels are drawn tightly together and little clots form in them, while, at the same time, you also get the advantage of the cautery; the glutinous, fibrinous exudation around the wire glues, as it were, the closed ends of these vessels together. With the Bryant operation you get none of these effects. To repeat his own expression, "the wire of the écraseur being screwed home only, as it becomes loose by cutting through the tissues."

It is evident, that in this case, the ends of the vessels are not drawn together and no clots form in them. If, when the wire is cutting itself loose, it should cut into the side of a vessel that is not constricted and with blood coursing through it it will be sure to escape by the side of the wire; when, if the vessel was first constricted and its blood circuit stopped, blood would not flow.

Fourth—This operation can be safely performed with ether, as the wire is continually imbedded in the tissues and need never come to a red heat, consequently the vapor of ether cannot ignite.

The battery used should be one that can be so regulated as to produce any grade of heat desired, and unless you have such a battery, the operation is liable to be a failure, for it is impossible to perfectly regulate the heat by the interrupter in the handle.

STRETCHING OF THE SUPRA- AND INFRA-ORBITAL, AND NEUROTOMY OF THE NASAL NERVE FOR NEURALGIA.

By FRED S. FULTON, A.M., M.D.,
New York.

THE history of the following case is important as illustrating first the benefits to be derived from operations on the nerves, for neuralgia of even chronic malarial origin, it being usually considered that neuralgia arising from this source offers about the least chance of relief of any of those originating in the many causes which give rise to this intractable affection; second, that the comparatively deep-seated location of nerves need not necessarily prevent operations upon them, and third, that after the operation the malarial poison seemed to manifest no tendency to further involve healthy tissue by any new explosion.

The patient, Mrs. G——, æt. 63, was admitted to Hahnemann Hospital, November 10th, 1885, having been for the past year or two at Dansville Sanitarium under treatment for persistent prosopalgia of the trigeminus. Her father's family had died of phthisis, which she herself had had when a young girl, and from which, after being given up to die, she made a complete and permanent recovery. Most of the ills that flesh is heir to had visited her. She had had typhoid, erysipelas, pneumonia, dyspepsia, and, for many years past, malarial fever which had been pronounced at first but had finally settled down into a form of dumb ague, manifesting itself by drowsiness, indisposition, nervous wakefulness, with generally marked periodicity, and, later, by neuralgia. The attacks commenced usually in the fall and extended through the winter. Her summers were generally free from

pain.   When she presented herself at the hospital, she complained of
an aching distress over the entire body, burning in the stomach which,
together with the pain, was aggravated after midnight.   The neuralgia
was periodic, though it might occur at any time.   It usually commenced
with soreness, redness and twitching of the upper lip, and extended
gradually over the ramification of the nasal nerve, shooting up the nose,
then lodging in the infra-orbital, and from there extending over the
entire side of the face and into the teeth.   The supra-orbital was
another favorite site of the pain, which radiated from there through the
eye, which would be exceedingly weak and sore, extending upwards
to the vertex and sometimes nearly to the occiput.   After several hours
the pain might abate or might increase until its severity induced tonic
convulsions with entire loss of consciousness.   The pain was sharp,
piercing, almost colicy in its nature and was followed by the most exquisite sensitiveness over the places where the various nerves affected
became subcutaneous.   The most careful and thorough dietary, and
electricity, applied by skilled specialists, had been tried without avail
at Dansville.   She was placed at once on *bell. θ* and *coloc. θ*.   She
came the latter part of November, and in a few weeks was entirely
comfortable and remained so during the winter, being able to go out
doors and take long walks which had been impossible for some months.
It was the most comfortable winter passed in years.   In the beginning
of April, '86, she again began to manifest symptoms of her old trouble,
and by the middle of the month was well advanced towards her former
deplorable condition.   At this time my term of service at the hospital
being ended, she came under the care of the most able physicians,
among whom were Profs. St. Clair Smith, J. M. Schley and E. V. Moffat.
Treatment was of no avail, the last prescription being that confession
of inability to help, *morphia*.   On July 5th she came again under my
care.   Hopeful of benefit from treatment which before had been
helpful, I renewed her former medicines, using all potencies, high
and low.   Many others as appeared indicated were administered, but
without result.   She went steadily from bad to worse, so that for
several days before I operated she suffered with the most painful convulsions, terminating in loss of consciousness for a varying length of
time.   On August 16th, '86, assisted by Dr. J. B. Garrison, I operated.
An incision was made at about the junction of the inner and middle
third of the supra-orbital ridge, immediately over the notch which
furnishes an exit for the nerve and accompanying vessels, and carried
obliquely upwards and inwards for about an inch.   A few muscular fibres
of the orbicularis palpebrarum were cut through, the tissue pushed apart
and the nerve discovered as a gray, glistening cord at the bottom.   This
was carefully raised on the handle of the scalpel and stretched towards
its peripheral extremity.   The force used would have been sufficient
to snap a straight extended piece of number forty sewing cotton, but
not enough to break the heavy number ten variety.   This was repeated
several times, when the nerve was found, stretched and pulled out
enough to require some reduplications to adjust it to its former bed.
The infra-orbital was next stretched.   A curved incision, about one
inch in length, with the convexity downward, was made a quarter of
an inch below the orbit.   One of the natural furrows was followed

which avoided any unnecessary scar resulting. The skin and fascia being incised, the orbicularis palpebrarum was pushed upward, uncovering the levator labii superioris and levator labii superioris alæque nasi, which were pushed aside with the handle of the scalpel. The nerve lay between them, but was much smaller and presented, instead of the gray, glistening appearance, a heavy, turgid, dark look, which might easily have lead to its being overlooked if any other structure had been in this location which could possibly have been mistaken for it. This was stretched in a similar manner, raising it entirely out of the wound, care being taken to stretch it behind the point where it divides into its terminal branches after its exit from the infra-orbital foramen. The nasal nerve was next attacked. An incision about an inch long was made over its course where it emerges below the nasal bone and becomes subcutaneous. After some careful dissecting with the handle of the scalpel, it was found and stretched. The wounds were then washed with a bichloride solution, 1 to 2,000, carefully cleansed and closed with silk. The patient rallied well, but next morning was nearly crazy, as all the vigor of the neuralgia had centered in the internal branch of the nasal nerve. The pain started at the junction of the nose and lip, shot up inside the nose, and followed the course of the nasal nerve into the eye. She was nearly frantic, and with true Spartan heroism demanded that that other nerve be removed. Accordingly, that afternoon I reopened the nasal incision, cut the cartilage of the nose close to the septum, to within about a quarter of an inch of the free border, opened the nasal cavity as much as possible and pushed down the mucous membrane from the wing of the nose. The hemorrhage, which was difficult to control, hindered materially. The nasal branch of the superior maxillary artery being cut just as it appeared below the nasal bone, retracted behind the bone and made it very difficult to secure. It was compressed temporarily with the forceps and later controlled by the application of the perchloride of iron. The nerve was then found and about three-quarters of an inch removed. The bleeding having been controlled, the edges of the cartilages entirely freed from the iron, the whole washed out with the bichloride solution, the lips were approximated by silk and the hole dressed with an antiseptic dressing of borated cotton held in the folds of bichloride gauze. The patient rallied well, and, after a few slight drawbacks, made a good recovery. Electricity was applied to the face and nose for several weeks before the operation with no apparent effect. It was continued, however, afterwards, as it lessened the soreness and allayed the irritated condition of the face and lips. On September 7th, she was well enough to go to the Catskills, where she has since remained. A letter received from her to-day (February 22d, '87), says in her emphatic, plain Saxon fashion, "I have been able to go to church every Sunday but two all winter, and I think that is very good for an old lady sixty-three, up in these snowy mountains, and my heart goes out continually in thanksgiving to the Good Father for all these favors, especially *no neuralgia.* Two different times I've had a very severe cold all over me, but as soon as I would get some relief from the cold, that old enemy of mine (malaria) would set in with all its malignant fury, as if determined to set the neuralgia all afire again, but he didn't succeed, and I think I am gaining in all of those malarial and neuralgic symptoms."

It might be well to add that before the operation was performed *quinine* was administered, after the remedies had proved of no avail, in doses varying from three to fifteen grains a day, and later *quinine* and *capsicum* were combined in five-grain pills in proportion of four to one. The administration of *quinine* had soon to be discontinued on account of the excessive prostration and despondency which it produced. It had no effect upon either the malarial manifestations or its outgrowth, the neuralgia.

———————

ABNORMAL ASSOCIATED MOVEMENTS IN THE FEET AND TOES IN NERVOUS DISEASES.—Prof. Strümpell says, when an individual not suffering from a nervous disease, lying in bed in the usual dorsal position, is required to draw up the lower limbs by flexing the leg upon the thigh and the thigh upon the abdomen, there is usually no associated movement at the ankle joint, or, if so, it is not of constant occurrence, and can be repressed voluntarily. But in many patients suffering from disease of the nervous system when the above-mentioned procedure is carried out, as soon as the thigh is lifted even a little the tendon of the tibialis anticus is seen to become prominent, the foot assumes the position of dorsal flexion of a greater or less degree, and the inner border of the foot is raised. If this result is well marked, the movement assumes almost the character of a tonic spasm, and the dorsal flexion, obliquely directed with the sole inward, is so great that it could only be done by an effort of the will after some trouble. In many cases, but not in all, this associated movement involves the long extensor of the great toe, and, at times, even the extensor communis. In such cases the tendons of these muscles are seen to be on the stretch, while the toes are correspondingly flexed in the dorsal direction. If the patient be requested to relax the muscles voluntarily, he, in most cases, is unable to do so; in some cases the foot can be held downward by special innervation of the calf-muscles. In general, the movement is limited to the side which has been put into voluntary action, but, in cases of combined system-disease of the cord, the associated movement appeared in both limbs, although only one side was voluntarily moved. Strümpell has seen this phenomenon in cases of cerebral hemiplegia and in spinal cord affection, presenting more or less completely a picture of the so-called spastic spinal paralysis. In hemiplegia the associated movement appears usually on the affected side, but, of course, will not occur if the limb is completely paralyzed, and yet, on the other hand, it has not appeared in cases in which voluntary dorsal flexion of the foot had been preserved. In two cases of unilateral lesion of the cord the author has observed the phenomenon on the motor-paralyzed side, and in one of them voluntary dorsal flexion of the foot was lost. Prof. Strümpell is unable to give an explanation of these facts, but thinks that the idea of an abnormal transverse conduction between neighboring nerve fibres cannot be wholly excluded.—*Neurolog. Centralb.*, No. 1, 1887.

EDITORIAL DEPARTMENT.

EDITORS.

GEORGE M. DILLOW, M.D., ... Editor-in-Chief, Editorial and Book Reviews.
CLARENCE E. BEEBE, M.D., ... Original Papers in Medicine.
SIDNEY F. WILCOX, M.D., ... Original Papers in Surgery.
MALCOLM LEAL, M.D., ... Progress of Medicine.
EUGENE H. PORTER, M.D., ... Comments and News.
HENRY M. DEARBORN, M.D., ... Correspondence.
FRED S. FULTON, M.D., ... Reports of Societies and Hospitals.

GEORGE G. SHELTON, M.D., ... Business Manager.

The Editors individually assume full responsibility for and are to be credited with all connected with the collection and presentation of matter in their respective departments, but are not responsible for the opinions of contributors.

It is understood that manuscripts sent for consideration have not been previously published, and that after notice of acceptance has been given, will not appear elsewhere except in abstract and with credit to THE NORTH AMERICAN. All rejected manuscripts will be returned to writers. No anonymous or discourteous communications will be printed.

Contributors are respectfully requested to send manuscripts and communicate respecting them directly with the Editors, according to subject, as follows: *Concerning Medicine, 21 West 37th Street; concerning Surgery, 256 West 57th Street; concerning Societies and Hospitals, 121 East 70th Street; concerning News, Personals and Original Miscellany, 461 West 71st Street; concerning Correspondence, 152 West 57th Street.*

Communications to the Editor-in-Chief, *Exchanges* and *New Books* for notice should be addressed to *102 West 43d Street.*

REVOLUTIONARY PROPOSALS.

PROFESSOR HENRY I. BOWDITCH has again been addressing himself to the problem of de-homœopathizing homœopathy. About a year ago he suavely invited the school to sink, with its distinctive name, into oblivion, and now he turns about upon his "regular" brethren, and proposes to them revolutionary proceedings. At the conclusion of his address on Homœopathy before the Rhode Island State Medical Society, he recommended the following programme:

1. "Let every State Society follow the lead of New York, and let the members be *allowed*, without injury to their status in these bodies, to consult with members of other legally constituted medical societies.

2. "Let members of either of these sects join our State Societies, provided they prove to the State examiners or censors that they have studied medicine a proper length of time, and are able to pass the examination required of all applicants for admission; and provided, moreover, they agree to cease to call themselves by any peculiar name, because they desire to enroll themselves as members of our time-honored profession.

3. "Let us endeavor to make the American Medical Association rescind the vote whereby it expelled the New York State Medical Society, simply because, by its resolutions, it intimated that the fight

between the regular profession and homœopathy had lasted long enough, and that hereafter consultations would be allowed to all legalized medical bodies.

4. "As interweaved and intimately connected with this controversy, let us, on all proper occasions, by all means in our power, endeavor to induce the American Medical Association to annul the illegal action of the Judicial Council requiring an annual signature by all the members to its so-called Code of Ethics, under the penalty of not being allowed to attend and take part in the friendly intercourse and scientific discussions of its meetings, a measure which tends to keep alive our divisions, and encroaches upon our individual rights of conscience, instead of promoting that harmony in the profession of America which the Association, by its power for good, might bring about at these annual meetings in various parts of the country."

One does not know which to admire most in these remarkable propositions,—the candor with which Professor Bowditch unbares the purpose of the New York Code, or the coolness with which he discloses the true inwardness of the "so-called Code of Ethics" of the American Medical Association. It will be noted that he admits (1) that entire freedom of consultation in New York was cloaked under the phrase, "Emergencies may occur in which all restrictions should, in the judgment of the practitioner, yield to the demands of humanity ; (2) that, for this late concession to the demands of humanity, the New York members were excluded from friendly intercourse and scientific discussions by their regular national organization ; (3) that those who respect the individual rights of conscience cannot consistently sign the annual agreement of the American Medical Association not to consult with members of homœopathic bodies. In openly advocating the position of the New York Codists, but stripped of all hypocrisy, Professor Bowditch inaugurates a sanguinary period within the ranks of the regular Knights of Medicine. How many "will be strung up by the heels, and have their throats cut," before the civil war is over, it would be idle now to calculate. The prospect, however, engages the lively interest of all who have already lost what Professor Bowditch feelingly designates as "status."

In thus coming up to the ground always occupied by the homœopathic members of a time-honored profession, namely, that of unre-

stricted privilege of consultation, without loss of status in medical
societies, or of friendly intercourse with their fellow-physicians, the
sagacious professor is both hindseeing and foreseeing enough to recognize that the rights of conscience and the spirit of the freeman
cannot be warred upon without inevitable defeat; that, in fact, the
time for rout is rapidly approaching.   He appreciates that irregular
over-riding and over-reaching of equity in medical, as in other, politics
alienates the sympathy of the American public, and, moreover, it is
apparent that he regards the success of homœopathy in securing the
good-will of the people as assuming alarming proportions.   The fight
has evidently lasted long enough for the discomfiture of the regulars,
and far too long for the benefit of homœopathy.   The bottom issue in
the fight, in whatever pretence disguised—the patronage of the public—
is being decided against the Medical League for the Suppression of a
Competing System of Practice.   Now, that the new system cannot be
suppressed, but has gained such power that it is passing from the
position of defense to one of taking the offensive, with something like
advantage in the favor of patrons, it is entertaining to witness the
growth of a yearning for the union of the schools, and of a more
lively sense of the individual rights of conscience.

Notwithstanding that we suspect that Professor Bowditch has
mapped out a strategic change of tactics with the same ulterior
motive, every true physician must wish success to him and his coad-
jutors in their efforts to assert the rights of liberty in consultative
practice.   Homœopathic physicians, in particular, having enjoyed
the inward satisfaction that there is in placing individual convictions
beyond the tyranny of "regular" dictation, can testify that, while
"status" is agreeable, it is but a flimsy prop in comparison with
manly avowal and assertion of the belief and of the rights of the physician.   It is pleasant and profitable to discuss the subjects which all
physicians of every therapeutic belief must have in common, without
restriction and without penalty—but there is the rub.   Professor
Bowditch should not, therefore, over-rate the temptation that there
may be in the invitation to become members of "our State Societies."
The regular organizations need to undergo a prolonged process of
regeneration before they can become permeated with the practice

of tolerance and friendly, fair discussion of the principles of the homœopathic method for the cure of the sick. Already members of a time-honored profession, there is no overpowering inducement to homœopathic physicians in being enrolled in the ranks of a self-styled body of regulars, condescending to receive their self-effacing brethren into the fold where they must observe silence upon the one thing in which they are most deeply concerned. And then, there is that peculiar name, with all the historic truth, future benefit to mankind, and self-respect which is bound up with it! What is to be done with that?

A word which has passed into all literature, and which must remain as long as there is any science of drug-therapeutics, cannot be abandoned by any agreement. So long as things are nouns, and nouns have names, the word homœopathy will endure; and moreover, as long as a body of physicians adopts a creed of unbelief, and demands abnegation and denial of the homœopathic name, perverting the words regular, unsectarian, rational, scientific to distinctive partisan use, so long the logic of discrimination and of circumstances must compel the acceptance of the descriptive title which defines the system of drug-selection and distinguishes a body thus cut off and set apart. In every sense of the word "homœopaths" are fully physicians, and, moreover, physicians broadly and essentially distinctive in the principle through which they learn and apply the uses of drugs. If the word homœopathic is misconceived, misinterpreted, misrepresented, the fault is not with them. If the word carries offensive criticism, it is because of the facts which are interwoven with the name and cannot be dissevered. History cannot be wiped out by an agreement to drop a word, nor can any word be dropped because it expresses offensive truth. That truth involves not only past protest against the harmful methods sought to be imposed upon all practitioners, and which have now been abandoned, but also against the present chaos of therapeutic principles, still harming while it drifts from one fashion to another.

Homœopathy is a definite principle in scientific drug prescription, and the organization of homœopathy is not only necessary for the perpetuation of the mass of truth it has already discovered and proven, but also for the development of methods and knowledge in the practical application of its principle.   Until its law of similars has been candidly recognized, accepted, and taken up to be worked out into its most practical use by all bodies of medical men, it has a large mission to fulfil in the evolution of scientific therapeutics.   Never more than now has it needed defense, promulgation, and development.   There is no shame connected with the name, and it has lost no power for good.   It represents a conviction in therapeutics resting upon scientific evidence, and it is not a mere sham for beguiling a livelihood from a confiding, silly public.   The name stands, and the physicians whose body of therapeutic convictions stands in the name, stand by it.

Meantime, disbelievers must agree to cease their league of suppression; the impartial law of the land must become the standard of regularity; the profession of medicine, in the scientific sense, must sink the ecclesiastical spirit of discipline for heresy; the practitioners of medicine, in the bread-and-butter aspect of their profession, must stamp out the trades-union animus against competition in business; members of the profession, in their individual relations towards each other, must employ the test of individual motive and merit instead of the arbitrary rules of restrictive societies; and physicians, in their humanitarian duties to their fellow-beings in distress, must be left free to follow their consciences, absolutely untrammeled, according to their best judgment of the circumstances which call for consultation, and irrespective of medical organizations and the names they bear. These principles of tolerance are too intimately connected with the homœopathic name to be surrendered.   When all the State Societies and the American Medical Association embody them in their written and unwritten law, and abnegate the creed of abnegation, then invitation to membership can come with grace and carry the hospitality of fraternal feeling to homœopathic physicians.

A BROADER LEARNING.

E ACH generation, as it passes away, bequeaths to its successor and heir a rich legacy of knowledge and wisdom.   This is added to by earnest workers, and in time, augmented by their diligence and patient zeal, is again handed down to a succeeding generation.   So the sum of human wisdom increases gradually but surely, and each

generation, in the aggregate, is somewhat wiser than those that preceded. If this be so, then it must follow that individual knowledge has
increased and that the intellectual condition of the average man is
better now than ever before. This ascent to a higher mental and moral
plane has wrought some curious and remarkable changes. The relations of things become altered, and from time to time a readjustment
is imperatively demanded. Perhaps in no department of human affairs
has the change been greater or more striking than in the profession of
medicine. The physician of our forefathers—pompous in manner,
mysterious in speech, rough and often uncouth in method, yet practical, for the most part, in thought and act, theorizing little, reading
little, working much, cultivating but slightly the ever-widening field
of medical learning, and often utterly ignorant of all other realms of
wisdom—these ancient disciples of Esculapius have nearly passed
away. And it must be so. For in the new adjustment, in the altered
environment, new men and new abilities are required. The physician of to-day must be prepared to face the requirements of the present. A prompt recognition of the signs of the times is essential to
professional salvation. Not only must he be master of his profession
in all its niceties and amenities, a careful student, a close reasoner, a
critical observer, simple in manner, gentle in speech, deft and skillful
in touch, an intuitive reader of hearts, but he must have applied himself to that wider learning which only comes from prolonged and
laborious effort. The physician no longer can be a man of one idea.
He is required to be a cultured man, a man of broad education, of
liberal learning, of trained mind. More and more the profession is
being pushed to the front to act as the vanguard of progress. It has
come to pass that a physician is judged by his ability and learning in
other fields quite as much as by the special knowledge which relates
to his profession. A well-known writer has portrayed the present
attitude of medical science toward the world of intellectual progress
so powerfully that we give an extract : "The profession of medicine
is, of all fairly lucrative professions, the one best suited to the development of intellectual life. Having to deal continually with sciences,
being constantly engaged in following and observing the operations
of natural laws, it produces a sense of the working of those laws

which prepares the mind for bold and original speculations and a reliance upon their unfailing regularity, which gives it great firmness and assurance. A medical education is the best possible preparation for philosophical pursuits, because it gives them a solid basis in the ascertainable. The estimation in which these studies are held is an accurate meter of the intellectual advancement of a community. Where the priest is reverenced as a being above ordinary humanity and the physician slightly estimated, the condition of society is sure to be that of comparative ignorance and barbarism; and it is one of several signs which indicate a barbarian feeling in certain aristocratic circles that it has a contempt for the study of medicine. The progress of society toward enlightenment is marked by the steady social rise of the physician—a rise which still continues even in Western Europe. It is probable that before very long the medical profession will exercise a powerful influence upon general education and take an active share in it. There are very strong reasons for the opinion that schoolmasters educated in medicine would be peculiarly well qualified to train both body and mind for an active and vigorous manhood. An immense advantage, even from an intellectual point of view, in the pursuit of medicine and surgery is that they supply a discipline in mental tension. Other professions do this also, but not to the same degree. The combination of an accurate training with imperative science, with the habitual contempt of danger and contemplation of suffering and death, is the finest possible preparation for noble studies and arduous discoveries."

COMMENTS.

A MODERN FABLE.—There was once an Ass that fed with some nobler animals in a large pasture. For a time all went well with the Ass and his soul was content within him. But, by chance, being chosen to office, he sought out all the fat and juicy places of the pasture and brayed, without ceasing, for more. Also his ears increased and waxed great. Now, when the other animals saw these things, they marvelled within themselves and said, "Surely this is an undoubted Ass; let us depose him from office." And they did so But he only brayed the more, and still sought out the fat and juicy places. And he communed with himself and said, "Lo! I am a disgruntled Ass and can no longer flap an official ear; how then shall I bray? Verily, I will seek fresh pastures!" Now, there was adjoining

another pasture, where different customs and methods obtained. And
the Ass drew nigh to the fence and held sweet conference with the
animals in the neighboring pasture.   And the Ass brayed and said
unto them, "Now, these many days have I desired to dwell with you,
and to cast in my lot among you."   But they said unto him, "Wilt
thou sever all other connections and obey our laws?"   And the Ass
said, "Yea, verily!"   But they further spoke and said, "Dost thou
acknowledge that thine former beliefs were but shams, and that thou
wert an Ass for believing them?" And he publicly acknowledged himself an Ass.   Then they permitted him to enter the pasture.   But he
communed with himself again in private and said, "If I go on the
other side of the fence I lose all on this side; if I stay here I lose all on
the other side; verily, I am an Ass! I will straddle the fence." And
he straddled it.   Now, when this thing was seen, the poor Ass was
maltreated and belabored on both sides of the fence at once, so that
he liked to have given up the ghost.   But he raised a tale of woe and
said, "Of a verity I am not the man who wrote the letter, but I am
the repository of medical science."   Upon this the stalwarts standing
near promptly kicked the Ass into the arms of a past *Era*, who extracted a stolen bray and restored it to its proper owners.   The Ass
then gave up the ghost.   *Hæc fabula docet* that straddling, as a fine art,
is not practiced except by Asses.

BOOK REVIEWS.

ORIFICIAL SURGERY, by E. H. PRATT, M.D.   Chicago: W. T.
Kenner.

This small book comes before us with a high-sounding title.   It is
remarkable in two ways—for the imposingness of its title and the
poverty of its contents.   Two features are commendable.   The author
calls attention to the neglected rectal pockets and papillæ, and cites
some interesting cases; the details of both, however, are so meagre
as to greatly impair their value.   In the treatment of hemorrhoids no
mention is made of the method which is, no doubt, the best, *viz.*: the
treatment by Kelsey's clamp and cautery, the author contenting himself with mentioning a few methods which are now being supplanted
by better.   The details and methods given are so meagre and unsatisfactory as to render them nearly useless.   The subject of rectal ulcers
is dismissed with the statement that they are generally syphilitic, and
can be cured with great ease and rapidity by the application of the
cautery and dilatation of the sphincter; the first of which statements
should be accepted *cum grano salis*, while the latter is in direct conflict
with the experience of nearly all surgeons.   No mention is made of
strictures of the rectum or the methods for their relief.   The treatment
of the diseases of the female sexual organs is a sort of parody on the
term "treatment."   There is scarcely anything in it, and what information there is would be quickly supplanted by better, by the perusal of
any text book published in the last half a century.   In short, the whole
work is one which belongs to a very undesirable class of medical
literature, the class which suggests authors as containing a fund of

information to be communicated upon some other occasion. Unless the book which the author states is in preparation is an infinite improvement on the present issue, we hope that the author will spare homœopathy the disgrace of its publication.   F.

A REFERENCE HANDBOOK OF THE MEDICAL SCIENCES, Embracing the Entire Range of Scientific and Practical Medicine and Allied Science. By various writers. Illustrated by chromolithographs and fine wood engravings. Edited by ALBERT H. BUCK, M.D., New York City. Volume IV. New York: William Wood & Company, 1887.

The present volume embraces topics from Icthyol to Milford Springs, and includes the important subjects, insanity, labor, larynx, kidney, liver and lungs, which are treated of with great fullness. There are, besides, innumerable shorter articles, judiciously allotted space according to their relative interest. Throughout the standard of scholarship is worthy of all praise, and in every way Vol. IV. is equal to its predecessors. The copious illustrations of themselves place the work above ordinary compliment, for they are faithful in drawing, really excellently engraved, and not the hackneyed reproductions with which one is familiar. The publication is of extraordinary utility and merit, to which one can turn with certainty for all sorts of out-of-the-way information, as well as to treatises, containing the latest advances in knowledge. We cannot commend it as highly as it is worth.

CORRESPONDENCE.

To the Editors of the NORTH AMERICAN JOURNAL OF HOMŒOPATHY :

IN this "city by the lake," whose medical population are pleased to call the "Vienna of America," life for its medical practitioners is full of the same bustling activity which is so characteristic of Chicago. All who practice the healing art in this atmosphere of tensive energy are compelled, *nolens volens*, to keep up with the madding crowd, or, his strength weakening, he is soon lost to sight and memory. In this mad rush, which shortens lives and rapidly produces both mental and physical exhaustion, neurasthenias of all forms abound. One cannot reside here without catching the infection for rapid work in every direction ; here the days pass unnoticed when promises for letters are made and the promise almost broken by deferred fulfillment.

Nearly 2,000 medical students annually attend the various medical colleges here—the majority of the colleges being grouped around the County Hospital, which furnishes abundant clinical material for the instruction of all. There are four allopathic, two homœopathic, one eclectic, a post-graduate school, and an ophthalmic college to supply medical pabulum for the students who desire to pursue their medical studies here.

Among practitioners of medicine in the city we find 883 regular and irregular physicians, 246 homœopaths, and numerous medical societies and clubs.

The dominant school, as regards numbers, is, of course, the allopathic, but the homœopathic practitioners have by far the larger number of our wealthiest and most influential families upon their lists. This extensive clientage is not the outgrowth of fashion, but the direct result of the good work which has been done in the past by the older homœopathic physicians, which has been ably supplemented by those of later years.

The homœopathic profession of Chicago, however, is sadly wanting in harmony, owing to the unfortunate complications which arose some years ago. This division in our ranks prevents our presenting that united front which would enable us to carry forward any scheme which might be considered advisable to advance the interests of homœopathy. It also lessens the respect which our scientific therapeutics should demand from the community.

I do not propose, at this late date, to discuss the *raison d'être* for two homœopathic medical colleges in this city; suffice it now, that both are in a flourishing condition, with an attendance during the session which has just closed of nearly 400 students, and with a graduating class from the Hahnemann of eighty-eight and from the Chicago of forty-six. The chairs in both institutions are well filled by excellent teachers and practitioners of homœopathy, whose names and fame serve to attract medical students from all over the world to listen to the practical instruction which their experience teaches.

Two homœopathic medical societies, The Chicago Academy of Homœopathic Physicians and Surgeons, and The Clinical Society, are well attended, and in their membership include the major portion of the city physicians. The Illinois State Society, which meets every alternate year in Chicago, this year holds its session at Joliet, in May. With 700 homœopathic physicians in the State, our State Society has been allowed to languish for some years, owing to a factional strife for leadership, which always results disastrously to any organization. During the last two years, however, a larger attendance upon its meetings and an increased interest in its welfare, is indicative of a future the profession may be proud of. The coming meeting at Joliet is already exciting much interest, and the promised attendance, together with the large number of topics for papers to be read which are announced, bids fair to make it one of the most interesting and successful meetings in the history of the society.

The hospitals of Chicago are exceedingly creditable to a city of its rapid growth and increasing population. Of those in which the homœopaths have an interest are, first, the Cook County Hospital, opposite the Chicago Homœopathic College, with its 850 beds, which are constantly filled. The attending staff consists of thirteen allopathic physicians and surgeons, together with seven of our own school. Every fourth patient received is assigned to treatment by the homœopathic staff. Each staff has its own corps of internes; and while no wards are exclusively under the control of either school of medicine, those under homœopathic treatment are grouped together at one end of the ward. The conduct of the members of the attending staffs, the internes and trained nurses is such as to prevent any professional clashing. Clinics are held bi-weekly by each staff and are crowded by the medical students from the various medical colleges located around the hospital. The clinical material, as may be supposed, is abundant, and cases of special interest are exhibited, by consent, in the clinics of both staffs.

The hospital of the Chicago Homœopathic Medical College is located in the college building, and has accommodation for twenty-five patients, which are filled during the college session by operative cases. The Central Homœopathic Dispensary, which has its clinic rooms also in the same building, and in the midst of several large allopathic dispensaries, has a daily attendance which taxes its large clinical staff thoroughly to look after.

Hahnemann Hospital is situated in the rear of Hahnemann College and located in the southern portion of the city. It has some forty beds, which are kept well filled during the year. The hospital contains a fine amphitheatre for holding the clinics in the hospital proper, and for the exhibition of cases, which are drawn from a large out-patient service.

The Half-orphan Asylum and the Foundlings' Home are entirely under control of the homœopathic profession ; and here, as elsewhere, the lessened death rate and shortened sick lists give evidence of the supremacy of the homœopathic law of cure.

At the close of last year one of our veteran practitioners of homœopathy, Professor A. E. Small, passed from our midst. At the funeral services held at the church of the New Jerusalem, the attendance of the profession was very large, the faculties and students of both colleges being present to do honor to the memory and good work of that pioneer of homœopathy, whose continued labor did much to advance the interests of homœopaths in Chicago and the West.

In closing this rambling epistle, I cannot refrain from mentioning the fact that I hear on every side words of commendation for your journal, owing to the high standing of the original articles which have filled its pages.   J. H. BUFFUM.

REPORTS OF SOCIETIES AND HOSPITALS.

HOMŒOPATHIC MEDICAL SOCIETY OF THE COUNTY OF NEW YORK.

THE regular monthly meeting of the Homœopathic Medical Society of the County of New York, was held in the reception room of the New York Ophthalmic Hospital, corner Third Avenue and Twenty-third Street, Thursday, March 10th, 1887, at eight o'clock.

Sixty-three members and visitors were in attendance.

The following were duly elected to membership: Drs. H. N. Fairbank Cooke, W. H. Jones, C. H. Laidlaw, John G. Moeder, A. R. McMichael, Mayhew Swift and T. C. Williams.

Committee on Diseases of the Throat and Chest, John W. Dowling, Chairman, reported four papers.

Dr. John W. Dowling read a paper on "Inspection, as an aid to Diagnosis in Diseases of the Circulatory and Respiratory Organs." He exhibited a number of patients to illustrate his remarks.

Dr. Malcolm Leal read a paper, "On the Necessity of a Differentiation between the Varieties of Croup, especially between the True and False."

Doctor Schley.—I do not know of any subject that interests the general practitioner more than the one on which this paper has been read. In my experience, it is not an easy matter to make a laryngoscopic examination in such cases, especially where the child is very young. A diagnosis is all the more important in such severe cases—first, as to prognosis and treatment—and when an accurate diagnosis can be made the intense fear of the family may be allayed. The treatment depends, of course, entirely upon what we find. In some cases of spasmodic croup, where an examination is impossible, I am frank to acknowledge that a diagnosis is not an easy matter, and at times absolutely impossible. In this country there is less membranous laryngitis than in more severe climates and in the northern parts of France and Great Britain. With us these severe cases, with urgent symptoms, are due, in the large majority of cases, to a condition of œdema.

In the case of paresis of the vocal chords in œdema or a spasmodic condition, I have perfect confidence in homœopathic remedies, but we must be sure of the pathological condition before we can, with certainty, quiet the mother and family. I have known of one instance, since living in New York, where the disease commenced primarily with all the symptoms of severe *spasmodic* croup, and was diagnosed as such on the fourth day by two competent physicians, where it eventually turned out to be a membranous condition, the child dying on the seventh day. Writers on this vexed subject seem to me to become mixed regarding the appellations of these different states.

Hoarseness in an infant is always a matter to be seriously considered. When you see a child on the third or fourth day of its sickness with such symptoms as Dr. McMurray has so well described, I do not think it possible always to say whether the patient is suffering from paresis glottidis, spasm, or a membranous laryngitis, or what will be the outcome of such a case, even though we see no membrane in the pharynx or nose.

It is in such cases that the use of the laryngoscope is a necessity.

Dr. Dillow.—I agree with the position taken by Dr. Leal, that a positive diagnosis between the different forms of so-called croup from the symptoms and pharyngeal appearances alone cannot be made without the aid of the laryngoscope. I have seen cases of pharyngeal diphtheria where the usual symptoms of laryngeal stenosis had existed during several days, but where the patient recovered without the appearance of membrane in the larynx. This especially needs to be considered in drawing conclusions as to the effects of remedies. The same error may sometimes occur where only supposed membrane exists in the pharynx. I remember well a case of this kind in which *lac caninum* gained much repute—the case of a girl of five, in whom alarming symptoms of obstruction of the larynx, with much fever, rapid pulse, almost toneless cough, stridulous breathing, had lasted without marked remissions for several days. An examination by candle-light showed apparently thick, tough, yellow membrane adhering to the tonsils and the walls of the pharynx, this opinion being concurred in by the three physicians present. *Lac caninum* was suggested and given as a last resort. The following morning the membrane had disappeared entirely, and the symptoms of laryngeal obstruction had vanished. A few months later it was my good fortune to treat the same child during an exactly similar attack, where I had full laryngoscopic facilities throughout. There was the same thick, tough deposit in the pharynx as before, but it was only adherent mucus, and the larynx, easily inspected, revealed only hyperæmia with some catarrhal swelling, and a narrow slit of a glottis, due either to paresis of the abductors or spasm of the adductors, both elements entering, as I then thought, into the case. There was the same sudden subsidence of distressing stenosis during a night after several days of continued symptoms as before, and no *lac caninum* was given.

There is another condition which may be confounded with membranous laryngitis, occurring rarely, but simulating the continuous character of the symptoms of obstruction with spasm. I have seen three cases, two of adults and one of a child, in which an acute catarrhal inflammation, confined mainly to the inferior surfaces of the true chords, had induced baggy swellings, not in the nature of serous œdema, but more like the thickening seen in chronic hypertrophy of the inferior surfaces of the chords. Below the free edge of the superior surfaces of the chords were seen the rounded swellings beneath, closely approximated, and thus shutting off all view of the trachea. In these cases there were present continuous stridulous breathing, worse on expiration, attacks of spasms of the glottis, and the cough and voice of croup. Mucus adhering to the edges of the swellings was found to be provocative of the paroxysms for breath, and being detached by coughing, differentiated between itself and the membrane of true croup. The swellings seemed to paralyze the power of the chords to separate to more than a very slight extent. The patients recovered from the attacks in from one to two weeks.

Dr. McMurray.—I shall not pretend to add anything to the very valuable paper and remarks that have been made. From what little experience I have had through life, I am disposed to congratulate Dr. Leal on his good fortune and success in the treatment of such cases. I know from experience the truth of what has been said of the extreme difficulties of the diagnosis of these different forms of croup, and, of course, that implies the uncertainty of prognosis. In the cases I have met with, there was one peculiarity—suddenness of attack. In a large proportion of those cases, the child is put to bed in apparently good health; shortly after it wakes up crowing and coughing and without making any noise at all scarcely. It is possible that the croup may commence that way, but generally it shows that the spasmodic character will be better in the morning. Now, my experience of true membranous croup is that it don't commence that way; not once in 500 times. You will usually find such cases commencing with a disturbance in the night—which you may be called to—but not of the extremely urgent character which you will find in spasmodic croup; child gets better, lies down and goes to sleep before morning. Towards the next evening, perhaps, that coughing will commence again; when that is so, and this occurs for a day or two in spite of remedies, I generally find you have got trouble. Now, I believe from that very fact that this differentiated condition, this false membrane, is the work of that very inflammation, which has commenced so gradually; that which was simply inflammation and swelling of the vocal chords results in the formation of the membrane; and I am very well satisfied that that is the true history of membranous croup in a great many cases. I am very glad to hear that there have been means found to avoid the necessity of resorting to tracheotomy. I have seen it employed a great many times, and have come to hold it in very great disrespect. I know that quite a number of years ago some of our very best surgeons abandoned the operation entirely.

Dr. Hallock.—I think the statement that serious forms of croup commence less suddenly is right. When they go to bed apparently well, have a sudden attack of croup at night, next morning they are better. I never feel satisfied or safe about a case like that until after the second night. If that passes well and the child is no worse, the case is one of spasmodic rather than true croup. If you will allow me, sir, I will relate, in this connection, my first experience in a case of spasmodic croup, and my use of aconite. I was called one night just after I began to use homœopathic remedies, in a great hurry, to the wife of my neighbor one door from me. When the door opened, I heard a hoarse cough and a curious noise which alarmed me, and the servant whom I met said to me : "Come as quick as possible." My impression was that I must give an emetic immediately in hot water. While waiting for the hot water—it did not come for some time—it occurred to me that I had in my pocket a little bottle of aconite. The woman was in great distress; could not lie down at all, and every once in a while made a noise which frightened the whole household. I put a few drops of the aconite in water in the usual way. I had used it once or twice before for fevers, and gave it to her. Before the girl got up stairs with the hot water, she had lain down and got to sleep. I waited to hear her cough again, but as she did not wake up, I left the medicine, so that if she got hoarser, she could take another dose ; and after leaving word for them to let me know her condition in the morning, I went home. The next morning, I waited half an hour ; the physician of the family was my most intimate friend, and with whom I had during several years exchanged business. I waited at my house, two doors only off, till the call of their doctor in the morning. I expected the doctor to come in, as we were on friendly terms. I waited for half an hour for the doctor, before going, but he did not come. I did not see the doctor as he did not call on me. In about a week from that time, we were driving through the street, and approaching each other in our gigs ; but upon seeing me, he was interested in looking to the other side of the street, and kept his eye there until I passed. I was surprised, but after that the doctor and myself never exchanged a word, although he was a very worthy man in every respect.

Dr. Deschere.—I think that a diagnosis between the different forms of croup is necessary, *not* for the mode of treatment as much as for the sake of prognosis. But the laryngoscope alone I can hardly consider competent. In case of children, where it is admitted only with great difficulty, it is possible that, looking into the throat of the child at the short moment that is given for exploration, you may not be able to see the membrane that is there. If the diagnosis, however, is made with the laryngoscope also, it only corroborates the correctness of the former. My experience coincides with that of Dr. McMurray, and besides I think it not so excessively difficult to make the diagnosis in marked cases without the aid of the laryngoscope. The entire course of membranous croup is different from the spasmodic form ; the continuance of the fever, of the hoarseness, of the cough with its characteristic bark, the difficult and sawing respiration, even between the paroxysms, etc., characterize the membranous variety sufficiently. If, in addition, I discover, on inspection, membranous deposits in the fauces, I do not want further evidence.

Dr. Berghaus.—I think that a great many cases that appear to be spasmodic, if treated by the laws of homœopathy can be prevented from turning into membranous croup. In all my practice I have had but one case in which operative interference was necessary, and it was a case of true diphtheria. It was a girl seven years of age, whose case was progressing very favorably, when suddenly croupy symptoms set in ; the case went from bad to worse, and the child became cyanotic. I called in Doctor O'Dwyer, the originator of intubation, to assist me. In a few seconds the tube was introduced. For five days the child kept the tube in the larynx with an occasional cough. Semi-solid food was given, and the difficulty seemed to be overcome when nephritis set in and carried her off; but the greatest boon was bestowed upon that child by having a tube introduced, and should I ever come across a case where surgical interference should be necessary, I should be in favor of intubation against laryngotomy.

Dr. Leal.—I have just a word to add. I did not mean to say in my paper that the difficulty lies in recognizing those cases of a purely spasmodic nature. Where the attack comes on suddenly and very severely, and dies away or disappears almost as quickly as it comes, it is usually purely spasmodic, and it is hardly necessary to make an examination of the larynx to show it. A membrane may appear in the larynx, however, after severe attacks of spasm; then the stenosis becomes more constant. I have seen cases of spasm where attacks would recur for several nights in succession. I was called in consultation recently to see a lady about thirty years of age; she had had attacks of spasm of the larynx and would become unconscious, when respiration would become re-established. There was not a trace of spasm as evidenced by the manner of breathing between these attacks. She had four or five attacks during the day and night; then they disappeared entirely. Such a case needed no examination to establish the diagnosis. But when the symptoms of laryngeal obstruction increase for two or three days, without intermission, then is the time when an examination of the larynx is necessary to tell whether the membrane is there. If the membrane is present in the trachea, unless it is also present in the bronchial tubes, you will not, as a rule, have any dyspnœa, except such as arises from spasm. I grant it is not an easy matter to examine children, but I claim that the difficulties are very much over-rated. The majority of children, if you know them, will submit to an examination, unless they have been fooled with and frightened before. There is no pain attending it, and a child's larynx is usually better seen than that of an adult; at any rate, you can get a fair idea of the trouble, sufficient, as a rule, to enable you to make a prognosis. It is, of course, impossible to say that membrane will not appear at some subsequent period.

Dr. Shelton read a paper on "A Possible Ætiological Factor in Diphtheria."

Dr. Deschere read a paper on "The Temptations of a Homœopathic Physician."

Then he said: This experience, I think, is very frequent with many of us. We ought always to try to be as firm as we can, and patients will have more respect for us. I think our brethren of the old school will ha e more respect for us if we do our best with homœopathic remedies.

RECORD OF MEDICAL PROGRESS.

ASTHMA is cured by oxalic acid according to Poulet.—*Lond. Med. Rec.*, February 15th, 1887.

CIRRHOSIS OF THE LIVER—RECOVERY.—Romain reports a case of recovery from cirrhosis of the liver in the *Arch. de Méd. et de Pharm.*, November, 1886. Probably the early institution of treatment led to the successful result.

TULIPINE is an alkaloid prepared mainly from the domesticated garden tulip, and is contained in all parts of this plant. One-third of a grain will kill a frog, and one and one-half grains will kill a cat. Death is caused by cardiac paralysis, but powerful nervous influence is apparent. In smaller doses it increases salivary secretion, and is both diuretic and laxative.— Nicot, in *Nouveaux Remèdes*, November 24th, 1886.

POSITION IN SLEEP, AND BRONCHITIS.—Dr. G. Nosovitch has examined 738 soldiers, and has found bronchitis in 235. In 97, the disease was left-sided; and in 66, both sided. The extraordinary frequency of one-sided localization led finally to the belief that the position of the body in sleep might act as a determining factor. Dr. N. therefore undertook observations for ten successive nights, on 612 sleeping soldiers, and found that 37.44% slept on the right side ; 33.17% on the left ; 23.07% on the back, and.6.29% on the belly.—*Lond. Med. Rec.*, February, 1887.

EXCISION OF CHANCRES.—Dr. Andronico claims to have entirely eradicated the syphilitic virus in four cases by excising the primary chancre. He believes that if the sore is situated in a locality such as the nymphæ or the prepuce, where excision is possible, and if the operation is performed within forty-eight hours, or at the very latest, three days, from the first appearance of the chancre, success may be hoped for. The operation, he says, is contra-indicated if a longer time than this has elapsed, or if the glands are enlarged.—*London Lancet*, February 19th, 1887.

RECTAL GASEOUS MEDICATION FOR EMPHYSEMA.—Pursuing the plan of M. Bergeon, MM. Renault and Shierry have employed lavements of carbonic acid gas in the treatment of emphysema complicated with catarrh. The number of observations has been but small. The general method of treatment was the same as that employed for the treatment of phthisis, but the sulphurous water was omitted. The results were remarkably satisfactory, especially as regards the relief of cough and shortness of breath, a daily lavement for a week or a fortnight being the usual course.— *London Lancet*, February 26th, 1887.

PUNCTURE OF THE UTERUS FOR ACUTE HYDRAMNOS.—Timaux reports the case of a woman 37 years old, who had had four normal labors. She thought she was in the fifth month of pregnancy and the abdomen was so distended that she had great difficulty in breathing. Finally operative interference became urgent, and puncture was made with an ordinary trocar. Fluid to the amount of seven litres was drawn off, when, as fœtal movements were felt, the process was stopped. The patient was much relieved and there is now no reason to suppose that pregnancy will not go to full term.—*Lond. Med. Rec.*, February 15th, 1887.

SALICYLIC ERUPTION.—Burning sensations in the skin, œdema of the eye-lids, and patches of bluish-red erythema, were noticed by S. Rosenberg to follow the administration of four grammes of salicylate to a seamstress. A bullous eruption appeared on the site of the erythema, as the result of continued use of the drug. Three days after the discontinuance of the drug the vessels dried up. A fresh experimental observation was made with a similar result. The urine gave a distinct ferri-chloride reaction. The inunction of salicyl ointment was followed by burning and red patches on the skin, with blueness of the face, and the urine showed the salicyl reaction.—*London Lancet*, February 5th, 1887.

RUPTURE OF ANEURISM INTO PERICARDIUM.—At a recent meeting of the Medical Society of London, Mr. Hugh Smith cited a case of rupture of aortic aneurism into the pericardium. It occurred in a washer-woman, aged forty-two, who died whilst working at the wash-tub. The specimen was exhibited, and showed dilatation of the first two parts of the aortic arch; the third part of the arch showed a sacular aneurism, which opened into the pericardium by a rent three-quarters of an inch in length ; as much as fifteen ounces of fluid and clotted blood were found in the pericardium. There was collapse of the left lung. During life signs of consolidation were noted at the apex of the left lung, but there was no laryngeal or pupillary signs.—*London Lancet*, February 12th, 1887.

THE MECHANISM OF EXOPHTHALMUS.—Dr. Durdufi found that after intravenous injection of cocaine, a stronger exophthalmus follows than after irritation of the peripheral end of the cervical sympatheticus. The fact that exophthalmus appears sometimes after the cessation of respiration and of the beating of the heart, shows that the grade of filling the blood-vessels cannot come here in consideration; we must also exclude the influence of the soft parts surrounding the bulbus and of the eyelids, as a bulbus, separated from all the parts, is still able to protrude. As, finally, exophthalmus may happen after division of the optic nerve and the external muscles of the eyes, he comes to the conclusion that it must be caused by the action of the other muscles, and he thinks that this is the case in morbus basedowii.—*Wiener Med. Presse*, No. 8, 1887, S. L.

STRYCHNIA AS AN ANTIDOTE TO ALCOHOL.—Dr. Jaroschewsky gave dogs a half to two ounces of 42–65° alcohol, and the latter dose caused a tottering gait and three ounces produced drunkenness; when such doses were given several times a week, they perished with symptoms of gradual emaciation, but when the dogs received with the alcohol two milligrammes strychnine for every ounce of alcohol, the animals stood five ounces of alcohol and they neither got drunk nor showed the strychine any injurious effect. After numerous experiments these conclusions may be made : (1) Strychnine neutralized the narcotic action of the alcohol. (2) Strychnine allows the introduction of larger doses of alcohol, so that its noxious effect may be prevented. (3) An increase of the doses of strychnine with parallel doses of alcohol reaches its maximum when the strychnine shows its toxic effect. (4) Its antidotal action has been shown on patients.—*Wiener Med. Presse*, November 8th, 1887.—S. L.

CHRONIC VALVULAR HEART DISEASE.—Sir Andrew Clark collects and tabulates from his private case records 648 cases of chronic cardiac valvular disease, the presence of which was not indicated by symptoms, and did not sensibly interfere with health. These patients all applied for relief of other conditions, of which dyspepsia, 275 cases, heads the list, being followed by rheumatism, 57; nervousness, 45; headaches, 35; bronchitis, 23; the gouty state, 22; eczema, 17; vertigo, 17; neuralgia, 17; catarrhal diarrhœa, 12; melancholia, 10; ague, 9; albuminuria, 8; anæmia, 8; pulmonary congestion, 7; hepatic catarrh, 7; renal calculus, 6; epilepsy, 5; and many other diseases, each of which did not occur in more than four cases. These last, with the ones quoted, give the following figures, if arranged according to vital system affected. Diseases or disorders of the digestive system, 326; nervous system, 134; rheumatic affections, 61; respiratory system, 47; skin, 30; gout, 23. Dr. Clark gives this *resumé* and the method pursued in arranging the cases, in the *Brit. Med. Jour.*, for February 5th, 1887, and in the following numbers of that journal appear the elaborate tables by which his paper was illustrated.

DYSLEXIE.—Berlin has observed six patients in whom this symptom appeared. It is characterized by the impossibility of reading more than three, four or five consecutive words. The patients read the words correctly, whatever the size of the print; but they cannot continue reading. They stop for an instant, and then resume, but with the same want of success. They have no affection of speech ; pronounce clearly words pronounced to them, and their intelligence is retained. Dyslexie has nothing in common with the visual hebetude of the ophthalmologists, for it is unaccompanied by any ocular trouble. It is a variety of aphasia, an incomplete and definite verbal blindness. The condition usually arises suddenly with various cerebral symptoms. The author has had four autopsies. In one case he found softening of the gray matter of the inferior parietal lobule. In the others the area of softening was not localized so precisely. There was always found important alterations in the cerebral arteries. The symptom always indicates a grave cerebral

lesion going on rapidly to death.—*Arch. Gen. de Med.*, November, 1886—
from *Edinb. Med. Jour.*, January, 1887.

A NEW PROCESS FOR DILATATION OF THE UTERUS.—Vulliet places the
patient in the knee-and-chest position, exposes the os uteri by means of a
Sim's speculum, and introduces into the cavity a tampon of cotton, which
is pushed in with a metallic sound.   Each tampon is previously dipped
into a solution of one part iodoform in ten parts of ether, dried and preserved in tightly-stopped bottles.   Tampons are introduced until the cavity
of the cervix is stuffed full.   After forty-eight hours the tampons are
extracted, and the operation is repeated, using more of the prepared
cotton.   The advantages of this method, says the author, are the rendering visible through all its length of the uterine cavity, with the ability to
operate therein and to see the results of operation.   Vulliet has employed
the method in case of cancer, of endo-uterine and parietal fibroids, and
in certain cases of chronic endo-metritis.   Labbe, Horteloup, Labbat, Porak
and Charpentier have all used the method and speak favorably of it.   Charpentier says that if the rules for antisepsis are followed, the method will
prove of great service in the treatment of certain pathological conditions
of the uterus.—*Jour. des Soc. Scientifiques*, October 13th, 1886.

HEPATIC PUNCTURE.—Dr. George Harley, *British Medical Journal*,
January 15th, 1887, gives full description of the methods used and precautions necessary to observe in puncturing the liver.   The precautions
he takes are as follows : "(*a*) Always commence the exploration either
with a fine aspirating needle, or an equally fine 7-inch long French exploring trocar, attached to a hypodermic syringe, which acts as an aspirator
and admits of at once perceiving whether pus, hydatid fluid, or blood is
to be dealt with ; so that, if need be, the instrument can instantly be withdrawn.   When pus is found, there is substituted a larger needle, to which
a rubber ball aspirator and syphon tube are attached.   (*b*) Never allow the
point of the exploring instrument to go anywhere near those portions of
the liver in which its large blood-vessels are normally situated.   (*c*)
Always penetrate the capsule at a part of the liver where the wound
orifice, after withdrawal of the instrument, can be brought into immediate
contact with the abdominal parieties, so as to admit of the opening into
the liver being firmly closed by direct pressure of a pad and bandage
applied to abdominal walls.   The external abdominal wound is closed
with a 2-inch square of plaster.

IODOFORM POISONING.—Dr. Wolowsky reported two cases of iodoform
intoxication.   A lady of about sixty suffered from carcinoma of the breast,
causing severe pains and insomnia.   As she was averse to an operation,
the ulcerating cancer was treated locally with iodoform, which diminished the pain and produced sleep, and she continually asked for a renewal
of the dressing, which she preferred to morphine.   In two months nearly
forty-three grammes were used up.   Suddenly gastritis, hæmatemesis,
and epistaxis appeared.   After four days, icterus, somnolence, dilatation
of the pupils and lassitude ; temperature 38.5 ; liver shrunken ; enormous
enlargement of the spleen.   The day following the patient failed to move,
lips compressed, the *rima* of the eyelids small, slight trismus, stertorous
breathing, death.
      The second case was that of an aged woman who, in consequence of
a fall, showed a wound, which for four weeks was dressed with iodoform.
She died with nearly the same symptoms.
      The picture of acute atrophy of the liver may be ascribed to the use of
iodoform, and such cases teach us to be careful in its continuous use,
especially with old people.—*Wiener Med. Presse*, No. 8, 1887, S. L.

EXTIRPATION OF THE THYROID GLAND.—Dr. Rogocritz describes the changes in the central nervous system after extirpation of the thyroid gland. He operated on rabbits, dogs and cats. Death happened after three days up to three months. In some cases depression, in others excitation of the central nervous system followed. The depression was often interrupted by spasmodic attacks, gradually increasing in intensity; the pulse fell, the temperature rose, often involuntary urination was observed. In the physical and sensitive sphere hebetude of the intellect, diminution of visual power, and paræsthesiæ appeared. The cause of death was an encephlo-myelitis subacuta. The changes in the central nervous system, found in necropsies, showed great similarity with those after intoxication with *arsen.* or *phosphor.*—granular degeneration of the nerve-cells, with partial formation of vacuoles—and are probably produced by changes in the blood, in consequence of the action of the products of the normal tissue-change upon the central nervous system, which is rendered inocuous in the normal animal by the action of the thyroid gland. In cases where they recovered, the hypophysis cerebri, or another organ, acted vicariously for the thyroid gland.—*Wiener Med. Presse,* No. 8, 1887, S. L.

HEROIC DOSE OF TURPENTINE IN CROUP.—In an obstinate and dangerous case of diphtheritic croup, which had extended into the larynx, after painting with boracic acid, and subsequently with a chloric acid application, without benefit, the child's condition becoming worse and worse, Dr. Lewentaner, of Constantinople, before resorting to tracheotomy, remembering a paper by Demlow in which turpentine was recommended in these cases, determined to give it a trial, and so administered, with his own hand, a teaspoonful of the pure *oleum terebinthæ,* giving after it some warm milk. In a quarter of an hour the labored laryngeal breathing had given way to normal respiration sounds. That night the child slept well, and was quite free from the brassy cough which had previously been present. The next morning he was quite lively, and was found playing with his toys. All trace of false membrane had disappeared from the pharynx, which merely presented a reddened surface. Convalescence was rapid and uninterrupted. The turpentine, however, caused an eruption of the face, trunk and extremities, having much the same appearance as the rash of measles, but of a brighter red. The spots completely faded in two days, and were followed by no sign of desquamation.—*London Lancet,* February 5th, 1887.

FOOD FOR INVALIDS.—By utilizing the results of the experiments of Dr. James Fraser on the relative digestibility of the chief albuminoid principles—*Lancet,* London, December, 1886, p. 1215—the following valuable deductions are obtained : "Beef tea, as ordinarily prepared, is of little nutritive value, but if the white of an egg be mixed with a cup of beef tea and heated to about 160° F., the value of the beef tea is greatly enhanced. Again, if minced raw beef be just covered with very weak hydrochloric acid (four drops of acid to one pint of water) and left to macerate for the night, the liquid strained off and squeezed out of the flesh by wringing in a cloth contains so much syntonin as to make it highly nutritious when neutralized ; such a liquid will remain clear after boiling to remove the raw flavor. In cases where the digestive powers are not in abeyance, one may give by mouth or by enemata one or more of the various forms of peptonised foods or fluids that are now in the market." The experiments with casein and gluten show that there are very few worse foods for a delicate stomach than the usual bread and milk. Whey is a mildly nutritious fluid, and easily digested. In cases where it is desired to feed the patient through the intestine, those substances found to be soluble in alkaline fluids, and therefore easily acted on by the pancreatic juice—as raw albumen, syntonin, or alkali-albumen—may be used alone or dissolved in some meat tea.—*Lond. Med. Rec.*, February, 1887.

DEATH FOLLOWING SOON AFTER WASHING OUT A DILATED STOMACH.—At a recent meeting of the Cambridge Medical Society, Mr. Martin brought forward the case of a patient who was admitted into Addenbrooke's Hospital under Dr. Bradbury, for stricture of the pylorus. He was forty-eight years old, and seven years previously had been an in-patient, with symptoms of pyloric ulcer. His stomach was now much dilated, and he suffered from flatulence, vomiting, pain and increasing weakness. He vomited large quantities of frothy fluid, containing sarcinæ. Ten days after admission it was decided to wash out the stomach. Soon after passing the tube into the stomach, the patient became very faint, so it was withdrawn. About two hours afterward he complained of stiffness in the jaws, with inability to open the mouth, and rigidity of the arms, which were strongly pronated and flexed, the thumbs being turned into the palms. The patient was conscious, and sweated profusely. The rigidity spread to all the muscles of the limbs and trunk, and the temperature rose to 103.4. He became pulseless and livid, the temperature rising to 107.2 before death, which occurred six hours and a half after washing out the stomach. Post mortem examination showed a simple stricture of the pylorus, with the scar of an old ulcer, and a much dilated stomach. There was no injury or abrasion of the mucous membrane. The other organs were healthy and no lesion of the brain was discovered.—*London Lancet, Jan. 8, 1887.*

CHYLOUS ASCITES.—At a meeting of the Harvein Society, Dr. Robert Maguire showed a case of chylous ascites, in a man aged forty-two, who had suffered from œdema of the feet twelve months before admission to the hospital, but this had subsided with rest in bed. Nine months later he was seized with sudden pain in the epigastrium, which, though less intense, lasted for five weeks. Two months later the abdomen began to enlarge. There was history of alcoholism, but not of syphilis, and the patient had never lived out of England. On admission there was general distension of the abdomen with fluid, enlargement of superficial veins and of spleen, but not of the liver. Two hundred and twenty ounces of milky fluid was removed by tapping. The fluid was slightly albuminous, contained a large amount of fat and peptones, and did not coagulate on standing. Fat globules, granular matter and leucocytes appeared under the microscope. In three weeks time, 218 oz. of similar fluid were removed; the fluid did not return, and there was then discovered prominence in the epigastrium with some increase in the liver dulness. Œdema of the legs still remained. Dr. Maguire diagnosed cirrhosis of the liver with some inflammatory material behind it, pressing upon the vena cava and the receptaculum chyli, causing rupture of the latter. It seemed very anomalous however, that lymph, which ordinarily flows under such very slight pressure, should, in these cases, accumulate to such an extent as to burst both the thoracic duct and the peritoneum. Dr. Ewart, commenting upon the case, believed that the collective force exercised by the muscular coats of the villi, might be sufficient to cause the rupture, although that exercised in each individual villus was very small.—*London Lancet, Jan. 1, 1887.*

DANGER IN CORROSIVE SUBLIMATE SOLUTIONS.— Concerning the large number of poisonings by the use of sublimate solutions, Lewin says : " The question is, ought this remedy to be employed in the treatment of wounded surfaces ? My answer is, no. I do not forget the great advantage which this remedy possesses as an antiseptic, but I hold that even one single fatal case occurring through its use outweighs a thousand healings by first intention through it. For the thousand cures could just as surely have been attained by an uninjurious remedy. Often enough the organism eliminates such a poison in many excretory ways, but we do not possess any criterion which will enable us to say beforehand whether, in any one individual, this will occur or not. So long as we do not know, if I may so express it, 'the personal toxic equation' of an individual, just so long we should not dare to place him in danger by a poison. I have often met the view that the washing out of a cavity or a wound is, as regards the absorption of the injected poisonous material, not analogous to the introduction of such poison into the stomach. In opposition to this view it may be shown that, although in the first mode a portion of the injected solution flows out, still, more readily yet than by the stomach, so much of the poison can be absorbed that a toxic state may follow. When only half a litre of sublimate solution of 1-1000 is injected into the uterus, it contains then half a gram, that is, five times as much as the maximal daily dosage. Even if 300 cc of this solution flows out, there remains for absorption still .2 gram, that is double the daily dosage by the stomach. Such a dose no one would dare to prescribe, either by the stomach or by the subcutaneous cellular tissue."—*Berlin. Klin. Wochens.*, No. 5, 1887.

SURGICAL MISHAPS—Reported by E. L. HUSSEY, F.R.C.S.E.—In 1861 a young lady applied to me with a small tumor behind the angle of the jaw on the right side. It was tough and almost cartilaginous under examination, and the skin was generally adherent over the surface. The case had been seen by the late Mr. Hester and Mr. Owen of Oxford, and by Sir H. Ackland. It was thought to be of a cystic nature, and the swelling had been injected with tincture of iodine. I cut through the substance in its whole thickness and endeavored to clear away the contents from each half; this could only be done to a very slight extent. The wound healed favorably. A second operation was undertaken some months afterwards. The skin was divided and separated without difficulty from the tumor. This now appeared to be about the size of a large walnut, and of a fibrocellular structure. I cut off the exposed part so as to clear the wound for a deeper dissection. Then forcing a hook in the remaining part, I endeavored to draw it forwards. This I was unable to do. The attachment was evidently very deep; the skull itself moved with the motions of the hook. I cut off, as deeply as I could, the part of the tumor which was transfixed by the hook, and closed the wound. This healed as favorably as after the former operation. The lady afterwards married, and she died from phthisis more than twenty years after the operation. There was not any fresh growth of the tumor. Being in communication with Mr. Caisor Hawkins at the time of the operation, I mentioned the case as a disagreeable piece of active surgery. He told me that Mr. Liston, in a similar case, found, upon the death of the patient, that the tumor had its origin in the base of the skull.—*London Lancet*, February 5th, 1887.

TUBERCULOSIS OF THE ŒSOPHAGUS.—At a recent meeting of the Medical Society of Vienna (*Progès. Méd.*, 1887, No. 6, Vienna Correspondence), Dr. Zemann, assistant to Professor Kundrat, read a paper on tuberculosis of the œsophagus, of which he distinguished four different forms. In the first the affection is propagated by direct extension from the bronchial glands or the lungs. In these cases the gullet may be perforated by direct ulceration, and frequently the contiguous portion of the trachea or bronchus is subsequently perforated; or the ulceration of the œsophagus may arise from tubercular deposit in its anterior wall. In the second variety the mucous membrane of the œsophagus is invaded by extension of tubercular disease of the pharynx or larynx, producing superficial ulcers, which are limited to the upper third. Instances were given of a still further propagation of the disease in the œsophagus of two patients who were suffering from strictures of the tube from corrosive poisoning. They were also the subjects of tubercular phthisis, and although the larynx and bronchial glands were free, yet caseous and yellow tubercles were found in the cicatricial tissue in the œsophagus. Bacilli were detected in these tubercles. The explanation evidently lies in the fact that ordinarily, from its thick epithelial lining, the œsophageal mucous membrane is protected from bacillary infection, and a protection which is destroyed by the action of corrosives. In both the cases it should be added, intestinal tubercle was present. The third variety is acute miliary tuberculosis, of which, however, only one case is on record, *viz.*, by Marotti. The fourth variety, also of great rarity, is infection of the œsophagus by sputum ; a condition probably only produced when the epithelium is more or less detached.—*London Lancet*, February 12th, 1887.

EXPULSION OF AN OVARY FROM THE RECTUM.—Tedford reports the following : Mrs. S., *æt.* 28, had three children and three miscarriages. By a mistake of symptoms, in November, 1885, a uterine sound was passed, without resistance, some four inches into the uterus, and on January 9th, 1886, a small fœtus was expelled. Considerable hæmorrhage occurred, but was checked in half an hour, and she rallied well. On January 14th, while seated upon the chamber, she was taken with tenesmus and a disposition to strain, and had severe pains in her abdomen. She could not resist the straining efforts until something was expelled through the anus. When seen she was lying on her side in bed, a red, cone-shaped tumor protruding from her anus. There was no hæmorrhage. The uterus was turned to the side and a little higher than natural. Examination per rectum showed the tumor to be attached to a pedicle which could be traced up to a rent in the bowel, through which it passed, as over a shelf. The tumor was a cystic ovary and was cut away after ligation of the pedicle. On the 17th a fluid tumor protruded and was in part removed, the remainder being replaced. The patient died and a *post mortem* examination showed that no omentum covered the bowels in front. The omentum was gathered into a mass on the left side near the crest of the ilum, and was greatly softened. The stump from which the left ovary had been cut had slipped out from the ligature into the pelvic cavity. The rectum and lower portion of the colon were firm to the touch, and intussusception was demonstrated. The ovary, covered by peritoneum, entered the bowel in the sigmoid flexure, and passed downward into the rectum, dragging the portion of bowel along the rent and opening again into the bowel below.—*Lond. Med. Rec.*, February 15th, 1887.

SULPHATE OF SPARTEIN.—Dr. Hans Voigt gives the results of his experiments made with *sulphate of spartein* in Nothnagel's clinic, as follows : 1. *Sulphate of spartein* acts in small doses as a stimulant to the heart, the contractions becoming greater in amplitude, the pulse fuller and higher, the arterial tension increased, and the pulse frequency generally lessened by some beats. 2. The action of the drug occurs quickly, in from three-quarters to one hour after taking, often continuing more than twenty-four hours, and during this time can be increased by a renewal of the dose. A cessation of the remedy for some days after it has been employed for several days is advantageous, as it then will act again more powerfully. It can be taken for a week daily without injury. 3. The rhythm of the heart's disturbed contraction is only restored in a few cases ; in severe disorders of the heart the feeble contractions become more extended, but not equally increased in strength. 4. The rate of respiration is at times increased, at times lessened, by the use of the remedy. 5. The renal secretion is frequently, corresponding to the increase in heart action, increased. 6. There often occurs a slight hypnotic effect. 7. Phenomena of intoxication, vertigo, headache, palpitation and nausea, occur only seldom. After its employment in small doses of from one to four milligrams, they were insignificant and transitory; if the remedy was repeated in spite of this, these phenomena disappeared. *Spartein* can properly be classed with infusion of *digitalis;* still its action appears to increase too rapidly, and is not permanent enough to be of service in severe compensatory disturbance; even through repeated doses the increase of the heart's action is not so continuous as under *digitalis.* It possesses a great advantage in its precise dosage and in its relative harmlessness; it is superior to the double combinations of *caffein, adonis vernalis* and *convallamarin.—Intern. Klin. Rundschau,* No. 1.

ANTISEPTICS IN MIDWIFERY.—Dr. Solovioff, of Moscow, reviews this subject in the *Proc. of the Moscow Physico-Medical Society,* Nos. 1 and 2, 1886, and concludes as follows: "1. In the very first place there stands the most careful disinfection of wards or rooms, of the practitioner, midwife, nursing staff, and instruments. The wearing apparel of the nursing staff should be disinfected by washing. Hands (especially under the nails) must be washed by means of a brush. The disinfection of linen, mattresses, etc., must be performed in stoves of a special construction (for instance, in Zlatovratsky's stove). 2. In the beginning of labor it is necessary to wash out the external genitals with a weak solution of corrosive sublimate, and during labor to make vaginal injections of the same solution every three hours. This rule should be insisted on, especially in lying-in-hospitals. 3. Intra-uterine irrigations are indicated in cases of retention of the placenta or fœtal membranes, as well as in cases of intra-uterine disease. 4. The following rules should be observed on irrigating with or injecting the sublimate solutions: (*a*) Not more than two litres of the fluid should be introduced at a time. (*b*) In disinfection for prophylactic purposes the passage of the fluid through the cavities should be as rapid as possible; in the cases of disease it should not last longer than three minutes. (*c*) After each irrigation the fluid should be removed from the vagina by pressing the perinæum backwards. When the womb is somewhat flabby the fluid retained should be pressed out of its cavity. (*d*) In uterine atony, anæmia, or renal disease, other disinfectants should be substituted for the sublimate. The same holds good in women who have never used mercurials. (*e*) Injections of corrosive sublimate should be performed by the practitioner himself; only in some exceptional cases being intrusted to an experienced nurse. (*f*) Only such irrigating apparatus should be used as gives an uninterrupted stream of fluid. (*g*) For prophylactic purposes a solution of corrosive sublimate, 1-5000 is sufficiently strong. In septic endometritis or pronounced infection, a 1-1000 solution may be used." The author quotes statistics to show the beneficial results of antiseptic irrigations, and gives his views as to the method of absorption in cases of poisoning.—*Lond. Med. Rec.,* February, 1887.

ACTION OF THE COMMON ALKALINE METALS AND EARTHS.—Dr. Curci says that:—Potassium, sodium, lithium, calcium, and magnesium form the three following pharmacological groups, according to their action in mammals. 1. The salts of potassium—muscular agents, at first stimulant, then paralyzing. 2. The salts of sodium and lithium—nerve agents, causing convulsions. 3. The salts of calcium and magnesium—paralyzing nerve agents. However, while they manifest these three principal types of action on the nervous and the muscular systems, they have an almost identical action on the heart and circulation. They all at first cause increase of the blood-pressure, with slowing and strengthening of the pulse, and then lowering of the blood-pressure, with quickening and weakening of the pulse, and finally paralysis of the heart. Dr. Curci finds that when the medulla oblongata, and therefore the vaso-motor centre, is destroyed, potassium, sodium, lithium and calcium produce increased blood-pressure, with slowing and strengthening of the pulse. Magnesium has no such effect. The first four, therefore, have a peripheral, magnesium a central, action. When the peripheral vaso-motor system is paralyzed by curare, sodium, calcium and magnesium do not increase the blood-pressure, or but very slightly; while potassium and lithium, as in the normal state, markedly increase the pressure and render the pulse slower and stronger. Sodium, magnesium and calcium, therefore, act on the peripheral vaso-motor nerves; while potassium and lithium act on the muscular fibre of the heart and blood ves-sels. Potassium in mammals acts more rapidly and energetically on the vessel and heart muscular fibre than on the voluntary striated fibre; but, speaking generally, it acts on all voluntary and involuntary mus-cles, while it has no direct or manifest action on the nervous system. In the Batrachiæ, on the contrary, potassium acts first on the nervous centres and then on the peripheral nerves; afterwards on the voluntary muscles, and, lastly, on the heart. This is probably due to the low temperature of the blood in batrachians. Curci finds that when frogs and toads are kept in hot water, until their temperature equals that of a mammal, potassium acts in the same way as in warm-blooded animals. In this experiment, many times repeated, the heart was ar-rested before the complete abolition of reflex and voluntary movement. The excitability of the myo-cardium is exhausted before that of the striated muscles. In batrachians, therefore, at a low temperature the nerve-tissue is more sensitive than the cardiac muscle to the action of potass; while at a high temperature this is reversed, and the heart be-comes more sensitive than the nerves, just as in mammals.—*London Medical Record*, October, 1886.

EXTIRPATION OF THE THYROID GLAND.—The dangerous result follow-ing the entire removal of the thyroid gland is now recognized by almost all surgeons. The earlier reports of the Swiss surgeons, Reverdin and Kocher, were quickly followed by reports from others substantiating the disastrous consequences of complete removal of the gland. The earlier experiments upon animals have been now collected and investigated because of the occurrence of the cachexia strumipriva. In the majority of these cases (in dogs) the animals did not survive, although exceptions to this were noted and results in opposition were obtained by some observers. Fuhr, of Giessen, has endeavored to clear up this confusion, and if his close analysis of facts is followed, his explanation will be seen to be in all probability correct. After reviewing the work of previous investigators, he considers the position and form of the thyroid in the dog, the animal upon which most of the experiments have been made, and then passes to the consideration of his own experiments. He removed from nine dogs the whole of the thyroid gland, and all except one died, with the typical nervous symptoms, by the 21st day, at latest, after the operation. Besides the nervous disturbance described by Schiff and others (tetanic rigidity, fibrillary contractions, tickling feeling), Fuhr also noted the frequent occurrence of purulent kerato-conjunctivitis. Through a further series of nine experiments he rejects the view that the severe phenomena following extirpation of the thyroid are caused by concomitant injuries during the operation, especially injury to the numerous nerves; as well as that which holds that the typical cachexia is due to destruction of the recurrent nerve, or to ligation of the thyroid artery. Incidentally to the latter he refuses to admit the regulation-theory of Schreger, Liebermeister and others that the thyroid gland serves as a regulating apparatus for the blood supply to the brain; for this theory is opposed to physiological experiment, to observations made upon man after removal of the gland, and is not in accord with the anatomical relations. Post-mortem section of a dog which survived total extirpation showed the existence of a small accessory thyroid amounting to about one-third of the whole mass. Following out these facts Fuhr found that a portion of the gland, amounting to at least one-third of the whole, was sufficient to keep the animal well, after removal of the remainder. If this residue was extirpated, no matter how long after the first operation, the animal died just as after total extirpation in the first place. The contradictory experiences of other experiments leads him to think that, through false anatomical ideas, other structures were removed and thus led to erroneous conclusions. He determined by microscopical examination that the gland removed by him as the thyroid was in reality that organ. He comes to this conclusion: The view that the so-called cachexia strumipriva of man depends upon the loss of the specific function of the thyroid gland, is more than probable. The disease does not attack all those from whom the gland has been removed, because very often a portion of the thyroid has been unintentionally allowed to remain, and so the patient has been protected from the cachexia. As a result of his studies he therefore condemns the total removal of the thyroid.—*Berlin Klin. Woch.*, *Jan. 10, 1887.*

NEWS.

APPOINTMENTS.—Hugh M. Smith, M.D., '76, and Edward Chapin, M.D., 78, have been appointed members of the Homœopathic Hospital staff, Brooklyn.

NEW HOSPITAL.—Still another new homœopathic hospital will be built this year. The good people of St. Paul have decided to put up one, have selected the site, and the erection of the building will be begun soon.

WOMEN'S COLLEGE.—The New York Medical College and Hospital for Women held its annual Commencement Exercises in Association Hall, Tuesday evening, April 19th. The hall was well filled with friends of the institution, and everything passed off in a most pleasant manner.

PHTHISIS.—In Great Britain one-fourth of all deaths are due to pulmonary consumption; in Paris, one-fifth; in Vienna, one-sixth. In our own country, as Dr. Edmund Andrews has pointed out, the disease diminishes as we recede from the sea. For instance, the deaths in Massachusetts are twenty-five per cent.; New York, twenty per cent.; Ohio, sixteen per cent.; Indiana, fourteen per cent.; Illinois, eleven per cent.; Missouri, nine per cent.; Kansas, eight per cent.; Colorado, the same; Utah, six per cent.; while on the Pacific Slope it again advances to fourteen per cent.—*Dr. Gilman, in Clinique.*

CHICAGO ALUMNI.—The annual meeting of the Chicago Homœopathic Medical College was held at the Grand Pacific Hotel, Chicago, February 23d, 1887. The following officers were elected for the ensuing year: President, W. F. Knoll, M.D., of Chicago; Vice-president, H. W. Danforth, M.D., of Milwaukee; Secretary, W. M. Stearns, M.D., Chicago; Treasurer, S. N. Schneider, M.D., Chicago. The Executive Board has in preparation a series of meetings for next fall and winter, when papers will be presented for discussion and addresses given by prominent men in the profession. W. M. STEARNS, M.D., Secretary.

318 *News.*

OPHTHALMIC HOSPITAL COLLEGE.—The annual Commencement Exercises of the College of the New York Ophthalmic Hospital were held on Tuesday evening, April 12th, in the Hospital building, Twenty-third Street and Third Avenue. Thomas C. Smith, President of the Board of Trustees, presided, and made the annual address. Dr. Henry C. Houghton, Dean of the Faculty, made an entertaining and suggestive speech. The address to the graduates was given by the Rev. Dr. McChesney. Five men received the degree of "Oculi et Auris Chirurgus," and three had conferred upon them "Certificates in Laryngology." At the conclusion of the Commencement Exercises lunch was served and the floor was cleared for dancing. The institution is in a prosperous condition.

HAHNEMANNIAN SOCIETY.—One of the most enjoyable events in the year to the students of the New York Homœopathic Medical College is the annual meeting of the Hahnemannian Society. An interested audience gathered at Association Hall, Wednesday evening, April 13th, to listen to the exercises of the society. An admirable quartette furnished music for the evening. The annual address to the society was delivered by Rev. T. S. Hasting, D.D. It is a great pity that all speeches on such occasions are not like Dr. Hasting's. There was nothing stale, flat or unprofitable about it; but, on the contrary, it was such a judicious mingling of wit and wisdom that the auditors regretted its brevity. The Class Poem was by Ralph Jenkins, M.D.; the Prognosis, by A. I. Thayer, M.D., and the "Send Off" to '87, by J. M. Woodruff, '88. The occasion was a most pleasant one and reflected great credit on the society and its officers.

THE GREAT PHYSICIANS AND THE APOTHECARY—A STORY WITH A MORAL ABOUT CONSULTANTS.*—Once upon a time a certain apothecary was called to attend a man who was sick of the fever and lay grievously ill and like to die. Now, it came to pass that the friends of this man, who loved and cherished him, were much desirous of having the benefit of an older and more experienced physician, who should say whether or no this man could be so treated as to recover, inasmuch as his apothecary thought him like to die. So this great physician came, and behold he talked learnedly and doctorally with the man's friends, and said: "Lo, this man is sore ill and I fear me for him; but verily, I will do all I can for him and watch over him." So this physician and this apothecary visited this man twice in the day, yea, and even oftener. But the apothecary waxed wroth and said to himself: "Lo, I have called upon this physician and he came, but now he goeth not away." So he consulted with the man's friends and they agreed that another great physician should be summoned to the sick man's bedside; albeit the apothecary who was a cunning man, thought by this means to get rid of the first physician, whose company he loved not. But, behold how a man may be deceived. This second great physician did even as the first, and now the two physicians and the apothecary waited on the sick man in the forenoon and again in the evening. And now the apothecary was sore vexed, and he cursed the day on which he was born, and he said in the bitterness of his heart: "I will arise and call on the very prince of physicians, for he is so great that he will surely send the other physicians away and leave me with the patient whom I am no longer able to advise! and in this wise I shall not lose my patient, neither shall I be sore angered as to heretofore." So he went thither and called him, and the prince of physicians came in a chariot drawn by two fiery steeds, and he pleased the friends of the sick man, and they said: "Verily, we are pleased with this great physician,"

* Founded on an actual occurrence in recent London practice.

and they told the apothecary, "Behold now, that this great physician comes, so have we no more need that you should quit your other sick people to see this man ! so prithee return unto thy house, lest you be wanted elsewhere." So this poor apothecary went his way—not rejoicing— and he told his wretched plight unto sundry of his brother apothecaries, who loved not the actions of these physicians, albeit great men of their day, and there was much bad language said on that day.—(*Hospital Gazette and Student Journal.*)

THE ALUMNI BANQUET.—One of the most successful dinners ever given by the Alumni Association of the New York Homœopathic Medical College was given on the evening of Commencement, at Delmonico's, April 14th, 1887. Early in the evening, the rapidly increasing numbers insured a large attendance, and when, at 8.30, the gavel of Pres. Norton called the assembly to order, the large parlors and anti-rooms were well filled. In the business meeting of the association more than usual interest was manifested by the members. It was decided that hereafter the executive committee shall prepare two tickets, each containing nominations for all the offices to be filled by the association at its annual meeting, and forward the same to each alumnus three months before such meeting. Drs. Fiske and Moffat, of Brooklyn, were appointed a special committee to take charge of the Alumni Lecture for the ensuing year. The election of officers resulted as follows: President, Dr. F. B. Mandeville, of Newark; Vice-Presidents, Dr. J. Lester Keep, Brooklyn, Dr. P. H. Mason, Peekskill, and Dr. L. P. Jones, Greenwich; Corresponding Secretary, Dr. S. H. Vehslage; Record-ing Secretary, Dr. Charles McDowell; Treasurer, Dr. Eugene H. Porter; Necrologist, Dr. Martin Deschere; Executive Committee, Drs. E. V. Moffat, A. B. Norton, W. W. Blackman, S. W. Clark, E. J. Pratt, and G. E. Tytler. At the adjournment of the business meeting, the association marched into the large dining-room, and there enjoyed literally a feast of good things. Music by an excellent orchestra enlivened the gastronomic proceedings, and for a time every doctor paid strict attention to that which appeared immediately before him. When the cigars appeared, Dr. George S. Norton, the retiring president arose, and in a graceful speech introduced the toast-master of the evening, Dr. Selden H. Talcott. As a toast-master, Dr. Talcott was an unqualified success. His impressive orotund delivery was em-phasized by the serenity of demeanor so characteristic of the man. The first toast of the evening, "Samuel Hahnemann," was drunk in silence and standing. Dr. Fiske responded to the "Alumni Association." Mr. Elihu Root, in responding to the "Law," made a most witty and entertain-ing speech and "brought down" the house many times. Rev. Dr. MacArthur made perhaps the most eloquent speech of the evening, in response to the toast "The Clergy." "The Ladies" were kindly and feel-ingly remembered by Dr. F. S. Fulton. "Our Boys" were portrayed by Dr. J. B. Dowling, and the "Class of '87" was extolled by Dr. B. W. Stillwell. Other speakers were, R. P. Flower, Dr. F. B. Mandeville, and Prof. Allen who responded to "The College." Dr. W. Tod Helmuth recited an original poem which delighted his auditors. Dr. Allen in his remarks gave a sketch of the college from the time of its founding more than a quarter of a century ago. He related its successes and discouragements, its trials and difficulties, and coming to the present time told of the effort making to raise a fund to put the college upon a firm and enduring foundation. He appealed to the alumni to help their alma mater in her hour of need. Several subscription papers were circulated among the alumni, and a little later it was announced that the amount raised by the association was nearly $10,000. Dr. Norton then introduced the incoming president, Dr. Mande-ville in an eloquent speech and shortly afterwards adjournment was had.

COMMENCEMENT EXERCISES.—Chickering Hall was filled to overflowing on the afternoon of April 14th, by a large and friendly audience assembled to listen to the Annual Commencement Exercises of the New York Homœopathic Medical College. On the stage, which was lined with flowers, were seated the faculty of the college, and distinguished invited guests. Among those present were Judge Cowing, R. P. Flower, George M. Clark, John T. Marshall, the Rev. D. Parker Morgan, and other prominent citizens. Salem H. Wales, President of the Board of Trustees presided. The members of the graduating class, forty-six in number occupied seats in the auditorium. The programme for the afternoon was a pleasing one. A glance at it told that there were no long orations to be delivered, no tedious speeches to be listened to. It was brief but effective. After prayer by Dr. Morgan, Mr. Wales introduced Dr. T. F. Allen, Dean of the college, who delivered the principal address. It has for some time been known that the trustees and friends of the college have been earnestly endeavoring to raise funds for a new college building and hospital. When Dr. Allen in his remarks referred to this effort he was listened to with the utmost attention and interest. He said in part : "The past year has been signalized by the erection and complete endowment by Mr. and Mrs. F. H. Delano, of the Laura Franklin Free Hospital for children, which has been placed in the charge of physicians and surgeons skilled in the practice of homœopathy. Our students are permitted to witness operations and study diseases in its wards, and although distant from the college and limited in its sphere is still a great help to us. The need of a free hospital in which medical students may witness the best methods of applying medicines for the cure of disease and of performing operations is sorely felt by the trustees and faculty of this college. Several years ago this faculty and their friends succeeded, chiefly by means of a large fair, in starting a surgical hospital, in which clinical instruction could be given. That institution was afterwards united with the Hahnemann Hospital of this city ; but recently the trustees of that institution have expressed their opinion that the interests of their hospital will not be advanced by the admission of medical students. We are therefore compelled to establish a new hospital and the faculty and their friends, knowing that homœopathy will be banished from the State should the college be obliged to close its doors, and knowing that to properly educate students we must have a free hospital for clinical instruction, are making a strong and united effort to obtain funds to erect and maintain. new college and hospital buildings. We have met with most encouraging success ; already two of our wealthy and large-hearted citizens have subscribed each $25,000, and similar subscriptions are confidently expected." Many other subscriptions have been secured and there is no doubt but that the full amount necessary will be obtained. The diplomas were then conferred upon the graduates by Mr. Wales. Dr. St. Clair Smith, President of the Faculty, awarded the Faculty prizes to the successful contestants. The first prize, a microscope valued at $100, was given to Edward D. Fitch, for general excellence throughout the three years' course. James Crook, Jr., received the second prize, a similar instrument, valued at $50. The Wales prize, a Helmuth pocket case of instruments, was given to F. W. Hamblin, by Dr. Helmuth. The honor men of the class were Benjamin W. Stillwell, John J. Russell, Walter W. Johnson, Samuel L. Jacobus and Russell P. Fay. The class valedictory, delivered by George B. Best, of Chatham, N. Y., was well composed and effectively delivered.

VOL. XXXV.   *JUNE, 1887.*   (Volume II, Third Series.)   No. 6.

NORTH AMERICAN
JOURNAL OF HOMŒOPATHY.

ORIGINAL ARTICLES IN MEDICINE.

OUTLINES OF A SYSTEMATIC STUDY OF THE MATERIA MEDICA.

By T. F. ALLEN, M.D.,
New York.

INTRODUCTION.— *Vascular Group.*

A THOROUGHLY practical and comprehensive course of study of materia medica is difficult to inaugurate and follow, partly because of the great number of books of reference required, partly on account of the time which one is rarely able or willing to devote to it, but more frequently on account of a lack of system in the work. The attempt to study isolated drugs with no attempt to group or classify under very general effects is like trying to study Botany by learning one plant at a time. He who would study Botany well, and take real pleasure in it, must master the characters of whole families and orders of plants, and either group the individuals or individualize his groups, always retaining in mind at least general characters for large groups and one or two peculiarities for individuals. This method I have found best for students in materia medica and shall attempt, in a series of articles, to follow it more or less closely. I shall attempt to form groups by first studying individuals, and shall begin with the simplest and most easily understood drugs. Before entering upon the study, however, a few words may be said concerning methods of work and books required. The first thing to be learned about any drug is its *absolute* effects—those which always follow large doses. To ascertain these we require works on Toxicology and all sorts of books and periodicals which furnish us experiments with large doses upon men (and also on animals). From these we obtain data which enable us to classify drugs by their pathognomonic affinities and lead to a very general and sometimes useful notion of their therapeutic properties. Having acquired information of this sort we must then seek out the individual peculiarities of the drug, and in order to do this we must examine experiments made with smaller doses, or watch the symptoms as they appear in one who has suffered from the more violent effects which have, in a measure, disappeared. Very little is, as a rule, gained by the systematic perusal of provings with small doses, even when they are presented in a narrative form; such symptoms appear in a very irregular fashion as compared with the natural sequence of effects of large doses. The individual peculiarities are found best (as a rule) by massing the symptoms in a schema and noting the frequent recurrence of symptoms and conditions under the various rubrics. But however found, the individual peculiarities are all-important and must never be overlooked. While one cannot prescribe rapidly and well for the sick *without* a schema (Hahnemannian), one cannot study the materia medica systematically or satisfactorily *with* a schema; and hence I advise the student to obtain first, the Cyclopedia now being issued by Drs. Hughes and Dake; secondly, some allopathic books which give the general physiological action of drugs, and lastly, Guernsey's characteristics; with these three one may begin. The very complex character of most drugs obtained from the vegetable kingdom makes it advisable to postpone their study to a later date, and take up first a substance, simple in its action and thoroughly understood, namely, AMYL NITRITE.

Amyl nitrite, obtained by heating fusel oil with nitric acid, produces, when its vapor is inhaled, flushing of the face, head and upper part of the body, with pulsating blood-vessels, rapid breathing and rapid action of the heart. These symptoms are due to a dilatation of the arterioles, caused by a temporary paralysis of the vaso-motor ganglia in the walls of these vessels. Sugar may also appear in the urine. The effects of the drug are usually quite transient, but in some cases the blood-vessels seem to be weakened for a long time. In my own case, for fully two years after experimenting with the drug, my heart was accustomed to beat violently on slight provocation, and, indeed, I was obliged to abandon entirely the use of tea on account of the palpitation which it caused, after proving *amyl nitrite*. These effects of this drug are absolute, and, so far as I am aware, there are no contingent symptoms characteristic of it. It may be noted that the external capillaries are chiefly affected, and that the dilatation is mostly confined to the upper part of the body; also, that the mental faculties are not impaired, but the effects are, like its therapeutic application, very general in character. Its therapeutics have been mostly physiological, that is, to produce in a patient the full physiological effect of the drug in order to relieve temporarily some (opposite) condition; for example, to dilate the capillaries and relieve the heart in angina pectoris, to relax spasm of capillaries in threatening epileptic convulsions. It does, however, (sometimes) cure permanently, according to the law of similars, the tendency to flushes, of women, at the menopause, and one case of Basedow's disease was permanently cured by it. In all these cases, however, there were no definite characteristics to guide the selection, and the prescription was made either because of the failure of other remedies, or on account of the lack of indications for other drugs.

The drug to be studied next is one most closely related to *amyl nitrite* both chemically and pathognomonically, namely, *nitro-glycerine* (glonoine of Hering). This substance (a glycerine in which three atoms of hydrogen are replaced by three molecules of nitrous acid) produces effects wonderfully similar to those of *amyl nitrite.* A minute quantity injected under the skin, rubbed on the skin, or touched to the tongue or lips, gives rise to the most intense flushing of the head and face, with terrible hammering in the head, synchronous with the pulse. This dilatation of the blood-vessels is not only superficial, but deep-seated, as shown by the ophthalmoscope, and the effects of the drug persist much longer than those of *amyl nitrite.* A perusal of the various provings will show that a most violent pulsating headache is produced by an almost infinitesimal quantity of the drug; that the headaches tend to rise up from the spine to the top and sides of the head; that they are particularly severe in the temples, and are generally aggravated by shaking the head. These head symptoms may be associated with nausea, with heaviness, and even numbness in the extremities, with palpitation, dyspnœa, and may be followed by neuralgias of a pulsating character. Our clinical experience with *glonoine* shows its usefulness to be confined to conditions associated with vaso-motor paresis, *characterised by a sensation of throbbing;* thus it is found extremely useful in the after-effects of sunstroke, the effects of suppressed menses, after-effects of shock, always with the peculiarity mentioned.

By the persistent sensation of pulsation *glonoine* may be distinguished from all the other members of the general group to which it belongs; indeed this persistent throbbing has determined its successful administration in neuralgias affecting remote portions of the body.

To these substances may be added, for the purpose of rounding out our group of substances which dilate peripheral arterioles, *ethyl nitrite, sodium nitrite, potassium nitrite,* and, indeed, many compounds of nitrous acid which seems to be the active agent in all these compounds. Workmen suffer, when making *sweet spirits of nitre* (ethyl nitrite, nitrous ether), from symptoms similar to those of *amyl nitrite;* and when taken internally in small doses, it causes flushing of the face, fullness of the head (like nitrite of soda), and also marked diuresis. These symptoms are often followed by perspiration and a fall of temperature, hence its former reputation as a refrigerant in fever. All these effects are transient and leave no permanent results. Even when used as a diuretic, it must be given frequently in small doses to secure the desired result. Lembke's provings show clearly the characteristic flushing heat of the face, rising from below upward (like *amyl nitrite*), followed by inclination to perspire. They also show increased secretion of urine, the rapid action of the heart, especially on making any effort, and general prostration.

The pains of all sorts in every possible part of the body are noted by Lembke in these, as in almost all his numerous provings, and are not to be ascribed to the drug taken. Doubtless this painstaking and conscientious prover experienced "barings," "stickings," "tensions" and "drawings" in bone and muscle, both while proving a drug and when in ordinary health.

At this point the student has two courses open to pursue :

1. Examine the alcohol series, beginning with the compounds of the monad radicals, *methyl alcohol* (wood spirit, found in wintergreen oil in combination with salicylic acid) ; *ethyl alcohol* (spirits of wine) and *ethyl oxide* (our common sulphuric ether); *amyl alcohol* (fusel oil) and follow with the dyad radicals, *oxalyl, lactyl, etc.*, bases of the organic acids up to uric acid ; and finally the triad, alcohol glycerine. After a review of what is known of the physiological peculiarities of these different substances (elementary), the student may take up the other ingredient of the three drugs considered in this first lesson, and examine the nitric acid series beginning with *nitrous oxide* (laughing gas) and running through the series up to nitric acid, noting the differences due to the varying amounts of oxygen, producing as we ascend the series greater stability in the compound and more lasting and different results. This course opens up an extremely interesting field of comparative study, but it will not prove so interesting to the general reader, and perhaps not so immediately practical as another method.

2. Examine and group all the drugs in the materia medica which show a predominating action on the *circulation* without producing marked organic disease (except so far as such disease prove secondary to the vascular disturbance), and without febrile reaction. It is possible to separate, in a measure, drugs which cause disturbance of

the circulation merely, from those which produce marked fever, though the vascular and febrile groups will certainly merge into each other.

Our "vascular" group will be easily and clearly subdivided into those drugs which effect chiefly the heart and those which effect the peripheral circulation, and these may again be variously subdivided. In this sort of work the best text book to follow seems to be Lauder Brunton.

At this point we must again call a halt, for it is not expedient nor practical to subdivide our groups too closely and go too minutely into the theory of drug-action as is done by Brunton and others, though every particle of information to be obtained from them is useful, and had we time (as some of our students have) we should carry out the scheme fully in this direction ; we propose, therefore, to seek sub-stances which possess a general pathogenetic similarity to *amyl nitrite* and *glonoine*, and whose effects are mostly shown upon the peripheral circulation, and in a manner similar to these drugs, namely, *arteriole dilatation.* This dilatation may, as we know, be produced by two different causes, direct stimulation of the heart or by direct paralyses of the arterioles, but the symptoms vary so widely that it will not be difficult to construct a distinctively vascular group (as contrasted with a cardiac group). Two marked examples of our group have been examined, namely, *amyl nitrite* and *glonoine*, to these we will add in general the acids, the nitrous compounds, all the alcohols, ethers and aldehydes, and a few other substances. We will omit the study of the alcohols, ethers and aldehydes, and proceed directly to the examination of the other members of our series.

(To be continued.)

THE FALLACIES OF POPULAR BACTERIAL RESEARCH.

By GEORGE W. LEWIS, Jr., A.M., M.D.,
Buffalo, N. Y.

I VENTURE to say that every science has suffered more or less in its earlier development from the unprincipled and unguarded asser-tions of a certain well-defined class of men, whose only prompter is an insatiate desire for notoriety, and whose only qualification that attracts attention to their sweeping statements is an established position in some other calling. I don't know that I should say "suffered from such assertions;" rather, perhaps, should it be benefited from them, for later on it is these very statements, far-reaching and groundless as they are, that serve, by their contrast, to strengthen and to disseminate the underlying principles of that science. It suffers only through the delay caused by the heaping on of so much trash, and the consequent sifting that is rendered necessary.

The striking features, however, of these so-called "new discoveries" and empty criticisms are (1) that they are not advanced, as a rule, until their supporters realize that the subject has assumed enough importance to warrant the attraction of popular attention to their statements, and (2) that the promulgators of the class of work to which I refer are as profoundly ignorant of their subject as the most superficial knowledge of it can well make them. I take it that Pope's expression, "a little knowledge is a dangerous thing," was meant particularly for this class of individuals. Nevertheless we all know that the more reckless and sweeping the assertion, the more certain is it to attract wide-spread attention, and this is the only object its maker desires. It matters little to most of them how soon it is disproved, so long as timely notice is taken of it. It may be taken as a well-based induction that the more careful the investigator, and the more complete his mastery over the endless practical difficulties which surround experimentation on his subject, the more certain are his experiments to give a guarded result, while extravagant and unfounded assertions are no less sure to crown the efforts of the unskilled.

These general remarks are intended as a preface to the subject in hand, for I don't believe that any science has ever suffered more for the cause of notoriety than has Bacteriology. The reason for this seems to lie largely in the fact that the science is being developed under very peculiar circumstances. In the first place, it is one of the few technical sciences in which the great mass of people takes deep interest. It is easy, therefore, for those possessed of only a superficial knowledge to play upon the popular mind. If no more harm were done there would be little cause for writing. But taking advantage of the combined deep interest, yet profound ignorance, of the masses, there has sprung up a vast number of self-styled discoverers, whose efforts, instituted solely for advertising purposes, bring little less than ridicule upon the Germ Theory of Disease. Private laboratories, fitted up with costly apparatus, are made to stand for extensive experimental research on the part of the owners, and in their own immediate circles, at least, no opportunity is lost to impress others with the idea that they are more or less closely identified with the onward progress of the science. Another cause that undoubtedly militates against the speedy uprootal of this sort of charlatanism is the impetus given it by the outbreak of an epidemic. Here a deal of notoriety is gained at the expense of popular fear.

Scarce, indeed, are the issues of even our most representative medical journals, in which more or less space is not given up to " new discoveries " in Bacteriology, always, of course, associating the name of Dr. So-and-So as the discoverer. Occasionally a few unimportant details, relative to the peculiar circumstances under which the discovery was made, and calculated solely to enlist the popular mind, are given. Very seldom is mention made of culture or inoculation experiments, but great stress is always laid upon the microscopic appearances of the organism, and the easy or difficult manner in which it takes the stain, and perhaps other comparatively worthless data. More often, however, we are simply informed that the discovery has been made, and, unfortified by details that would assist subsequent observers in confirming the experiments, all else is left as the work of a prolific imagination.

Now and then the monotony of " new discovery " trash (this word in lieu of a better one) is varied by a vigorous and wordy attack upon some demonstrated and generally accepted organism. It seems unnecessary to add that the success or failure of such attacks, depends largely, so far as the desired notoriety is concerned, upon the ability of the ones who make them to replace the blighted (?) remains of the old theory, with a new discovery. Sometimes the devices resorted to and the claims made are, to say the least, unique.

A fair sample of the indefiniteness which invariably characterizes such work is seen in the following, which appeared in the editorial columns of the New York *Medical Record* of February 26th, 1887, and upon which the editor passed a very just criticism. The article has reference to the report of the Cholera Commission despatched to Spain last year by the combined action of the Royal Society, the University of Cambridge, and the Association for the Promotion of Scientific Research. The commission consisted of Drs. Roy, Graham, Brown and Sherrington, and a review of their report is thus given in the journal named:

" Twenty-five typical cases of cholera were examined, either immediately, or at a short interval after death, with the result that Koch's Comma Bacillus was not discovered in the intestinal canal in all cases. In some this microbe was present in great abundance, in others it was far less conspicuous, while in many undoubted cases, where death occurred before the reaction stage set in, it could not be detected at all. These observations were confirmed by the result of plate cultivations in gelatine and agar-agar. Moreover, it was found that, when present, the Comma Bacilli were collected either on the surface of the mucosa, or so close to it as to suggest a penetration of the epithelium after death; but in the majority, the organism could not be found in the mucous membrane or in any of the tissues or organs. These results, which are directly·opposed to Koch's, are considered to be conclusive against the Bacillus having a pathogenetic relation to the disease, but it is suggested to be the cause of the premonitory diarrhœa, which is held, not to be a mild attack of Asiatic cholera, but only a predisposing condition. Having satisfied themselves that the Comma Bacillus is not the cause of cholera, these investigators similarly dismiss the claims of Emmerich's straight Bacillus to that distinction, and also state that they were unable to recognize Klein's straight Bacillus in any of their preparations."

I have also read a copy of the original report and the above is as concise a review of it as can be given.   Here we have a good illustration of the broad assertion, unsustained by reliable evidence, to which I have referred in the first part of this paper. The report is based upon an examination of only twenty-five cases. Compare this with Koch's three years of uninterrupted study in cholera-infected localities, before a single utterance was given to the world. The commission is frank to acknowledge that its report is somewhat premature, further investigation being needed, especially in the line of artificial cultivation. Its hasty dismissal of Koch's theory is unwarranted and savors strongly of English prejudice. Its reasoning, too, shows a lack of familiarity with Koch's views. Now listen to the indefinite character of what might naturally be expected to follow. " After much research another fungus was discovered which is believed to be pathogenetic. It consists of granular masses and a delicate mycelium which could not be stained without difficulty, and which was pronounced by Messrs. Vine and Gardiner to belong to the Crytridiaceæ, a class which includes many rapidly-growing and virulent parasites of vegetables. The difficulties of its detection may have led to its being overlooked by former observers; while the objection of possible after-contamination is met and refuted."

The criticism offered by the editor is as follows :   " It is, we venture to say, highly improbable that the researches above described will have much weight against the long-continued and careful observations of a trained mycologist like Koch."

The societies represented by these four men are the leading organizations of Great Britain in scientific investigation, but I doubt if much reliance is placed by them in the report of this commission. Their proceedings are usually both definite and trustworthy, but here both characteristics are lacking. Is there a single sentence in the whole report that conveys the slightest clew to assist subsequent observers in confirming their views ?   Not one that I can detect. They say the new fungus consists of granular masses and a delicate mycelium which cannot be stained without difficulty. They even go so far as to classify the new fungus. Now, what fungus, pray, does not consist of granular masses, and a more or less delicate mycelium? These are the two known characteristics of all fungi. With regard to the difficult staining I shall have occasion later, in speaking of the tubercle organism, to refer to its unreliability as a primary factor in diagnosis. It is valuable only as a confirmatory measure. Moreover, it is not by any means a constant quality in the same organism. Subject, for example, several cultures of a given bacterium to different conditions of temperature and nourishment, each one maintained at the same throughout its growth, and you will be sure to notice degrees of stain-taking. This is perhaps less noticeable in the Tubercle Bacillus on account of its limits of temperature being more closely defined.

The position which Bacteriology occupies to-day in its relation to health and disease has been gained solely through perfected methods of studying minutely the life histories of the various organisms known to us, and yet, the implicit confidence which is placed by many in microscopic appearances as a basis of diagnosis in bacterial affections clearly indicates the utter unreliability of a large proportion of the work done in this field. For the purpose of ascertaining beyond all doubt whether a micro-organism is actually the "*causa causans*" of a disease, Koch has laid down the following postulates, which are strictly adhered to by all careful workers :—(a) The micro-organism must be found in the blood, lymph or diseased tissues of man, or animal, suffering from, or dead of the disease. (b) The micro-organisms must be islolated from the blood, lymph or tissues, and cultivated in suitable media outside of the animal body. These pure cultivations must be carried on through successive generations of the organism. (c) A pure cultivation thus obtained, must, when introduced into the body of a healthy animal, produce the disease in question. (d) Lastly, in the inoculated animal the same micro-organism must again be found. These steps naturally suggest a sequence in the various processes which must be adopted in a practical study of micro-organisms associated with disease.

Notwithstanding the axiomatic character of these postulates, and, in reality, the short time required for the execution of the necessary steps in each, we are every now and then led to believe from articles in our own journals that more speedy, and quite as trustworthy, diagnoses can be made from microscopic examinations of the discharges peculiar to the diseases in question. This is particularly the case with Tuberculosis. The methods of treating the sputum previous to the examination are both varied and numerous, each having its devotees; but they all unite in a dependence upon difficult stain-taking as the one strong point in the diagnosis. Biedert, whose plan, as given in the *Medical Record* of March 19th, is perhaps the latest, claims that the smallest number of bacilli, if present, can be detected. The essential features of his method are as follows : A tablespoonful of the suspected sputa is added to twice that quantity of water, and fifteen drops of a strong solution of soda. This mixture is boiled until it becomes quite fluid, and then diluted with about two ounces more of water. After being again boiled the mixture is nearly homogeneous and free from lumps and particles. If, on cooling, a thin fluid does not result, more water may be added. A conical vessel now receives the mixture, and after two or three days the supernatant fluid, having deposited its bacilli, can be decanted. The sediment, after energetic stirring, can now be examined in the ordinary manner. This method is open to additional objection on account of the dangers of after-contamination.

From the comparatively healthy mouth there have been isolated various micro-organisms that, so far as known, have no pathological significance. Any uncleanly condition, arising from laxity in the use of the brush or toothpick, whereby animal and vegetable matters are exposed to the process of decomposition, greatly increases the number and character of these organized bodies. The saliva, too, teems with living creatures, which, like the above, under the microscope, bear a close resemblance to each other. How then, I ask, can a trustworthy diagnosis be made from microscopic examinations of sputum, which contains, besides the possible Tubercle Bacilli, numerous other bacteria of like form and appearance? It will, no doubt be claimed that a sufficient distinction can be arrived at through the staining peculiarities of the tubercle organism. Here, however, I would say that at least two of the non-pathogenic forms from the human mouth (Weinhawer's Bacillus and Babe's Bacillus) with which the writer is acquainted, can only be stained successfully by adopting some one of the methods recommended for the Tubercle Bacillus. In fact, several of the species found in the mouth were not discovered till late, on account of the difficulties experienced in staining them. Reference has been made, moreover, to the inconstancy of this quality of stain-taking, owing to the influence of different conditions of temperature and nourishment upon their organization. If the Tubercle Bacillus possessed distinctive microscopic characteristics like the Anthrax Bacillus, for example, there would be cause for placing some reliance in its appearance, but unfortunately it has no characteristic under the microscope that is not shared equally by other bacteria the field of vision.

If the discovery of the Tubercle Bacillus is to have any real value from a therapeutic standpoint, it is essential that it be detected in the incipient stage of the disease. To do this requires not only a very exact primary method, but all the available checks that can possibly be interposed in the various steps necessary for its confirmation. The one respect in which all micro-organisms differ is their manner of growth. Here, then, is manifestly the starting point from which every reliable diagnosis of bacterial disease must proceed. Other measures of whatsoever sort are to be regarded as subservient to this, and to be of value only so far as they confirm the steps already taken.

Before closing this paper I wish to speak of the importance of maintaining an even temperature throughout the growth of the organism. It is a feature in bacterial study too often neglected, and one which, if allowed to pass unheeded through successive generations, is certain to result in more or less pronounced modifications as regards structure and development. It is a question, too, whether intentional neglect in this respect will not, in time, check, or even destroy permanently, the pathogenetic tendencies of many of the bacteria. Every organized body has its normal limits of temperature, beyond which it cannot pass without suffering. It is a factor in their well-being next in importance to suitable nourishment. There is little doubt that these unicellular bodies are quite as sensitive to changes in temperature as are the most complicated and highly developed of the vegetable kingdom.

HODGKIN'S DISEASE.*

By EDGAR V. MOFFAT, A.M., M.D.,

New York.

LAST summer, while in care of another physician's practice, I was so fortunate as to have charge of a case of Hodgkin's disease; and as it is rather an unusual opportunity for the general practitioner, I venture to make it an excuse for presenting the subject to you this evening.

I could only gather a fragmentary history of the case, for certain features in the course of the disease had passed unnoticed. I only saw it for a short time, almost at its worst, and have recently learned that three months thereafter the patient died; but I do not know the

* Read before the Homœopathic Medical Society, County of New York, April 21st 1887.

mode of death or the condition immediately preceding. Still, there are interesting and practical lessons to be learned from those few weeks' observations.

Another case at present under my care differs so widely from the first, that instead of detailing these histories, I will give a brief general description of the disease, which will enable us to see more clearly the interesting features of our cases.

Though certain general features of this disease were known long ago and mentioned by several authors, Dr. Hodgkin, of Guy's Hospital, London, gave its first general clinical history in 1832. At the suggestion of Dr. Wilks, in 1878, it was called and has since been very commonly known as *Hodgkin's Disease.*

But among better and descriptive names we have Progressive Glandular Hypertrophy; Adénie (by Trousseau); Adenia, or Adenosis; Lymphadénie (Ranvier), or Lymphadenoma or Lymphadenosis; Lymphatic Anæmia (Wilks); Pseudoleukæmia (Wunderlich); Malignant Lymphoma (Billroth); Lymphosarcoma (Virchow), etc.

Of all these terms, Lymphadenosis seems the most applicable, as showing the general tendency to growths of the lymphatic glands.

Nothing whatever is definitely known regarding its cause. It is not hereditary, and males are much more frequently affected than females.

The disease may be defined as a more or less general enlargement of the *lymphatic glands*, with later developments of progressive anæmia. Remember, never *true* glands, only adenoid tissue, is affected.

From an unknown cause certain lymphatic glands, generally the cervical, first become enlarged, with, however, no pain or visible impairment of health, unless from pressure or other mechanical cause. The area of infected glands increases generally very slowly, involving any or all of the axillary, inguinal, bronchial, mesenteric, retroperitoneal, those of the anterior or posterior mediastinum, etc. Curiously, the mesenteric and inguinal glands are less prone to enlargement than almost any others. Wherever we have a normal presence of adenoid tissue, as in mucous membrane, liver, kidney, stomach, intestines, etc., the same hyperplasia may be seen. The spleen becomes affected, generally enlarged, with disease of the malpighian follicles. When this appears, we have anæmia established. If the spleen pulp be hypertrophied and the malpighian follicles are mostly affected, as is generally the case, there will be no increase of white corpuscles in the blood, but anæmia, with diminished number of the red.

Anatomically, we find two varieties of enlarged glands, the *hard* and the *soft*, though clinically the distinction is unimportant, as the course of the disease is about the same in each case, and we may find both varieties or transition stages in one patient, or the same gland may at different times show both formations. The enlargement is first seen in a single gland; this soon extends to others of the group till they may each become as large as a hen's egg, forming a continuous matted lobular tumor; generally they are freely movable under the skin, there being little or no periadenitis.

On section the soft variety (soft almost to fluctuation) shows a grayish red or whitish surface, exuding a milky juice; the boundary between cortical and medullary zones, except in the smaller nodules, is lost, and the lymph channels in the gland nearly obliterated; no change however is seen in the afferent or efferent lymphatic. Microscopical sections show a vast increase in the number of lymph corpuscles composing the adenoid tissue; they crowd the gland, infiltrate the septa and capsule, and even the trabeculæ of the stroma. Besides are seen many giant cells. In this soft variety there is no fibrous induration or hyperplasia of the stroma; all the activity seems to center in the nuclei, making it one of cell proliferation. Very rarely does this burst, penetrate the capsule and invade surrounding tissues.

In the hard variety of lymphoma, the section shows more white and glistening, no juice exudes, the lymph channels are not so obscured and the walls of the vessel are quite thickened. The microscope shows an increased cell proliferation here, too, but a far greater tendency to sclerosis of the capsule, septa and reticulated trabeculæ. There is a decided tendency in the embryonic reticulated stroma to become true fibrous connective tissue; but even a hard gland may show spots identical with the soft variety.

There is no histological appearance here of the sarcoma or of a cancerous formation. The applicability of Virchow's term "lymphosarcoma," lies in the tendency to secondary developments in distant organs or localities, like the sarcomatous metastatic formations. Yet the structure may sometimes resemble to a certain extent the small, round cell sarcoma. The malignancy referred to in Billroth's "Malignant Lymphoma," is seen in the fatal tendency of the disease and the new formation of these tumors in spite of all treatment.

As to symptoms, cause and duration, there is great variety in different cases. The onset is generally very gradual; simple enlargement of the superficial glands of the neck alone being noticeable perhaps for several years, or there may occur longer or shorter periods of quiescence and even subsidence of the glandular swellings, either spontaneously or as the result of treatment. In other instances the internal glands may first become involved and the patient show pressure symptoms, or even die before the external glands present any of the characteristic lesions.

The disease may run its course in three or four months, or in as many years. One of my cases died after about three years and a half, and in the other there has been slowly progressing glandular enlargement for seven years, and as yet the general health is very fair.

As to symptoms; if we bear in mind that the glandular tumors vary in size, often being larger than a cocoanut, and that scarcely a region in the body is exempt from their possible development, we may have most varied effects from pressure on nerves, blood-vessels, bronchi, trachea, œsophagus, intestines, ureters, pelvic organs, etc. As they are not essential, we class them all under pressure symptoms. Fever, either continued or remittent, is common in advanced stages, and, if at all high, is a grave sign ; pneumonia a dangerous complication, and pleuritic effusion from pressure a common condition. Toward the end insomnia may be inveterate, or, more rarely, we may see somnolence. The anæmia becomes marked, with great exhaustion, fatty heart, anæmic murmurs, a tendency to ulceration of mucous membrane and general failure of nutrition; these precede the end, which, if not from suffocation, starvation, or other pressure effect, may come with collapse.

From involvement of the kidney, parenchymatous nephritis may ensue.

A true splenic leucæmia may be present as an intercurrent malady, but, in most instances, forms no part of Hodgkin's disease proper. We miss the hæmorrhages, the diarrhœa, and the great enlargement of the spleen, with the marked increase of leucocytes seen in the leucæmia.

The anæmia need not necessarily produce pallor, for, as in both of my cases, glandular masses pressing on the jugular vein give the face a red, bloated look, very much like that of an habitual drunkard.

There are many phases of the disease we cannot touch upon, but bear in mind its main features — progressive *general* enlargement of the lymphatic glands, frequent involvement of the spleen, with final establishment of severe progressive anæmia.

The prognosis is almost universally *bad*. A very few cases have been reported cured, but the vast majority die in a few months, perhaps, or in a few years at farthest. The average is a little over a year.

Neither physician or patient should be lulled to security by the subsidence of all symptoms, for such periods of remission may appear and last a year, but the disease is almost sure to recur. Or, at times, the glands may become temporarily softer and smaller, without apparent cause, and these facts should always be borne in mind in weighing the efficacy of any course of treatment.

The glands may grow much smaller shortly before death.

The diagnosis is generally easy if the superficial glands be affected, or if sufficient time have elapsed to show the development of the case. Until it can be observed that the enlargement is *progressive*, a diagnosis is impossible, for *simple* lymphoma presents all of the essential features of malignant symptoms in its earliest stages—but the simple remains always a local trouble, while the malignant, in time, becomes general.

Syphilis may resemble the early features of Hodgkin's disease, but in the former we have the history, the especial involvement at an early stage of the occipital and the epitrochlear glands, and, in syphilis, they do not tend to form the massive tumor, nor the *uncomplicated* glandular enlargement of Hodgkin's disease.

Scrofula may be much more difficult to differentiate, but the scrofulous glands are prone to suppuration or caseation, while both of these conditions are very rare, indeed, in Hodgkin's disease. In scrofula the induration is most apt to begin about the angle of the jaw; in malignant lymphoma, in the anterior, or especially the posterior triangle of the neck. The scrofula rarely tends to the general induration and the new formation of adenoid tissue in most unusual localities, as may often be seen in lymphadenosis.

In rare cases the bronzing of the skin with pronounced anæmia will suggest Addison's disease; but this is seen in Hodgkin's disease only where enlargement of the retroperitoneal glands involves the solar plexus; and enlargement of other glands will generally decide the case.

The differential features of leucocythæmia have been mentioned, namely, the *early* enlargement of the spleen (which occurs late in Hodgkin's disease), and the increased proportion of leucocytes in the blood.

True sarcoma and carcinoma will be differentiated by their progressive developments and destruction of adjacent tissues.

As to treatment; thus far general experience shows *arsenic* to be the only drug which has any marked influence in this disease. The old school advises pushing Fowler's solution until twenty or twenty-five-drop doses, three times a day, are reached, or until poisoning symptoms appear, when the dose should be diminished and again increased as tolerance is established. In the later stages *arsenic* seems the homœopathic remedy for many cases, and certainly is most useful. *Phosphorus* has been tried with but slight benefit. I find no reliably reported success from other remedies, though *merc. bin.*, *nitric acid* and *conium* appear to have helped my cases somewhat. *Arsenic*, however, rendered better service than all the others. The *baryta* preparations seem worthy of trial in the early stages. Excision, except in the earliest stages, is useless; and even then it will not help statistics, for an accurate diagnosis cannot usually be made at that period.

Having thus given a general idea of the disease, let me mention some points in the course of my cases.

CASE I.—First—the one still living. This is a lady of 42, married; two children, the youngest about 14 years old. Without apparent cause, there appeared, seven years ago, an enlargement of the glands at the apex of the right posterior cervical triangle. It was painless, the glands very hard and freely movable. There has been a very slow but sure extension, first filling up the triangle, then extending under the trapezius and anteriorly, next into the axilla and down toward the breast. Since appearing in the axilla, there has been severe neuralgic pain in and about the breast, evidently from nerve pressure. Within the past two years the glands in the opposite axilla have become involved and are encroaching upwards on that side of the neck. The inguinal glands are still free, and I cannot determine the existence of internal tumors, though their presence is very probable. The glands are firmly matted together and immovable, though the skin is freely movable over them. She is rather feeble, somewhat anæmic, but able to attend to her duties as usual. I can find no trace of scrofula about her. The point of interest in this case is its slow development, it being one of the longest, if not *the* longest, on record, I think. *Conium* has seemed to hold the glandular growth in check, but on account of the uncertain nature of the disease, I cannot say that it really has been a factor.

CASE II.—The other case was a man of 42, married, of good family history, but who for years had been a heavy drinker.

Three years and a half ago the disease began in the neck as usual, and spread rapidly, with early development of anæmia. At this time he was seen by some eminent New York physician, who prescribed Fowler's solution of *arsenic* and pushed it to the extreme limit of tolerration, indeed to pretty sharp poisoning. As a result (probably), the swelling disappeared, he became able to travel, went to the Carlsbad springs, and for a year counted himself entirely cured.

On resuming his business, however, the trouble returned worse than ever. I cannot trace the steps of his relapse, but give you his condition while under my care.

From adenoid deposits under the skin, his head and face looked abnormally large. The nodules ran all through the scalp, around and in front of the ears, in the cheeks. The face, as I mentioned, from jugular obstruction, was red and bleary, conjunctivæ injected, mucous membrane of mouth involved in the deposit in the adenoid tissue of the submucosa, so the tongue was swollen, the gums swollen, bleeding, teeth falling out, sense of taste absolutely lost from pressure on gustatory nerves, tonsils swollen, and in the site of a lost tooth ulceration began, which spread with alarming rapidity, attacked the alveolar arch of the superior maxilla so that necrosis ensued, with loss of large pieces of bone. Packing with iodoform and washing with carbolized calendula finally checked the ulcerative process. The nasal fossæ were pretty well filled with the growth, so the sense of smell was gone, nasal breath impossible and a thin, acrid coryza was constant.

The neck, axillæ, back and skin here and there over the body were affected, the tumors on the back looking like wens. The spleen was moderately enlarged, but the groins comparately free from infection.

From the condition of the mouth I prescribed *merc. bin.* with temporary benefit and I thought the glands were a little better under it; as this improvement failed I gave him *nitric acid*, with better results, though very soon after that the fever, which had run pretty constantly at 102 degrees, suddenly went to 105 degrees with severe dyspnœa, and pneumonia developed in the lower lobe of the right lung. This, for a man in his condition, was a very dangerous complication, but he weathered it after a time. After this the dyspnœa reappeared without increase of fever, which had returned to 102 degrees, and I found that from pressure of a mass of enlarged bronchial glands about the root of the lung, and of those in the posterior mediastrum, an extensive pleuritic effusion was forming. This could not be checked. I did not consider it wise to perform paracentesis, so it continued while I saw him, but it seemed to cease at a certain point and he grew accustomed to it, breathing with the left lung.

Inveterate insomnia now appeared and threatened to completely exhaust the patient. Homœopathic remedies failed me, or rather I failed with them, so resorted to *morphine*. At once this gave relief, the patient grew stronger and better in every way, having from six to eight hours sleep each night.

About this time a slight diarrhœa appeared, the thirst increased, patient was constantly restless and complained of exhaustion. Fowler's solution of *arsenic*, three drops three times a day, was now administered, with decided benefit, but the condition did not altogether subside. Coming in one day I saw him with a plate of meat before him. which he seemed to relish, and, for some time after, in answer to inquiries, his wife said he was eating well; so my suspicions were diverted. But still he grew weaker, and on one occasion I caught the expression of his eye—a peculiar, wild, restless, almost fierce, almost insane expression, which I remember having seen in one or two cases of starvation. The pulse was 160, feeble and fluttering. Inquiries as to exact amounts eaten showed that the wife's idea of "eating well" was most inadequate, and our patient was actually starving. A diet list, feeding every two hours to the limit of his digestive powers, soon wrought a wonderful change—the diarrhœa and sleeplessness improved, the strength picked up, pulse fell, and he seemed like himself again.   This, with a similar experience in a different case and connection, taught me a useful lesson—to take for granted, in giving directions, that the attendant knows absolutely nothing, and make instructions and questions most explicit.   With smell and taste gone, of course, there was no relish for food, and because the patient did not wish more, the attendant took it for granted he did not need more.

The *arsenic* was continued, with slight though steady improvement, until the return of the physician whose place I was taking. Since then I simply know that he lingered until January, then died. It is to be regretted that no autopsy was held, for it was certainly a marked and instructive case of Hodgkin's disease.

In closing, Mr. President, allow me to make a plea for a revision in our nomenclature.   In this paper I have used the ordinarily accepted terms, for it would seem pedantic, under the circumstances, to do otherwise.

But the term "lymphatic gland" is a misnomer.   A gland is an epithelial structure having a definite secretory power ; yet the "lymphatic glands" have no epithelium in them, and so far as we know, have no true secretion.   Hence, Dr. Prudden's term of "*lymph-node*" is far more applicable.

Then another closely-allied misnomer is the term, "adenoid tissue."   This consists of a fine reticulated stroma, closely packed with lymph corpuscles, reminding one of ova in a shad roe.   But "adenoid" means gland-like ; yet this tissue has none of the characteristic epithelial feature of a gland—in fact, it contains no epithelium whatever.   It is the tissue of which lymph-*nodes* are composed ; hence, might be called lymphoid tissue instead of "adenoid."   An adenoma, or glandular tumor, is never composed of adenoid, but of epithelial tissue.

Our technical terms are full of inaccuracies, but here is an opportunity to correct at least two errors.

MACKENZIE'S CONDENSER may be much increased in its illuminating power by painting the inside of the cylinder with zinc white, mixed with gum water.—*Journal of Laryngology*, May, 1887.

THE RELATION OF THE PHYSICIAN AND THE SANITARIAN TO HEREDITY, WITH STATISTICS AS TO IT.*

By LABAN DENNIS, M.D.,
Newark, N. J.

(Concluded from page 277.)

THE most complete and exhaustive presentation of the facts of heredity accessible to English readers, that has fallen into our hands is the very able work of Th. Ribot, on "Heredity" (Appleton & Co.), translated from the French. This author has drawn largely from all the prominent writers on this and kindred topics, such as Lucas, Spencer, Darwin, Buckle, Burdach, Maudsley, and a host of others, so that his book is a miniature cyclopædia of most interesting and valuable facts to be carefully studied by everyone concerned for the well-being of the race.

In his introduction he calls attention to the facts of physiological heredity, showing how children resemble their parents in external structure, in general appearance, in the limbs, the trunk, the head, even in the nails and the hair, but especially in the countenance, expression or characteristic features. Strangely, too, children may undergo such metamorphoses as shall cause one to resemble at one time the father and at another time the mother. Heredity may also be traced in the complexion of the skin, the shape and size of the body; thus, obesity has been known to make its appearance under all the disadvantages of hard labor and poverty. So, too, the transmission of peculiarities in the form, size and anomalies of the osseous system, as in the proportions of the cranium, thorax, pelvis, vertebral column, and even the smallest bones of the skeleton, are of daily observation. Even the heredity of excess or defect in the number of the vertebræ and the teeth has been seen. The circulatory, digestive and muscular systems obey the same laws which govern the transmission of the other internal systems of the organism. So, too, heredity regulates the proportions of the nervous system. This is evident in the general dimensions of the brain; it is often apparent in the size and even in the form of the cerebral convolutions. It also regulates the fluids as well as the solid parts; the blood is more abundant in some families than in others, and this superabundance may transmit a predisposition to apoplexy, hemorrhage and inflammation. The same may be said with regard to the bile and lymph. So, too, fecundity,

---

*Read before the N. Y. Medico-Chirurgical Society.

length of life, and those purely personal characteristics called idiosyncrasies are hereditarily transmitted. In some families the hair
turns gray in early youth, and the vigor of the physical and intellectual faculties fails prematurely. In some, immunity from contagious
diseases is a well-established fact. Heredity may transmit muscular
strength in the various forms of motor energy, as seen in the families
of athletes, prize-fighters, wrestlers and oarsmen. Some are possessed
of exquisite dexterity and grace of movement, as shown by the
transmission of a talent for dancing. So, too, peculiarities of voice
with its defects, as stammering, speaking through the nose and lisp-
ing, the possession of great powers of singing, and the absence of all
ear for melody, are transmissible. Even extreme loquacity seems to
run in families. Dr. Lucas mentions the case of a servant girl who,
when dismissed for incessant talking, not only to others but to dumb
beasts, to inanimate things, and even aloud to herself, said to her
employer: "It is no fault of mine; it comes to me from my father;
the same fault in him drove my mother distracted, and one of his
brothers was like me." The transmission of anomalies of organization
is a well-observed fact. Thus, horny excrescences of the skin running
through five generations have been observed; so, too, albinism, rickets, lameness, hare-lip, and all deviations from the normal type are
seen. It is a disputed question whether these variations remain
fixed or return gradually to the normal type. In proof of the latter
may be mentioned the case of the Colburn family, in which each
member had six fingers and toes. The anomaly continued through
four generations.

The ratio of normal to abnormal was, in the first generation, 1 to
35; second generation, 1 to 14; third generation, 1 to 3¼; showing
a return to the normal type taking place very rapidly.

On this same point Dr. Gull says: "The strength of modern
therapeutics lies in the clearer perception than formerly of the great
truth that diseases are but perverted life processes, and have for their
natural history not only a beginning, but a period of culmination and
decline. The effects of disease may be for a third or fourth generation, but the laws of health are for a thousand."

Ribot points out, too, that even peculiar habits and modes of physical exertion are transmissible.

The bulk of his work, however, is taken up with the consideration
of the heredity of intellectual and moral qualities. Thus, in his first
chapter, he points out how natural instincts in men and animals are
transmitted. In the next, how sensorial qualities, those of touch,
sight, hearing, smell and taste, whether defective or in excess, are

handed down through generations. In another he considers the gifts of memory with all its peculiarities, and shows how it is heritable. In the next he takes up the work of the imagination, as in writers, poets, painters and musicians, citing numerous cases of its hereditary character. In the fifth he considers the powers of the intellect, as exhibited in men of science, philosophers, economists and men of letters. In the sixth he treats of the sentiments and their abnormal variations, the passions, showing the heredity of general sensibility, of antipathies, of the sexual appetite, of dipsomania, of moral tendencies and their opposites, gaming, avarice, theft and homicide. In the seventh he considers the heredity of the will, the two classes of the mind active and contemplative, the transmissibility of the active faculties in statesmen and soldiers. In the eighth he takes up the heredity of national characteristics and in the ninth morbid psychological phenomena, such as insanity, hallucination, suicide, homicidal monomania, demoniacal possession, hypochondria, presentiments, mania, dementia and general paralysis. In part second he considers the laws of heredity; in part third the causes, and in part fourth the consequences, thus giving a complete statement of the relations of heredity to individual and social life, such as must furnish food for thought to all intelligent men of whatever station in life.

This brief sketch of the views of scientists as to the hereditary relations of families may be appropriately supplemented by a statement of the conclusions at which medical men have arrived as to the transmission of diseases.

A rapid glance over the pages of Carpenter, Ziemssen, Reynolds and Pepper shows that heredity is accredited with more or less influence in the production and development of alcoholism, cerebral anæmia, angina pectoris, aneurism of the aorta, asthma, atrophy, progressive muscular; hyperæmia, brain; hemorrhage, brain; hypertrophy, brain; calculi, renal; chorea, chlorosis; cancer, intestines, kidney, liver, stomach, uterus; convulsions, infantile; catarrh, stomach; dementia paralytica, diabetes, dyspepsia, epilepsy, gastritis, gallstones, goitre, gout; heart, dilatation, fatty, rupture of; hæmophilia, hay fever, hepatic congestion, hypochondriasis, hysteria, insanity; leucocythæmia, splenic; lymphadenosis, meningitis, cerebral, tuberculous; migraine, neurosis, stomach; neuralgia, neuropathic predisposition; paralysis, progressive muscular atrophy, phthisis pul., pseudo-hypertrophy, muscles; rheumatism, spasm of the glottis, somnambulism, tabes dorsalis, spinal irritation and syphilis, affecting mucous membranes, bones, joints, glandular structures and the nervous system.

Thus is presented an outline of the evils to be avoided in hereditary descent. We have said that physicians heretofore have been laboring on the side of nurture; they have taken the human being, as brought into the world, and have endeavored to correct the evils found, with but slight reference to the doctrine of prevention. Sanitary science at the present day is bringing into greater prominence preventive medicine, as contrasted with curative medicine. We may appropriately ask ourselves, therefore, in view of the importance of this subject, what the profession can do to ward off these evils, and to develop a stronger and nobler race upon the earth.

Says Mr. Galton: "Man finds himself somehow in existence, endowed with a little power and intelligence; he ought, therefore, to awake to a fuller knowedge of his relatively great position, and begin to assume a deliberate part in furthering the great work of evolution. He may infer the course he is bound to pursue, from his observation of that which it has already followed, and he might devote his modicum of power, intelligence and kindly feeling to render its future progress less slow and painful. Man has already furthered evolution very considerably, half unconsciously, and for his own personal advantages, but he has not yet risen to the conviction that it is his religious duty to do so deliberately and systematically."

We are met here, however, by another difficulty. Evolution among *races* has been governed by the principles of the "survival of the fittest."

Says Mr. Greg: "The abler, the stronger, the more advanced, the finer, in short, are still the favored ones; succeed in the competition, exterminate, govern, supersede, fight, eat, or work the inferior tribes out of existence." As instances, we may mention the Indians of Antilles, the red man of North America, the South Sea Islander, the Australian, and even the New Zealander.

This principle of natural selection holds good also in the case of *nations*, examples of which are the Greeks overpowered by the Romans, and they, in turn, by the rude Northern warriors.

But when we come to the case of individuals in a people, or classes in a community, the principle would appear to fail, and the law is no longer supreme. Civilization, with its social, moral and material complications, has introduced a disturbing and conflicting element. It is no longer the strongest, the healthiest, the most perfectly organized. It is not men of the finest physique, the largest brain, the most developed intelligence, the best *morale*, that are favored and successful in the struggle for existence; rather often those emasculated by luxury and those damaged by want, those rendered reckless by squalid poverty, and those whose physical and mental energies have been sapped, and whose characters have been grievously impaired by long indulgence and forestalled desires. Respect for life has preserved thousands with tainted constitutions, and frames weakened by malady or waste. "Brains bearing subtle and hereditary mischief in their recesses are suffered to transmit their terrible inheritance of evil to other generations, and to spread it through a whole community." Security for property, with its transmission and enjoyment, has enabled many an unworthy and incapable possessor and inheritor to take precedence over others in many of the walks of life, to carry off the most desirable brides from less-favored, though nobler rivals, and make them the mothers of a degenerating instead of an ever-improving race. Thus both the upper and the lower classes of society are unfitted to carry forward the improvement of mankind. Both marry as early as they please, and have as many children as they please—the rich, because it is in their power; the poor, because they have no motive for abstinence—and scanty food and hard circumstances do not oppose, but rather encourage procreation. "It is the middle classes—those who form the energetic, reliable, improving element of the population, those who wish to rise, and do not choose to sink, those, in a word, that constitute the true strength and wealth and dignity of nations—it is those who abstain from marriage, or postpone it." (Greg). Mr. Galton also says: "Again, there is a constant tendency of the best men in the country to settle in the great cities, where marriages are less prolific and children less likely to live. Owing to these several causes, there is a steady check in an old civilization on the fertility of the abler classes. The improvident and unambitious are those who chiefly keep up the breed. So the race gradually degenerates, becoming, with each successive generation, less fitted for a high civilization, although it retains the external appearance of one ; until the time comes when the whole political and social fabric caves in, and a greater or less relapse towards barbarism takes place."

Thus the tendency in communities of advanced civilization to multiply from their lower rather than their higher specimens, constitutes one of the most formidable dangers with which that civilization is threatened. The counteracting influences, it is to be hoped, will be found in the spreading intelligence, the matured wisdom, the ripened self-control, in the social virtues which that civilization nurtures and in which it ought to culminate. (Greg).

One other cause of the numerical failure of the higher types is to be found in the fact already alluded to by Mr. Galton, on discovering that the children of scientific men are not as numerous as those of their own fathers, namely, that cerebral development tends to lessen fecundity. It would seem, therefore, that herein lies one of the greatest dangers of a high order of civilization. The answer is so admirably given by Mr. Herbert Spencer, in his "Principles of Biology," that we give it in part as quoted by Mr. Greg :

"The necessary antagonism of inviduation and genesis not only fulfills with precision the *a priori* law of maintenance of race, from the monad up to man, but insures the final attainment of the highest form of this maintenance, the form in which the amount of life shall be the greatest possible, and the births and deaths the fewest possible. The excessive fertility has rendered the process of civilization inevitable, and the process of civilization must inevitably diminish fertility, and at last destroy its excess. From the beginning, pressure of population has been the proximate cause of progress. It produced the original diffusion of the race. It compelled men to abandon predatory habits and take to agriculture. It led to the clearing of the earth's surface. It forced men into the social state ; made social organization inevitable, and has developed the social sentiments. It has stimulated to progressive improvements in production, and to increased skill and intelligence. It is daily thrusting us into closer contact and more mutually dependent relationships. And after having caused, as it ultimately must, the due peopling of the globe, and the raising of all its habitable parts into the highest state of culture; after having brought all processes for the satisfaction of human wants to perfection ; after having, at the same time, developed the intellect into complete competency for its work, and the feelings into complete fitness for social life, the pressure of population, as it gradually finishes its work, must gradually bring itself to an end."

Having thus briefly stated a few of the elements of the great problem before us, what we, as physicians, should be studying is, not merely how to relieve the suffering which comes into the world, and prolong the lives of the wretched and miserable as well as of the healthy, but how to secure that a larger proportion of those born shall come as of right to the possession of an inheritance of health, long life, energy, well-balanced sensitiveness of organization, self-reliance and enthusiasm, which go to make the difference between one fitted to advance the world in its upward course, and one ever dependent on humanity for even a tolerable existence. Dr. Holmes has said : "There are people who think that everything may be done, if the doer, be he educator or physician, be only called ' in season.' No doubt; but *in season* would be often a hundred or two years before the child was born, and people never send so early as that."

Let us now begin to save a few of the unborn.

What, then, are some of the methods whereby this is to be accomplished?

Man at the present is the outcome of past centuries of animal life upon the earth, the foremost product, "the heir of untold ages and in the van of circumstance." As no naturalist can tell how any improved species originates, but has learned to seize the happy product, multiply, propagate, and still further develop it, so we should humbly and patiently study the conditions which seem to have produced any marked and noble stock in the human family, perpetuate and nourish the individuals, and encourage them to beget their like by suitable marriages, that their offspring may be a permanent possession on the earth.

Mr. Galton says : " It is hardly necessary to insist on the certainty that our present imperfect knowledge of the limitations and conditions of hereditary transmission will be steadily added to ; but I would call attention again to the serious want of adequate materials for study in the form of life-histories. It is fortunately the case that many of the rising medical practitioners of the foremost rank have become strongly impressed with the necessity of possessing them, not only for the better knowledge of the theory of disease, but for the personal advantage of their patients, whom they now have to treat less appropriately than they otherwise would, through ignorance of their hereditary tendencies and of their illnesses in past years, the medical details of which are rarely remembered by the patient, even if he ever knew them. With the help of so powerful a personal motive for keeping life-histories, and of so influential a body as the medical profession to advocate its being done, and to show how to do it, there is considerable hope that the want of materials, to which I have alluded, will gradually be supplied."

Accordingly, he has prepared a "Life History Album," which, with a "Record of Family Faculties," is a veritable *multum in parvo*, so convenient and comprehensive that most intelligent families would be only too glad to have them brought to their notice for prompt and continuous use.

May we not, then, with the aid of these life-histories, arouse in every family an approach to some adequate appreciation of the immense value of the knowledge so acquired, both to the individuals themselves for the right governing of their lives as they come to maturity, and also to guide in the selection of appropriate companions whereby to propagate such qualities as shall most enrich the world?

Instruction may be given to parents and teachers in the matter of the several diatheses, and so children may be taught to recognize and shun that most wide-spread and pernicious one, the strumous, which now destroys more lives than any dreaded plague or pestilence. The effects of the intermarriage of families and of persons of like temperaments should be pointed out. Simple books in plain, untechnical language, like Fothergill's "Maintenance of Health," which has a chapter on the subject of inheritance, could be placed in the hands of all moderately-educated families. The careful study of Ribot's "Heredity" would greatly profit any intelligent household.

The subject should be insisted on as a vital matter of study in all higher schools in which physiology and hygiene are taught. Happily, many of our State Legislatures are being aroused to the overwhelming importance of the latter subject.

Thus, both in the family life and in the school, the growing youth would be taught to regard themselves as parts of a great system of rational beings, fitted by heredity to carry on certain works, and urged so to adjust themselves to their environment that the best of which they are capable may be accomplished, and the resulting offspring be enabled to start on a slightly higher plane. If physicians and sanitarians will set this before them as the ideal standard up to which the family and the school must be brought, the two most important agencies for the elevation of the race will be won.

In the furtherance of this scheme, likewise we believe that the family physician should be, and if it were properly carried out, would become, more and more the trusted counselor and adviser of those under his charge. Matrimonial alliances would be more especially subjects for his wise and affectionate judgment. If it is the physician's duty, in common with all philanthropists, to protect the helpless, relieve the suffering and prolong the lives of the sick and diseased, it is more imperatively his duty to prevent, by all legitimate means, the birth of such into the world. Thus, he may aid in hastening, as Mr. Greg says, that "day when, as the moral tone of society advances, and men rise to some larger and more vivid perceptions of their mutual obligations, the propagation of vitiated constitutions, as well as of positive disease, will be universally condemned as culpable, and possibly prohibited as criminal. Some classes and communities have already, from time to time, reached this slight rising ground in social virtue, in reference to the three fearful maladies of insanity, leprosy and cretinism. Surely a further progress in knowledge and reflection, and a somewhat wider range of sympathy, may extend the list to scrofula, syphilis and consumption. I can discern no reason, beyond our own halting wisdom and deficient sense of right, the strange ignorance of some classes, and the stranger senselessness of others, our utterly wonderful and persistent errors in political and social philosophy in nearly every line, why a very few generations should not have nearly eliminated from the community those who ought not to breed at all, and have taught prudence to those who ought to breed only in moderate and just proportions."

Business enterprises, changes of residence and occupation, with all the complicated effects of climate, food and clothing, and the relative value of new social relations, should be thoroughly discussed by families with the physician. They *will* be when life, in its highest and best sense, becomes "more than food and the body more than raiment."

We can only suggest a few ways in which the specialist may be helpful to society in this work. For example, Dr. J. S. Billings (Art. Hygiene, Pepper's Syst. Med.) says : "The importance of taking into account hereditary influences is well illustrated by the care which is taken to obtain information with regard to them in well-conducted life insurance companies. The medical examiners of such companies have their attention specially called to this matter, and the following extract from a manual of instructions shows how it is regarded from a business point of view : 'If consumption· is found to have occurred in the family of the applicant, he is to be regarded not insurable under the following circumstances, *viz.* :

	Years of age.
If in both parents, not insurable until	40
If in one parent, not insurable until (except for 10 ten-year endowments, then 20 years)	30
If in two members, not parents	35
If in one member, brother or sister (except for 10 ten-year endowments, when peculiarly favorable)	20

"If apoplexy, paralysis or heart disease is found to have occurred in any two members of the applicant's family, he is to be regarded as insurable only upon the endowment plan, the term of insurance to expire prior to his reaching the age of fifty years. If insanity shall have so occurred (in two members), a provisionary clause is essential, and is attached to the policy by the company."

We ask, why should not such facts, the results of long years of work by medical examiners, be more generally published through the press, till the fathers and mothers of the country realize them as thoroughly as do the directors of insurance companies? If a life is not insurable, what is its marriageable value? What a burden of suffering and unrequited toil, sickness in the progeny and blasted hopes in the parents, will result from the union of such with others equally vitiated !

The hereditary transmission of diseases of the eyes, heart, lungs, nervous system, kidneys, digestive viscera, blood and generative organs should be constantly kept before the profession by specialists, and such facts and figures as may be made comprehensible to the laity should for their guidance, be given to the press, and so spread broadcast through the land.

We believe that the pulpit should likewise be urged by the medical profession to contribute its share to the general good, in the preaching of a religion of humanity which should condemn disobedience of physical law as equally culpable with infractions of the moral code. In the light of this truth, the reckless imposition of disease, early blight, hopeless wretchedness and premature death upon helpless and inoffending offspring should be regarded and taught as a most heinous crime against man and God. The possession of the globe by a strong and noble race, and its conversion into a paradise, should be regarded as among the legitimate aims of the earthly life, and not merely the speedy transfer of that race to new and untried conditions in a life to come.

We are happy to see that some of the clergy, already aroused to the importance of this matter, are writing and preaching upon it.

The conclusions at which we arrive, then, from this hasty review may be summed up as follows:

In determining the mental and physical characters and efficiency of man, nature is more potential than nurture. Great powers of body and mind seem to run for generations in families. Early marriages favor the rapid multiplication of those engaging in them. Hence they should be encouraged in the strong, discouraged in the weak.

Defects of constitution descend to posterity even more certainly than their opposites. It becomes man's duty, therefore, systematically to favor the evolution of a higher race. Suitable matrimonial alliances are among the most powerful agencies for the accomplishment of this purpose. In this process the best and strongest races and nations have survived in the past, but civilization has introduced into society elements favoring the rich and the poor, worthless classes; and the increasing demands of that civilization have made the intellectual less fertile, thus putting a check upon the growth of the best classes in society, which only intelligent and educated forethought can counteract.

Our duties are, then, to cultivate and perpetuate the nobler types of mankind. To do this we should encourage increase of knowledge among families by inducing them to write and study most diligently their life histories, and to govern their family alliances accordingly.

Teachers, also, should be instructed in their value and importance, that schools may become propagators of this class of truths.

The family physician should at once put those under his charge upon their guard as to certain hereditary evils to be avoided, and hold up to view the constitutional qualities more to be desired than wealth and social position.

Specialists should see that the press teems with the facts and figures which show the pitfalls and the prizes of life.

The clergy should be urged to preach that the heavenly life must begin in the right use of the earthly, and that men are best fitted to die when best prepared to live.

CONGENITAL CYANOSIS, WITH REPORT OF THE OLDEST LIVING CASE RECORDED.*

By WILLIAM C. LATIMER, M.D.,
Brooklyn, N. Y.

IT is neither the importance of the subject, nor the frequency of its occurrence, but the rare and peculiar case we have to report, that leads us to select this subject for your consideration this evening.

CONGENITAL CYANOSIS (*morbus coeruleus*).—Blue disease has come to be described as a disease by itself; this, however, is wrong, it being simply a symptom of a congenital malformation of the circulatory system.

Dr. Eustice Smith (Wood's Ref. Hand Book of the Medical Sciences) says: "The malformation may be one of several forms, the most common consisting in a constriction of the pulmonary artery, and a deficiency in the septum of the ventricles ; the aorta communicating with the right ventricular cavity. The heart is always enlarged, especially the right side."

Cazeaux, Gilchrist, and the general teaching of anatomists, state the cause to be non-closure of the foramen ovale or foramen of Botel.

"Edmonds, quoting from J. Lewis Smith's Diseases of Children, gives a table of 162 cases examined post mortem, in which neither of the above causes were present in a single case."

---

*Read before the Homœopathic Medical Society of the County of Kings, April 12th, 1887.

Among the other causes we again quote from the last named authority.

1. Pulmonary artery absent, rudimentary or partially obstructed, ...   97 cases.
2. Right auriculo-ventricular orifice impervious or contracted, ...   5
3. Orifice of the pulmonary and the right auriculo-ventricular aperture impervious or contracted,   .   6
4. Right ventricle divided into the cavities by a supernumerary septum, ...   11
5. One auricle and one ventricle,   .   .   .   12
6. Two auricles and one ventricle, ...   4
7. A single auriculo-ventricular opening ; inter-auricular and inter-ventricular septa incomplete, .   .   1
8. Mitral orifice closed or contracted,   .   .   .   3
9. Aortic and left auriculo-ventricular orifices impervious 'or contracted, ...
10. Aorta absent, rudimentary, impervious or partially obstructed, ...   3
11. Aorta and pulmonary artery transposed,   .   .   14
12. Venæ cavæ entering the left auricle,   .   .   .   1
13. Pulmonary veins opening into the auricle, or into the venæ cavæ, or azygos veins,   .   .   .
14. Aorta impervious or contracted above its point of union with the ductus arteriosus ; pulmonary artery wholly or in part supplying blood to the descending aorta through the ductus arteriosus,   .   .   .   2 ¨

The conditions above enumerated cover the previously mentioned 162 cases.

With this diversity of conditions to produce a single visible symptom, we think the following definition best suited to our subject :

Any congenital malformation of the circulatory system which prevents a free and perfect oxygenation of the blood; or causes mixture of venous with the arterial blood in or as it is leaving the heart.

The length of life in most of these cases is short.

In a table of 186 cases by J. Lewis Smith, the length of life attained was as follows :

17 lived less than one week ; 10 lived more than one week, but less than one month ; 12 lived more than one month, but less than three months ; 11 lived more than three months, but less than six

months ; 17 lived more than six months, but less than one year ; 12 lived more than one year, but less than two years ; 21 lived more than two years, but less than five years ; 21 lived more than five years, but less than ten years ; 41 lived more than ten years, but less than twenty years ; 20 lived more than twenty years, but less than forty years ; 4 lived more than forty years.

Thus showing that 54 per cent. died before reaching the fifth year ; and 87 per cent. before the twentieth year, while only 2 per cent. lived past the fortieth.

The condition usually presents itself at, or within a few hours after, birth ; unless the malformation is slight, when it may not manifest itself for several years.

' The late Dr. Flint stated, a short time before his death, that so far as he remembered, the case hereinafter reported, was the only similar case he had ever seen over 41 years of age.

We have taken the liberty of trying your patience with this extended list of statistics and outline of a condition intra-uterine in its origin, and for which no cause has yet been found, in order that the singular manifestations in the case now to be reported may be fully realized.

In August, 1832, Mrs. W., of New York, was stricken with cholera. At the time she was about eight months pregnant; her physician, the late Dr. Willets, decided that his only hope of saving her life was by inducing delivery. What the peculiar conditions were that brought about this decision we are unable to learn.

The fruits of this conception proved to be twins, girls; one dead when delivered, the other supposed to be; but prolonged and persistent efforts at resuscitation were finally rewarded by success, and she still lives.

From the beginning she was dubbed the blue baby, and still holds her title thereto. When well and quiet, her skin, lips and mucous membranes generally are nearly normal; while the least agitation, excitement or sickness will cause the skin to assume shades varying from normal to that of one suffering from the bite of a rattlesnake, while the lips will become blue, the countenance drawn and death-like, the blood settle under the nails, often causing those unaccustomed to the attacks to think she is surely dying. The action of the heart is as variable as the conditions just mentioned, sounds of every variety being heard on applying the ear to the chest. It is not uncommon for her to have convulsions at these times, lasting from five to twenty minutes, and often repeated; have seen her have twenty within two hours; during their continuance she will roll her head from side to side, force it backward until the occiput touches the spine, pound it with her fists, unless held, and if, as sometimes happens, she is alone and falls on the floor, will beat it against the floor, wall, or anything that comes in contact with it, at the same time uttering complaints of pain in her head until all consciousness is lost. In the intervals between the convulsions her tongue will run without limit, and any secret committed to her keeping is revealed, while any orders or directions given by her physician and disobeyed, share the same fate. During this talking she is unconscious of all her surroundings, and any attempt to arouse her is rewarded by an active convulsion. She undoubtedly has attacks of convulsions during sleep, as she often complains of soreness about the head on waking, and the palms will show imprints of the finger tips. In from three to twenty-four hours after an attack she will, except for a little soreness, be as well as usual.

She will care for the sick, or assume responsibilities for weeks without any trouble, but the moment the strain and excitement are relinquished she is sure to have an attack. Undue excitement coming suddenly will sometimes produce the same result.

Not the least interesting feature of this case is a recurring abscess. It first appeared when she was six months old, pointing between the seventh and eighth ribs, right side; it was poulticed and opened in anterior axillary line; from that time until she was twenty-four years of age, it opened from once to three times a year, all the openings being within a radius of two inches; during this time she was under the care of the late Dr. Van Winckle, of New York. In 1857, she moved to Brooklyn and came under the care of the late Dr. Nathaniel Ford; the abscesses appeared as usual, but he allowed them to break internally and discharge through the bowels. From 1857 to 1862 their recurrence under his (Dr. Ford's) treatment was not quite as frequent, yet averaged more than once a year; at times the pus and blood regurgitates into the stomach and is vomited.

Another singular manifestation in the case is an annual attack of cholera, occurring in August, as a reminder of her birth-day; the symptoms seem nearest those of *veratrum*, but this remedy has no effect, and in spite of all remedies, with one exception hereinafter mentioned, it has run a regular course of five to twelve days.

She came under the care of the writer in February, 1882. Since that date the abscess has formed four times; broken internally each time and been accompanied with regurgitation and emesis; during this time she has had an attack of pelvic cellulitis, with formation of abscess upon the right side, which opened through the vagina. At this time there was considerable hemorrhage, and it was feared for several days she would not survive the shock; she made a good recovery.

She menstruated regularly from her fifteenth year until nearly her fifty-second, except when pregnant; since that time she has passed through the menopause, the last three menstruations being 195, 93 and 162 days apart; were very profuse and long lasting.

She married when about thirty years of age, and the fruit thereof is one son, now twenty-two years old, well formed and healthy. Her labor was normal, but placenta was retained five hours, and she nearly perished from hemorrhage before it was removed; recovery slow.

In the fall of 1883 she was carefully examined by the late Dr.

Flint, of New York, who pronounced the foramen ovale open, and the case the oldest he had ever met.

The next point of consideration will be : what remedies have done for this peculiar case.

Previous to 1882, the treatment had all been allopathic, and, to use her own words, had accomplished nothing ; it had not prevented a single abscess, relieved a single attack of cholera, or prevented a convulsion. During the time she has been under homœopathic treatment, the abscesses, omitting the pelvic one, have been less than one a year ; passed one season, 1886, without the choleraic attack; the convulsions have become less frequent and severe, notwithstanding she has during this time passed through the menopause as before stated, a critical period even to those in perfect health.

The action of remedies has been in keeping with the case ; subject to attacks of bronchitis from the slightest cold, in which the larger bronchial tubes alone seem involved, accompanied by chest pains and cough, which seemed well covered by *bryonia*. This remedy was first tried in the 3d ; result, immediately thrown into convulsions, and no relief of the chest and bronchial symptoms. In succeeding attacks the remedy was tried in higher potencies until the 30th was reached, and each time with the same result, at that point the remedy was abandoned, and others studied and tried, with the result of finding that *bell.* 3d ; *kali bich.* 1st and *merc. sol.* 3d, used according to the respective stages of the disease, and accompanying symptoms, have given the best results of any used, and produce less disagreeable aggravations.

For the convulsions, *bell., cicuta* and *cuprum met.* studied and tried as follows : *bell.* 30 ; *cicuta* 3 and 30, and *cuprum met.* 30 ; the latter with the best results, often cutting short an attack if placed upon the tongue during a convulsion ; and if begun early, that is, when symptoms of their approach are first felt, warding it off, a dull headache lasting twenty-four to forty-eight hours taking its place.

For the choleraic attacks *camphor, arsenicum, veratrum* and *opium* have been tried and found wanting, except as before stated. She passed 1886 without an attack. Just before it was due she began taking *veratrum alb.* 2c, and continued it until the time for it had passed. She also spent the time in the country; which accomplished this result I leave you to form your own opinions.

When the attacks of convulsions are coming on; the headache, dull eye, with flashes of red light, quick and variable pulse, mottled skin, anxious expression, with great mental anxiety, have led to the study of *ars. alb., phos.* and the *snake poisons* and the trial of all except *naja*, and each found to produce no effect.

I have watched the case carefully under many and varied circumstances for five years ; I am not prepared to affirm or deny the diagnosis of Dr. Flint ; in fact I believe that only a post mortem will fully decide the location of the malformation ; while an abscess so located as to reform and open upon the surface for a time, and then internally, without more serious results, has been a puzzling question to all who have seen the case, while none seem willing to name structures involved thereby. If any one can shed any light upon this peculiar case, in any of its parts, we shall be most happy to have them do so.

ORIGINAL ARTICLES IN SURGERY.

TWO CASES OF SARCOMA OF THE LONG BONES.*

By WM. TOD HELMUTH, M.D.

THE study of bone tumors is possessed of great interest to the practical surgeon, especially those neoplasms which are known as malignant. The ordinary osteoid homologous tumors are benign, embracing the varied forms of mature connective tissue, as found in the skeleton and elicited in the exostoses. The primary malignant tumors ought all really to be classed as sarcomas, that is, if we accept the epithelial origin of carcinoma, for, with the exception of the upper jaw, no epithelial elements enter into the formation of bone, every constituent, even to the endothelial lining of the vessels, belonging to the connective tissue. The difference, then, between innocent and malignant osteoid tumors is found in the fact that in the former the connective tissue is mature and complete, and in the latter immature and embryonic. It may be stated as a fact, that the more the tissue resembles the embryonic or imperfectly developed structure, the greater the malignancy of the growth. The very vexed question regarding the classification of tumors need not be entered upon in this place, as there is no end to opinions regarding the methods of *origin* of tumors, nor to the shades of difference that are continually being found by every microscopist.

The operating surgeon must make his diagnosis *before* the tumor is cut out. The microscopist, in most instances, renders his decision *after* the removal of the neoplasm. The clinical classifier must be entirely influenced by the presenting symptoms, while the variety, position, shape and arrangement of cells are the guides for the microscopist. My own opinion is, that if the latter gentlemen in different portions of the world, do not desist from adding new varieties to the already overstocked tumor classifications, the confusion which now exists will soon be worse confounded.

---

* Read before the Homœopathic Medical Society, County of New York.

The microscopist, however, can and does materially assist the surgeon in two ways:

1st. When he can examine a portion of the tumor before operation, as frequently is possible in cystic, villous, papillomatous growths, and those others found in the accessible cavities.

2d. By comparing the results of his investigation of post-operative specimens with the clinical symptoms, as noted by the surgeon, thus enabling the latter, should a similar case present, to be more precise in diagnosis and accurate in prognosis.

But, unfortunately, men often attempt a classification of the neoplasms found in the human body, who rarely, if ever, see a tumor in its original position with its appearances, its natural history, its remote and local symptomatology. The enthusiastic microscopist may have a hundred thousand slides arranged in his boxes and is ready to demonstrate his favorite classification to any one having the time and patience to examine them. The specimens, it is true, are all there, but where are the patients? The clinician, on the other hand, sees the growth in its bed—the human body; he observes the symptoms, objective and subjective, which are presented by it ; he marks the inroads it is making on the constitution upon which it is thrust, and he desires to know what it is, whence it came, and whither and with what result it is going; and this, too, before his patient is dead, or mutilated or crippled. Microscopists, as a rule, care little for the patient, or care for him only in the degree in which he fulfills the programme assigned him by the character of the cell which is found in his tumor. If the cell predicts death, there is an undefined satisfaction in seeing him die; if, on the contrary, the forecast is restoration to health and no return, then the recovery is hailed as a triumph of the oracle.

In presenting these cases, I shall give as nearly as possible the naked eye appearances of the tumors and their clinical manifestations, to assist others in making diagnoses correctly, while the tumor is in the body and the patient alive, in order that a fair prognosis may be made and the advisability of operative measures considered.

Let me here say, however, to those who have still lingering in their minds the ancient definition of "sarcoma" as defined by Abernethy of old, *i.e.*, "those non-malignant tumors which are fleshly in their feel and often harmless, excepting from pressure," that speaking from a tolerably large experience, it is my belief that, with few exceptions, all the so-called sarcomata, no matter whether appearing in the soft or hard structures of the body, are malignant, indeed, in some instances more so than the lower forms of carcinomata; they kill more quickly than epithelioma; they invade every structure with amazing rapidity, and though they rarely present the one great clinical characteristic difference between themselves and the carcinomata, *vis.*, "*infiltration,*" the symptoms of general adynamia are as well marked.

The sarcomas affecting the jaws will not be considered here, although I may mention a fact in this connection : That in six cases of removal of the upper maxillary bone, five were myeloid and one encephaloid, and that the average duration of life from the removal of the tumor until the death of the patient was from three to eighteen months ; that of three cases of extirpation of the lower jaw, two were for sarcomas, and both died within the year.

Sarcomas of the long bones are not of frequent occurrence, and are generally central, the sub-periosteal being even less often met with.

The former are more frequently found about the articulations, where the cancellated structure preponderates, and far away from the nutrient artery. In their commencement, especially at the epiphyses, the diagnosis is very difficult. Even gummata have been known to simulate them, while cold or scrofulous abscess of bone, and that tubercular enlargement known of old as "white swelling," often present a remarkable similarity to them. The diagnosis, however, between the innocent and the malignant growth can sometimes be made out. If a tumor occurs in any of the long bones and grows *rapidly*, is painful, has an uneven consistency with smoothness of surface, and enlargement of the subcutaneous veins (to which latter I attach great importance), with the absence of the ordinary symptoms of inflammation, the case may generally be diagnosed, but, unfortunately, there are chronic inflammations of bone and accumulations beneath the periosteum which so resemble tumors that the diagnosis becomes at times impossible, especially when it is remembered that all the symptoms of inflammation may be present in the progressive sarcomas, as in one of the cases about to be detailed. On the other hand, a very important characteristic should be remembered—that in the neoplasm proper the suppurative process is almost *nil*, while it may proceed in the healthier structure covering the growth. Suppuration, caries and necrosis certainly result from a prolonged inflammatory process in bone. Another point in the diagnosis of these tumors is of importance, and that is, whether they are central or sub-periosteal. Both varieties are malignant, and kill in about the same space, but there are some differential points which may assist the surgeon.

1. The sub-periosteal tumors are less frequent.

2. They occur much earlier in life, the average age being about twenty-two years.

3. They grow with greater rapidity than the central.

4. Their malignancy is much greater.

5. They implicate the lymphatic glands.

6. They have no bony capsule, as often, though not invariably, do the central neoplasms.

7. As a rule the joints are not invaded.

8. There is no pulsation in the sub-periosteal.

9. There may be a tendency to calcification, but the liability to fracture is much less in the periosteal than that found in the central tumors.

10. There is a peculiar radiation noticed in the sub-periosteal round-celled tumors ; after section it seems to start from certain capillary formations, and to run from thence in distinct lines, often at angles, into the very substance of the bone.

The two cases that I present are offered to show how readily the diagnosis may be made out in the one case, and how difficult it is to establish the nature of the disease, when inflammatory action exists at the same time with a growing sarcoma.

CASE I.—G. C., aged fourteen years, subject to malarial fever, and had taken large doses of quinine and Fowler's solution. When brought to me I found him emaciated, sallow, with an "ague cake" of large size, and giving all the evidences of poor nutrition and exhausted nerve force. On the lower third of the left humerus and the outer aspect of the bone was a smooth, ovoid, elastic swelling, the skin being tense, with a slight reddish blush, and a fluctuating spot here and there upon the surface. The pain in the part was not continuous, but intermittent in character, occurred chiefly toward evening and at night. Here and there over the surface the subcutaneous veins were somewhat enlarged. The elbow-joint was not involved, although the growth extended to it. An incision into one of the fluctuating spaces brought nothing but a profuse flow of venous blood, which, however, was soon checked. I made a circular amputation above the upper third, which was attended with no trouble in any way. The wound healed without an untoward symptom, but in four weeks glandular enlargements appeared above the clavicle, which increased rapidly. The boy's health, although he could go about from time to time, gradually failed ; symptoms of utter adynamia followed, with death in twenty-two months after the amputation.

On section the tumor presented here and there small portions of cartilage imbedded in the growth, the entire thickness of the shaft of the bone was destroyed, and marked radiating structure was discovered (which rested in a matrix of pulpy formation). Specimens of the tumor were not microscopically examined. But I believe it was a sub-periosteal, round-celled sarcoma; of this, however, I cannot be sure, but it was doubtless a sarcoma, and certainly it killed the patient. The age, the point of development, the trabeculated appearance to the naked eye, and its chondrification, would be the clinical evidences and the nature of the tumor.

How lymphatic enlargement appears with sarcomata in the long bones it is difficult to explain, but it may be that the sarcomatous disease existed in a latent form simultaneously with that developed in the bone, and that as soon as the more pronounced affection was removed, the glandular growths were produced.

The next case is one which possesses many interesting points. The record has been prepared for me by Dr. Knight.

CASE II.—The patient was a youth of fourteen years of age, and came under my observation in September last. Two years previously he had fallen from a horse, severely injuring the right leg. A short time thereafter a tumor appeared above the external malleolus, gave but little pain, except at night, and was accompanied with some swelling. After several careful examinations, the fluctuation was so apparent that I concluded that a cold abscess was forming, probably the result of the injury, and therefore had warm applications made to the part. I was very much in doubt as to the character of the swelling, and therefore recommended an exploratory incision. Esmarch's bandage was applied, and a long cut, extending along the middle and lower third of the leg, was made; after the skin had been cut through, the healthy peronei muscles showed themselves; on holding these aside with retractors and cutting down upon the bulbous mass, the knife entered a cavity containing a large quantity of grumous blood and some laminated membrane. This cavity seemed to have been a diffuse aneurism occasioned by the rupture of a vessel of the third caliber, perhaps a vein, at the time of the accident. A large amount of broken-down tissue was removed, but I could recognize neither bony lacunæ, nor spiculæ, nor chondroid formation. There was a profuse hemorrhage, but the cavity was stuffed, the wound approximated, a decalcified bone tube was put in, and the minutest antiseptic precautions taken. Things went well for about a week, when the temperature rose rapidly, reaching 105°; suppuration appeared in the lips of the wound, and on cutting out the sutures the parts gaped and showed me a tumor containing a cavity which contained fungoid granulations. The whole appearance then was one of a developed sarcoma, and the removal of the limb was recommended. I pause here to call attention to the fact already alluded to, that a sarcoma, when associated with inflammatory action, may be mistaken for an ordinary bone disease, and that even after exploratory, or, indeed, deep incisions, complications may occur to perplex the surgeon. Through the very center of this tumor was a large pocket entering the bone and sending a diverticulum to the other side of the leg. A counter-opening was made and thorough drainage effected; the temperature went to 99° and varied from that to 102°. At the urgent request of the boy's mother, the operation was deferred for a few days, to see if any improvement could be effected, and, indeed, his appetite in a measure returned, he sat up in bed, was cheerful, and there was no increase in the growth; in fact, it appeared to diminish; but a diarrhœa, with a rise of temperature, determined an immediate amputation. Every precaution was taken to have a perfectly antiseptic operation. It was hoped that the leg might be taken off in its upper third, but upon sawing the bone it was found to be so diseased that a knee amputation had to be performed. A long, square flap of skin was dissected off anteriorly and a short one posteriorly. The patella was left in. The flaps were held together by silver sutures, secured by lead buttons, and sewn about the edges with a continuous cat-gut suture. Bone drainage tubes were left in each angle of the wound and an air-tight antiseptic dressing was put on. Immediately after the operation the temperature fell to nearly normal. On the third day it rose to 104°. The dressing was opened and about an inch of the anterior flap found to be gangrenous. This diseased tissue was removed with the scissors and the flaps brought together by adhesive plaster. An open dressing was now put upon the stump and the flaps healed rapidly. The patient was discharged December 5th. A few days before he left the hospital a small oval tumor was discovered upon the right side at the vertebral margin of the seventh rib. An examination of the amputated leg showed the muscular tissue much broken down and destroyed. The fibula was about three times its natural size, with trabeculated cavities filled with broken-down grumous tissue, and here and there very much honey-combed. The fibular side of the tibia was also involved. Microscopical examination by Dr. Fulton showed the growth to be a round-celled, sub-periosteal sarcoma.

The subsequent history is as follows : For a while the patient continued to gain, the stump healed perfectly and he went out several times. On January 27th, after returning from a drive, he complained of feeling much exhausted. He took to his bed then and never left it alive. The tumor on his side began to grow rapidly, spreading over the abdomen and back, projecting at least a foot from his body. Another tumor soon appeared in his groin, and two weeks before he died one in the stump. The growth was very painful, and for a month or more obliged the boy to sit upright all the time. The growth finally involved the lungs, and for a while before the end he had no pain, but simply a distress for breath. Patient died April 19th, 1887, or in about ten months from the appearance of the disease.

The peculiarities of this case first consist in the cavity containing venous blood and *débris*, which is sometimes found in alveolar, and sometimes in granular celled or myeloid central tumors, and which, from the profuse blood supply, often give rise to pulsation, and have been denominated aneurism of bone. The second consideration, in view of the facts, is this : Would the boy have lived longer if he had not been operated upon? No doubt he was sarcomatous in diathesis. The immense tumor on his ribs, existing without inflammation and without pain, the extension of the disorder to the lungs and the abdomen, and finally to the stump, which was perfectly healthy in every respect after the amputation (the condyles of the femur being carefully inspected by several surgeons present), all point to such a condition, and if the leg had been left upon the body, would the other neoplasms have developed? This is a question for serious consideration, and the case is worthy of report, from its beginning to its ending presenting many unique symptoms.

NEURASTHENIA VASOMOTORIA. — Professor Rosenbach, of Breslau, considers this affection a pure neurosis of the heart, without any organic change—a symptom of general neurasthenia. We meet it most during puberty in anæmic and nervous constitutions. Excessive bodily or mental exertions, or from the cramming of students; excessive use of stimulants—tea, coffee, alcohol, tobacco; mental depressing motions, leading to melancholia, are of value in relation to ætiology. The stage of excitation is followed by one of depression. During the former we meet rapidly alternating hyperæmia, especially of the face and hands; paræsthesia of the skin, chest and upper extremities; hyperæsthesia in the cardiac region, with præcordial anguish and sensation of palpitation; sleeplessness; loss of appetite; constipation; frequent inclination to urinate. The function of the heart is hardly ever increased; the pulse beats more frequently. In the second stage paleness prevails, with despondency and lassitude. The sensation of palpitation in the heart and arteries is, notwithstanding the decreasing power of the heart and weak pulse, a lasting one; the general reflex-irritability abnormally increased; headache, vertigo and fainting present. Differentially, diagnostic points are: the age, the ætiology and the absence of all organic changes in the heart; the continuity of the symptoms; whereas, in real affections of the cardiac muscle, or of the cardiac blood-vessels, the attacks set in paroxysmally; the absence of all symptoms of stagnation; the slight changes (deep sighing) in the breathing, notwithstanding the sensation of subjective dyspnœa. When lasting too long, or improperly treated, this nervous debility of the heart may pass into real affections of the muscle and blood-vessels of the heart; but, after all, this is rarely the case. Our chief duty will be to remove the *causa noxæ*, which often means mental treatment and bodily nutrition.—*Centralblatt für Klin. Medicin*, 48, 1886.—S. L.

EDITORIAL DEPARTMENT.

THE AMERICAN INSTITUTE AND ORIGINAL WORK.

LAST year at Saratoga foretold a large attendance at this summer's meeeting of the American Institute of Homœopathy. The general satisfaction with the accommodations provided and an abundance of the side attractions which pleasantly supplement the more serious work of a convention will undoubtedly gather a still greater number, to enjoy a short vacation in a delightful resort of fashion. There is the promise of many papers, and, in general, confidence of success under the management of President Orme and his associates in office. So far as the present traditions of procedure and methods in organization will permit there is the best reason for anticipating an unusually profitable meeting. The question arises, however, what initiative in methods will be taken to improve the quality of papers, to infuse interest and vigor into the scientific meetings, and to incite original investigation? For it may be taken for granted that the success of meetings is not to be gauged by the number in attendance, or the number of papers, or the social satisfaction, but by advance in intelligent purpose to attain the fundamental objects of the organization.

With the methods in vogue during the past few years and with the general tendency of all organizations to become less definite in purpose as they increase in size, it is a question whether the customary machinery of the Institute is not in need of improvement. The plan of sectional meetings will undoubtedly provide more time for the individual bureaux; but there is also the danger of its dividing the Institute into as many special societies, which will swamp the main object of the body as a whole. The committee having the plan in process of maturing are evidently alive to this disorganizing tendency, and further remark would be premature. What requires particular attention is the present plan of confining the bureaux to assigned topics, of allotting portions of the field chosen to members of the bureaux, and of excluding all papers not relating to the special subjects agreed upon at the beginning of the year. Such a plan gives the semblance of systematized collective work, it is true, but it has resulted mainly in collated papers, reflexes of old-school writers, mostly stale. Original investigation being directed by individual bent, and not following along lines of assignment, it is a question whether the transactions would not contain more profitable matter if there were more volunteer papers growing out of individual predilections, suggested not by the special subjects of medicine in which the writer is reputed to be interested, but by voluntary choice of topic upon which he may feel he has something substantially of his own to contribute. As it is, the members of bureaux have prescribed tasks to get through with, *con amore* or not, and those not members of bureaux feel that their coöperation is not invited, or if invited, that attention will be given them after the members of the bureaux, which, in view of the large number on the list, is effectively discouraging. If the bureaux were understood as committees to secure papers as well as to prepare them, as winnowers, not necessarily producers, as more the middlemen of the Institute, it would, we believe, be decidedly more encouraging to spirited and original work. We are aware that there are reasons in favor of the customary plan, which have grown out of experience, but no reasons can outweigh the fact that it has substituted collative imitation for original investigation. There is undeniable truth in the strictures of our well-advised contemporary, *The Hahnemannian Monthly:* "The effect of these rules is to lower the Institute in its scientific work to the level of the college lecture-room and laboratory * * * and directly discourage original research and independent observation."

Again, it would appear that the Institute might be more interesting while in session if some plan were devised by which selected papers alone could gain the honor of attention. To grant a reading to every paper, skeletonized to the juiciness of bone and whether or no calculated to call out valuable thought in discussion and interest the meeting, is not intelligent economy of the brief hours at disposal. The life and movement of a medical assembly depend upon the general interest taken in the subjects, upon their novelty and the adequacy as well as pith with which they are presented, and upon the character of the discussion which follows. More than two or three papers with an instructive debate cannot be crowded into the time allotted to the bureaux, whether in general or sectional meetings, More especially should there be intelligent planning for discussion. Every discussion needs to be led by men prepared to seize the salient points and start the current of debate in the right direction. There might be some sort of an executive board, whose duty it should be to select the papers and to secure the leaders in discussion; or the bureaux might severally assume this responsibility, each for its own portion of time.

There is another point which should lie very close to the heart of every member who believes that there are greater possibilities in homœopathic therapeutics than are now developed. It is the proud boast of the school that it has the only rule by which the curative use of a drug is certainly learned from its properly observed effect upon the healthy human organism. But the experimental work carried out by the Institute during the past few years is a practical disclaimer of the vital efficacy of this belief. The study of the materia medica as it is and the effort to make it what it ought to be constitute the very elixir of life of homœopathy. The most needful subject for agitation just now is involved in questions which we have previously suggested : How can the American Institute become in verity an American investigating Hahnemann of the latter half of the nineteenth century? How can the Institute be organized into an experimental body of national proportions, having as its essential object the reformation and augmentation of the materia medica upon the basis of collective accurate, conclusive and adequate experiments? And how can' the onus of work, heretofore laden upon a few in committees, be distributed by them, not as heretofore to a few fitful volunteers, but to the many, actually organized to carry out to finality systematic investigation? Such questions may seem Utopian, but homœopathic therapeutics would derive more benefit from the Institute if ideal yearnings stirred up more desire for perfection. Let us hope that the formative spirit of the Institute, after brooding so long in lethargy, will seize the resources of the school for experimental drug science and direct them into channels where they may flow together, a mighty stream of usefulness. And even if it should be deemed impracticable to organize efficiently for systematic research, it surely is more in the power of the Institute to stimulate directly individual drug research and therapeutic study. It would be no difficult matter to secure endowments for prizes for the best provings during the year, for the best original study in the existing materia medica, and for the most valuable addition to the treatment of disease by the homœopathic method.

A GRAPHIC CASE.

IN the *North American Review* for May, 1887, there is an interesting article upon "Beecher's Personality," in which the writer, Dr. W. S. Searle (his physician), gives an exquisite instance of drug-action according to the law of similars. Mr. Beecher, it will be remembered, was a patron of homœopathy.

" 'Emotion with me works inward, not outward, often till it seems as if there were a vast gulf formed by it within me. My intellectual efforts are intuitional, to a large extent. A sermon seems spread out before me like a picture, into which my brain seems to open out, and inspired by which I preach. All this is customary and normal, but latterly, as a result, I think, of mental strain, there has come upon me a peculiar experience, which I clearly recognize as illusional, but which, nevertheless, is very real to me. I retire at night and sleep well until about 4 A. M., when I am startled from a sleep which has been dreamless by hearing my name called, and I lie awake, hearing, distinctly and with apparent realty, voices calling me in the sweetest and most inviting tones. Nothing of terror is experienced : on the contrary, my moral state is the most blissful and entrancing. I seem to be on the very borders of Heaven. Now, while this is the case, my judicial reasoning self lies there, perfectly aware that this is all hallucination, and the outworking of an overwrought and overstrained brain. I seem to have a double existence, as if another self were beside me in the bed—one perfectly sane and recognizing the other as abnormal, and the other under the full sway of these illusionary perceptions—as well satisfied with their reality as if they truly existed. Now, I have yet four weeks of labor before I can go to grass for the summer's rest, and I want to be sustained so far as may be during them.

" 'Something of the sort has come to me when in a fever. Then, my being has seemed to become a noun of multitude, my feet seemed a tenement-house full of insubordinate tenants, whom I endeavored to control in vain. Each separate part of me was an individual, and all in discord. But the most curious imagination has been that I was a locomotive, all fired up, and impatiently waiting for the engineer who would come to start me '

"To some it may be interesting to add that this hallucination was quickly dispelled by the administration of Cannabis Indica, or Haschish, as it is called in the East. To all, it is an autobiographical exposé of the workings of this marvelous intellect, and the sensitiveness of this harplike organism, while it also demonstrates the sound substratum of common sense which recognized at once the cause of his condition, and sought in medicine for its cure."

We may also add that it likewise demonstrates Mr. Beecher's good sense in seeking the homœopathic method for its cure.

MIDDLETOWN STATISTICS.

THE Sixteenth Annual Report (Jan. 12th, 1887,) of the State Homœopathic Asylum for the Insane, at Middletown, N. Y., furnishes interesting reading and convincing testimony of the superior relative efficacy of pure homœopathic treatment conjoined with intelligent hygiene. In Superintendent Talcott's statement there are most instructive practical suggestions which every practitioner would gain by knowing. Attention is called to the advantages of early treatment in the Asylum ; to the important plan of hospital treatment of the insane; to proper food ; to diversion after rest; to the preventable causes of insanity ; to school training for the insane, and to leading indications for homœopathic remedies. We regret that our rule, not to reprint from other journals, published reports and transactions—a rule which, by the way, was established to secure novelty in the papers upon our original pages—must prevent republication of many portions worthy of the widest perusal. The report should be in the hands especially of the homœopathists of other states, where there are no homœopathic asylums for the insane. Dr. Talcott, by his executive talent and gift in working out the indications for the selection of the similar, has rendered a great service to humanity through homœopathy. Recent graduates should appreciate the wide field which he has been opening for them; for, with the demonstrated success of the New York Asylum, other states will follow the example of New York in rapid order. We need, in advance, a full force of physicians, carefully trained in the management and homœopathic treatment of insanity, so that the pretext which enabled the old school to catch our Michigan neighbors napping may never again be used with even the semblance of belief. The Middletown Asylum is not only a great pioneer in its work, but an opportunity for education which young physicians cannot value too highly.

It will be remembered that the percentage of recoveries on the whole number of discharges during 1886 was 50.95, the best record which the Asylum has yet had. We subjoin, as still more clinching, Table No. 3:

SHOWING PERCENTAGE OF DEATHS ON WHOLE NUMBER TREATED.

	Whole number treated.	Deaths.	per centages.
1874,	69	4	5.79
1875,	152	11	7.23
1876,	195	14	7.17
1877,	228	14	6.14
1878,	284	15	5.28
1879,	283	15	5.30
1880,	311	13	4.18
1881,	340	15	4.41
1882,	391	20	5.11
1883,	410	18	4.39
1884,	423	21	4.96
1885,	486	27	5.55
1886,	568	17	2.99

AN IMPORTANT UNDERTAKING.

D R. RICHARD HUGHES, has described our materia medica as "a *rudis indigestaque moles*, a picture in which one cannot see the wood for the trees, and which bears no resemblance to anything upon earth." Whatever the resemblance, the description accords with the feelings of practitioners, dropped into the midst of the woods to clear out a system of study and art of selecting for themselves. And, as such constructive power is unfortunately the gift of only a few, the average man fails to acquire a satisfactory grasp of the materia medica. There is nothing which he desires to know systematically so much, and nothing which eludes his endeavor more. Discomfiture necessarily results in discouragement, and discouragement in apathy and alienation. A simple, salient materia medica, with outlines firmly and tersely sketched, and confusing minor details omitted, is a consummation devoutly wished for, the most practical kind of boon to homœopathic prescription. It gives us great pleasure, therefore, to call attention to the first of a series of articles, which will appear in our pages from month to month, upon "Outlines of the Materia Medica," by Dr. T. F. Allen. His preëminent fitness needs no comment. In his gift of seizing broad distinctions and power of tersely composing them, as well as in his comprehensive knowledge, both of his subject and the needs of the student and practitioner, will be readily recognized the assurance of a most notable contribution to our science and literature.

CHANGE OF BUSINESS MANAGERS.

W ITH the May number, Dr. George G. Shelton resigned the position of Business Manager of this journal, and Dr. Arthur B. Norton was appointed to fill the vacancy. Dr. Shelton has labored, at much personal sacrifice, to inaugurate and establish the JOURNAL upon its present basis, and, having been largely instrumental in achieving it, his other duties could no longer permit the expenditure of time required for the transaction of our business, He retires with the thanks of the Directors, who would express their appreciation of his valued services, which have been without remuneration, and performed with energy and devotion. The fact that the JOURNAL is now upon a self-supporting financial foundation is sufficient testimony of their confidence in his management.

The attention of readers is directed to the address of our new Business Manager, who will attend promptly to all communications.

COMMENTS.

SOCIETY OBLIGATIONS.—This is emphatically an age of organization. Without it concerted action is impossible, and progress, if not absolutely prevented, is retarded. The work accomplished by the leading homœopathic bodies in this country during the past thirty years can hardly be too greatly estimated. By this work, the feeble and struggling handful of homœopathic physicians fifty years ago have become to-day a compact and powerful organization. Only by united effort, by societies and other organizations, can that public recognition be obtained which insures equality before the law and defeats the perennial attacks of a disintegrating sect. Added to this power of offense and defense, inherent in every body of associated men, are the advantages that naturally come from association—the advancement of professional knowledge, the encouragement of scientific study, and the stimulation of mind, produced by contact with the brightest and best intellects. That society work is and has been of the highest importance ; that its results are tangible and valuable, no physician, unless besottedly ignorant, will attempt to deny. But, while all are willing to share in the benefits, but few are found willing to come in the vanguard of workers, and share in the burden and heat of the day. Some, vaguely aware that a society meeting is to be held, have no thought of attending. Others, too indolent to furnish papers, or take part in discussion, sneeringly criticise the proceedings at a safe distance. Still others—and these are the pure and noble patriots—cry out in distress that the organization is in the hands of a ring, and they cannot countenance such proceedings. Well, gentlemen stay-at-homes, in the name of Aristides the Just, what would you have? If the papers are dull and prosy, or too long drawn out, why do you not write better and brighter ones? If the discussions drag, or are flat and unprofitable, why do you not inject new life in 'the debate? If the organization is really in the hands of a clique, why do not you attend and vote it down? If you are so anxious to grasp the beneficial results, why do you lurk so far in the rear? And if you do attend a society meeting, do something while you are there. Make your presence known—your influence felt. The man who, returning from a society, boisterously proclaims the meeting a failure, and regrets his loss of time in attendance, announces his own incapacity for social work, and creates a justifiable suspicion that he contributed nothing towards the success of the meeting. Let there be a representative gathering at Saratoga. The time and place are favorable, and an enjoyable programme will be offered.

TOLERANCE.—Dr. Lilienthal mildly inquires in one of our exchanges why he should be written down an ass for holding certain opinions, and intimates, indirectly, that he has received some of the vulgar abuse the ignorant controversialist delights to shower upon his more intelligent and courteous opponent. The venerable doctor seems surprised at his treatment, and his inquiry, translated, may read, "Why are the pages of certain homœopathic journals disfigured by coarse and offensive personalities?" The inquiry may well be made, for of late the pages of some of our exchanges have been so besmirched with impudent familiarity and vulgar epithet, that one is seized with a desire to take the tongs and consign the offending periodical to oblivion, or the ash-barrel. This manner of argument is the natural result of an ignorant or intolerant mind. Mr. Beecher once said, that bigotry is "most contemptible from a human standpoint, and disgraceful from the standpoint of Christianity." Mr. Beecher was undoubtedly right. It has been said that tolerance is "the willing consent that other men should hold and express opinions with which we disagree, until they are convinced by *reason* that these opinions are untrue." Tolerance, then, does not merely mean the forgetting of differences, but the clear recognition of them, and the hearty acceptance and use of them. Perhaps if some of our esteemed contemporaries should use a little reason in place of invective, they might find it fully as effective.

DR. BRUNTON SQUIRMS.—Dr. Lauder Brunton's work entitled, "Therapeutics, Pharmacology and Materia Medica," has reached a third edition. There is no marked change in the body of the work, it is as decidedly homœopathic as ever, but the preface has been remodeled in a vain attempt to explain why his book smacks so strongly of homœopathy. A desperate attempt. But the Doctor flounders bravely along and finally gets helplessly mired. In sheer desperation, probably, he undertakes to define a homœopathic medicine, not what it is, but what it is not. Listen: "The mere fact that a drug in small doses will cure a disease exhibiting symptoms similar to those produced by a large dose of the drug does not constitute—is not a homœopathic medicine." The homœopathic school in this country has labored under the impression that this was just what did constitute a homœopathic remedy. Dr. Brunton acknowledges that his "Index of Diseases and Remedies," was chiefly compiled from Dr. S. V. L. Potter's work on "Comparative Therapeutics." Dr. Potter is a member of the American Institute of Homœopathy, and has actively participated in the proceedings. The Dr. will have to explain again.

A NEW RULE.—Something must be wrong with the morality of the Harvard student. It is probably that he does not always tread the path of rectitude and peace. At least it may be inferred from the new rule lately promulgated by the Harvard Faculty. They now require that in all cases in which the college has heretofore required a physician's certificate to the fact of illness of absent students, such certificates must specify the cause of illness, in order that the Faculty may be able to judge of the validity of the excuse for absence. There can be no doubt but that such a rule is a mistake. It steps between the patient and the physician, and requires the latter to violate confidence reposed in him. Moreover, the Faculty assume the power of sitting in judgment on the physician's opinion as to the severity of the disease and its required treatment.

BOOK REVIEWS.

TRANSACTIONS OF THE INTERNATIONAL HOMŒOPATHIC CONVENTION, 1886. London: E. GOULD & SON, 1886.

TRANSACTIONS OF THE HOMŒOPATHIC MEDICAL SOCIETY OF THE STATE OF PENNSYLVANIA, 1886.

TRANSACTIONS OF THE MASSACHUSETTS HOMŒOPATHIC MEDICAL SOCIETY, 1886. Boston, 1887.

TRANSACTIONS OF THE HOMŒOPATHIC MEDICAL SOCIETY OF THE STATE OF NEW YORK, 1887. Part I.

The proceedings of the International Convention occupy a volume of 274 pages, thoroughly edited and presented in the original languages in which the papers were prepared. Considering the haste with which the Convention was organized at the last moment by the energy of Dr. Hughes, the contents are interesting, though small in bulk. Abstracts of the principal papers having previously appeared in our columns, no special mention need be made. The general character of the transactions are commendable in being distinctively homœopathic, in this respect furnishing a model for our own societies. It is to be noted, also, that scrapped collations from books are conspicuously absent. The Transactions, while disappointing from the standpoint of what they might have been had our Belgian colleagues worked with purpose and will are, thanks to Dr. Hughes, of genuine value in a library as a record of the status of homœopathy in various parts of the world, and as containing instructive papers which are by very many too few. The paper and print are excellent.

Massachusetts sends out a thin volume of 185 pages, containing nothing in the way of collective investigation or original matter worth noting in review. It is not a creditable record of serious society zeal; and, coming after its predecessor of 1885, which showed some activity in homœopathic research, it is disappointing, especially so as representative of a State supposed to be foremost in New England energy.

But if Massachusetts is lank of contents, New York is stricken with poverty. The general make-up has an impecunious suggestiveness, a slip-shod, down-at-the-heel sort of air which betokens utter dispiritment. It has the merit of putting in a prompt, if disreputable, appearance. There must be something radically at fault either in the organization or traditional methods of the society. The officers of the past year were zealous and capable, and if there had been a due appreciation of obligation upon the part of individual members to the interests of homœopathy, or even a proper pride in a respectable appearance before the world, we would have been spared this reflec-

tion upon the Empire State. Evidently the society's large and capable
membership needs to be aroused to a due sense of the fitness of
things, and all members should fall to with a will to remove disaffection
and apathy, first in themselves and afterwards in others. Without
including in our criticism the few who contributed papers, it is to be
hoped that this will be the last misrepresentative issued by the
society.

The Transactions of Pennsylvania offer varied contents, which furnish much interesting and instructive reading. All the Bureaus present
full reports, and the papers are homœopathic in their therapeutic bear-
ings. There are no contributions in new drug research, but there is
evidence of attentive study of our materia medica. The therapeutics
of hemorrhages, collectively elaborated, is of noteworthy value. The
volume, as a whole, is well edited, and the most creditable of all the
State Society Transactions.

A PRACTICAL TREATISE ON OBSTETRICS. Vols. I., II., and III.,
by A. CHARPENTIER, M.D., Paris. Illustrated with lithographic
plates and wood engravings. These are also vols. of the
"Cyclopedia of Obstetrics and Gynæcology" (12 vols.), issued
monthly during 1888. New York : William Wood & Co.

Vol. I treats of the *anatomy of the internal and external genital organs,
menstruation, fecundation, normal pregnancy and labor,* and comprises
507 pages of text and illustrations. The latter (267 wood engravings
and 4 colored plates) have the merit not always attained in medical
works, of being clear and readily understood in their relation to parts
to which they refer; in the chapters on *anatomy* they afford objectively
a better understanding of the medical features of the female pelvic organs and contiguous structures than any other work on obstetrics we
have seen, though many cuts are not original, but taken from works
some of which are familiar to the American profession.

In the remarks on *"the management of the normal puerperium"* the
position taken by the editor against the *routine* practice of using vaginal injections during this period ; against the advised delay (eighteen
to twenty-four hours) in putting the child to the breast in all cases,
and his suggestions about dressings of the vulva are all logical and
commendable.

Vol. II. contains 381 pages, illustrated by 45 wood engravings and
2 colored plates, and treats, under the general title "PATHOLOGY OF
PREGNANCY" of (1) *disease affecting the pregnant woman, independent of
the gravid state;* (2) *diseases of pregnancy;* (3) *disease of the ovum ;* (4)
disease of the fœtus ; (5) *miscarriage,* and (6) *extra-uterine pregnancy.*
Many pages in this volume evidence the good work done by the
editor in the way of corrections and additions to conform with present
knowledge and belief on these subjects. His note on erosion under
ulcerations (?) *of the cervix during pregnancy,* p. 32, and reference to
Figs. 11 to 7 by Nieberding, on the succeeding page, will be generally
accepted as correct.

Vol. III. contains 348 pages, including 248 wood engravings, and
treats of "THE PATHOLOGY OF LABOR," in two divisions: (1) *"maternal
dystocia,"* and (2) *"dystocia due to the fœtus."* A third chapter deals

with "*ergot and its uses.*" The conclusions arrived at by the author
limiting the use of *ergot* to "hemorrhages of the puerperium," are
eminently wise and far in advance of the ordinary practice of using
ergot in this country at that date (1882). The routine habit of giving
a dose of *ergot* before leaving a patient after confinement is condemned. On this point the author seems to be in advance of the
editor, who rather favors this use of *ergot* (Vol. I., p. 502).
Most practitioners now, we believe, accept Pajot's law, "as long
as the uterus contains anything, be it child, placenta, membranes,
clots, never administer *ergot;*" we also believe that an added number
of physicians each year will agree with Dr. Reamy, of Cincinnati, that
"*ergot* not only closes up the uterus, but likewise interferes with the circulation within it, and therefore interferes with the process of involu-
tion and must lay the foundation for sepsis."

The three vols. taken together (Vol. IV. not yet issued) indicate that
the work will be a valuable addition to the literature on obstetrics
heretofore printed in English. Too much cannot be said in commendation of the enterprise of the publishers who continue to place
standard works within the reach of the great majority of the medical
profession in this country. D—N.

A TEXT-BOOK OF PATHOLOGICAL ANATOMY AND PATHO-
GENESIS, by ERNST ZIEGLER, Professor of Pathological Anatomy
in the University of Tübingen. Translated and edited for Eng-
lish students by Donald MacAlister, M.A., M.D., F.R.C.P., etc.
Three parts complete in one volume. New York: Wm. Wood &
Co., 1887. Octavo. Pp. 1091.

The immense amount of observation and learning packed into
these pages in practical form for the systematic instruction of un-
dergraduates renders the work of equal value to practitioners. Having
passed through four German editions in four years, it is now within
the reach of American readers, who will appreciate it as fully as it has
been in the author's nation, where it has become the standard. The
translator has produced a text of clearness, almost faultless, in which
he has preserved the objectivity of style so characteristic of the original.
It is, generally speaking, the best book to study from and refer to; full
up to the times, accurate, succinct, copiously illustrated, systematically
arranged, and thoroughly indexed. The citation of authorities in
whose works the subjects can be more fully followed up is not the
least valuable portion. A marked merit lies in the definiteness, direct-
ness and completeness with which all that is attempted is expressed.
Dr. MacAlister, by adding matter in brackets and careful revision, in
which he had the assistance of Professors Klein and Greenfield, with
other eminent English pathologists, has materially supplemented the
original.

A COMPEND OF ELECTRICITY AND ITS MEDICAL AND
SURGICAL USES, by CHAS. F. MASON, M.D. Philadelphia: P.
Blakiston, Son & Co., 1887. Pp. 100. No. 3. Medical Briefs.

This is a very brief, rudimentary manual, designed for students.
As an introduction to the study of the subject it will be found useful.

CORRESPONDENCE.

To the Editors of the North American Journal of Homœopathy:

The eleventh meeting of the California State Homœopathic Medical Society took place May 11th and 12th, and as the Y. M. Ch. S. had a large meeting in their own hall, we met in the large lecture room of the college, and the audience filled the room to the utmost. In fact, the homœopathic school is booming, like everything else, just now, on this coast, and over thirty new members were enrolled the first evening, after having passed the scrutiny of the censors. Where did those new members come from? "Go west," said Greeley, and these young men from the east did not stop "go west," till the Pacific commanded a halt. But our young men from the east need not be afraid to come; there is plenty of room on this Pacific coast, and there is still many a nook and corner left where a homœopathic physician would do well. This even holds good in the larger cities, only it takes a much longer time to get a foothold, and the expenses are as large as they are in New York or Philadelphia. But *revenons à nos moutons.*

All the business, even to the election of officers for the ensuing year, is done the first evening, and thus the following days can be dedicated to the real work of the session—a wise plan, which ought to be followed even by the American Institute, as thus all log-rolling is more easily prevented. I am most happy to say that genuine homœopathy grows here luxuriantly and the tenets of the *Organon* are more strictly adhered to than it is with the members of many older societies. Still, great liberty is everywhere allowable, as long as it does not degenerate into license. The first paper in the morning was read by Dr. Martin, on the limitation of zymotic diseases, especially typhoid and cholera, and he took the affirmative side of the question, when treated homœopathically from the start. Dr. Worth believes in mercury and kali bichrom. in diphtheria, and hardly ever uses anything else. That this brought on a long discussion may be imagined, as we do not treat generalities, but want every case to be strictly individualized. Ledyard, who is a strong adherent of the high potencies, gave cases from practice, and the general applause which followed showed that California homœopaths do not consider them moonshine. Similar cases were reported by Mr. Neal, especially on delirium tremens, a disease of the coast, where alcohol has still too many adherents. The most interesting paper was that of G. H. Martin of Honolulu, on the climate of the Hawaiian Islands, which have every variety of climate, from semi-tropic to snow, and he warned the physicians not to send their phthisical patients to the Islands. I hope to see his interesting paper in full in one of our journals.

The same carelessness everywhere—these bureaus without a paper, for which the chairs are to blame. Mrs. Dr. Ballard read a paper on the care of new-born infants, but it fell dead on these grown-up M.D.'s, who rather wished to listen to the report of surgery. In fact, clinical medicine and surgery are the favorite topics in western countries, where the physician is so often forced to use his own ingenuity in treating accidents, and the treatment of gunshot wounds (everybody, nearly, carries his revolver in his trousers) took up nearly the whole afternoon.

Everywhere the tail-end of bureaus is slaughtered, and there is no help for it; their only hope is in the next year, when they will stand at the head. As everywhere, most work is done by the few, and the *oi polloi* have no time nor inclination for literary labor.

Still, I am glad to have convinced myself that homœopathy is flourishing on the coast; that surgery is carried out by most of our men without intruding on their allopathic neighbors; that the school, started here with small beginning, is steadily growing in favor with the public, and the output, to use a miner's expression, is bright.

SAN FRANCISCO, May 14th, 1887.   S. LILIENTHAL.

REPORTS OF SOCIETIES AND HOSPITALS.

HOMŒOPATHIC MEDICAL SOCIETY, COUNTY OF NEW YORK.

THE regular monthly meeting of the Homœopathic Medical Society of the County of New York, was held in the reception room of the New York Ophthalmic Hospital, on Thursday evening, April 21st, at eight o'clock.

President Beebe in the chair.

Drs. Geo. B. Dowling and Isabella M. Pettit, were elected members of the Society.

The Committee on Clinical Medicine, Lewis Hallock, M.D., Chairman, reported four papers.

Dr. Hallock then read the first paper of the evening on "Epidemic Diarrhœa and Dysentery."

Dr. Dearborn :—I have not seen much about these cases of diarrhœa and dysentery that led me to suppose they were epidemic in their nature, but, so far as I have been able to inquire into these cases, they have seemed to me to be of the nature of catarrhal disturbances, and, in most of the cases, to result from the violent changes of temperature. The patients were affected with catarrhal disturbance of the small or large intestines, instead of the more ordinary rhinitis. As to the one *symptom*, diarrhœa, these cases *seem* to be very much alike, and perhaps for this reason might be attributed to epidemic influences. Against the epidemic nature of these attacks stands the facts that the conditions of each individual who had this disease were different, and that no one remedy seemed to meet these cases, and that indications were pretty well distributed over the various remedies for cases of diarrhœa. I have seen them show indications for *phytolacca, bryonia*, or *nux vom.*, which is not often a remedy in diarrhœa, but in these cases it acted very promptly. I saw some mention of cases of epidemic diarrhœa in Chicago, by Dr. E. M. Hale, in attacks beginning with acute coryza, and the catarrhal trouble extending to the stomach and bowels, and characterized by profuse watery evacuations morning and evening *only*. Dr. Hale named *cotoin* 2x as a prompt and satisfactory remedy. The most noticeable features of these attacks of winter diarrhœa that I have observed, have been the *sudden onset* and *short duration* of the affection under the use of an appropriate homœopathic remedy. My cases have averaged less than three days duration, quite in contrast with cases of summer diarrhœa or dysentery lasting six to ten days.

Dr. Fulton:—Several cases of this kind have come under my care this winter. In a neighboring town also many cases have occurred of a nature similar to those spoken of. All of these cases of diarrhœa were characterized by the same symptomatology. They were ushered in by a violent nasal catarrh, which was very soon followed by the diarrhœa, which was painless, abundant, and occurred mainly in the early morning. The disturbance of the alimentary track disappeared in a few days, leaving in its stead a more or less vigorous bronchitis; with troublesome cough, which was very persistent. The trouble partook more of the nature of an old-fashioned influenza, being characterized by a more acute catarrhal condition of both the digestive and respiratory tract, with fever and prostration. The bronchitis which remained was more troublesome to relieve than the preceding diarrhœa. In my cases sulphur was of the greatest service.

Dr. Leal :—I have noticed a few of these cases, and one point struck me as common to all of them, and that was a very decided prostration. I think in about eight or ten of the cases which I have seen within the last four weeks, the majority of them developed catarrhal symptoms. In some, after the diarrhœa ceased, the catarrhal symptoms still held on. In one case the diarrhœa began very suddenly with pain, and was checked almost immediately by giving *podopyllin* ix, which was the one remedy that seemed to cover the symptoms in the majority of cases. In three cases which I now recall, one dose was given at the time of the visit, with directions to repeat it after each stool ; and in all these three cases there was no more trouble, nor need for repetition of the remedy.

Dr. Dearborn :—I was in the presence of eight or ten medical gentlemen some weeks ago, when they all volunteered to give the remedy they had found most useful, and there were only two who named the same drug. Most of them had different remedies, and they each based the remedy employed upon the character of the attacks; the same fact is apparent in the experience of those given here to-night, and, as I said before, this at least confirms me in the feeling that the attacks are somewhat due to individual and temporary causes, rather than to a general epidemic influence.

Dr. Moffat read the second paper on " Hodgkin's Disease, with Cases."

Discussion, Dr. Dowling.

Dr. Fulton :—Among the different names given by Dr. Moffat, which are considered to apply to this affection, is that of lympho-sarcoma, first used by Virchow. As applied, however, by the German physician and understood by most surgeons, it represents quite another disease from Hodgkin's. Lympho-sarcoma is a malignant affection of perhaps one gland or a chain of glands, and does not generalize itself throughout the entire glandular system, in the manner which is characteristic of Hodgkin's disease. Generalization occurs, but it is the generalization of malignancy as seen typically in sarcoma and carcinoma. The microscopic appearance is also very different from that of simple enlarged glands. I have one very fine microscopic specimen of lympho-sarcoma taken from a tumor of the jaw and neck, which was removed by Dr. Wilcox from a colored man. The bulk of the tumor is composed of small, round-celled sarcoma corpuscles, held together in a net-work of fibrous and myxomatous tissue, while scattered throughout the specimen were ducts, oval in shape, and lined with perfectly formed columnar epithelium. These were the characteristic features. Just how they came in a lymph node, which is not epithelial in its nature, I am not prepared to state, but I have seen the same characteristic columnar epithelium in an enlarged lymph node taken from the mesentary of a man who died from scirrhus cancer of the liver. It would seem that malignant infection of the lymph nodes starts the development of cells, which, while seen in other portions of the body, are entirely atypical when referred to these bodies. I have seen the same development in lympho-sarcoma of the testicle in a speci-men while studying with Dr. Heitzman. These characteristics, together with the fact that lympho-sarcoma cause the destruction of bone and all other tissues adjacent to it, are sufficient to distinguish it from Hodgkin's disease.

Dr. Dearborn:—I have only seen one case of Hodgkin's disease in private practice, and I only saw it twice. It was fatal, as they all are. I remember during my course of study to have seen two or three cases in the hospitals. I do not remember how the cases were treated. In some of these cases the disease had been traced to primary local injury. That, I believe, is the only exciting cause to which this disease has been traced. It is important in cases where some glands are affected to make a positive diagnosis from other glandular affections, and in many cases this is impossible until the case has progressed. Though the disease is rare, this difficulty in making an early diagnosis gives it greater clinical interest.

Dr. Schley then read a paper on " A Valuable Remedy in the Cure of Organic Heart Disease."

Dr. A. R. McMichael:—There has been only one case of heart trouble in which I have had occasion to use the *iodide of sodium*, and that was one of dilatation without hypertrophy. Attacks of angina occurred daily. *Iodide of arsenic* was prescribed every two hours and continued two weeks, with relief, when the *iodide of sodium* was tried in five-grain doses three times a day, the relief was immediate, and continued as long as the patient was under its influence; as soon as it was discontinued, which was after a two weeks' trial, the pains returned, when the *iodide of arsenic* was given again, and continued several weeks. Although the relief was not immediate, it was more permanent.

Dr. Cowl:—With reference to the idea that angina pectoris is simply a functional disorder, it strikes me that though we may not discover any organic lesions about the heart such as we find, however, in the majority of cases, we may take the ground that the patient who suffers from angina pectoris would not do so unless there were some local trouble. There may be disease of the heart which we do not discover *post mortem*, although in the majority of cases angina pectoris is attributable to some marked trouble about the heart, rather than to some irregularity about the nervous system.

· Dr. Dillow:—The remedy belongs to the class whose use has been derived from clinical observation rather than therapeutic law, and it is by no means clear as yet that it really cures any organic disease of the heart. In other words, it belongs to the class of empirical remedies whose *modus operandi* and sphere of application have not been determined. The theories cited to explain its action are very speculative, and when pressed back to their ultimate meaning, explain nothing. Certainly this is true with regard to the so-called absorbent action, the word absorbent express-ing a supposed fact of disappearance of morbid products rather than any explanation of *modus operandi*. The chemical theory is even more vague, the imaginary reactions occurring being entirely unknown. Where they occur, what they definitely are, belongs to supposition and not science. We must remember, then, that dealing with an empirical remedy, we cannot come to anything like positive conclusions unless we have a large number of cases from which to form a deduction either as to its efficiency, its mode of operation, or sphere of application. It will probably turn out with the *iodide of sodium* as with other drugs empirically used, that it will appear to act in one case and fail in another, for reasons which cannot be determined. I apprehend that after the first flush of its introduction is over and the evidence comes to be sifted, it will not prove so curative as is now promised. And if it should prove to be curative, its action is as likely to be homœopathic as any other, for all that now appears to the contrary.

I would ask the author of the paper what effect the *iodide of sodium* had upon the coincident kidney affections where these existed, and whether the renal manifestations were probably secondary to the cardiac lesions ?

Dr. Schley:—In the first place I differ with Dr. Dillow. Medicine, as I hold it, is more or less empirical. We do not understand *how* medicines act in the large majority of cases, even under the laws of homœopathy. The *iodide of potassium* does *not* cure all cases of syphilis in the tertiary stage, unfortunately, nor would the *iodide of sodium* cure *all* cases of angina pectoris. In Dr. Henri Huchard's nine cases of angina pectoris five were cured; the others were relieved, or indifferently affected. As to the changes noticed in those suffering from nephritis, if there were any, it was for the better. Dr. Huchard detected *iodine* in the urine. The causes of angina pectoris are still very obscure, and in replying to Dr. Dowling as to its pathology, I would cite five cases recently tabulated by Dr. Gowers, observed during life by him, and where an autopsy showed, in *three* cases, a dilatation of the ventricles filled with blood; in two cases a contracted ventricle, nearly empty. This would speak against a *local* vaso-motor paresis. In all of these cases organic trouble was present in the valves, muscles and coronary arteries, either anterior or posterior. But there is another condition of angina, which is purely nervous. Such patients die suddenly, and no organic disease is found *post mortem*. Persons die apparently from angina pectoris in two ways— the one from a sudden paralysis of the heart, the other from local vasomotor spasm. In reply to Dr. McMichael as to the continuance of the treatment, I would say that, in my opinion, such cases are to be kept under the influence of the drug for an indefinite length of time, whether the cause be a nervous or organic one, and I lay especial weight upon the fact that all my patients had palpable heart trouble. Dr. Dowling's case in Albany was evidently not one of angina pectoris. The case I mentioned first, continues to improve; she still continues to take the *iodide of sodium*, and I propose to let her continue it. The dose administered now is three or four grains nights on retiring.

Dr. F. J. Nott then read a paper upon "The Temperature Curve in Typhoid Fever."

Dr. Clark :—As far as the old school observations go, it seems to me that the older writers noticed an even curve in the temperature, but later, like Pepper, when they get nearer to homœopathy in their treatment, the temperature curve changes, for we all know that a well-selected remedy (homœopathic) will *modify* the fever.

Dr. Cowl :—Dr. W. J. Martin, of Pittsburgh, Pa., reported 100 consecutive cases of typhoid fever without a death in the *Hahnemannian Monthly* some three years ago, and makes a statement similar to that of Dr. Nott concerning the temperature.

Dr. Schley :—Dr. Dowling's idea is quite correct, that these typical cases do exist. They are frequently met with in Germany and Austria. Liebermeister, while professor at Tübingen, undoubtedly saw many such instances. I, myself, in Prof. Bamberger's wards in Vienna, have had the opportunity to see and study them. I have observed their running the usual course of fourteen to twenty-one days, the temperature gradually rising until the crisis is reached. In New York my experience has been somewhat similar to Dr. Nott's. This modification is due here, I think, to climate, plumbing and method of treatment employed. And I would state again, Mr. President, as I have often done before in this Soci-

ety, that I am still of the opinion that the course of typhoid fever cannot
be checked any more than that of an uncomplicated croupous pneumonia.
Meeting adjourned at 10.50.

RECORD OF MEDICAL PROGRESS.

THE COCCUS OF TRACHOMA.—Dr. E. Schmidt is stated to have succeeded in finding Sattler's micro-organism of trachoma, which, he says,
is very similar to staphylo-coccus pyogenes. By a culture of this coccus
he succeeded in inducing granular lids in dogs and cats.—*London Lancet*,
April 30th, 1887.

COMMON SALT IN MIGRAINE.—Dr. Babow, of Berlin, finds that half a
teaspoonful of common salt, taken as soon as the premonitory symptoms
of an attack of migraine begin to show themselves, will frequently cut it
short in about half an hour ; similar treatment has also been proved of
service in epilpesy, as was remarked some years ago by Nothnagel; the explanation being probably in both cases that a violent reflex action is set
up.—*London Lancet*, May 7th, 1887.

A CASE OF CHRONIC DIPHTHERIA.—Luigi Concetti observed in a boy of
five years a case of nasal diphtheria, which lasted for months, but failed to
show decisive symptoms of the disease, so that the doctor considered it at
first a catarrhal rhinitis. During the initial stage, and twice afterwards,
febrile symptoms appeared, caused by the absorption of infectious material stagnated in the nasal cavity. Towards the end of the disease paralysis of the velum palati set in. There was never a symptom of diphtheritic deposit in the fauces or larynx. During the same time three children
of the same family were attacked by the disease, and one little girl of
fourteen months succumbed to it. Cases of chronic nasal diphtheria are
frequently observed during an epidemic, and are too often diagnosed as
a simple catarrhal rhinitis, and we ought to be, therefore, more careful
and consider even the mildest case of rhinitis, under such circumstances,
suspicious.—*Prog. Med. Wochenschrift*, 11, 1887.—S. L.

ON LEAD-PALSY.—Oscar Yierordt (Leipzig), found in the autopsy of a
clear case of lead-palsy only severe degeneration of the serous radicles,
less so of the medianus, and hardly any of the ulnaris. After studying the
literature of lead-palsy, he speaks against the supposition of a purely
central origin; he would rather consider it a motory-trophic neuritis or
myo-neuritis, believing that the chronic action of lead may be described
as a poison which simultaneously affects the cell of the anterior cornua,
peripheral motory-nerve fibers, the end plate and muscle fibrillæ. As the
motory-trophic impulse is thus ignored and the nervous conduction—on
account of the affected nerves—retarded, the whole system suffers primarily
in the peripheral parts most distant from the central parts. The affection
progresses towards the center, and when the patient lives long enough,
may attack the ganglia of the anterior cornua. The extensors are more
frequently affected, because in general they perform the most labor.—
Arch. f. Psychiatrie 18, p. 48.—S. L.

TEA AMBLYOPIA.—We read in a contemporary that M. Molchanoff, a
Russian, who is reputed to be the wealthiest tea merchant in the world,
has arrived at Paris from Hankoy with the intention of placing himself
under the treatment of Dr. Charcot and an experienced French ophthalmic
surgeon. The great tea magnate is suffering from amblyopia, which, it is
said, is the result of the prolonged practice of tea-tasting. It is not
unlikely that tea taken in excess might produce amblyopia similar in char-

acter to those toxic amauroses which result from the abuse of alcohol, tobacco, opium and quinine; but we are not aware that this form of amblyopia has been particularly described. Wecker does not mention it in the last volume of his large work just completed, and it is not mentioned in the "Real Encyclopedia," nor in the "Gräfe Sämisch Handbuch." Tea is hardly indulged in in this country to a sufficient extent to produce any marked effects upon the nervous system, but it is undoubtedly a sedative and acts powerfully upon the heart.—*London Lancet*, May 7th, 1887.

HODGKIN'S DISEASE.—At a recent meeting of the Sheffield Medico-Chirurgical Society, Dr. Porter showed enlarged supra-renal capsules from a case of Hodgkin's disease. The patient, a woman aged fifty-one, had suffered from enlarged glands on both sides of the neck ; the original enlargement on the left side occupying most of the posterior triangle. There was also a large mass of mesenteric glands forming an abdominal tumor, and smaller enlargements of the axillary and inguinal glands. The tumor on the left side of the neck had, from pressure, given rise to great pain up the side of the neck and face and down the left arm; and the external carotid and radial pulses were barely distinguishable. There was also œdema of the left hand, and the arm became ultimately useless. One symptom had been, flushing and profuse perspirations, at first more or less limited to the left side of the face, due to pressure on the sympathetic. The patient died of gradual exhaustion. At the *post mortem*, the tumors were found to be entirely glandular. There was some enlargement of the right lobe of the liver and of the spleen, but no lymphoid nodules or bands apparent in either organ. The supra-renals were very large indeed. No enlargement of the intestinal solitary glands was found.—*London Lancet*, April 30th, 1887.

THE NERVES OF TASTE.—Schiff has succeeded in keeping alive for a long time animals in which he had divided the trigeminus and facial nerves (and also the acoustic) within the cavity of the skull. From these animals (dogs) he deduced the following results : 1. Division of the trigeminus between the brain and Casserian ganglion destroyed the sensation of taste on the anterior portion of the tongue. 2. Division of the facial within the vault of the cranium had no influence upon the sensation of taste. 3. Division of the first and third branches of the trigeminus was without influence, while division of the second branch of this nerve above Meckel's ganglion destroyed the sensation of taste of the two anterior thirds of the tongue. 3. Injury to the facial during its course through the petrous bone likewise destroyed the sensation of taste to the same degree. 5. In certain cases division of the lingual nerve above its anastomosis with the chorda tympani produced also partial lost of taste. Schiff sums up: The taste fibers go from the lingual, partly through the chorda tympani, partly through the lesser superficial petrosal nerve to the facial, and in this to the geniculate ganglion which they then leave in order to pass through the greater superficial petrosal nerve to the spheno-palatine ganglion (Meckel's) and from this point they go out with the second branch of the trigeminus to get into the trunk of the fifth.—*Neurolog. Centralbl.*, April 1st, 1887.—O'C.

THE VARIETIES OF THE REACTION OF DEGENERATION AND THEIR DIAGNOSTIC AND PROGNOSTIC SIGNIFICANCE.—Dr. R. Stinzing, of Munich, has endeavored to give more precise distinctions between the different modifications of the reaction of degeneration, and, as far as possible, to classify them from a clinical point of view. Out of eighteen observations on the conditions of electric irritability in suitable cases of peripheral or spinal paralyses he was able to form four groups which he has arranged in a series according to the severity of the degeneration. In the first group (the highest grade) he found : Reaction of degeneration with *total loss* of electro-irritability ; in the second group: Reaction of degeneration *with partial* (faradic) irritability of the nerves; in the third group he brought together all the middle grades of degeneration, reaction of degeneration with retained irritability, but with sluggish response on the part of the nerve to faradism. Accordingly, the galvanic contraction from the nerves may be either prompt or sluggish. The fourth group embraces, finally, the lightest forms of RD with prompt contraction from the nerve, the usual partial RD. In estimating the grade of RD the writer holds, and correctly, the behavior of the affected nerves towards the current as being more decisive than that of the muscles ; the more closely the nerve-irritability approaches the normal for both kinds of current the more favorable is the prognosis. And in the same sense, sluggish, contraction is a better sign than absence of irritability.—*Neurolog. Centralbl.*, March 1st., 1887.—O'C.

THE JUGULAR HUM.—The unreliability of the well-known *bruit de diable* or jugular hum, as a sign of anæmia, was pointed out by Weil, whose objections have been disputed by Guttmann, but are now sustained by Dr. Reinhold Apetz (Virchow's Archiv., Bd. 107, Hft. 3). The results of the auscultation of 660 individuals, of whom 115 were anæmic, 161 "barely" anæmic, and 384 "not anæmic," was to show that the murmur was detected in the proportion of 35 per cent. of the first class ; 46 per cent. of the second, and 39 per cent. of the third. Without following the writer through his analysis, which corresponds fairly closely with the similar observations of Weil, it may be interesting to cite the conclusions at which he arrives. These are to the effect : 1st. That venous murmurs detected in the internal jugular vein under all circumstances depend in the first place upon the age of the affected individual ; the murmurs becoming less frequent with advancing age. 2d. That venous murmurs detected by turning the head to the other side are of no value in the diagnosis of anæmia, but have only a physiological importance. 3d. That some pathological importance specially belongs to the true murmurs detectable when the head is kept straight in the upright position ; when they occur loud and continuous in individuals of twenty to sixty years of age, yet they are generally too insignificant to be of value in the diagnosis of anæmia. 4th. Under no conditions do the venous murmurs have any special diagnostic value in chlorotic and other anæmic states.—*London Lancet*, April 30th, 1887.

CARBOLATE OF MERCURY IN SYPHILIS.—Dr. Karl Shadek, of Kieff, being anxious to try the effects of carbolate of mercury, which has been strongly recommended in syphilis by Professor Gamberini, requested M. H. Brandt, a pharmacist in Kieff, to prepare some for clinical use. This he did by precipitating a very dilute solution of bichloride of mercury with a concentrated alcoholic solution of carbolate of potassium. A yellowish precipitate was obtained, which, after being frequently agitated with the liquid for twenty-four hours, assumed a whitish appearance. It was filtered and washed with distilled water till the washings showed no traces of chloride. It was then transferred to a fresh filter paper and dried under a bell jar. In this way a nearly white, tasteless, amorphous substance was obtained, which was scarcely acted upon or dissolved by cold, but was readily soluble in boiling hydrochloric acid. The name given to it by Dr. Shadek is "hydrargyrum carbolicum oxydatum," and he has been using it in his private practice for several months. At first he gave it in the form of pills, one of which, containing about an eighth of a grain, was ordered three, or occasionally four, times a day. It was well borne, and did not interfere with the digestion. In some cases the treatment was continued for six or eight weeks without producing colic or other disagreeable symptoms. The total number of syphilitic cases in which it was given internally was thirty-five—twenty-six men, six women and three young children. In five of these there was swelling of the gums and salivation. Mercury was found in the urine after the third dose. Its therapeutic value was especially remarkable in macular and tubercular syphilis and in syphilitic psoriasis of the palm and sole. Syphilitic rash and slight relapsing forms yielded to the treatment in from two to four weeks; in syphilitic affections of the mucous membrane and in papular and pustular eruptions, from four to six weeks were required. Multiple enlargements of glands were little affected by it. In the case of children of from two to four years old, doses of about the fifteenth of a grain were well borne twice daily.—*London Lancet*, May 7th, 1887.

THE ANALGESIC INFLUENCE OF THE ANODE.—Dr. Niermeijer (Holland) reports the case of a man whose arm was torn out close to the shoulder by a machine. There were violent pains in the stump which did not cease after amputation of a part of it, or, later, after exarticulation. The patient complained of pains in the whole of the absent extremity and had the feeling as if it bent at the elbow at a right angle ; was pressed tightly against the chest, and as if the fingers were in constant motion. The pain extended over the whole scapular region, the trapezius muscle and the greater part of the pectoralis major, and the skin of this whole region was extremely sensitive to pressure. In all the painful parts there was a slight degree of muscular atrophy with lessened faradic reaction and a slighter difference between the anodal closure contraction and the cathodal on this side as compared with the other. The brachial plexus was extremely sensitive to pressure above the clavicle. Niermeijer tried the application of the anode, stabile, upon the brachial plexus and the joint, a moderate current being employed three times a week for some minutes, a rheostat being in the circuit. After a week, the patient was able to sleep quietly, the sensation of finger-motions had become less ; after the second week the pains had almost entirely disappeared, the hyperæsthesia had decreased, and in the next week the pain had wholly gone. The patient still had the feeling that the absent arm was bent at the elbow to the utmost degree, and was in the position of extreme adduction, with fingers immovable, and a burning sensation in the hand and at the shoulder-joint, but this also disappeared. Niermeijer had already had good results from this same application in some cases of prosopalgia and nervous tinnitus ; it is necessary that the patient should be some time under the influence of the anode without any change in the current strength. Later, the patient suffered from a blow upon the enucleated shoulder-joint and felt, as a result, pain in the wrist-joint of the amputated extremity, with a feeling of painful flexion of the joint. After four applications with the anode, stabile, this also disappeared.—*Neurolog. Centralbl.*, April 1st, 1887.—O'C.

NEWS.

SOCIETY MEETING.—The Wisconsin Homœopathic Medical Society will meet at Waukesha, June 22d, 1887.

THE PERISCOPE.—The St. Louis *Periscope* has ceased to be. It died very hard and fought valiantly for life. It will be missed among our exchanges.

RECEPTION.—The members of the Missouri Institute of Homœopathy, during their stay in St. Louis, were handsomely entertained one evening by Dr. J. Martine Kershaw.

PERSONAL.—James A. Freer, M.D., formerly on the staff at Ward's Island Hospital, has recently been appointed on the staff of the National

Homœopathic Hospital at Washington, D. C. He has also been appointed on the staff of the New Dispensary.

PERSONAL.—Dr. Malcolm Leal has removed to "The Albany," 222 West Fifty-second Street. Dr. Alton G. Warner has resigned his position as House Surgeon in the New York Ophthalmic Hospital, and has removed to 113 Henry Street, Brooklyn, N. Y.

A NEW INSANE ASYLUM.—The good people of Minnesota are evidently bound to have homœopathy in their midst. It is stated that a new hospital for the insane is shortly to be built, and is to be in charge of homœopathic physicians. We hope there will be no mistake about this one.

MARRIAGE.—On Wednesday evening, June 1st, Mary Edith Wellington, of Brookline, Mass., and Dr. Edgar V. Moffat, of New York, were united in matrimony. . Dr. Moffat's many friends in New York and Brooklyn join in wishing him and his accomplished bride a prosperous and happy future.

A MERITED HONOR.—Dr. W. H. Dickinson, of Des Moines, Iowa, was recently elected President of the Iowa State Board of Medical Examiners. Dr. Dickinson has been for some years a member of the Iowa State Board of Health. He is an alumnus of the New York Homœopathic Medical College, Class '65·

SOCIETY NOTE.—At the May meeting of the New York Society for Medico-Scientific Investigation, papers were read as follows: On "Abdominal Section," by Dr. Knight; "Notes on some Peculiar Effects of Narcotics," by Dr. Beebe ; "The Relation of the General Practitioner to Antisepsis," by Dr. S. Wellman Clark.

INTERESTING QUESTIONS.—The following topics will be considered by the American Public Health Association at its next meeting. 1. The Pollution of Water Supplies. 2. The Disposal of Refuse Matter of Cities, 3. The Disposal of Refuse Matter of Villages, Summer Resorts and Isolated Tenements. 4. Annual Diseases Dangerous to Man. The Association meets at Memphis, Tenn., November 8th, 9th, 10th, 11th, 1887.

AN ENGLISH DINNER.—Our homœopathic brethren in England evidently know how to provide and enjoy annual dinners. The Hahnemann Dinner of the British Homœopathic Society, in commemoration of the birth of Hahnemann was exceptionally successful. The dinner was presided over by Dr. Roth, the President of the Society. Among the speakers were Drs. Roth, Yeldham, Blackely, Hughes, Pope and Major Morgan and Mr. Cameron.

KINGS COUNTY SOCIETY.—At the thirtieth annual meeting of the Homœopathic Medical Society of Kings County, held May 10th, 1887, the following officers were elected for the ensuing year: President, J. L. Moffat, M.D. ; Vice-President, W. C. Latimer, M.D. ; Secretary, H. D. Schenck, M.D. ; Treasurer, Hugh M. Smith, M.D. ; Necrologist, Elizabeth M. Clark, M.D.; Censors, E. Hasbrouck, M.D., H. Minton, M.D., H. M. Lewis, M.D., W. M. Butler, M.D., and E. Chapin, M.D. Interesting addresses were made by Prof. T. F. Allen, M.D., of New York, and the retiring President, J. L. Moffat, M.D.

OBITUARY.—Dr. E. A. Lodge, one of the oldest and best known of the homœopathic physicians of Detroit, died January 25th, 1887. He was born in London, England, May 6th, 1822. Coming to Detroit in 1859, he rapidly built up a large and lucrative practice, which he retained until compelled to relinquish it by failing health. For many years he was the editor of the *American Homœopathic Observer*. He also established the first homœopathic pharmacy in the west. He was an active and consistent Christian, a devoted father and an estimable citizen. He leaves a widow and eleven children—six sons (three of whom are physicians) and five daughters.

THE BOSTON FESTIVAL.—The Semi-Centennial of Homœopathy in New England was celebrated in a fitting and successful fashion on the 12th of April, in Boston. The attractions of the evening were numerous and varied. In the large hall where was served the "high tea," were found the many decorated and tasteful tables, each presided over by a mistress and her fair aids. In the smaller hall Col. Charles R. Codman and Dr. Selden H. Talcott delivered notable addresses. In the concert hall a promenade concert was given by a full orchestra of fifty pieces. Over five thousand people were in attendance, among them Gov. Ames and his staff. The financial result was very gratifying, $4,500 being secured. We congratulate our Boston brethren upon their success.

THE NEW COLLEGE.—It may now be considered as definitely settled that the New York Homœopathic Medical College will have a new building. It will have much more than that. An entire block has been purchased on the eastern Boulevard, between Sixty-third and Sixty-fourth Streets. The dimensions of the plot are 177 ft. x 231½ ft. In the center of the lot will stand the college building proper, 75 ft. x 110 ft., thoroughly equipped, in every way, for the very best of medical teaching. On the south-east corner will stand the Medical Hospital, 55 ft. x 75 ft., four stories in height. The Surgical Hospital, of equal dimensions and height, will be placed on the north-east corner. It will contain a fine operating-room and amphitheater, extending through two stories. In the rear of the lot, on Sixty-fourth Street side, will be found the Maternity Hospital, and the opposite side, on Sixty-fifth Street, will have apartments for nurses and a training school. The friends of homœopathy in the city are enthusiastic, and determined to richly endow the college, and make it the leading clinical school in the world. The grounds and building will cost over $500,000, most of which is already secured. An endowment fund of $1,000,000 is to be secured later.

OBITUARY, DR. DETWILLER.—The late Henry Detwiller, M.D., of Easton, Pa., had the distinction of making the first homœopathic prescription in Pennsylvania (1825), of practicing medicine for a period longer than the alloted three score years and ten of the Psalmist, and of closing a life of activity up to within three weeks of his death at 92, the oldest homœopathic physician of the United States. He was born in Langenbruch, Switzerland, and educated in medicine at Freiburg, Baden. In addition to extensive success as a practitioner, he achieved a large fortune by business sagacity, and, moreover, pursued studies in natural history. He collected the *flora sauconensis,* an herbarium of the Upper and Lower Saucon, and a museum of the fauna of Pennsylvania representing, with few exceptions, the entire animal life of the State. He was a member of the Medical Faculty of the Homœopathic Healing Art, at Allentown (1836), assisted at the organization of the American Institute of Homœopathy (1844), and of the Homœopathic Medical Society of the State of Pennsylvania, and was a corresponding member of the National Historical Society of Basil, his native canton. His family consisted of four daughters, three sons, all of whom were physicians, twenty-seven grand-children, twenty-one great-grand-children, and two great-great-grand-children. He was a consistent member of the German Reformed Church, and was greatly revered for the worth of his character. Of his sons, Drs. Wm. and John J. Detwiller survive him.

At a special meeting of the Lehigh Valley Homœopathic Medical Society, held at the office of Dr. Doolittle, Easton, April 25th, at which

there was a full attendance, the following resolutions were passed:
"WHEREAS, After a long and useful life, it has pleased Divine Providence
to remove from us Dr. Henry Detwiller, an ex-president of this society;
Resolved, That in his death this society has lost a faithful and a most useful
member. *Resolved*, That while we most deeply deplore his loss, we are truly
thankful that he was allowed to live so many years among us. *Resolved*,
That by his seventy-two years of active practice, his great devotion to his
professional duty, his kindness and courtesy to those of us who came in
professional contact with him, he has established among us for himself a
perpetual remembrance and left us an example worthy of emulation.
Resolved, That we extend to the bereaved family our sincere sympathy.
Resolved, That we attend the funeral in a body. *Resolved*, That a copy
of these resolutions be sent to the family of the deceased, to each of the
papers of this city, to the NORTH AMERICAN JOURNAL OF HOMŒOPATHY,
and to the *Hahnemannian.*—E. D. DOOLITTLE, M.D., F. J. SLOUGH, M.D.,
DANIEL YODER, M.D."

DR. TALCOTT'S ADDRESS.—From Dr. Talcott's eloquent and suggestive
address, delivered at the Boston Semi-Centennial, we make the following
extract: " To recapitulate—Here, then, are some of the achievements of
Samuel Hahnemann: 1. He portrayed the true nature of disease and
described it as a disturbance of vital force. 2. He enunciated the law of
similars embodied in the doctrine, '*Similia Similibus Curantur*'—a law
upon which scientific medicine is inevitably based. 3. He inaugurated
the plan of proving drugs upon the healthy before using them as medicines for the sick. 4. He discarded polypharmacy as unscientific. 5. He
adopted the plan of using the single remedy for the safe and speedy cure
of disease. 6. He made war against blistering, bleeding, purging, administering emetics and all forms of unnecessary depletion. 7. He defined
medicine in a manner comprehensive enough for all time. In his
'Lesser Writings,' he states: 'A knowledge of diseases, a knowledge of
remedies, and a knowledge of their employment (that is for the cure of
disease), constitute medicine.' That definition has not as yet been improved
upon. 8. He reduced the size of the dose until all danger of aggravation
from the dose was removed. He proved the possibility of successful
treatment by the administration of medicines in minute quantities; and
when that fact was determined, there was a gradual abandonment of the
'kill or cure' doses of the ancients. Who can estimate the influence of
such a man, who wrought during an eventful life such miracle-like
achievements? He developed a philosophy as comprehensive, as bene-
ficient, as far-reaching in its conception of usefulness as the prodigious
philosophies of Aristotle, of Plato and of Lord Bacon. This man worked
alone, unaided, uninspired, save by his personal sense of the possession
of a mighty and glorious truth. With that truth in his soul, he rose like a
giant from the ranks of the people, seized the masses of antique theory
and uncertain conjecture by which he found himself surrounded and
hurled them into the yawning gulf of a well-earned oblivion. He portrayed with the clearness of sunlight the folly of old-time methods of treating the sick by rash and blindly heroic means, and he proved the powers
and effects of drugs upon himself ere he ventured to administer them as
medicines to the sick. He covered Europe with the evidences of his
marvelous medical skill! He swept back the tide of long and bitter persecution by the sublime triumphs of his art! He kept up the glorious carnival of his succssful practice until he was crowned with surpassing
honors in Paris; and he rested not until, by the grandeur of his achievements, the city of Leipsic, from which he had been driven as a fugitive
and a vagrant, erected a stately monument to his name—a monument that
remains to this day as a fitting memorial to his magnificent and imperish-
able memory."

VOL. XXXV.   *JULY, 1887.*   (VOLUME II, Third Series.)   No. 7.

NORTH AMERICAN
JOURNAL OF HOMŒOPATHY.

ORIGINAL ARTICLES IN MEDICINE.

OBSERVATIONS UPON THE TEMPERATURE IN TYPHOID OR ENTERIC FEVER.*

By FREDERICK J. NOTT, A.M., M.D.,
New York.

IT HAS been my fortune to see a good deal of enteric fever during the past year or two, and as I have been much impressed by the irregularity of all the typhoid manifestations, and especially of the temperature, it may be of some interest to refer, in a very brief manner, to a few observations made upon the course of this particular symptom.

During my early studies in medicine the idea was impressed upon me that the most characteristic symptom of typhoid fever—the one symptom upon which alone a diagnosis could be surely founded, and without which the diagnosis must, necessarily, be doubtful—was the course of the temperature.

Such was my confidence in this very prevalent doctrine, that during my first year of practice I refused persistently to recognize the true condition of a patient who evinced almost all the classical symptoms of enteric fever, because the temperature pursued an erratic course; and, when I came to sign the death certificate, was forced to do some considerable violence to my conscience by attributing the sickness and fatal issue to acute meningitis. Looking back upon such an incident in the light of some experience, I can see how blinded I had been by the teachings of the schools and text-books.

---

* Read before the Homœopathic Medical Society, County of New York, April 21st, 1887.

Now, in order to demonstrate the general medical opinion upon this subject, I will offer a few quotations from well-known authorities :

Wunderlich says (Medical Thermometry, p. 246) : "In forms of disease with protracted pyrogenetic stage the rise of the temperature happens thus : It begins to ascend in the evening ; in the morning it moderates again, to rise again considerably the following evening. It may thus happen that the normal temperature is again reached in the morning of the first day, or even that the initial stage is interrupted by a still longer interval free from fever."

"In this type the initial stage lasts three or four days, but seldom more than a week. If the temperature is not high by that time the illness will remain slight and quickly pass away ; if the temperature, on the other hand, rises to a considerable height, we must not expect so sudden a termination to the illness."

"This type occurs most constantly in typhoid, and so much so that the diagnosis can be based upon the initial stage alone (the other symptoms being conformable.)"

Liebermeister says, "that in typhoid the febrile movement has * * * a typical and cyclical course. To each separate period corresponds a certain degree of fever, and the separate periods are so far limited that, in uncomplicated cases, they do not exceed a certain duration."

"The diagnosis of typhoid can usually be made from the fever curve alone ; and this is true not only of the simple cases, but also of the obscure and complicated ones. In mild typhoid the temperature curve corresponds exactly to that in severe cases, with the difference only that it runs about one degree lower."

Most of the English and American writers follow the German authorities implicitly.

Jürgensen says, "that in milder typhoid the initial period of Wunderlich is almost entirely wanting, and during the height of the disease the temperature varies greatly. In a great majority of cases the usual picture of the well marked form is to be observed. Deviations, however, are observed here also. The third stage, characterized by its steep curves, is almost entirely wanting."

Pepper, of Philadelphia, in his treatise, says : "The febrile movement, however, rarely follows a perfectly typical curve, and I consequently find, in looking over the temperature sheets of a large number of cases, very few which bear, except during the first period, anything more than a general resemblance to the sheet which Wunderlich has prepared as typical."

This statement of Dr. Pepper, which is really only the American of Dr. Jürgensen's carefully worded acknowledgment, is in exact accord with my own observations. As a matter of fact, I have yet to see a typical case of typhoid, and am rather inclined to doubt its existence outside of the books, which are much too apt to tell us what we ought to instead of what we do find. No two cases of the disease are alike. The description of one will not fit another. Certainly no disease is characterized by a greater tendency to variation and irregularity. One often reads and hears what is denominated a clinical picture of the patient, or a clinical history of the disease, and it is generally an hodge-podge of impossible combinations.

To justify these statements, I exhibit the records of six cases of typhoid taken at random from my note-books. Of these cases, two died and four recovered. In no one of these cases does the temperature curve correspond to the classical description of its proper course. The nearest approach to it, strange to say, is in the mildest case of all, in which, during the first week, the rise and fall of the curve is quite characteristic, although, even in this case, the highest point is *not* reached, contrary to the dictum of Wunderlich, until the second week, upon the ninth or tenth day, after which the temperature declines by lysis to perfect convalescence.

In four of these cases, one of which was fatal, the temperature is lower during the second than the third week. That, of course, is all wrong.

In three cases, two of which were fatal, the temperature was higher in the third than in the second week. Surely such a state of things would prove deceptive to a disciple of the German nosologists.

In two instances, both of which recovered, the temperature was higher, or quite as high, at my first visit as at any time during the entire illness. In one case, 105°; another, 104°; a third, 103°; a fourth, 102½°; a fifth, 102°; and the sixth, 101°, was recorded at my first visit.

Of course, in considering these facts, we must remember the great probability that many patients with typhoid are not under observation during the first week; but I cannot think that I did not see any one of these six during the initial period.

I have seen several patients who were, in my opinion, threatened with typhoid fever, because of a gradually increasing remittent fever, associated with various pains and malaise, and who were quite ill enough to desire observation. These people were quite rid of fever, and convalescent in four or five days; and a reconstructed diagnosis permitted nothing more ponderous· than influenza, or catarrhal fever. So, if so much discomfort and constitutional disturbance are produced by an evanescent catarrh, how much ought to develop during the first week of typhoid? Surely, quite as much, at any rate. And, consequently, we ought to, and probably do, see more patients during the first week of typhoid with a high temperature, which has not developed by easy ascent, but suddenly, than the sticklers to the rail-fence temperature dogma would like to admit. It is possible that hospital enteric fever of the German type is different from that which prevails in private practice in New York, but I do not think so. Neither can I understand how we can entertain the idea of an apyretic typhoid, and rely upon our thermometers to indicate the character of the disease.

The difficulty is just here. As in many other matters concerning so-called scientific observation, the authorities have formulated an hypothesis, and attempt to make the disease fit the theory. In actual experience, typhoid fever is simply a name for a specific inflammation of certain localities in the intestine, which inflammation is generally manifested, among other symptoms, by elevation of the temperature, which is subject to more or less regular remissions and exacerbations. Just as erysipelas may occur without redness of the integument, and just as pneumonia may not cause rust-colored expectoration, so may typhoid fever fail to produce some of its most characteristic symptoms.

My conclusion is, that we must be wary lest we attach too much importance to any one symptom in making up our diagnosis in any given case, and that especially we must be prepared for cases of enteric fever in which the temperature curve is as irregularly developed as any other symptom. The temperature of typhoid is by no means so regular as it has been pictured; and though I grant that in many cases, perhaps in a majority, the chart will show that the development, increase, continuance and decrease of the temperature, coincide pretty closely with the rules so carefully enunciated, still I am satisfied that the exceptions are so numerous as to seriously weaken the pathognomonic value of the symptom.

SIEGESBECKIA ORIENTALIS.—" Siegesbeckia is a shrub, the green parts of which have quite a reputation in the mauritius as an alterative, and its preparations are given in syphilis, gout, scurvy, etc." Dr. J. Hutchinson in the *Brit. Med. Jour.*, for June 25th, describes the use of tincture of siegesbeckia and glycerine in equal parts applied night and morning for the cure of ring-worm.

OTITIS MEDIA HÆMORRHAGICA.

By K. B. BULLEL, M.D.,

Bombay, India.

CASES of pure and simple otitis media hæmorrhagica, I think, are rare. Dr. Roosa mentions two cases, and Burnett only makes a passing allusion to the disease in his work on diseases of the ear. This is, in itself, a sufficient inducement to me to place the following case before the profession :

Mrs. C——, aged 42, mother of nine children, and of good health, was placed under my treatment for an acute attack of pain in the left ear. Previous history—she has been suffering from the pain in the ear for the last ten days. The pain at first was of an intermittent nature and confined to the ear only. For the last two days it has been very severe, constant, and radiating all over the left side of the head and face. Complained of a feeling of fullness and acuteness of hearing on the affected side. The act of mastication and deglutition aggravated the suffering. The parts were very sensitive to touch. There was occasional paroxysmal aggravation of the severity of the pain.

Along with these symptoms there were slight pyrexia and insomnia. On examination I found the left tympanic membrane uniformly congested and slightly bulged at the anterior and inferior quadrant. Right membrane was slightly indrawn. Naso-pharynx congested. The severity of the pain and the bulged appearance of the membrane induced me to suggest the operation of paracentesis, with a hope that that would relieve the suffering of the patient. The operation was performed at once. To my surprise, there was a gush of blood through the puncture in the membrane and through the side of the nose, and nearly two drachms flowed freely. The intensity of the pain and the sense of fullness were immediately relieved. From this time on, until complete recovery of the patient, which took nearly a week, there was not a drop of blood or muco-purulent matter that escaped through the puncture in the membrane; the latter closed in five days. Subsequent examination of the urine showed no trace of albumin in it. It is nearly four weeks now. On examination of the ear I find no trace left as to where the membrane was punctured. In my opinion this case can be called a pure and genuine " Otitis Media Hæmorrhagica."

———————

BACTERIAL ORIGIN OF RHEUMATISM.—Dr. Mantle—see *Brit. Med. Jour.*, June 25th, 1887—believes that rheumatism is produced by the agency of a bacterium, which he thinks in most cases enters the system through the lymphatic structure of the tonsil.

EPIDEMIC DIARRHŒA AND DYSENTERY.*

By LEWIS HALLOCK, M.D.,
New York.

THE extensive prevalence of diarrhœa during the latter part of the past winter must, I think, have been noticed by every active practitioner. In the heat of summer and autumn we expect to see frequent cases of diarrhœa, not only in children and infants, leading to cholera infantum, but often also in adults, tending to the chronic disorder or to decided dysentery. But in the bracing atmosphere of winter its general prevalence to such a degree as to deserve the character of an epidemic is certainly noteworthy and almost phenomenal. The disease in summer is usually attributed to the relaxing effect of the season, to imprudent exposure, to evening dews and chills, to careless sea-bathing, insufficient clothing, indulgence in ripe or unripe fruits, etc.

In winter, however, these conditions are changed, and the cause must be sought elsewhere. It will be remembered that the months of January and February last were unusually wet and stormy, and the weather so variable that a period of three or four days seldom occurred without some marked change in the temperature or humidity of the atmosphere.

This unusual character of the season was doubtless the cause of the prevalent diarrhœa, which, in the number of cases occurring (with perhaps the exception of measles), far exceeded those of tonsillitis, diphtheria, scarlatina, or other usual epidemics of late winter and early spring.

The disease has generally been of a mild form, lasting from two to six or eight days and yielding readily to appropriate remedies, as *cham., dulc., china., mercurius,* etc.

Adults of both sexes have been the most frequent sufferers, the disease in this respect contrasting with the diarrhœa of summer, which all know has it subjects mostly among infants and children. The number of discharges has varied from three or four in twenty-four hours in the mild cases, to fifteen and twenty a day in others. After the first two or three bilious evacuations the discharges usually became aqueous, often profuse, then less frequent, more bilious and offensive,

---

*Read before the Homœopathic Medical Society, County of New York, April 21st 1887.

followed in a few instances with tenesmus, but in no case becoming bloody or dysenteric. The usual colicky pains preceding each discharge were mild, and abdominal tenderness to pressure slight and soon relieved. A few of the adults supposed their attacks due to fatigue; others to sudden cold or some error of diet, but most admitted of no cause and knew of no reason for the attack. Like other forms of epidemic disease the symptoms usually appeared with little premonition, and in the absence of any known exciting cause seemed wholly due to some change in the atmospheric condition affecting the whole community.

The most noticeable feature of the epidemic was *not* its severity, but its unseasonable prevalence in the *cold* instead of the warm season of the year. Recent reports of similar sickness in Albany, Philadelphia and Washington confirm its right to the character of an epidemic if not the title of winter cholera which some have given it.

A similar frequency of diarrhœa in a milder form was noticed in the city last year, and caused the remark that *severe* epidemics of cholera, diarrhœa and dysentery were often preceded by such unusual symptoms, indicating the probable increase of intestinal disorders in the following summer. No such results, however, followed, until the unusually variable weather of the past winter. In both its extent and severity, however, the recent epidemic has exceeded that of the previous year.

Diarrhœa of an epidemic character, excepting when premonitory of Asiatic cholera, as it was in this city and elsewhere, in the form of cholerine, before its arrival in the malignant form, is less frequent than its related and more dreaded disorder, epidemic dysentery.

Medical history abounds with descriptions of epidemic and contagious forms of *this* fearful disease, and when occurring in camps, jails, on shipboard, or in other confined and crowded situations, is but little less fatal or alarming than the dreaded form of Asiatic or malignant cholera. Happily the increased attention to hygienic care and prevention, by cleanliness, ventilation, disinfection and other precautionary measures of the present day, almost confine the knowledge of such pestilential dysentery to the records of its ravages in former years. But dysentery of a *less* serious form occasionally prevails as an epidemic in locations usually favorable to health, and even in the pure and open air of the country.

One of these epidemics it was my fortune to see during my medical pupilage many years ago at the east end of Long Island.

This city was suffering its last serious visitation of yellow fever, and great numbers of the population, to escape from the pestilence, left for the country. I also left and spent the compulsory vacation with a relative physician located between Riverhead and Southold, and in his company saw much of country medical practice. The most serious disease encountered was dysentery, of a type far more severe and fatal than any I have since witnessed. The attack usually commenced with diarrhœa, lasting only twelve to twenty-four hours, followed by fever, tenesmus and frequent bloody stools. In some cases diarrhœa was unnoticed, and the disease began suddenly and violently with severe colic pains, great prostration and frequent discharges, so profuse that fatal collapse ensued on the second or third day of the disease. One instance of this hemorrhagic form I witnessed in an able-bodied farmer of middle age, in which the blood had saturated through both the beds on which he lay and extended in a stream across the floor of the entire room. This exhausting hemorrhage was the characteristic feature of the epidemic and the chief cause of the great mortality. In the cases where bleeding was less profuse, recovery was slow and tedious, in others a low enteric fever of a typhoid form ensued, from which some survived, but most succumbed. Adults of both sexes were the chief victims and but few children were attacked. So far as I can recall its history the disease lasted about two months, and was mostly confined to the two towns, or rather to the country from ten to twenty miles in extent, between the towns of Riverhead and Southold, lying on the north side of the bay dividing the east end of Long Island.

Various theories of the *cause* of this fearful epidemic were suggested. Some attributed it to the unusual cold and wet summer, others to an unknown miasma, but the general verdict charged it to offensive emanations from decaying fish caught in large quantities in the adjacent bay, and spread for manure on almost every farm along the road, rendering the atmosphere offensive to all, and often producing nausea and vomiting in persons traveling from one town to the other. This specious explanation, though accepted by many, was rejected by others, for the reason that the same cause had long existed before, without any such effect, and I may add that it has continued annually to the last few years in which the fish have been caught away from the shore and so used that the effluvia no longer exist; yet during the long years before and since that memorable season no epidemic of a similar character has been known in that vicinity. The cause, though probably of local origin, remains undetermined and adds another example of the often unexplained and mysterious origin of epidemics.

THE USE OF MYDRIATICS.*

By ALTON G. WARNER, M.D.,

Brooklyn, N. Y.

I MUST beg the indulgence of the gentlemen present who are ophthalmic specialists, for attempting to treat a subject which is to them very trite and commonplace.

The other gentlemen may think that the subject belongs only to the specialist; but I shall only attempt to make a few suggestions in regard to the use of mydriatics in general practice.

The agents at our command for producing mydriasis, or dilatation of the pupil, are *sulphate of atropia, sulphate of duboisia, sulphate of daturine, hydrobromate of homatropine, hydrobromate of hyoscine* and *hydrochlorate of cocaine.*

If a drop of one-half per cent. solution of *atropine* be instilled into the eye the first indication of dilatation of the pupil begins, on an average, in fourteen minutes. The maximum dilatation is reached in about thirty-five minutes. It remains at its height for twenty-six hours, and normal contraction returns at the end of four and one-half days. With the same concentration of *duboisine* we get the first indication in eight minutes, and the maximum dilatation in nineteen minutes. The maximum dilatation persists twenty-four hours, and normal contraction is reached in four days.

Daturine is seldom used. No such careful experiments have been made as with the above drugs, but its action is more feeble, and also more irritating.

Homatropine, used also in the one-half per cent. solution, causes beginning dilatation in nine minutes, and maximum in thirty-three minutes. The height of the mydriasis persists three hours and the pupil becomes normal in twenty-four hours. *Hyoscine* produces a much more powerful effect. The maximum effect is reached about as soon as with *duboisia,* but it does not persist quite as long.

The action of *cocaine* is variable. A slight amount of dilatation occurs in from five to ten minutes and this disappears in an hour or so.

There has recently been introduced a new drug called *scopoline,* which is said to be superior to *atropine.* It has not been used in this country, and little is known of it.

---

* Read before the New York Society for Medico-Scientific Investigation.

These agents are believed to produce a paralysis of the filaments of the motor oculi distributed to the sphincter iridis, and also an irritation of the sympathetic fibres which supply the dilator of the pupil. In addition, they cause paralysis of the muscle of accommodation.

This latter concerns us only in a negative way; for with paralysis of the accommodation for the purpose of testing refraction, we, as general practitioners, have nothing to do. We must, however, bear this fact in mind when dilating the pupil for other purposes; for if it be necessary and allowable for the patient to use his eyes, he will not thank us for depriving him of his power of accommodation for several days.

Another use of mydriatics is to dilate the pupil for the purpose of making an ophthalmoscopic examination of the fundus oculi. It is desirable that every physician, especially if out of reach of a specialist, should be able to use the ophthalmoscope sufficiently to recognize affections that he may or may not safely treat. Be the examiner ever so expert, he will find many conditions in which he obtains a more satisfactory view of the fundus by dilating the pupil. For this purpose *homatropine* is to be preferred, for the reason that its effects pass off sooner. *Cocaine* may be used, but we are not so certain of a maximum dilatation. As a means of diagnosis, and as a therapeutic measure in the treatment of corneal and iritic affections, we have the most essential use of mydriatics.

There is no more frequent error than that of mistaking an iritis for a conjunctivitis and treating it accordingly. There are many cases of iritis in which the dull color of the iris, the pain and the peri-corneal injection may not be sufficiently marked to attract attention, and the immobility and irregularity of the pupillary margin may pass unnoticed; meanwhile, plastic exudation is going on and adhesions are formed between the iris and the lens capsule. If the practitioner is *certain* that he is dealing *only* with conjunctivitis, he does not wish to annoy the patient with a dilated pupil. This is the result of using most of the eye-drops sold by druggists. But unless iritis can *absolutely* be excluded, it will be safer to instil a drop of *atropine, duboisine,* or *hyoscine,* and so confirm the diagnosis. If synechia is shown, the further use of the mydriatic is indicated.

We shall not speak of the treatment of the case as to rest, heat, remedies, etc. The great essential is to dilate the pupil and keep it so. For this purpose we may use *atropine, duboisine,* or *hyoscine.* The effect of the other mydriatics is not sufficiently powerful or enduring. The amount of the drug and the frequency of its use will depend upon the density and duration of the adhesions. In mild cases a few instillations may suffice, but in long-standing cases we may require hourly applications. In such cases we must be governed by the ability of the patient to tolerate the drug. If pushed beyond a certain limit, the poisonous effects of the drug appear and its use must be stopped. Any of the above-mentioned agents will be better tolerated if the patient is in bed. We can also guard against the ill effects, to a certain extent, by being careful to incline the patient's head outward and holding the finger over the lachrymal puncta. This prevents rapid absorption by the lachrymal apparatus. A better effect will be obtained by making applications as often as every hour, and stopping as soon as any symptoms of poisoning are manifest. If the patient tolerate the use of the drug thus frequently for a day or two, and the adhesions still remain, it is better to suspend its use for twenty-four hours and then begin again. It will be found at times that the synechia has given way during the interval, or the pupil can be dilated with a rush upon second trial.

Atropine is most frequently used, in a solution of four grains to the ounce; it has the advantage of being cheaper than the others and will usually accomplish the desired end. At times, however, its continued use induces a follicular conjunctivitis which may be very persistent. *Duboisia* will often be tolerated by patients in whom *atropine* produces a conjunctivitis. Also, we find that some patients who become delirious from *atropine* will tolerate *duboisia*. If there be no bad effect from the *atropine*, there is little use of substituting *duboisia*, for it is not so enduring.

It is rather in mild cases of chronic iritis, after operations, that we use *duboisia*. The symptoms of *atropine* poisoning are well known. The dry throat is usually the first symptom and should warn us to stop the drug. If pushed further, we get the flushed face and delirium with great desire to escape. It is needless to say that *opium* antidotes *atropine*. In poisoning from *duboisia* the throat becomes *very* dry. The patients are excited, but weak and trembling. They manifest a frequent desire to get out of bed, but are more easily controlled than when under the influence of *atropine*.

Hydrobromate of hyoscine, if used in a one per cent. solution, acts very powerfully upon iritic adhesions. There are few patients, however, who can tolerate its continued use. Often, from a single drop, the patient loses control of his legs, his mouth becomes dry, his speech thick and his ideas confused. Patients have frequently said to me that the sensation at the time was that they were paralyzed. Strong coffee relieves the symptoms, but camphor is probably the best antidote. Some persons exhibit a surprising degree of toleration for *hyoscine,* but so great is the difference in patients in this respect that when frequent applications are made they should be carefully watched by a nurse lest poisoning occur. The same remark applies to *atropine* or *duboisia.*

In the wards of the Ophthalmic Hospital we had recently three cases of specific iritis under treatment with *hyoscine.* These cases, occurring at the same time and being treated with the same solution, will serve to illustrate the degree of tolerance. All were in bed. One (male) had *hyoscine,* one per cent. solution, hourly for three days, when the synechia gave way. No symptoms of poisoning occurred. The second case (female) had the same solution hourly for *two weeks* without any constitutional effect and with very little effect on the adhesions. The other eye then becoming affected, the drug was used every two hours in *both* eyes for *two weeks* longer. No adhesions remained in the second eye, and no drug symptoms occurred at any time. The third case (female) had this solution every two hours for one day, when she became delirious. The use of the drug was stopped, but the delirium lasted over forty-eight hours. The patient talked incessantly and picked at the bed-clothes. She would not stay in bed, but was too weak to go about much. She was not violent, unless opposed. During this time she would not swallow anything for fear of being poisoned.

I will not detain you with cases of *atropine* poisoning. They are, of course, frequent in hospital practice. If symptoms of poisoning appear, the patient must be watched lest he escape from the room. A strait jacket may be required. Even after sleep is induced by an hypodermic of *morphine,* the patient may awake still delirious and suddenly disappear. This once happened in my experience, but fortunately, on reaching the street through a window, the man recovered and went home without harm.

Old solutions are more apt to poison than fresh. In corneal infiltrations and ulcerations we may use mydriatics to keep the iris at rest and prevent complications, and for the calmative effect upon the cornea. *Atropine* or *duboisine* will here have the preference. An application two or three times a day will probably suffice. In corneal affections the use of *eserine* has been substituted by many for that of *atropine.* This should always be the case when any glaucomatous symptoms exist, for increased tension is always a contra-indication to the use of mydriatics.

THERAPEUTICS OF SPINAL IRRITATION.

BY F. F. LAIRD, M.D.,

Utica, N. Y.

(*Concluded from page 286.*)

Scuttelaria lat.—"This remedy should be thought of where muscular twitchings, choreaic spasms, and general irritability of the muscular system are markedly manifest. Sleeplessness or sleep disturbed by dreams of a frightful nature, general emotional disturbance and extreme susceptibility to pain and impressions of all kinds. In many cases of 'general nervousness,' traceable to spinal anæmia, this remedy is useful." (Kershaw.)

Secale.—The well-known physiological effect of *ergot* in producing anæmia of the brain and spinal cord has led to its successful use in spinal irritation. The writer has been most successful with *secale* in spinal irritation dependent upon sub-involution of the uterus. "In paralysis or paresis of the lower extremities, paralysis of the sphincter vesicæ, sciatica, irritable uterus and numbness and tingling of the lower extremities, it is useful." (Kershaw). *Extreme aversion to heat ; during sleep can bear only the lightest covering.*

Sepia.—This drug, although barely mentioned in the literature of the subject, is one of our most potent remedies, owing to the extreme frequency with which spinal irritation is associated with derangements of the female sexual system. The sooner physicians learn to recognize the fact that spinal irritation in women is, in the *great* majority of cases, but a reflex symptom of uterine or ovarian irritation, the more will *sepia* be used and appreciated. Functional derangement of the liver, manifested by the characteristic symptom, "*putrid urine, depositing a pinkish, adherent sediment,*" is generally present.

Silicea.—Stiffness of nape of neck *with headache.* Weakness in back and a paralyzed feeling in lower extremities. Stiff, sore feeling down right side of spine, then across loins and over right hip. *Burning in back while walking in open air and becoming warm. Throbbing in back. Constant aching pain in center of back. Stiffness and pain in small of back when rising from a seat. Pain as if beaten in small of back at night. The coccyx is painful as after a long carriage ride ; stinging in the bone which is also painful to pressure.*

Very sensitive, starts at least noise. Vertigo and headache ascending from nape of neck, RELIEVED BY WRAPPING UP THE HEAD WARMLY. *Soreness of scalp.* Painful sensitiveness to sound, with roaring in the ears;

difficult hearing of the human voice (PHOS.) DIFFICULT EXPULSION OF
STOOL WHICH SEEMS TO SLIP BACK INTO RECTUM. ALWAYS GREAT COSTIVENESS
IMMEDIATELY BEFORE AND DURING CATAMENIA. *Finger nails rough and yellow.*
OFFENSIVE SWEAT OF FEET WITH RAWNESS BETWEEN THE TOES; burning of soles.
ICY-COLD FEET, EVEN IN BED. COLDNESS OF LEGS AS FAR AS THE KNEES, EVEN
IN A WARM ROOM. ALWAYS COLD, EVEN WHEN EXERCISING. *Unhealthy skin,
every little injury suppurates.*

Aggravation—DURING NEW MOON ; *from motion.*

Amelioration—From warmth in general.

Prescribed upon the above indications, *silicea* will be found a grand
remedy. One case in which spinal irritation and offensive foot-sweat
alternated was speedily cured by this remedy. Following the hint
of Dr. C. C. Smith, that "when *cina* fails in vermiculous affections,
silicea is generally the remedy," the writer has had signal success in
four cases of spinal irritation in children, dependent on worms, and
markedly aggravated at the time of the new moon.

Sulphur.—*Stiffness with cracking of cervical vertebræ.* Tearing, tension, drawing and sticking in cervical muscles. *Stiffness, now in back,
now in hips, painful on turning over in bed; he was obliged to hold his
breath.* Heaviness in back and lower extremities in the morning on
rising. *Bruised feeling in back and in spinal muscles.* Burning between
scapulæ. *Tension and bruised pain between scapulæ and in nape of neck,
extending to shoulder on moving the head. Pain in small of back compelling patient to walk bent. Violent pain in small of back only on stooping, tension as if everything were too short; the pain extends over abdomen to pit of stomach and as far as the knee.* Aching, tensive pain in
back, driving patient out of bed in the morning. *Stitches in small of
back.* Aching pains in sacrum, worse from 2 to 5 A. M.

Vertigo and congestive headaches with HEAT ON VERTEX. *Feeling of
suffocation, wants doors and windows open.* HOT FLUSHES FOLLOWED BY
PERSPIRATION AND DEBILITY. GONE, EMPTY FEELING IN STOMACH AT 11 A. M.
Weakness in chest during evening while lying down. DIARRHŒA, DRIVING
PATIENT OUT OF BED IN THE MORNING; PAINLESS AND EXCORIATING ANUS.
Burning in vagina causing great restlessness. SOLES OF FEET HOT, PUTS
THEM OUT OF BED TO COOL THEM. PATIENT ALWAYS WALKS OR SITS BENT
OVER. Says Kershaw: "An extremely useful and often indicated
remedy. There is generally *great tenderness of the cervical vertebræ
and excessive soreness of the scalp* so that combing the hair or even
touching the head is painful. These are reliable symptoms and point
strongly to *sulphur as the remedy.* * * * Neuralgia especially affecting the left supra and infra-orbital regions. Neuralgic pains affecting
the left superior maxillary nerves and left ovary alternately. * * *

Deeply-seated infra-orbital pain aggravated by percussion of the cervical vertebræ."

The sulphur patient is lean, stoop-shouldered and almost invariably presents this highly characteristic symptom: SHE CAN ASSUME ANY POSITION EXCEPT STANDING STILL. She can, perhaps, walk a mile in perfect comfort, but if compelled to stand stationary in a crowd for five minutes, all her symptoms are markedly aggravated.

Tarantula.—Prof. Farrington summarizes the action of this remedy in the following masterly manner: "The patient is nervous, restless and compelled to keep constantly in motion. The headaches are violent and are sometimes relieved by rubbing the head against the pillow. Indeed this hyper-sensitiveness of the peripheries of the nerves seems to be a general characteristic; for the patient is comfortable only when rubbing the hands together, moving the legs, etc. The spine is often exquisitely sensitive, while trembling and *ennui* show the general exhausted condition. Choreaic symptoms are well marked. Hysteria is clearly pictured even to the deceptions which such persons are prone to practice." *General hyperæsthesia, extreme nervousness* and *marked hysterical symptoms are the prominent indications.*

Tellurium.—*The spine from the last cervical to about the fifth dorsal vertebra became very sensitive, and the seat of a peculiar sense of irritation, which made the prover dread having the part touched, or even approached;* this dread was disproportioned to the actual sensibility of the part when pressed or rudely touched, for this sensibility was not really very great; from the vertebræ above mentioned a peculiar irritation seemed to radiate upwards into the neck, outwards into the shoulders, and forwards through the thorax to the sternum; the distress caused by this sensation was aggravated by fatigue, but only partially relieved by repose.

The above carefully described symptoms were obtained by that conscientious observer, Carroll Dunham, and should be put to clinical test.

Theridion.—"Is suited to hysterical women whose minds are very much excited. Time seems to pass very quickly. Patient is very talkative. She is subject to headache, which is usually situated over the left eye, and is aggravated by the heat of the sun and by very slight noises. Even a person walking across the floor of the room renders the pain unbearable. The headache is associated with vertigo and nausea, both worse on closing the eyes. The spine is very irritable, with great sensitiveness between the vertebræ. So great is this hyperæsthesia that the patient sits sideways in a chair in order to avoid the pressure against the spine. Every sound penetrates the teeth and through the whole body."—Farrington.

This spider poison closely resembles the tarantula, but is distinguished by *marked aggravation from slight noises, which cause or intensify headache, vertigo and nausea.* The last three symptoms are also *worse from motion.*

Zincum.—"Both spinal and cerebral anæmia, with great depression of spirits, profound melancholia, loss of memory, inability to think or do any mental work, general languor of the body and atrophy of muscular substance. Cerebral depression, rendering the patient stupid. Neuralgia about the root of the nose, vertigo, with tendency to fall to the left side, soreness of scalp, and general amelioration of the symptoms when out of doors. General agitation of the whole body, with constant movement of the feet, points to this remedy. Trembling and weakness of the lower extremities, making the walk uncertain and staggering, are indications for its use. Choreaic twitching and epileptiform convulsions are also symptoms curable by means of this remedy."—Kershaw.

Always feels best during the menstrual flow. Aggravation of all symptoms from wine.

ORIGINAL ARTICLE IN SURGERY.

TUMORS OF THE BLADDER.*

By F. E. DOUGHTY, M.D.,

New York.

IT is only within a very recent period that neoplasms of the bladder have received, either at the hands of the pathologist or surgeon, anything like the amount of attention their importance demands.

The almost invariable difficulties that surrounded their early detection, and the impossibility of our art to remove them, even when their presence was established, have no doubt been the chief factors in producing this state of affairs.

We can then, with just pride, mark another advance in our science and art, in the improved methods of their recognition and treatment, and thus extend our aid to this class of suffering humanity. In entering upon the subject that is to engage our attention for a few minutes, we desire to state once for all, that we purpose treating only of

---

*Read before the Homœopathic Medical Society, County of New York.

such growths as have their origin in or involve the walls of the bladder, thus excluding those familiar outgrowths from the prostate which find their way into that viscus.

Tumors of the bladder can neither be called of common or rare occurrence. As we have intimated it is only very recently that they have attracted much attention. Up to this time no individual has had a sufficiently large number of cases come under his immediate observation to enable him to obtain more than general data in regard to them.

Perhaps Sir Henry Thompson has had the ripest experience, and he has also availed himself of the unique advantages presented in the preserved specimens in the museums of England. His views should therefore be closely studied, even though we find them not quite in harmony with other well-known writers.

The preserved specimens show that malignant growths occur about as frequently as the non-malignant; yet, Sir Henry's personal experience does not confirm this. Mr. Coulson considers the malignant formations as being most frequently encountered, and Dr. Gross seems also to hold the same opinion.

As regards the physical conformation of these neoplasms, a considerable proportion present a single outgrowth from the vesical wall, more or less pedunculated. Some are broad and sessile, with possibly two or more lobes ; occasionally two or even more separate tumors are met with in the same bladder.

The point of origin varies as regards the vesical parietes, though on the whole they seem to manifest a predilection for the lower half of the viscus.

Great diversity obtains as to their structure ; at times they are soft, filamentous or fimbriated ; or, again, they are firm and solid. Those which are attached by means of a narrow neck, or pedunculated, present themselves only in the minority of cases, as about one in six or seven cases ; the same is equally true of the sessile form. Between these two extremes fall the majority, with a tendency toward the sessile rather than toward the pedunculated.

Whether men or women are most predisposed to this disease is an open question, as some emphatically state that they occur more frequently in men, while others take the opposite position.

The facility for confirming a diagnosis by means of digital exploration of the bladder offered in women may account for the opinion that they are more prone to be thus affected.

In spite of the difficulties that surround the nomenclature of tumors in general, including those of the bladder, we can readily make two grand divisions, the malignant or heteroplastic, consisting more or less of elements never found in the tissues of the healthy bladder; and non-malignant, innocent or homœoplastic growths, *i. e.*, those made up only of elements identical with normal bladder tissues.

As regards the first division, we may say that such growths are usually secondary in their development, either as metastatic deposits, or as extensions of a similar growth from neighboring parts.

Primary carcinoma of the bladder is regarded by Dr. Gross as among the rarest of surgical affections.

This view is not shared by many others, and we must admit that such primary developments do occur, and not as infrequently as Dr. Gross would have us believe, for Heilborn alone describes seven such cases. The same lack of concord obtains in regard to which variety of carcinomatous formations occur the oftenest.

Thus, Thompson and Gross consider the epithelial form as most common, while Grant and Coulson give to the encephaloid variety the first place.

Scirrhus is also occasionally encountered, but no doubt many cases of so-called scirrhus are nothing more than the firm infiltrating form of epithelioma, characterized by a dense stroma of fibrous tissue.

As curiosities, one occasionally meets examples of melanotic and colloid tumors.

The old term "villous cancer" is now about obsolete, and the growth to which it was given is now regarded as wholly innocent in its nature. But it must be remembered that not infrequently carcinomatous neoplasms become covered by a kind of villous growth, similar to the villi observed on the chorion, made up chiefly of blood-vessels.

Such tumors are especially prone to involve the base of the bladder between the openings of the ureters and the internal meatus. However rich these tumors may be in villi, and so resemble the simple villous tumor, they are distinguished by involving all the vesical tissues, and in possessing those histological elements characteristic of carcinoma—features wanting in the simple form. A carcinoma may occur as a circumscribed solitary tumor, or a local mass, polypoid in shape, projecting into and perhaps nearly filling the bladder, or in the form of nodules; or as a diffuse infiltration of all the tunics of the bladder, so as to convert them into a dense mass, from one-quarter to one or even two inches in thickness.

These tumors, when of long duration, usually are in a state of ulceration and offer a rough, ragged, foul surface; or the ulcer may be covered with long and swollen villous excrecsences, or occupied by soft, broken down, pultaceous *débris*.

Sarcomas, using this term in the sense in which it is now employed, are exceedingly rare, as up to a recent date, Sefleben's case was the only one on record.

Turning now to the innocent or homœoplastic neoplasms, we find that they may be divided into four classes.

· 1st. Mucous polypi. This form has thus far been observed chiefly or only in young children, and they resemble the soft polypi—myxomata—so frequently met with in the nasal passages.

2d. Fimbriated papilloma, or, as sometimes called, " villous " growth. The essential feature of this formation is a structure in which the vesical mucous membrane is developed into papillæ.

These papillæ are long, extremely delicate processes, sometimes hair-like and arranged side by side ; or again, bifid or branched.

Generally they are disposed in a group arising from a circumscribed base which contains other and more solid structure than the processes themselves.

As a rule only one such growth is found, but occasionally more, or even the entire lining membrane may be covered with them.

3d. Fibro-papilloma. In this variety we find also the fimbriated processes just mentioned, but they are less numerous, as well as shorter, and do not constitute the major part of the growth which is more solid, and made up of unstriped muscular fibres and connective tissue.

4th. Tumors of a transitional type, as Sir Henry Thompson calls them. They resemble the last form; the basic structures are still the normal vesical tissues, but are peculiarly arranged, and contain, moreover, irregular cellular elements which are foreign to normal tissue. The term transitional seems most appropriate, as they resemble benign growths, yet possess elements characteristic of sarcoma.

It may be remarked in passing, that any vesical neoplasm may become encrusted with phosphatic salts, and so convey the impression that a calculus is present instead of a tumor.

Symptoms.—The manner in which the symptoms appear varies ; sometimes they are sudden in their onset, or develop gradually.

The tumor may have existed for some time and have given no evidence of its existence, until sudden hemorrhage, or retention of urine occurs, due to the tumor becoming accidentally displaced, or from its having reached a certain size, or from the rupture of blood-vessels. Sometimes the first manifestation is a sudden attack of pain, either in the region of the bladder or in the back and loins, soon followed by hæmaturia and painful micturition.

Much more frequently, however, the symptoms appear gradually. At first a sense of uneasiness, gradually increasing to pain, is experienced in the region of the bladder, back or loins. This may be intermittent or continuous, and of varying intensity. Ere long irritability of the bladder is added, marked by increased frequency of micturition and tenesmus.

The degree of irritability varies greatly ; the calls to empty the viscus recurring every hour, or even every few minutes, and the contractions of the organ producing only slight pain, or most intense agony.

From the presence of a clot or fragment of the tumor in the vesical orifice of the urethra, or from the tumor itself impinging against the same, sudden and complete retention of urine may occur.

As we have seen, hæmaturia may be of sudden development and the first symptom to attract attention. If the disease manifests itself slowly, hæmaturia soon becomes added to the other symptoms enumerated above. It may be copious and intermittent in character, or less free and continuous. In cases of fimbriated papilloma the urine is almost continuously tinged with blood ; less so in the fibro-papilloma, and still less so in the transitional forms.

The examination of the urine in a suspected case will many times render most valuable information, and should never be omitted ; for while it may fail to afford any positive evidence of vesical growth, it will serve to exclude other diseases of the genito-urinary tract and so narrow down the diagnosis by exclusion.

Occasionally the unaided eye may detect small, slightly translucent, semi-gelatinous fragments, which under the glass appear made up of spindle-shaped nucleated cells, some short and broad, others elongated and acquiring the character of fibres.

Again, villi, or portions of them, will pretty surely be found if such a tumor is present, especially if the specimen subjected to examination is obtained (as it should be) by injecting the bladder with water and removing it by means of the aspirator and evacuating tube, such as are used in litholapaxy ; for by such a procedure one can scarcely fail to detach some of the villous processes if they are present.

In case of malignant disease, *débris* of various kinds, with purulent material, will also be present.

Rectal digital exploration gives negative results in cases of soft tumors, and but little can be learned of a positive nature from the use of the searcher.

In the hard varieties, however, the sound may render most valuable information, its excursions being limited by the tumor.

In this brief review of the symptoms of neoplasms of the bladder, we find no single, or even combination of symptoms, which can be regarded as diagnostic or pathognomonic, for they all may be present in greater or less degree in other affections.

Of them all, the most important is the hæmaturia, and we must determine first whether the blood has a vesical or other origin. If the stream of urine starts clear, or only slightly tinged with blood, and toward the end of the act of micturition it becomes bright red from admixture of fresh blood, the source of the bleeding is, undoubtedly, vesical. If this point is determined, and if we can, by proper examinations, exclude calculus, prostatic disease, stricture and traumatisms of the bladder and urethra, the presence of a tumor is highly probable, even though the urinary analysis, vesical and rectal explorations fail to furnish additional positive light. To remove all doubt, another and crucial examination is at our disposal, not to be made, of course, unless the weight of evidence points in the direction of tumor; but, on the other hand, not to be omitted when such evidence is present. We refer to digital exploration of the bladder. This is very easily accomplished in the female through the urethra; but its mere facility of accomplishment should not lead us to indulge it without decided reasons, for indiscriminate dilatation of the female urethra not infrequently results in permanent incontinence of urine. When, as we have said, the indications exist, it should not be omitted.

And these remarks apply equally well to the male. By means of median cystotomy the forefinger can, in the great majority of cases, be passed readily into the bladder, and if at the same time, the fingers of the disengaged hand be deeply pressed downward behind the pubes, or introduced into the rectum, pushing up the base of the bladder, every aspect of the vesical wall can be brought into contact with the intromitted finger, and thus not only the presence of a tumor determined, but also its attachments and physical features may be thoroughly appreciated.

In cases complicated with great prostatic hypertrophy or obesity, when the finger would not be long enough to enter the bladder from the perineum, then epi-cystotomy, or supra-pubic incision should be made. Indeed, some prefer this operation to the perineal in all cases.

Treatment.—Surgical measures only are of avail, and consist of the removal of the neoplasm, or as much of it as is possible or prudent, through the perineal or supra-pubic incision, or, in the female, through the urethra, or a vesico-vaginal incision.

If the tumor proves to be very large and sessile in character, then epi-cystotomy should be made, even though the perineum had previously been opened for exploration, for by the former procedure much more room and more direct access can be obtained to the vesical contents.

The removal is effected by means of forceps especially constructed for this purpose, with which the growth is twisted off, if it is possessed of a neck, or is bitten and twisted off piecemeal, if sessile, or is removed by ecraseur or ligature. In case of villous tumors, scraping or curetting must be resorted to.

In a large proportion of such operations the results are most satisfactory and recovery is perfect. Of course, such procedures are attended with danger, more or less, according to the nature, size and attachment of the growth, but, without operation, death is almost inevitable, and only after great and prolonged suffering, while the mortality from operation is not higher, if as high, as from lithotomy, except in malignant cases, or when the tumor has involved a great portion of the vesical parietes. Hence, the earlier the true condition is appreciated and surgical aid invoked, the better chances the patient has not only of surviving the operation, but of making a complete recovery.

In conclusion, we would crave your indulgence for the very imperfect manner in which we have presented our subject, of which imperfection no one can be more conscious than the writer, and we can only offer as an apology, lack of time, due to unavoidable circumstances.

EBERTH'S RODS IN TYPHOID STOOLS.—In the *Vratch*. No. 22, Drs. Shpolansky and Strojanoff report results of examination of stools in ninety-six cases of enteric fever. In ninety of these the typhoid bacilli were found. Of those examined eighty-eight recovered and eight died. In one of the latter no bacilli could be detected in the stools during life. In one of three convalescent patients examined no bacilli were found after the temperature had finally returned to the normal range. In the other two, the microbes were still daily discovered for nine and fifteen days respectively after the defervescence.—*Brit. Med. Jour.*, June 25th, 1887.

EDITORIAL DEPARTMENT.

EDITORS.

GEORGE M. DILLOW, M.D., ...	Editor-in-Chief, Editorial and Book Reviews.
CLARENCE E. BEEBE, M.D., ...	Original Papers in Medicine.
SIDNEY F. WILCOX, M.D., ...	Original Papers in Surgery.
MALCOLM LEAL, M.D., ...	Progress of Medicine.
EUGENE H. PORTER, M.D.	Comments and News.
HENRY M. DEARBORN, M.D., ...	Correspondence.
FRED S. FULTON, M.D., ...	Reports of Societies and Hospitals.

A B. NORTON, M.D., ... Business Manager.

The Editors individually assume full responsibility for and are to be credited with all connected with the collection and presentation of matter in their respective departments, but are not responsible for the opinions of contributors.

It is understood that manuscripts sent for consideration have not been previously published, and that after notice of acceptance has been given, will not appear elsewhere except in abstract and with credit to THE NORTH AMERICAN. All rejected manuscripts will be returned to writers. No anonymous or discourteous communications will be printed.

Contributors are respectfully requested to send manuscripts and communicate respecting them directly with the Editors, according to subject, as follows: *Concerning Medicine, 21 West 97th Street; concerning Surgery, 256 West 57th Street; concerning Societies and Hospitals, 121 East 70th Street; concerning News, Personals and Original Miscellany, 461 West 71st Street; concerning Correspondence, 152 West 57th Street.*

Communications to the Editor-in-Chief, *Exchanges* and *New Books* for notice should be addressed to *102 West 43d Street.*

DR. BRUNTON'S DISCOMFORT.

IN its June issue *The Monthly Homœopathic Review* takes up the explanation with which Dr. Brunton prefaces the third edition of his "Pharmacology, Materia Medica and Therapeutics." It will be remembered that in former editions Dr. Brunton had appended an Index of Diseases and Remedies, many of the remedies recommended as useful being taken, without acknowledgment, from homœopathic sources. On being pressed for an explanation in the columns of the *Lancet*, Dr. Brunton advertised an answer in the preface to the forthcoming edition of his work. It is this answer which the *Review* takes up *seriatim*. In the reply Dr. Brunton is shown, by his own confession, to have had no proper sense of responsibility for the reliability of the therapeutic recommendations in his index, or of that honor, sometimes felt by authors, which leads them to acknowledge the sources from which they derive their information. In short, Dr. Brunton's apology is that he took, unacknowledged, from the books of other men, but mainly from Dr. Potter, what they, in turn, had taken from homœopathic text-books, with or without acknowledgment. The *Review* maintains that "Dr. Brunton's *Index* contains indications that more than thirty per cent. of the applications of remedies named therein have been derived by some one or other from homœopathic treatises." The pity in Dr. Brunton's case still is, that after apologizing for not having acknowledged, until forced to do so, his indebtedness to Dr. Potter, he should still claim that *apis* is the only homœopathic remedy which, to his best knowledge, he has not expurgated from his present edition. As the *Review* says, Dr. Brunton's "best knowledge" is of "a singularly poor sort," a sort, we would add, so poor that it would bring the blush of shame to an author in any other department of honest literature.

But it is not to Dr. Brunton, as an apologist for his plagiaristic conscience, that we desire to direct attention. His preface, in addition, contains an attack upon homœopathy as a system of quackery which has called forth from the *Review* an aggressive defense from which we extract, not only because it is an interesting example of good dialectics, but also because it so fairly and ably states the broadest basis of homœopathy. Dr. Brunton writes :

"It is not the use of a single drug at a time, of a small dose, of a globule, nor even, as we have already seen, of a drug which may produce symptoms similar to those of the disease, that constitutes homœopathy. The essence of homœopathy, as established by Hahnemann, lies in the infinitesimal dose and the universal application of the rule *similia similibus curantur*. But the infinitesimal doses are so absurd, that I believe they have been discarded by many homœopaths. To such men all that remains of homœopathy is the universality of the rule *similia similibus curantur*, and the only difference between them and rational practitioners lies in the fact, that the latter regard the rule as only of partial application."

The *Review* goes on to comment as follows :

"With regard to the infinitesimal dose, Hahnemann had worked out the evidence in support of the rule of similars as the basis of drug-selection long before he arrived at the conclusion that medicines were most advantageously and successfully used (when prescribed homœopathically) in infinitesimal quantities. So that such doses cannot be said to be any part of the 'essence' of homœopathy. Having in the previous sentence implied that the rule *similia similibus curantur* does not constitute homœopathy, he now says that it is its 'universal application' that does so. And, in the next, he tells us that 'rational practitioners'—these, we suppose, are in Dr. Brunton's view restricted to those who are of Dr. Brunton's way of thinking—that 'rational practitioners' 'regard the rule as only of partial application.' It is not, then, according to this authority, that, as the *Lancet* said a few weeks ago, the law of similars is 'a fantastic notion;' but on the contrary, it is a true rule of drug-selection, though only true within a limited area. It is believing in its general, or as Dr. Brunton misleadingly puts it, its 'universal' application, that constitutes a man a homœopath.

"If by 'universal' Dr. Brunton intends to signify that in every possible condition for the relief of which a physician or surgeon may be summoned, this rule is held to be applicable, he is mistaken, and is, therefore, 'open to correction,' as he suggested at the commencement of his remarks he might be found to be. Hahnemann, in his earliest days, restricted its application to chronic diseases. Further experience proved its advantage in prescribing for acute disease, while in the note to paragraph 67 of the last edition of 'The Organon of the Healing Art,' he still points out some conditions in which antipathic measures must be resorted to. *   *   *

"That Dr. Brunton allows that it is of 'partial application' as a guide to the selection of drugs is, so far, a matter for congratulation. It is the first occasion on which, so far as we remember, a prominent teacher of medicine has acknowledged as much. Hitherto it has been denounced by admirers of Dr. Brunton as a 'fantastic notion,' and a notion of this kind can hardly be regarded as one of even partial application. If it is of partial application, we should like to know how partial this application is to be, in order to constitute its applier a 'rational practitioner.' The first duty of a physician is to relieve his patients' sufferings by the best, safest, and quickest means known to him—not to someone else. If a physician called to a case does not know and has no means of ascertaining what medicine is homœopathic to the condition, however much he may believe in the abstract truth of homœopathy, he necessarily falls back upon a palliative. Here, then, is one limit to the universality of the law—the knowledge of materia medica possessed by the physician. Again, in order that a medicine may be used homœopathically, we must have a record of provings of experiments with it before we can apply it. It may be that we may meet with cases to which the action of no known medicine corresponds. Here, again, we must fall back upon a palliative. Then sufferings may be induced by purely mechanical causes— which no medicine whatever, administered on any principle, would remove.

" How far, then, is this rule applicable ? Here experience alone can answer. Dr. Brunton's experience is limited—hence he says its application is partial. We had thought, before we were made acquainted with the source of ' The Index of Diseases and Remedies.' that his experience of homœopathy was limited to about one-third of the conditions met with in practice, but as this ' Index' is now stated to have been compiled from the experience of others, we have no means of estimating Dr. Brunton's. Those who have made a thorough, careful, practical, clinical study of homœopathy find that it is applicable in nearly every case they are called upon to prescribe for ; that it furnishes the means of ascertaining a directly curative, specifically acting drug, such as no other principle does. Relief may be, and doubtless is often given by medicines acting upon the antipathic, or even the allopathic principle—but a directly curative or specifically acting remedy cannot be found through either. Cases treated homœopathically, when cured, are cured directly; such as are treated antipathically, when cured, are cured indirectly.

"Conscious, apparently, that the degree of extent to which the law of similars is applicable, is a very feeble reason for denouncing it as ' certainly bad,' Dr. Brunton proceeds as follows : ' At first sight this difference may seem to be only slight, but it is not so in reality ; for while the rational practitioner, refusing to be bound by any ' pathy,' whether it be allopathy, antipathy or homœopathy, seeks to trace each symptom back to the pathological change which caused it, and, by a knowledge of the action of drugs on each tissue and organ of the body, to counteract these pathological changes, the homœopath professes to be in possession of a rule which will enable him to select the proper remedy in each case by a consideration of the symptoms without reference to the pathological condition. He may thus dispense with anatomy, physiology, pathology and pharmacology. All that is necessary is a list of morbid symptoms on the one hand and a list of the symptoms produced in healthy men by various drugs on the other.'

"In the first place, we can assure Dr. Brunton that a homœopathic physician is simply 'bound' to do the best he knows for his patient. He believes that homœopathy, wherever he can bring it to bear, enables him to do that best, but he is in no way pledged to treat his patient homœopathically if his case, or his knowledge of materia medica, does not admit of homœopathy being applied, or of his applying it. The gentlemen styled by Dr. Brunton ' a rational practitioner' is at liberty to treat his patient homœopathically, but, according to the present standard of medical ethics, he is ' bound' not to say that he does so, not to admit the homœopathicity of his prescription ; if he does this and is at the same time a hospital physician, the secretary of the institution to which he is attached may be instructed by his colleagues to write to him and request him not only to desist from admitting that he practices homœopathically, but from doing so at all, or resign his position !.

" Then the rational practitioner 'seeks to trace each symptom back to the pathological change which caused it.' Probably so, and his homœopathic brother does so likewise, and further, it must be admitted that both not unfrequently do so in vain, and, as often as they do fail, they seek to cover up their failure in a cloud of hypothesis.

" Of the manifold advantages of a correct interpretation of symptoms it is needless to write. They are admitted on all sides. . . . A correct pathological interpretation enables us to form our diagnosis ; this guides us not only in our prognosis, but in directing our patient to suitable diet and regimen, to appropriate climate and occupation, to the general hygiene suitable to his condition and to the group of medicines from among which the one most homœopathic to his state will be found. It is in the answer to the question—Which member of this group is most homœopathic to the individual case before us ?— that the value of the particular symptoms expressive of the morbid condition in that particular patient becomes so marked. And yet, again, how many cases there are of the pathological nature of which we at present know but little, and how many others are there regarding which the knowledge we have, or think we have, is more or less purely hypothetical ? By comparing the totality of the symptoms observed in disease with those produced by drugs, we are able to select medicines which do cure. This may seem very absurd to those who never tried to find a remedy in this way, though why it should do so we do not exactly see ; but those who have made the experiment have over and over again been abundantly satisfied with the result. No physician, whether he practices medicine upon a scientific or a merely empirical basis, can dispense with anatomy, physiology and pathology for the simple reason that drug-prescribing is only one part of his duty. Still less can the homœopathist do without pharmacology. Had it not been for the work of Hahnemann we should never have heard of pharmacology to-day ! Hahnemann possesses the clearest title to be regarded as the Father of Pharmacology. Dr. Brunton defines pharmacology as 'a knowledge of the mode of action of drugs upon the body generally, and upon its various parts.' Hahnemann was the earliest physician to acquire and publish a considerable mass of knowledge of this kind. *Fragmenta de Viribus Medicamentorum Positivis sive in sano corpore humano observatis,* published at Leipsic in 1805, was the first work which ever conveyed any real knowledge of the mode of action of drugs upon the human body generally and upon its various parts! A work regarding which Dr. Waring (*Bibliotheca Therapeutica,* vol. I, p. 65) says : ' However much one may be inclined to differ from the inferences or conclusions drawn by the author from his facts, all must admire the zeal and labor bestowed by Hahnemann in his investigations as set forth in this work.' And now, forsooth, homœopathists are told that they 'dispense with' pharmacology! The real truth is that without pharmacology, homœopathy would be non-existent, simply because it would be practically impossible. This is another point on which Dr. Brunton is 'open to correction,' as he modestly suggested that he might be found to be.

"Further, we should like to know how, when 'a rational practitioner has traced all the symptoms of his patient back to the pathological change which caused them,' he proceeds 'to counteract' them? Does he do so homœopathically, antipathically or allopathically? He must do so in one way or the other, when he uses drugs—which does he employ?

"In the next paragraph Dr. Brunton tells us how it comes to pass that homœopathy is quackery. 'It is' he writes 'the falsity of the claim which homœopathy makes to be in possession, if not of the universal panacea, at least of the only true rule of practice, that makes homœopathy a system of quackery ; and yet this arrogant claim constitutes the essence of the system.' Dr. Brunton would have occupied these four or five pages of his preface to much better purpose had he, instead of dealing in mere denunciation, demonstrated the falsity of the claim which he says is made for homœopathy. The claim we make for homœopathy is, not that it is the only true rule of practice in all instances—this will depend upon the nature of the case to be treated, as we have already shown—but it is the only rule by which we can discover specific remedies for individual cases. And as specific remedies, where applicable, are those which are more directly, more quickly and more frequently curative than any others, it is the best and safest rule of practice.   *   *   *

" He also adds to the sentence we have quoted that any man who 'regards the rule *similia similibus curantur* as only of partial and not of universal application, has no right to call himself a homœopath.' We maintain that any man who regards the law of similars as of partial application is a homœopath, so far as he goes, whatever he may call himself. And, further, we may say that, while no one is in honor bound to call himself anything, a man who practices homœopathy and denies that he is a homœopath, is, in the present state of professional feeling, a good deal of a coward. If a physician knows that a certain doctrine is true in relation to a certain number of cases, it is his duty to say so, and to act up to what he knows openly, and when this doctrine is denied *in toto* by some, decried as a 'fantastic notion' by others, and brusquely put aside as 'all humbug' by many more, the man who knows that it is a doctrine of practical utility in any number of cases, however limited, is false to his profession if he refuses to say what he knows, and when his refusal to do so is based upon a fear of the loss of professional status, he becomes, as we have said, a coward.

"Dr. Brunton says further, that if we have renounced the errors of Hahnemann's system we ought not to retain its name.

"What is Hahnemann's system? As we understand it, it is as follows :—

" 1. The study of drug action upon the healthy human body.

" 2. The selection of specifically acting remedies upon the principle of *similia similibus curantur.*

" 3. The administration of medicines in doses smaller than will excite their physiological action.

" 4. The prescribing of medicines singly and uncombined.

"This is homœopathy, and Hahnemann's method of carrying it out. If there are errors here, we should be glad to know what they are. We see none.

" 'A medical man,' we are told, ' is bound to do the best he can for the good of his patient; it is obvious that although he may employ baths or packs as a mode of treatment, he cannot, without becoming untrue to his profession, throw aside all other means of treatment and become a hydropath.' A physician, who is known as a hydropath, is, we have always understood, one who has endeavored to develop the use of water as a remedial agent to the greatest extent to which it is capable of being developed ; but he does not, therefore, 'throw aside all other means of treatment.' The homœopath stands in a similar position in one respect, and yet a different one in another. The hydropath, as such, deals with only one remedial agent. The homœopath, as such, points to a rule by which all drug remedies may be employed in a certain direction. Neither does he throw aside all other means of treatment. The means of treatment at our disposal are not restricted to drugs ; they are not even limited, in the use of drugs, to such as act specifically. But when we know that a specifically acting drug is a curative agent of the highest power

—when we have reason to believe that homœopathy provides the only known method of discovering such curative agents—then in endeavoring to do our utmost for the good of our patients, we are first of all bound to seek for them through homœopathy.　To say or to imply that a homœopath throws aside all other means of treatment, is to state what is well known to be contrary to fact.　＊　＊　＊

"Few things can strike the reader of this, the latest endeavor to place homœopathy in the category of quackeries, more forcibly than the change—the total change—in the method of doing so, from any which has preceded it during the last sixty years in this country.　In 1827 Mr. Spry, in the 'Edinburgh Medical and Surgical Journal,' declared the doctrine of homœopathy to be 'visionary;' and Dr. James Johnson, in the 'Medico-Chirurgical Review,' termed it 'preposterous.'　The Provincial Medical and Surgical Association, in 1851, resolved that it was 'completely at variance with science and common sense.'　Ridicule in every form that the imagination could suggest has been applied to it by writers in the medical press from that time to the present; and now Dr. Lauder Brunton acknowledges that it is of 'partial application.'　Dr. Wilks, six or seven years ago, at the College of Physicians, protested against the idea of there being any doctrine in therapeutics.　To-day an examiner at the college not only admits the existence of doctrine in therapeutics, but also allows that homœopathy is a therapeutic doctrine of 'partial application.'　All definition of the word 'partial' he carefully avoids.　Homœopathists have been denounced by every epithet that could express moral and intellectual degradation; now our baseness is restricted to believing that homœopathy is not only a doctrine of partial, but of general application !

"To such trivial dimensions as these, to such unsubstantial proportions as these, has the opposition to homœopathy been whittled down !"

THE AMERICAN INSTITUTE, 1887.

THE American Institute of Homœopathy has rounded out another year's work, in a session noted for good management, and occupied with much work of the average sort of interest.　The meetings in sections fairly justified their inauguration.　The number of papers read was so great as to almost suffocate attention and discussion, but it is scarcely to be expected that a first year's experiment should be flawless. There can be no doubt but that the plan of sectional working has come to stay, and that, in the near future, suitable methods will be developed by which the best papers, that is, those calculated to excite the liveliest immediate interest, will alone be read, and then followed immediately after reading, by well-planned, animated discussions to which will be assigned an appropriate share of time. The session of 1887 can, then, be noted as moving toward the evolution of more attractive meetings. It is to be regretted, however, that there was not more deliberation over the still more important matter of inciting a higher order of original papers and independent work, especially in our materia medica and therapeutics.

The chief feature of the meeting we have not yet noted, the position taken in the Presidential address, and unanimously endorsed by the Institute. It is certainly no new position, but an emphatic reaffirmation of the old, which always appears to be ever new. After reviewing the various shifting grounds which have heretofore served for maligning and ostracizing physicians avowing the rule of similars, President Orme took up the present fashionable pretext, to wit, that homœopathy constitutes a "sect" and bears a "sectarian" name. He ably showed that the term "regular" is as sectarian as the word homœopathic, that "sects" are not sinful, but have their place and use in the evolution of progress, that the fundamental law of the land recognizes the rights of sectarianism, as natural and inalienable, being of direct benefit to the people, that, if homœopathy is a "sect," it is broad, tolerant and liberal, and that, in no proper sense of the word, can "sectarian" be applied to homœopathy by way of reproach. " Homœopathists, then, having no thought of relinquishing their distinctive title, under present conditions, what is the true basis of harmony ? First, the Golden Rule ; second, the acceptance, by the profession at large, of the definition adopted by the American Institute of Homœopathy, of the term 'regular physician ;' third, the recognition and co-operation of the members of the different schools under the above conditions." The address closed with suggestions as to the adoption of resolutions to which attention is directed in other pages of this issue.

The resolutions, in effect, dispel the mistatements, stale, sterile, slurring and untruthful, which have formed the capital of the "sect" that is a "sect" in order to suppress all other "sects." Resolution seventh declares that homœopathists will continue to be a "sect" until their work shall have been accomplished in securing a proper consideration of the doctrine of *similia similibus curantur*." With the President's address preceding this resolution as explanatory of its meaning there can be no objection, but, dissociated from its connection as it will be, we cannot but think that the wording is unfortunate, capable of being twisted to a perverted meaning. For the word "sect" has been borrowed from theology for its offensive suggestions, not its most candid meaning, and the word, "doctrine," associated as it is with the evidence of things not seen, does not properly apply to a principle, theory, law or rule of prescription deduced from positive knowledge and scientific experiment. Homœopathy, being as broad as the whole realm of the various sciences included under the general term, medicine, and being, moreover, a scientific system of therapeutics, has nothing in common with narrowness, intolerance, bigotry, fanaticism and exclusiveness; and, as an organization among medical men, it is a party for the establishment of certain principles of freedom in medical practice and organization, including the proper use of a name, The word "sect" has no proper application to politics or science. We fear that the Institute has blundered in inconsiderately permitting a *mal apropos* designation, employed in medical warfare for the sole partisan purpose of affixing odium and fallacious suggestions.

The election of officers was a step forward. President A. C. Cowperthwaite has executive force, the oratorical gift, and, what is more important, the dominant interest in homœopathic therapeutics which is needed to keep our national body moving in its distinctive direction. With Pemberton Dudley to second him as General Secretary, the next meeting will be marked with red letters, and more than ordinarily initiative in better methods and higher work.

COMMENTS.

WHO ARE DEGRADED ?—"Our correspondent knows as well as we that the use of the term 'homœopathic' is considered by the whole world, outside the sect which it distinguishes, as in bad taste and *degrading to all who use it.*" (Italics ours). The preceding is taken from the reply signed "Ed.," of *The New York Medical Times,* to a correspondent in its June issue. What constitutes use of the term "homœopathic" the "Ed." does not explain ; but, by way of comment, we append what seems to us a very conspicuous use.

SENIOR EDITOR—Trustee of the New York *Homœopathic* Asylum for the Insane, President of the staff of the Ward's Island *Homœopathic* Hospital, attending physician to the Hahnemann Hospital (whose charter reads that "all patients in said hospital shall be under the professional care of physicians and surgeons skilled in and *practicing under the homœopathic system of medicine*)," member of the *Homœopathic* Medical Society of the County of New York, of the *Homœopathic* Medical Society of the State of New York, and of the American Institute of *Homœopathy.*

JUNIOR EDITOR—Member of the Medical Society of the County of New York (whose by-laws read : "That the Comitia Minora be directed to recommend no applicant for admission to membership unless he be a graduate from a medical college in good standing, or a licentiate of a regular unsectarian State or County Medical Society of this or any other State ; or, if *his diploma or license be of a sectarian character, unless the applicant declare in writing his or her abnegation of sectarian principles and practice.*" Attending Physician and Secretary of Staff to the Ward's Island *Homœopathic* Hospital.

Now, these two gentlemen, in fact constituting *The Medical Times,* we feel it in order to ask: If all who use the term "homœopathic" are thus degraded in the eyes of the world, how much degraded below this degradation must be those who cling to the honors and privileges of the homœopathic sect, using, misusing and abusing it all at the same time?

Degrading is, however, a little larger word than we would strictly apply, even in deference to the *Times,* but what the word should be our neighbor can no longer afford to ignore. The question of most pressing interest just now is not whether homœopathy should keep its honored name, but whether there is any name for the public conduct of the editors of *The Medical Times* as related to the "sectarian" honors and trusts which they hold.

RETIREMENT OF DR. ARNDT.—In the May number of *The Medical Counselor and Michigan Journal of Homœopathy,* we find the valedictory of Dr. H. R. Arndt and the salutation of Dr. D. A. McLachlan. After many years of service—years in which illness and death in his family have added to the strain of overwork in our literature and in private practice—Dr. Arndt feels "the imperative need of perfect rest from care and work." There will be wide sympathy for him in his bereavement and ill-health, and the heartiest wishes for his restoration.

In welcoming the incoming editor we express the hope that he will carry on the *Counselor* in the same spirit of candor, courtesy and devotion which have made its pages heretofore a strong force in the homœopathic school. The *Counselor* has been vigorous and able, and, in the first number under its new management, it gives promise of continuance in well-doing.

BOOK REVIEWS.

ANÆMIA, by Frederick P. Henry, M.D., Prof., etc.   Philadelphia : P. Blakiston, Son & Co., 1887. 16mo., pp., 136.

This is a clear-running, brief description, with judicious commentary, by one who has observed exactly to good purpose, and assimilated the literature of anæmia.   While it might be fuller in exposition, it covers the ground as well as could be expected in a reprint of a series of papers contributed to a journal, "The Polyclinic."   Its perusal will tend to the employment of more exact methods in diagnosis, to the more frequent counting of blood-corpuscles and estimating the percentage of hæmaglobin, especially in the lighter forms of secondary anæmia and the earlier stages of the more profound primary varieties.   The latter are well differentiated under the titles of Chlorosis, Anæmia Lymphatica (Hodgkin's Disease), Leucocythæmia, Anæmia Splenica, and Pernicious Anæmia.   The Toxanæmias are but barely suggested.   In general method the handling is systematic and the style good, while the book is printed in elegant form and bound with good taste.

OXYGEN IN THERAPEUTICS, by C. E. Ehinger, M.D.   Published by W. S. Chatterton & Co., Chicago, 1887.

This little work of 149 pages is well worth perusal.   It presents in a clear, explicit manner, the cases to which the oxygen treatment is applicable, the method of preparation and application of the gas, the apparatus necessary for its successful use, the fallacy of the noted compound oxygen craze, and the accessory measures necessary to render the treatment most effective.

Many cases from actual practice are given to show the practical results.   It is not a pretentious work, but it succeeds admirably in doing what the author intended, namely, to furnish practical and reliable information, in sufficient detail, to be entirely serviceable to any one desirous of employing the treatment, and, in addition, to show that it is a valuable remedial agent in the treatment of many affections of the respiratory and alimentary tracts.   F.

TAKING COLD, by John W. Hayward, M.D., M.R.C.S., L.S.A.   Published by E. Gould & Son, London, England.

This little book is intended by the author as a family guide for domestic prescribing.   It contains a short, popular description of the various diseases resulting from cold, followed by a concise statement of the ordinary homœopathic treatment for such ailments.   It is not intended for the profession, but would be a reliable guide for family use in ordinary cases.   F.

REPORTS OF SOCIETIES AND HOSPITALS.

AMERICAN INSTITUTE OF HOMŒOPATHY.

THE American Institute of Homœopathy began its fortieth annual session at Saratoga Springs, June 27th, 1887. The meeting was called to order by the President, Dr. F. H. Orme, Atlanta, Ga. After the address of welcome by Dr. S. J. Pearsall, of Saratoga, to which the President responded, Dr. Orme delivered the annual address before the Institute, in which he reviewed the progress of homœopathy during the past century and year; the position gained; the respect accorded to the new school; upheld a liberal sectarianism as essential to the well-being of medicine; hailed the era of approaching toleration, as evidenced in the writings of the more advanced thinkers of both schools, and advocated the harmonizing of the different elements of our own and other schools. He offered the following recommendations for action by the Institute: That the American Institute most earnestly endorses the improvement of homœopathic therapeutics and all other departments of medical science; that the imputations cast upon the early homœopaths were the result of ignorance and prejudice and are unworthy of our school; that the charge made by the American Medical Association that members of the homœopathic school " practiced upon an exclusive dogma to the rejection of aids furnished by experience and the allied sciences," is entirely devoid of foundation in fact; that the later charge that homœopathists traded upon a name is a positive calumny; that the present position of the medical profession, that it is blame-worthy for homœopathists to concert together under a denominational name, thus constituting a "sect," is a flimsy pretext; that the division of medicine into schools results from the unwillingness of other members to thoroughly examine into the doctrines of the new school; that it is advisable for homœopathists to continue to form a sect until the proper consideration by others of the doctrine of *similia similibus curantur* be obtained.

Drs. W. T. Helmuth, B. W. James and G. A. Hall were appointed a committee to consider the above recommendations.

Dr. E. M. Kellogg, Treasurer, then offered his report.

Dr. J. C. Burger presented the report of the Executive Committee, recommending some slight changes in the rules governing the sectional plan.

Dr. T. F. Smith, Chairman of the Bureau of Statistics, reported the following: Number of medical societies reporting, 123; number of medical societies not reporting, 27; number of national societies, 5; number of sectional societies, 2; number of state societies, 31; number of local societies, 112; number of hospitals, houses, etc., reporting, 43; number of hospitals, houses not reporting, 14; the hospitals report a bed capacity of 4,239; whole number of patients treated, 13,862; number cured, 5,935; number relieved, 4,471; number died, 910, showing the very low mortality of 1 5-10 per cent.; number of dispensaries reporting, 34; number of dispensaries not reporting, 12; number of patients treated therein, 142,629; number of prescriptions, 376,886; number of colleges reporting, 14; number of students, 1,171; number of graduates during the past year, 372; number of alumni, 7,732; number of journals, 24.

Reports from delegates from the different societies and hospitals were next heard.

Dr. A. R. Wright, of Buffalo, said they had a hospital in that city, of seventy-five beds, with an average of fifty patients. A training school for nurses was being maintained with great success.

Dr. T. F. Allen, New York, reported for the Laura Franklin Free Hospital for Children. It was built by the Astor family and presented to the homœopathic profession with an endowment of about $300,000. It was opened last December, since which time they had treated 112 patients and lost four. It was under the charge of the Sisterhood of St. Mary, and contained between fifty and seventy-five free beds. Also a free hospital was being built in connection with the Homœopathic Medical College of New York. The site has been purchased, paid for, and a balance on hand of about $150,000 or $200,000, with which to commence operations. Already ten beds had been endowed at $5,000 each.

Dr. M. J. Chapman, Pittsburgh:—They have a hospital with 200 beds. They had treated during the year 1,114 patients; 867 were cured; seventy-three improved; twenty-three unimproved; sixty-seven died, making a gross mortality of six per cent. Deducting the cases which were practically moribund on admission, the real mortality was two per cent. A large dispensary is connected with the hospital, and also a training school for nurses.

Dr. H. C. Allen, Ann Arbor:—Their hospital was filled. A new hospital was to be built at Detroit. $200,000 had been donated by two prominent citizens of that city. They proposed to erect a hospital equal to any in the country.

Dr. Horace Packard, Boston:—The Massachusetts hospital was doing magnificent work. It is out of debt; has received $50,000 in donations, and has $80,000 invested.

J. B. G. Custis, Washington:—The National hospital was succeeding. It had thirty-three beds and about twenty patients.

TUESDAY MORNING.

After some preliminary business, the Institute listened to the report of the Committee on Drug Proving, which was presented by Dr. L. Sherman, Milwaukee. Two provings of *adonis vernalis*, in ten grain doses, had been made; eleven provings of *chininum arsenicosum* in the first and sixth trituration, in one grain doses, and also of the sixth and thirtieth dilution; thirteen provings of *lilium tigrinum*, in five and ten grain doses of the crude material.

Dr. Martin Deschere, New York, was appointed on the Bureau of Drug Proving to fill the place of Dr. E. M. Hale, Chicago, whose term expires this year.

The Committee on Pharmacy next reported. Dr. C. W. Butler, Chairman, stated that their experiments had been in two directions: first, to ascertain the physical properties of drugs; second, to discover the pathogenetic properties of drugs. Twenty-one provings of *merc. sol.*, in different potencies, had been made to determine the drug power of different preparations. A summary of the results was given by Dr. C. Wesselhoeft, Boston. The medicines were distributed in boxes marked 1, 2, 3, 4. No. 1 was *sac. lac.;* the others were first and thirtieth cent. and a precipitated preparation of *merc.*, with ninety-nine parts of *sac. lac.* One prover had violent symptoms, such as diarrhœa, influenza, catarrh, etc., from *sac. lac.* One had no symptoms from *sac. lac.*, or from the thirtieth. The symptoms obtained from the different preparations of *merc.* did not materially differ from each other. None, however, are obtained from the thirtieth. The pathogenetic effects were shown mainly upon the intestinal canal, less so upon the bronchial mucous membrane. Two provers were made violently sick.

Dr. C. Wesselhoeft then presented a paper on "Why Trituration Makes Drugs Darker." A paper read last year by Dr. L. Sherman, gave some important facts regarding the ability to sub-divide metals by trituration. In these experiments it was shown that metals became darker when ground for a long time with sugar of milk, leading one to infer that the increase of color was due to the greater comminution of the metal. To test the accuracy of these experiments, Dr. Wesselhoeft instituted the following experiments. He first ground thirty grains of the first decimal trituration of copper for 100 hours in a wedgewood mortar. It became much darker. He then ground an equal quantity of *sac. lac.* for 100 hours. Long before the time had expired the *sac. lac.* had assumed the same dark color. He then ground an empty wedgewood mortar with an ordinary pestle for 100 hours, producing a dark dust in the bottom of the mortar, which readily washed off and made a dark solution. By forcibly rubbing the pestle over a wedgewood or porcelain mortar, a dark line will be produced, which, when continued, forms an impalpable, dark powder, which, when mixed with the trituration, gives it a dark color. This change in color occurs, to any marked degree, only when small quantities of medicine are triturated. When greater amounts are ground, the change in color is much less marked. Dr. Wesselhoeft, therefore, holds that the color is due to the kind of mortar used and to the smallness of the quantity triturated. A porcelain mortar produces much less change from rubbing away of its own substance than a wedgewood. The author holds that there is a limit to the divisibility of insoluble materials by trituration.

Dr. L. Sherman then gave a summary of two years' work in this department. Before commencing, he said he could not accept the results of Dr. Wesselhoeft's experiments. He was aware that wedgewood mortars produced the result mentioned, but that the best porcelain material did not, providing there was sufficient material used to constantly engage the pestle, so that the mortar shall not itself be triturated. He had ground *sac. lac.* for 100 hours by this method in porcelain mortars without the least darkening of the trituration; also different metals ground, while they produced a darker color for longer trituration, each had its own distinctive color and were not uniformly a dark, dingy color, as they would be if the change were due to the presence of material from the mortar. The following were the conclusions reached: 1. That all the various metals grow darker the longer they are triturated. 2. The darker color is not due to oxidation, as it occurs in gold, platinum, etc. *Sac. lac.*, triturated for 100 hours in porcelain mortars, does not grow darker, if there be enough sugar to constantly engage the pestle. Each metal, also, has its own distinctive color after trituration. The finer the precipitate the darker the color. 3. The darker the color the finer is the division of the particles, as shown by the microscope. 4. The Hahnemannian period for the trituration of metals is long enough to reduce only the softest metals; a much longer time being required than is ordinarily supposed. 5. The rapidity of the sub-division diminishes with the length of time of trituration, almost the entire reduction being effected in a comparatively few hours. Samples of *merc. viv.* were presented, which had been ground up to twelve hours. Little change took place after the second hour. With increased trituration insoluble drugs become more suspensible. 6. In cases of *merc. viv.* all samples purchased were found to be too little triturated. 7. The British method of trituration is not so good as the Hahnemannian. The former gives forty minutes to the first decimal and forty minutes to the second decimal trituration. The Hahnemannian method gives sixty minutes to 100 grains. 8. Triturations of 1,000 grains of *merc. viv.* for 10 hours cannot be distinguished from the trituration of 100 grains for one hour, showing that the time must be proportioned to the amount triturated. 9. Trituration of 100 grains for ten hours shows it to be much better sub-divided than when prepared after the Hahnemannian method. 10. *Cupr. met.*, as purchased in market, was uniformly found to be deficient as regards the sub-division of the particles. These preparations, when ground in proportion of ten hours to 1,000 grains, became much darker. Dr. Sherman does not believe that trituration does not reduce the finest particles of matter. The change in color, the test by subsidence and the microscope all show that this change can go on indefinitely.

The report of the Committee on Medical Education was next presented by its Chairman, Dr. T. Y. Kinne, in which he said: This institution should shake off its lethargy. It stands between the student and the college faculty. The subject of medical education was properly divided into preparatory, collegiate and post graduate. The student must be thoroughly educated before entering college. The colleges are in advance of the profession in their appreciation of the necessity of this measure. The colleges are not on an equal footing regarding their courses of study and preliminary requirements. A graded course and preliminary examinations should be insisted upon by this Institute as binding upon all colleges.

Dr. Kinne offered resolutions, which provoked a lengthy discussion, after which the following motion was passed: That three members of the Inter-collegiate Committee should meet with a like number from the Committee on Medical Education, consider the subject and report next year to the Institute a comprehensive system of medical education.

Dr. Millie J. Chapman, Pittsburgh, then presented the Bureau address on Obstetrics, in which she gave a hasty review of the complications of gestation, the advantages of early treatment, and the good results obtained by the administration of homœopathic remedies.

Dr. L. H. Willard, Allegheny, read the Bureau address on Surgery, in which was given an excellent *resumé* of the advances of surgery in the last year or two. Regarding fractures of bones, he did not consider the old-fashioned sand-bags as sufficient, but believed that better recovery was obtained by the use of splints and bandages. In brain and abdominal surgery great advances had been made, as also in the supra-pubic operation for vesical calculi. This was becoming the most satisfactory method of treating stone in the bladder. The quadriceps extensor femoris, when ruptured, had been wired through the lower one-third, securing immediate union and a serviceable muscle. In orthopœdic surgery, the removal of bone and open section in tenotomy were coming more to the front, owing to perfected antiseptic measures. He believed that the prominence and progress of homœopathy was due more to the surgeon and surgery than to any other cause.

TUESDAY AFTERNOON.

The Bureau of Surgery considered hip-joint disease. L. H. Willard, Allegheny, Chairman, presented the first paper on "The Etiology, Diagnosis and Prognosis in Hip Disease." He believed that the disease resulted from both a strumous diathesis and from traumatism. Phymosis also is said to cause it; but he doubted if it ever caused true hip-joint disease. Symptoms were persistent or intermittent limping. If the disease were in the acetabulum, the pain would be referred to the knee; if in the head of the bone, it would be in the hip itself. There was heat and inflammation; leg was thrown forward; the gluteal fold was obliterated ; weight of body was borne by the sound limb, and there was fixation of the joint by the muscles. Fever was worse at night. Limbs jerked during sleep. In second stage there was an aggravation of the symptoms of the first stage. Leg was forward; greater fixation of the pelvis. Pain was worse than before and more unbearable at night; relieved by extension. The stage varied from a few days to weeks. The third stage was a stage of suppuration, with necrosis of the head of the femur and acetabulum. The leg is adducted; shortened. Pelvis tilted; knee thrown over the sound leg; dislocation of the head of the bone backward upon the dorsum ilii, with one or more discharging sinuses leading down to necrotic bone. In the congenital dislocation we have shortening, normal mobility; no fixation. Pain on motion of the trochanter; abscess over the part; no pain in the knee; no deformity, and usually a rheumatic history. The prognosis should be guarded. It is favorable in a child of good general health, and more so in the first stage. If inflammatory products are deposited, there will be ankylosis. If the disease progresses to the third stage, there will be necrosis, and we must then operate.

"The Pathology of Hip Disease," by Dr. W. L. Jackson, Roxbury, Mass., was then read. Most cases originate in the bone; less frequently, if ever, in the synovial membranes and articular cartilages. If the disease originates in the acetabulum, it starts in one or more of the ossific centers or nuclei, or in the cavity itself. If in the femur, its starting point is usually at the osseous nuclei, along the epiphaseal line on the lower part. The recognized causes are an inflammation of the joint, extravisation of blood into the bone or cavity, and tuberculosis. The bone may become calcified or carious. The abscess usually breaks into the cavity of the joint, exciting articular inflammation, which rapidly destroys the membranes and cartilages of the joint. The latter are sometimes entirely detached from the bone and float as foreign bodies in the cavity of the joint. If the disease starts in the synovial membranes, the free border of the bone first ulcerates; if in the bone, we get ulceration of the deeper surfaces, with great thickening of the synovial membranes. The cartilages are gradually worn away from the bone, which in turn becomes softened, the head at times becoming detached from the shaft of the bone. A new joint may thus be formed between the head and the pelvic bone. When the disease starts in the acetabulum, the pus may perforate into the pelvic cavity and open anywhere. If it originates in the head of the femur, the most frequent opening is just back of the great trochanter, or it may burrow to the knee. When the head of the bone escapes back upon the ilium and forms a new socket, the acetabulum becomes filled with inflammatory products and obliterated,

"Therapeutics of Hip Disease."—Dr. John E. James, Philadelphia. The first thing to be done is to place the patient in bed, give him rest and extension. A weight and pulley attached to the leg is the best method. The amount of weight must be determined by the relief of the pain. The remedies, particularly in scrofulous cases, are :*calc. carb.* and *phos., merc., phos. stram., fluoric acid, bell., bry., arn., puls.* In the second stage, with much effusion, must aspirate as soon as possible and as often as it refills. Fixation, with extension and counter-extension, are the most applicable here. The remedies are *bell., rhus, stram., arn.* In the third stage resection or excision is demanded as soon as suppuration is established. The patient should have a good, strong, nutritious diet, with fruits, cod-liver oil, and exercise in the open air. *Rhus* acts best on the right hip and *stram.* has remarkable control over the disease in the left. In addition to the above, *silic.* and *hepar* are very valuable.

Mechanical Treatment.—Dr. G. A. Hall, Chicago. In this paper Dr. Hall described the various appliances used, including the splint of Harris, Sayre, Davis, Taylor, Thomas; Hutchinson's shoe, Darrach s wheel crutch, Hamilton's splint, etc. In the early stages the patient should be put to bed and mechanical treatment applied. In a very young child he has used, with success, a foot splint, retained *in situ* by bandages or plaster-of-paris. In older children he uses either a Hutchinson's shoe with crutches and a weight of lead upon the diseased limb, or a Thomas's splint, or both combined. Taylor's and Sayre's splints do not accomplish the objects desired. All splints allowing movement in the joint and endeavoring to relieve the cotyloid cavity from the weight of the body have been failures. Best treatment is to keep patient in bed for first few weeks and then use Hutchinson's shoe, with lead on the diseased limb for extension.

"Operative Treatment of Hip-joint Disease."—Dr. Wm. Tod Helmuth, New York. If the bone is dead or liable to die, it should be removed. Latterly the operation is not called for as frequently as before, on account of the improved appliances for the earlier treatment of the disease. Of all these, Dr. Helmuth has had the best results from the use of Hutchinson's shoe. Operation is called for in the third stage where the bone is dead, as evidenced by the probe. In performing the operation, the part is first scrubbed with a 1 to 2,000 solution of *merc. cor.*, which is also injected into all the sinuses, a saturated solution of iodoform and ether is next poured over the leg, the patient placed on the well side. The knife is entered at the superior spinous process of the ilium and carried down in a curved line about four or five inches. The incision is carried to the bone, dividing the periosteum, if any be left. This, together with the muscles, is pushed back by the periostitome, a chain saw passed under the bone to be removed, and the bone severed. Then, by grasping the head with a heavy bone forceps, with a few nicks of the knife and periostitome the bone is easily twisted from its connections. The dead bone in the acetabulum is then removed with the gauge, the wound filled with the balsam of Peru, closed with deep and superficial sutures, a drainage tube inserted and the whole covered with many layers of the bichloride of mercury gauze, rubber tissue or oiled silk, and tightly secured by a roller.

Dr. N. Schneider, Cleveland:—Hip disease is caused by a peculiar diathesis. Patients suffering from phymosis have this diathesis, which causes the joint trouble. In order to be sure of hip disease, the patient must exhibit constitutional symptoms and fixation of the pelvis. In the treatment rest is the great factor. Nature can do more than we can with splints. In order to overcome the excessive muscular contraction, the child should be put to bed and extension, by weight and pulley, applied to the leg. If patient must get up, use Hutchinson's shoe. When patient is convalescent and is able to walk, then splints are useful and will prevent traumatism. Homœopathy greatly lessens the number of fully-developed hip diseases.

Dr. J. H. McClelland, Pittsburgh:—Most cases are either acute or chronic; the former is traumatic, begins in the center and spreads to the surface; the chronic is just the opposite. The causes are mainly traumatic. The patient should be placed at once in bed. The best results are obtained by simply fixing the joint. Dr. McClelland does not believe much in weight and extension. *Stram., bell., merc., hepar, silic.* were the best remedies. Wood, wool and cotton combined make the most absorbent dressing.

Dr. S. B. Parsons, St. Louis:—All cases of distension of the capsule are not hip disease. The latter is nearly always tubercular in character, as is white swelling; night sweat, hectic fever, cough, etc., will follow. Dr. Parsons has operated upon sixteen cases of hip-joint disease in the third stage. Of these fourteen recovered entirely. One died two months afterwards and the other six months. Every patient received an oil bath every day, Phillips' wheat emulsion of cod-liver oil, but no stimulants.

Dr. J. E. Jones, Westchester, Pa., places a stout plaster-of-paris splint on diseased hip and a Hutchinson's shoe on the other. The patient walks about on crutches during the day, and extension is applied at night by the weight and pulley.

Dr. J. C. Morgan, Philadelphia:—Tuberculosis is the consequence and not the cause of articular disease. It is begotten by the original inflammatory disease. The absorption of these cheesy matters, which are deposited in the joint, is the cause of the generalization of tuberculosis. In these cases will get amyloid degeneration of the liver, kidneys, spleen and all organs. *Stram.* has proved exceedingly useful in very many cases of disease of the *left* hip. It acts also on the right side. *Lycopodium* also is indicated when the patient wakes at night with very great ill-humor and pain.

Dr. Wm. B. Van Lennep, Philadelphia, wished to enter a plea for early operation. Exsection should be performed as soon as suppuration becomes fully established. The results are very much better.

Dr. S. F. Wilcox, New York, believes that in some cases apparatus is of great assistance. Has seen one case in the third stage cured by apparatus. If the patient is placed in bed and extension applied the disease may often be aborted. He presented a modification of Taylor's splint, which was designed to obviate the necessity of the patient walking directly upon the cross-piece. The brace was similar to Taylor's, except that about five or six inches from the bottom was a curved bar at right angles to the splint, which extended back of the leg to the corresponding point on the inside. To this bar was attached an upright extending down to the floor and parallel with the main shaft. These had rubber pads in the end, upon which the patient walked, and also rubber straps for extension.

Dr. Fred. S. Fulton, New York :—In some cases where operation was not considered advisable, either on account of extensive involvement of the sacrum, coccyx, or pelvic bones, or where a movable joint was already being formed by nature, he adopted Prof. Billroth's method of injecting into the sinuses a solution of glycerine loaded with iodoform. The sinus or cavity was filled with the solution and then sealed up as tight as possible with adhesive plaster. It would usually stop the suppurative process and gradually restore it to a healthy condition.

Dr. M. O. Terry, Utica, N. Y., had had one case of hip disease from purely reflex trouble. Before splints are applicable counter irritation with the thermo-cautery is of great value.

Dr. Wm. Tod Helmuth, New York, regards hip disease as resulting simply in dead bone. Tuberculosis is rare in his experience. The bone is like any other which has necrosed.

Dr. A. Claypool, Toledo, cited a case of simulated hip disease, in which he cut down for the purpose of exsecting. He simply removed what dead bone appeared, inserted a drainage tube and gave *symphytum* externally and internally. The case entirely recovered.

Dr. G. A. Hall, Chicago :—If the pain is in the knee, or just back of the knee, the disease is always internal. Believes that tuberculosis is usually a consequence and not a cause of the disease. Does not believe much in apparatus. Sayre's and Taylor's splints do not accomplish the objects desired. The perineal band is an abomination. Rest is the great factor. In young subjects can do almost anything, but in those over twelve or fifteen the operation is apt to prove fatal.

Dr. J. C. Morgan, Phil., advocated the use of adhesive plaster in place of the ordinary perineal band. The plaster can be applied under the buttock, one strip overlapping the other. It does not slip or excoriate. If the patient is given a bath with castile soap and alcohol, excoriation will be prevented. Lateral displacement of the uterus by pressure on the sacral nerves will simulate hip disease.

Bureau of Obstetrics.—Dr. E. V. D. Pardee presented a paper on "Nervous Complications of Gestation." In the vomiting of pregnancy relief can be given by elevating the hips and shoulders; also by a linen compress saturated with French brandy strapped over the gastric region, with adhesive plaster, which acts mechanically on the muscles to keep them quiet, and will greatly help at times. Spoke of a case of itching which occurred at the period of viability. It would continue till gestation was completed. The mother should prepare for the child's reception. It develops the maternal love, particularly when the child is not wanted. It gave no time to mope and brood.

Dr. Geo. B. Peck then read his paper upon "The Accidental Complications of Gestation." The comparison of the treatment of allopathic physicians with those of this school showed disastrously for the former. He spoke of the various complications of the puerperal state, such as hysteria, chorea, epilepsy, cholera, typhus, yellow, intermittent and typhoid fevers, scarletina, measles, variola, heart disease, pleurisy, emphysema, pneumonia and phthisis.

In sixty-seven mothers suffering from phthisis, twenty under the care of one practitioner were benefited, all their children being plump; that successive pregnancies averted the disease in the case of another ; that seventeen under the care of two physicians improved until after delivery, which was followed by a rapid development in five; that nine other patients are living and that two more lived two years. All children were living and well. Twenty-five per cent. of phthisical mothers will die the first year after confinement.

Dr. T. F. Allen reported the case of a lady in her second pregnancy who had fallen down stairs near the eighth week. In falling she fractured her leg. This was attended to, but the mother was greatly in fear that the child would have club feet. When born no mark was upon the child save a horribly bruised nose and a lip which looked as if it had been in recent conflict with a pugilist.

Dr. T. L. Brown:—He believed that in many instances too much medicine was given. The patients suffered from drug sickness instead of any positive ailment. He cited the case of a lady who had been treated for years for all conceivable diseases, but without permanent cure. When she came into his hands he concluded that she was suffering from drug poisoning, and so placed her on large-sized blank pellets. She began to improve and has entirely recovered.

Dr. Wm. Owens reported a case of supposed tumor, which proved to be a fecal accumulation. Upon its discharge the tumor disappeared.

Dr. Gause said that some months since he was consulted by a husband concerning the supposed pregnancy of his wife. All the symptoms of pregnancy were present. After a certain time they all disappeared. They had again reappeared. The doctor was anxious to see if they would again subside as before.

Dr. B. W. James cited two cases which occurred in his practice fifteen years ago of left-sided tumor in the ovarian region, complicating pregnancy. Much alarm was felt. One patient was delivered at full term of a healthy child after a normal labor. The patient is still living and the tumor has disappeared. The second case caused much trouble. It came down and produced obstruction. After delivery everything went on all right. The tumor has re-appeared and is continually growing.

Dr. T. L. Brown called attention to the statement he saw recently that t e pulse of pregnant women was the same, standing, sitting, or lying down.

Dr. P. Dudley said he had made the experiment in forty-eight young men, in whom he had found the pulse to be the same whether they stood, sat, or lay down.

Dr. H. T. Wilcox reported the case of a fibroid tumor of many years standing. She used electricity and caused its entire disappearance.

Dr. T. F. Allen reported an amusing instance of a physician who had married late in life and presumed that pregnancy had set in. Another physician being called in found it a mistake. The infant's trousseau was disposed of for between $700 and $800.

Dr. G. Custis called attention to *argentum nitricum* in albuminuria. He had found it eminently serviceable in many cases.

Dr. H. C. Allen said that in such cases of intense itching as those mentioned by Dr. Pardee, the late Dr. H. N. Guernsey had directed him to look for a scrofulous diathesis, and, to get at the bottom of this, to give a dose of *psorinum*, to be followed later by a dose of sulphur.

In Dr. Allen's experience this advice had proved of great aid to him.

Dr. Weaver detailed the case of a woman who suffered from albuminuria during gestation. In this case convulsions set in after the child was born. They were directly traceable to the renal disorder. The evils of albuminuria do not always cease with the termination of gestation.

Dr. Culvert closed the discussion with the narration of the case of an elderly lady who married a gentleman of seventy years of age. The patient was brought to her bed with the usual symptoms, but full term passed with no result. Eighteen months from supposed date of conception the fœtus was born, weighing but one pound. The question arose then, was it a fœtus or a full term child carried beyond term and become atrophied? The subsequent pregnancy of this same patient had pursued a similar course.

The bureau then adjourned.

TUESDAY EVENING.

The Bureau of Clinical Medicine, Dr. J. W. Dowling, New York, Chairman, next reported.

Dr. Dowling read a paper upon "Diseases of the Kidneys and Bladder," in which he cited a case of albuminuria of twenty-three years' standing. At present albumen and casts do not always mean serious disease. The nicer points are of no great importance. Symptomatology is the great thing. He cited the case of John Morrissey, whose life had been lengthened ten years by a rigorous diet and abstinence from alcohol.

"Nervous and Ophthalmic Complications of Renal and Bladder Diseases.' Dr. Clarence Bartlett, Phil.:—The nervous affections of the kidney in which albumen and sometimes casts are excreted, are produced by prolonged overwork, epileptic convulsions, cerebral tumors and allied troubles. Vesical neuroses are frequently caused by over sexual indulgence. Retinitis follows kidney diseases, and is often the first symptom which leads the patient to regard himself ill. It is diagnosed by the ophthalmoscope and the chemical and microscopical evidences of kidney disease.

Paralysis and convulsions are due to apopletic attacks. The blood-vessels become hard and inelastic and rupture easily. Syphilis and Bright's disease are the most frequent causes of hemiplegia. Paraplegia is more infrequent. Dr. B. cited a case of recurrent convulsions due to Bright's disease, in which successive spasms occurred, each preceded by a diminution in the amount of urine excreted. The third one proved fatal. The kidney was found contracted. Uræmic coma may be slow or rapid and is characterized by quiet breathing in place of stertor.

"Heredity as a Factor in the Etiology of Bright's Disease," Dr. A. L. Kennedy, Boston. In this paper the supposed heredity of Bright's was traced through its connection with gout, rheumatism and allied disorders.

"Nephritis as a Necessary Consequent upon Senile Changes," Dr. J. M. Schley, New York:—In advanced age the kidney is often called upon to eliminate large quantities of uric acid, which irritate the kidney and cause Bright's. There is also a tendency toward the breaking down of glandular tissue and toward the development of connective tissue, which gradually obliterates the renal structure. The large granular kidney is most frequently followed by heart disease and apoplexy, the latter of which is very rare after the parenchymatous variety.   There are certain conditions of the system which precede the elimination of large quantities of albumen, which should tell us much.   Dr. S. considers the microscope as the only reliable means of reaching a correct diagnosis.   His conclusions were as follows:

Few persons, male or female, reach the stage of profound senile changes in this section of the country without manifesting some form of nephritis; also that after we pass the age of forty-five we meet with changes in the kidneys, and the higher we climb on the ladder of age the more frequent are these morbid conditions found.   After seventy it is one of the greatest rarities to find a healthy secreting kidney.   If we should examine such cases carefully we would find disease where health seemed to exist.   By appropriate diet and clothing such troubles may be held in abeyance for years.   The microscope is the surest medium to rely on for a diagnosis and prognosis.

Dr. T. F. Allen, New York:—Of all the mercurials *merc. prot.* is most frequently indicated in renal diseases.   *Merc. cor.* is rarely indicated.   Sub-acute nephritis, with lithæmia often calls for *colch.*   Inability to stretch out the legs on account of pain in the kidneys, and coldness in the pit of the stomach, and nausea, alternating with pain in the back of the head, are the main indications for *colch.*   Picric acid relieves the head symptoms.

Dr. Geo. M. Dillow, New York:—It is very rare to find a healthy kidney in a person over seventy years of age.   Senile nephritis is properly arterio-sclerosis, resulting in atrophied kidney, the arterioles undergoing the hyaline-fibroid change, thus impairing the blood supply and causing degenerative changes in the glandular substance proper.   In the case of the contracted granular kidney there is a strong liability, during the acute inflammations, to sudden death.   When the kidneys are diseased a complicating pneumonia may run its course with but little rise of temperature and with but the slightest cough.   Dr. D. cited the case of a man who had a complicating pneumonia, pleurisy of both sides, with effusion, endo- and pericarditis, yet the temperature scarcely rose above 100.   The diminution in the amount of urine excreted by the aged is most important.   It is usually observable two or three days before death.   The most important consideration in the examination of urine is the amount of total solids eliminated.   We must associate the quantity of urine excreted during the twenty-four hours with the specific gravity.   To calculate the total solids multiply the last two figures of the specific gravity by $2\frac{1}{3}$, the co-efficient of Hæser, which gives the number of grammes of solids for every 1,000 cubic centimeters of urine; two healthy kidneys should eliminate between sixty and seventy grammes of solids per day.   In Bright's disease there is almost always a great diminution of total solids excreted.

Dr. J. C. Morgan, Phil.:—In about four-fifths of the cases the elimination of total solids is diminished about one-half.   A person weighing 150 pounds, with good exercise, should eliminate sixty grammes daily.   Reason for this diminution lies in the liver and diet rather than in the kidneys.

Dr. Geo. M. Dillow, New York:—In interpreting the amount of total solids we must consider the individual case.   If the patient is on a slop diet the total amount will probably not exceed thirty grammes.   If such a patient were only eliminating ten grammes it would indicate danger.   Meat diet will increase the total solids, but may not reduce the inflammation.   As a rule the ordinary urinometer, for such estimates, is not reliable.   The most reliable ones are manufactured by Tagliabue, of New York; Hicks, of London, and Codman & Shurtleff, of Boston.

Dr. J. W. Dowling, New York:—Meat diet is injurious unless a large amount of hot water is taken in connection with it. Kidney disease is only a feature in a general process. Arterio-capillary fibrosis comprehends the entire ground.

WEDNESDAY MORNING.

The Committee on Medical Literature reported the homœopathic journals published in this country. Dr. T. F. Allen moved that the *Medical Times*, published in New York City, be stricken from the list of homœopathic journals, as being a constant and bitter opponent to all the interests and advancement of the school. This was seconded by Dr. Pemberton Dudley, of Phil., and Dr. G. E. Sparhawk, and carried by a unanimous vote.

Dr. S. P. Hedges, Chicago, Chairman of the Bureau of Gynæcology, presented the Bureau address, in which he introduced a new speculum, which acted on the principle of a Sims' with the patient on her back. It retracted the perineum and did away with one assistant. He recommended Hank's dilator for rapid dilatation; Miller's uterine repositor, the urethral clamp for confining cocaine in operations on the urethra; the pessary made by Drs. Hamilton and Skene, of England, for urethrocele and incontinence of urine; Sims' pessary for retroversion, and the electric light for vaginal examination. He described the operation of Grailey Hewitt for conical or elongated cervix, which consists in removal of a small piece of mucous membrane from the posterior lip and bringing the edges together; the new operation of Dr. Wm. Tod Helmuth for retroversion of the uterus by stitching the fundus to the abdominal wall; the introduction by Drs. Marssey and Beebe, of pins for use in lacerated perineum; Alexander's operation of shortening the broad ligaments; Emmet's button-hole operation on the urethra; rapid dilatation for the cure of dysmenorrhœa; use of electricity in extra-uterine pregnancy; removal of the ovaries and tubes for uterine fibroids; hysterectomy for same condition—he regarded this as too dangerous to be advised; laparotomy for acute and suppurative peritonitis, abscess in abdominal cavity, intestinal wound, and intussusception of the bowels.

Dr. H. recommended the use of ethyl bromide as an anæsthetic, as being safe, prompt and free from the gastric disturbances of ether.

Following this was the Bureau address on Ophthalmology, Otology, and Laryngology, by Dr. C. H. Vilas, Chicago. Dr. Vilas not being present, it was read by Dr. Geo. S. Norton.

In the attempt to transplant eyes from the rabbit no successful case had been reported. Washing out the vagina before delivery with *merc. bichlor.* will often prevent ophthalmia neonatorum. Enucleation is the best method of treatment in sympathetic ophthalmia. In his cataract operations he no longer pays any attention to strict or limited antisepsis, and does not hesitate to subject his patients to exposure from sewer gas, erysipelas, or small-pox. No bad results have followed. The healthy secretions of the eye are not injurious. He used boracic acid for purulent otorrhœa.

The Bureau address on Pedology was then read by its Chairman, Dr. C. D. Crank, Cincinnati, in which he mentioned the ground to be covered in the sectional meeting.

WEDNESDAY AFTERNOON.

The Bureau of Gynæcology, Dr. S. P. Hodges, Chicago, Chairman, reported.

The first paper, by Dr. Ed. T. Blake, London, was upon "Dilatation of the Cervix." Dilatation is either immediate or delayed. The former is sudden, violent, but without rupture; the latter is slow, by tents or rubber bags.   Dilatation by cutting is not advisable.   He uses Palmer's dilator. Molesworth dilator is the best in pregnancy.   Bougies are not much used in Europe.   Of those employed Prof. Hager's, which are gauged from one-twelfth of an inch to one inch, are the most popular.   Tents are falling into disuse.   They should be rendered perfectly aseptic before use. They are tedious and apt to produce inflammation.

"Hot Water as a Topical Application," Dr. R. Ludlam, Chicago.   The merits of hot water are that it is safe, available, effective, and does not interrupt the action of remedies.

Its employment was first introduced by Dr. T. A. Emmet, of New York.   It can be applied either by a syringe, as an irrigating douche, in the shape of a sitz bath, locally to the abdominal walls, or by hot sponges to the cervix.   The *modus operandi* of this agent is first as a vaso-motor stimulant, narrowing the caliber of the blood-vessels; second, by the peculiar action of moist heat upon the peritoneum in relieving suffering and aborting inflammation; third, by its action on cellulitis in aborting suppuration; fourth, by its anæsthetic effect on the nerves of the vagina in relieving neuralgia.   It is useful in every form of pelvic inflammation or neuralgia, and can be used with safety when the doctor is away.   It will stop intra-pelvic hemorrhage, allay the pain and hasten the suppuration of an abscess, or stop bleeding, whether it be *post partum* or from cancer. When used to excess it may devitalize the tissue and cause suppuration, thus weakening the patient, favoring leucorrhœa and making chronic a pelvic inflammation.   Dr. L. does not recommend it as a specific for all troubles, but it is one of our best and safest remedies.

"Surgical Treatment of Uterine Disorders," Dr. L. A. Phillips, Boston.   Dr. P. first made a strong plea for a more liberal attitude to be taken by the profession generally upon this subject.   In order to make it a success we must have an absolutely correct diagnosis, unity of purpose in all branches of the profession, and our operators must be equal to the best. The conditions demanding surgical treatment are severe laceration of the cervix and perineum, with their characteristic symptoms; epithelioma of the cervix in its incipient stage; polypoid and fibroid growth should be curetted or cut away; the uterine appendages may be removed, or hysterectomy be performed in cases of large fibroids; Alexander's operation offers a cure for some of the worst cases of retroversion; while ovarian and tubal diseases must be treated by abdominal section with its appropriate operation.   These cases cannot be relieved with medicine and should be operated upon at once.

"Intra-uterine Medication and Intra-Uterine Stem Pessaries," Dr. C. B. Kenyon.   The treatment of increased glandular activity is often treated by violent caustics, which destroy the membrane and glands.   Many symptoms follow in the train of such treatment.   The failure to cure with intra-uterine applications is because they are not made thoroughly enough. The best method of application is by the cotton pledget wound around an applicator, and carried to the fundus, or by gelatine medicated bougies. In order to cleanse the cavity previous to application it is wiped out with cotton and injected by means of a uterine syringe with listerine.   If pus is present, the peroxide of hydrogen, in proportion of five drops to a drachm to each patient, followed by listerine, is employed.   He uses *pinus canadensis, arg. nit.* and *iodoform*.   In order to dilate and medicate the uterine cavity he uses small bits of cotton tied to thread; these are passed into the cavity and allowed to remain forty-eight hours.   It is perfectly harmless.   Has treated fifty cases and in only two was there the least trouble.   No pain is experienced except at the first, which soon passes away, and relief follows.   Regarding intra-uterine stem pessaries, he does not find two cases a year which demand their use; these are usually cases of arrest of organic or functional development of the uterus or ovaries. They should never be used where there is any tendency to inflammation or pain. They should be removed if they excite any discomfort. The stem should be a half-inch shorter than the uterine cavity. The comfort of the patient should determine the length of time it should remain in place.

"The Local Action of Iodoform, Iodine and Allied Medicaments," Dr. O. S. Runnels, Indianapolis. Glycerine has a depleting effect and is useful in hyperplasia, sequelæ of inflammation, sub-involution, etc. Iodoform and iodized phenol are largely composed of iodine. They quicken the function, soften adhesions and indurations, and excite uterine contractions. Iodine is absorbed into the circulation very rapidly and, no doubt, exercises a constitutional as well as local action. The latter is the better stimulant. Tannic acid is an astringent. *Pinus canadensis* is very valuable in catarrhal discharges. *Calendula* is a great healer, relieves swelling and is a germicide. In old ulcers *glycerole of calendula* or *hydrastis* will excite granulation. The latter drug is indicated by cachexia, weak muscles, and obstinate constipation.

"Uterine Electro-therapeutics," Dr. B. Frank Butts, Philadelphia. The faradic current is useful in neuralgic conditions, as ovaralgia, and when a stimulant effect is desired. The galvanic is more like a chemical reagent; it has a greater effect in producing organic changes; it alters the atomic condition of inflammatory products. The effect of a moderate current is to hasten tissue change; of a strong current, to kill tissue. The positive pole is the most destructive, and may kill tissue by hardening and inspissating it; the negative disintegrates, has a fluidifying effect, and is more applicable to all neoplasms. By moistening a piece of canton flannel and using it over the electrode, will get a diffusion of the current; if use simply the bare metal plate, the charge becomes a powerful superficial current.

Electricity will excite uterine contractions and is applicable in uterine hemorrhages. Galvano-puncture is applicable only to large tumors, and is attended with danger. In excessive menstruation the positive pole should be used over the abdomen and the negative in the vagina; in amenorrhœa it should be reversed. Extra-uterine pregnancy is best treated by the faradic current. No deaths have resulted from its use. In interstitial pregnancies, electricity will sometimes change the position of the fœtus and render it normal.

Dr. Phil Porter, Detroit, had prepared a paper on "Pessaries and their Applications," but owing to the length of the preceding ones, he did not read it.

Dr. J. K. Warren, Worcester, Mass :—The positive pole of the galvanic current should never be used upon a mucous surface, it will produce a slough. Electricity should be used frequently and for a very short time, in order to get its best effects. If the part is moistened with any medicament, and the battery applied, will get a medicinal effect at once. Cocaine and other agents can be used most satisfactorily this way.

Dr. Smith :—Remedies should be differentiated. He uses locally whatever he gives internally.

Dr. T. C. Comstock :—Does not believe in intra-uterine medication. Has used all the remedies spoken of, and does not think he has done any great harm. That is the most he can say. Applied chromic acid to one case, and it went into an almost fatal collapse. He very seldom uses pessaries now, and never an intra-uterine stem. He also operates on the cervix less frequently than formerly. In strictures of the urethra and stenosis uteri, nothing is as good as electricity.

Dr. O. S. Runnels, Indianapolis :—In the use of the hot douche, the recumbent position should be insisted upon. At least one gallon should be used at a time; half a cup of salt added to the douche gives a tonic effect. The hips should be elevated. The syringe should have no hole in the end of the nozzle ; the douche should not be too long continued or it will produce a relaxation. If the hot water does not answer, gradually change to cold water in much less quantity.

Dr. N. Schneider, Cleveland :—Prolapse of the uterus is often due to sub-involution of the vagina, caused by a laceration of the vagina just within the vulval orifice. Such cases require to be sewed up and the vagina restored to its normal caliber. Pessaries should only be used to support the uterus until the vagina is able to do so.

Dr. H. T. Wilcox, St. Louis :—Believes that the dress of women has much to do with uterine disorders. No weight should be borne from the hips, and there should be no pressure upon the waist.

Dr. Phil. Porter, Detroit :—We should not entirely condemn the use of pessaries. We should all understand the principle of their application, as much harm is done by physicians who are forced to use them without understanding their *modus operandi.* Only one or two pessaries have a true underlying principle. Does not believe in intra-uterine stems. He uses only the closed lever pessary of Hodge. They are the only ones he recommends. Vagino-abdominal pessaries are a curse to womankind.

The Eye, Ear and Throat.—The Bureau of Ophthalmology and Otology met in the upper club room at three P.M., Dr. George S. Norton, of New York, presiding. Papers were read as follows :

"Sarcoma and Carcinoma of the Choroid," by C. H. Vilas, of Chicago.

"A Clinical Study of the Verbascum Thapsus," by H. P. Bellows, of Boston.

"Fibroid Polypi of the Nose and Throat," by Dr. E. H. Linnell, of Norwich, Conn.

"Importance of the Ophthalmoscope in the Diagnosis of the Diseases of the Brain," by Geo. S. Norton, of New York.

These papers were discussed by Drs. Jos. E. James, Geo. S. Norton, E. H. Linnell, A. M. Cushing, B. W .James, Clarence Bartlett, A. B. Norton and John C. Morgan. At 5.30 P.M. the bureau adjourned.

Bureau of Pedology,—Dr. C. D. Crank, Chairman of the Bureau of Pedology presented his paper, the main argument of which was that it was a mistake to treat eczema *per se,* but to treat the patient, and the eczema will take care of itself. In support of this position the essayist cited a number of authorities even of the old school. "Empiricism," he said, "is a confession of ignorance ; education is the remedy."

Dr. B. F. Dake, the secretary, read the following papers : "Infantile Eczema; its Ætiology, Diagnosis and Pathology," by himself ; "The Therapeutics of Infantile Eczema," by Wm. E. Leonard, M.D., of Minneapolis, Minn. ; "The Skin Diseases of Infancy and Early Childhood; External Treatment," by Philip E. Arcularius, M.D.; "Suppressed Infantile Eczema," by T. C. Duncan, M.D., of Chicago ; "The Relation of Vaccination, Dentition, and Eruptive Fevers to Infantile Eczema," by Wm. H. Bigler, M.D., Phila. Dr. Wm. Owens read a review and critique of all the foregoing papers, whereupon discussion ensued.

Dr. Gregg Custis reported that he had had some cases of eczema, but had learned to leave off the external treatment suggested in one of the papers ; he also found that washing was injurious ; he did not wish to be understood as championing uncleanliness, but that the daily washing all over each day of an infant with eczema was a grievous mistake. He believed that the paper by Dr. Dake, was the ablest presented, and that it was dangerous to suppress an eczema by topical applications. He had found *lycopodium* one of his principal remedies.

Dr. Beebe did not believe that any of the papers clearly established whether eczema was a parasitic or a constitutional disease. If it be a parasitical disease, undoubtedly outward applications would be of benefit. He had found vaccination an aid in clearing up an eczematous condition in a child. He questioned whether vaccination had ever been followed by syphilis.

Dr. Boyer had noticed that when eczema was suppressed it usually had a deleterious effect upon the mucous membrane, showing itself either in a cough, a catarrh, a diarrhœa or possibly an inflammatory condition resulting in asthma. He used white castile soap for cleansing and followed immediately with sweet cream. He also made use of a preparation of tar externally.

Dr. Vandenburg claimed that no bad effects had followed from the use in his practice of topical applications, and recited several cases. He had good results from the mecurials.

Dr. T. F. Smith has had quite a number of infantile eruption cases, and he had found that washing except for cleanliness was injurious. He discountenanced the use of ointments. He had found *graphites* an excellent remedy in the majority of his cases.

Dr. Dudley said that the fear of suppressing a disease had never been to him the bug-a-boo that it was to others. He would not say, however, that diseases when suppressed did not reappear at other points in subsequent times, but thus far his outward applications had not so resulted. He gave a case of strangury which was unmistakably traceable to a previously suppressed eruption.

Dr. Schley, who had been a pupil of Hebra, of Vienna, had no fear of results from outward applications to eczema.

Dr. T. L. Brown believed that many of these cases would get well of themselves if properly dieted and made to take fresh air and exercise. He used an application of boiled lard, which had given him good results.

Dr. Custis said that the difficulty with the specialist was that he never saw the results of his outward application. A patient troubled with an eruption goes to the specialist and is apparently cured, and that is the last the specialist sees of that case. When, however, later on, the patient comes down with some other trouble that can be directly traceable to the dermatologist's application, he goes to his old physician for treatment.

Dr. H. C. Allen recited a case of a physician, a lady, who had sent to him for treatment of her intermittent fever. The medicine sent cured the fever but brought to the surface an old eczema that had been suppressed years before by an old school physician. From the time of the suppression the lady had not had good health, but as soon as the eruption reappeared her health began to mend and is now rapidly improving.

Dr. Sturtevant believed that it was necessary to make a correct diagnosis before attempting a prescription. He used some local applications usually the *mercurius corrosivus.*

Dr. Owens confessed that he used external as well as internal treatment in eczema, and he had had good results. He mentioned an instance where a patient has had eczema in summer and rheumatism in winter for the past ten years; therefore was obliged to believe in the metastasis of eczema.

Dr. Dake related an interesting case which had been partially deaf. On inquiry he learned that the patient had been treated for eczema years before that, and succeeding the treatment had become deaf. By using the proper homœopathical medicine, Dr. Dake had now succeeded in restoring the hearing and in curing the old eczema.

Dr. Schley closed the discussion by adhering to his views as formerly expressed that he had seen no bad results follow from the local application of remedies.

The Bureau of Materia Medica was opened by its Chairman, Dr. H. M. Hobart, Chicago, by a paper on the "Physiology of Sleep." The cause of sleep is understood to be a demand for an increased amount of oxygen, lack of cerebral excitement, lessened blood supply to the brain. The deepest sleep occurs in about the first hour, when it becomes lighter for an hour, and then nearly as deep as before. From this time it becomes gradually less profound until morning. The effects of sleep are the universal renewal of tissue, slowing of the respiratory and cardiac movements, sinking of the temperature and diminution of glandular activity.

"Coma, delirium, and other forms of Abnormal Somnolence," Dr. Geo. W. Winterburn, New York:—Several cases were detailed, one of a man, an artist, who was cured by *sepia* 200; one a lady affected with coma, who had widely dilated pupils, cured by *bell.* 200; a man who had had measles, and who took afterward an inordinate quantity of beef tea which he could not digest. He became comatose. *Ars.* 12 relieved him. For lethargy he uses *phos. acid, plumb., cicuta.*

"Remedies for Ordinary Sleeplessness," Dr. Geo. W. Winterburn :— He detailed the symptoms which would indicate *sulp., bell., hyos., stram., sepia, puls., calc. carb., phos., coffea, ac., ignatia,* etc.

"Insomnia from Reflex Causes," Dr. S. C. Cowperthwaite :—In such cases remedies were applicable on account of their covering the totality of symptoms. He grouped them according to the organs to which they were most applicable.

"Sleeplessness from Brain Trouble," Dr. T. F. Allen, New York :— Treatment in these cases is slow and unsatisfactory. Opium and chloral are worse than useless. They must have long hygienic treatment and change of location. *Coffea, cannabis indica* and alcohol have been most useful. The latter he gives a few drops in water, a few sips to be taken every hour or two.

"Dreams—Remedies for, Dr. S. Lilienthal, San Francisco :—The conclusion was that dreams were rather unsatisfactory to treat. *Ac., verat. vir., zinc., am. carb., conium, kali nitricum, nux vom., merc., phos., plat., and puls.,* were cited as being most applicable.

Dr. T. F. Allen :—The way to treat insomnia is to send them away and give them proper hygiene.

Dr. J. C. Morgan, Phil.:—*Magn. phos.* is a great brain nutriment. Uses it in the twelfth and thirtieth. In hyperæmic condition in students and brain workers, *gels.* does best. In drunkards, *ac.* and *gels.* give excellent results. Dreams are at times good indications in prescribing. He cited the case of a man who constantly dreamed about water, who was entirely cured by *verat. vir.* This was succeeded by turbulent restlessness in the morning, which was dispelled by *hyos.; kali brom.* is also a valuable remedy.

Dr. Geo. S. Norton, New York :—Much sleeplessness is caused by errors of refraction which proper glasses will cure.

Dr. H. C. Allen, Ann Arbor:—The most prominent cause for insomnia is in the excessive use of coffee, liquors, etc., in brain workers.

Dr. Chas. Mohr, Phila., cited the case of a woman who worried much and could not avoid thinking of death the moment she lay down. *Crotali* cured her. *Bryonia* cured another case of insomnia brought on by money losses.

Dr. Cushing :—In drunkards, *cannibis indica* will generally cause sleep.

THURSDAY MORNING.

The resolution of Dr. T. L. Brown, of Binghamton, which read as follows : that "This Institute condemns the action of any college which graduates an unsuccessful candidate from another school, unless he attends at least one full course of lectures at the college where he applies for a degree," was adopted.

Dr. T. L. Strong, New York, presented his report on foreign correspondence. Dr. O. S. Runnels presented the report from the International Convention, held last year at Basle, Switzerland. The convention will meet in this country in 1891.

President Orme appointed Drs. I. T. Talbot, of Boston; J. P. Dake, of Nashville ; J. W. Dowling, of New York ; B. W. James, of Philadelphia ; R. Ludlam, of Chicago ; O. S. Runnels and T. C. Comstock, of St. Louis, as a standing committee to make arrangements for this convention.

The Special Committee on Pharmacopœia presented its report through Dr. A. C. Cowperthwaite, in the absence of Dr. Dake, Chairman, recommending that Drs. Lewis Sherman, J. W. Clapp and F. E. Boericke, be appointed a committee to confer with the committee of the international convention, the British pharmacopœia to be the basis for a new one.

The Bureau of Psychology was reported by Selden H. Talcott, M.D., in the absence of the Chairman, Dr. H. B. Clark, of New Bedford, Mass. The doctor read a paper on "Habits which tend to the Production of Insanity."

Dr. J. D. Buck, of Cincinnati, read a paper on "The Physio-philosophy of Habit."

The Bureau address on Anatomy, Physiology and Pathology, was presented by Dr. J. C. Morgan, of Philadelphia, Chairman, who gave a brief outline of the work for the past year.

The Institute then proceeded to the election of officers with the following result :

President, Dr. A. C. Cowperthwaite, Iowa City, Iowa ; Vice-President, Dr. N. Schneider, Cleveland, Ohio; Treasurer, Dr. E. M. Kellogg, New York ; General Secretary, Dr. P. Dudley, Philadelphia, Pa. ; Provisional Secretary, Dr. T. M. Strong, New York ; Board of Censors, R. B. Rush, M.D., Salem, Ohio ; R. F. Baker, M.D., Davenport, Iowa ; T. F. Smith, M.D., New York, N. Y. ; H. B. Clarke, M.D., New Bedford, Mass. ; Mary A. B. Woods, M.D., Erie, Pa.

After a warm discussion over Niagara Falls, Lake Minnetonka, Minn., and St. Clair, Mich., Niagara Falls was selected as the place of meeting in 1888.

Sanitary Science.—The Bureau of Sanitary Science met in the main assembly room at three o'clack, Dr. H. E. Beebe, presiding. The following papers were read and discussed.

"Ocean and Seashore Climate,' Bushrod W. James, M.D., Philadelphia, Pa. "The Study of High Altitudes in Relation to Disease," A. S. Everett, M.D., Denver, Col. "Observations on Florida Climate," H. R. Stout, M.D., Jacksonville, Florida. "Influence of Climate in Bronchial Affections," Charles E. Jones, M.D., Albany, New York. "Influence of Climate in Pulmonary Affections," Joseph Jones, M.D., San Antonio, Texas. "Influence of Climate in Disturbances of the Nervous System," William Owens, M.D., Cincinnati, Ohio. "Influence of Climate in Diseases of Alimentary Canal and its Appendages,": G. H. Wilson, M.D., Meriden, Connecticut. "Influence of Climate in Disturbances of Circulation—Secretion and Excretion," George M. Oakford, M.D., Lexington, Kentucky.

The discussion was participated in by Drs. Beckwith, B. W. James, Stout, Dudley, Brown, Jones, Fisher, Kinne, Adams, Gorham and Nickelson.

The Bureau of Pathology, Anatomy and Physiology convened in the afternoon. Dr. J. C. Morgan, Phil., Chairman.

The first paper was by Dr. F. Park Lewis, upon "The Pathology of the Blood in Malarial Diseases." The existence of a separate malarial bacillus is disproved. The blood, however, of those suffering from malaria is full of pigment which is formed in the blood, and fills the capillaries and tissues of the brain full in very severe cases. These granules are enclosed in a hyaline membrane, which is incorporated within the red blood corpuscle. Of these there are four different forms, the crescent, oval, spheroid and ciliated. These *plasmodia malariæ* are small, and in the algide stage difficult to see, as they are not pigmented; they have an amœboid motion. The crescents are very numerous in cases of pernicious malaria ; they are not constant, however. The plasmodia occur in intermittents and the crescents in remittent or malarial cachexia.

"Neurasthenia as a Cause of Malaria," Dr. S. Penfield, Danbury, Conn.:—In this paper an analogy was drawn between these two diseases as to their symptoms and origin, and the deduction made that the former was the cause of the latter.

"Pathological Processes in Malaria," Dr. Wm. Owens, Cincinnati :—In this paper Dr. Owens discarded all the previously advanced theories, and advocated that the real cause of malaria was to be found in the incessant rythmical movements and daily fluctuation of temperature. It is primarily a neurosis and acts through the sympathetic system. Malaria is found in all places and altitudes from 63 deg. north to 57 deg. south latitude, providing there is a change of temperature of about 15 deg. or 20 deg., occurring in the twenty-four hours. Outside the above limits and conditions, little malaria is found. The primary pathology is functional. The organic changes, such as enlargement of the spleen, liver, etc., result from functional disturbance of the fluids. From this cause get enlarged spleen; amyloid liver, sallow skin, granular kidney, fatty heart, shortness of breath, cachexia, degeneration of the blood corpuscle, and anæmia.

"The Differential Diagnosis of Fevers," Dr. W. H. Dickerson, Des Moines, Iowa :—The characteristic symptoms of other fevers were given. The malaria bacillus will assist in diagnosing malaria. He mentioned much that Dr. Lewis presented as diagnostic of intermittent or remittent fever.

"Special Relation of Malaria to the Eye, Ear and Throat," Dr. A. Wanstall, Baltimore:—He mentioned keratitis, ulceration of the cornea as a result of malaria, citing several cases of conjunctivitis, keratitis, iritis, strabismus, amaurosis, tinnitus aurium, and otitis media and externa, resulting from this cause and cured by such remedies as *quinine* and *china arsenicosa*.

"Congestive Forms of Malarial Diseases," Dr. J. C. Morgan :—Dr. Morgan believed that malaria was due to a peculiar dampness which pervaded certain localities, assisted by heat and causing decay of organic matter. The congestive forms were due to irritation or paralysis and were very malignant. The greater the venous congestion, the lower the temperature ; where this is very great, death may occur in a few hours, or from the least over exertion. The malignant forms cause great cachexia and sloughing of tissue. Death may come suddenly, even when the patient is apparently convalescing. The chronic or scorbutic cases are most apt to die this way. A clot forms in the heart and stops the *vis a tergo*, resulting in tremendous venous engorgement, producing infarctions in the spleen or liver. The pernicious cases are either algid or febrile, generalized or local, cause cardiac paralysis and may prove fatal in thirty-six hours. In the insidious form the brain is stupid, with great weakness, burning in the stomach, may simulate cholera ; at times get almost constant tenesmus and stool which is bloody, and consists of shaggy mucus and epithelium. The nature of the locality and the periodicity of attack should discover the real nature of the disease. A rapidly fatal pneumonia or cerebral apoplexy with coma may supervene, or the patient may quietly sleep into death with little pain or fever. The periods of the exacerbation of all malarial fevers are not stated correctly in the books. They are on the sixth, fourteenth, twenty-second and forty-second days.

Dr. Clarence Bartlett, Philadelphia:—A similar parallel might be drawn between neurasthenia and any other form of disease, and a like relationship established. He cited the case of a gentleman who suffered from high fever, choleraic symptoms every third day, who failed to be relieved by ordinary treatment, but recovered under the use of *sulphate of cinchonidium.*

Dr. Geo. S. Norton, New York:—We should be careful of our diagnosis of malaria. Everything that is periodic and relieved by *quinine* may not be malaria, and all diseases following malaria may not be proper sequelæ but result simply from impairment of health. To call a disease malarial, it must be periodic when periodicity does not belong to the disease. He cited a case of malarial strabismus cured by *quininum arsenicosum.*

Dr. A. R. Wright, Buffalo :—Changes of temperature alone do not sufficiently account for the production of malaria, and must have in addition, heat, moisture, and decaying vegetation. Changes of temperature alone affect other organs than the abdominal viscera, while malaria primarily acts on these. These three essential conditions may exist where but little rain falls.

Dr. W. H. Dickenson :—Heat, moisture and decaying vegetation are the prime factors in the production of malaria. While the West was a new country and presented these conditions, malaria was always present, but now that it is settled malaria has given place to typhoid.

FRIDAY MORNING.

The Committee on Medical Legislation, Dr. A. F. Sawyer, Chairman, reported favorable legislation in New York, Pennsylvania, Minnesota, and unfavorable in Michigan.

The following resolution, moved by Dr. O. S. Runnels, was passed, *Resolved,* That not more than one half of the time of a bureau be consumed in the reading of papers, and that the papers of those who are present be first read, after which, if time allow, those of absent members may be read. The committee on the Transactions reported that they favored the publication of the Transactions in its present form. It was so ordered.

Dr. H. D. Paine, New York, necrologist, then presented the memoirs and biographies of those who had died during the year. The following is the list, which is much smaller than usual.

Dr. H. Detwiler, Easton Pa.; Dr. A. E. Small, Chicago, Ill.; Dr. H. B. Eaton, Rockport, Me.; Dr. Rollin P. Gregg, Buffalo, N. Y.; Dr. C. Th. Liebold, New York, N.Y.; Dr. David Cowley, Pittsburgh, Pa.; Dr. Chas. Bossart, New York; Dr. J. P. Dake, Nashville, Tenn.; Dr. R. Sargent, Philadelphia.

Memorial remarks were then made by different members, among whom Dr. R. Ludlam paid a most touching tribute to Dr. A. E. Small, and Dr. Geo. S. Norton to Dr. C. Th. Liebold.

The following chairmen of bureaus were appointed by the President. Organization, etc., T. F. Smith, M.D.; Surgery, John E. James, M.D.; Obstetrics, George B. Peck, M.D.; Clinical Medicine, George E. Gorham, M.D.; Gynecology, Phil. Porter, M.D.; Pedology, B. F. Dake, M.D.; Opthalmology, etc., Joseph E. Jones, M.D.; Materia Medica, A. R. Wright, M.D., Psychological Medicine, J. D. Buck, M.D.; Sanitary Science, H. R. Stout, M.D.; Anatomy and Physiology, W. von Gottschalck, M.D.

Committee on Pharmacy, Lewis Sherman, M.D.; Medical Education, T. G. Cumstock, M.D.; Medical Literature, Pemberton Dudley, M.D.; Medical Legislation, J. H. McClelland, M.D.

There were 186 physicians in attendance and 132 visitors. Of the physicians, 59 came from New York, 28 from Massachusetts, 28 from Pennsylvania, 12 from Ohio, and 10 from Illinois; California sent 3; Florida, 1; Georga, 1; and Canada, 1.

The Institute then adjourned to meet at Niagara Falls next year.

RECORD OF MEDICAL PROGRESS.

MALIGNANT PUSTULE.—The *Paris Médicale* of January 29th, publishes notes of three cases of malignant pustule treated successfully by Dr. Rivas, who applied a paste composed of quinine powder (*sic*) and essential oil of turpentine. The powder and essence were employed in sufficient quantities to form a soft paste, which should often be renewed, as it dries quickly.—*Lond. Med. Rec.*, May 16th, 1887.

UNSATISFACTORY RESULTS OF UNILATERAL REMOVAL OF THE UTERINE APPENDAGES.—Mr. Lawson Tait, in the *Brit. Med. Jour.* of June 4th, quotes twenty-six cases to show that in those cases where unilateral removal of the uterine appendages for unilateral disease was insufficient, because, sooner or later, in thirteen cases, recurrence of the disease on the opposite side has rendered, or will render, a second operation necessary, while in only three of the twenty-six was there evidence of unimpairment of function in the unaffected side.

CORROSIVE SUBLIMATE IN PHTHISIS.—Dr. J. L. Porteous reports, in the *Edin. Med. Jour.*, May, 1887, three cases of phthisis, all in first stages, one with laryngeal complication, all relieved entirely of symptoms by use of corrosive sublimate solution, inhaled from a "finely-dividing spray producer." One dram of the solution being inhaled at a sitting, and the application being repeated every four to six hours. No other remedies were used, and in the only case where diet is mentioned, buttermilk was used. The doctor neglects to state the strength of the corrosive sublimate solution, and also the length of time the spray was used at the short intervals, though the treatment was continued from one to four months.

NOMENCLATURE OF SKIN DISEASES.—Dr. Robert Liveing, in an address delivered before the Medical Society of Middlesex Hospital, published in the *Brit. Med. Jour.*, May 7th, 1887, concludes : 1. That when two skin diseases coexist, they are generally quite distinct, and should be called by their well-recognized names. 2. That diseases are not natural, and do not follow the laws of natural development. 3. That it is very doubtful whether hybrid or crossed diseases exist at all, and that certainly there is no sufficient justification for a hybrid nomenclature. 4. That syphilitic skin diseases differ from ordinary skin diseases in their etiology, pathology and treatment ; and that this difference should be fully recognized in our nomenclature. 5. That medicinal rashes are not diseases of the skin, but simply eruptions, and should be so named.

TREATMENT OF HAY FEVER.—Sir Andrew Clark, in the *Brit. Med. Jour.*, June 11th, 1887, writes that he has used, for local application to the mucous membrane of the nose and upper pharynx in cases of hay fever, a mixture of "glycerine of carbolic acid one ounce, hydrochlorate of quinine one dram, and a two-thousandth part of perchloride of mercury. Heat will be required to dissolve the whole of the mercury." This is applied, after cleansing the nostrils, to the mucous membrane of the nares and posterior surface of the soft palate. The application is often disagreeable, but results in relief in the majority of cases, and in several cases one application has been sufficient. In most, however, several applications, made every second or third day, have been necessary. Sir Andrew says he has used this local method for over twenty years, and finds it as good as any of the less radical methods.

ANATOMICAL REASON FOR THE PREPONDERATING INFLUENCE OF THE LEFT CEREBRAL HEMISPHERE.—Prof. Gerhardt holds, in a lecture on the diseases of the cerebral arteries (*Berl. Klin. Wochensch.*, No. 18, 1887), that the functional predominance of the left cerebral hemisphere, as evidenced by the location of the speech center, by the general occurrence of right-handedness, and by its greater proneness to disease is due to the larger blood distribution to that side than to the right hemisphere. The left carotid artery ascends almost perpendicularly so as to form an elongation of the ascending aorta, the right carotid being given off from the arteria innominata. The right vertebral artery is given off by the subclavian after the latter has described its arch and become horizontal, but the left vertebral arises from the apex of the subclavian's curve. Thus there results as between the two vertebrals as well as the carotids an advantage to the left side.—O'C.

POISONING BY PENNYROYAL.—Mr. Girling, in the *Brit. Med. Jour.*, June 4th, reports case of a woman, æt. 40, who took one ounce of the essence of pennyroyal for suppressed menstruation. About an hour after, Mr. Girling found her in a state of extreme collapse. " The face was pale, cold and bedewed with beaded sweet, and the hands and feet were cold and clammy. She lay apparently unconscious; could at first be roused by shaking and shouting to her, rapidly sinking, however, into a state of profound coma. The pupils were of normal size and responded to light. The action of the heart was exceedingly weak, irregular and fluttering ; the pulse at the wrist being scarcely perceptible. The first sound of the heart was almost inaudible, while there was distinct reduplication of the pulmonary second sound. There was jactitation and feeble retching, with much salivation, but no vomiting and no purging. Temperature, 97 deg. F. Breath smelt like peppermint." An emetic followed by stimulants produced good results and the patient recovered.

ALBUMINURIA.—Professor Grainger Stewart at the June meeting of the Royal Society, at Edinburgh, presented the results of his investigations on the discharge of albumen from the kidneys of healthy persons. His conclusions, according to the *Brit. Med. Jour.* of June 11th, are as follows : " That there is no sufficient proof that albumen is normally discharged from the kidneys ; that albuminuria is much more common among presumably healthy people than was formerly supposed, tests having demonstrated its presence in nearly one-third of the population ; that the frequency of albuminuria increases as life advances; that it is more common among persons whose occupations involve arduous bodily exertion than among those who lead easy lives; that albuminuria frequently follows the taking of food, especially of breakfast, which more than any other meal increases the percentage of albuminuria ; that moderate muscular effort rather diminishes than increases albuminuria ; that it is often produced by violent and prolonged exertion; that cold bathing produces or increases albuminuria in some individuals, and that the existence of albuminuria is not of itself a sufficient ground for the rejection of a proposal for life insurance."

ELECTRICITY AND LACTATION.—Gubb, in the *Lond. Med. Rec.* for May, reports Aubert's and Becquerel's two cases in which lacteal secretion was suppressed—in one case from a pneumonia, in the other from mental emotion. In the first case, after a fortnight's suppression, mild faridization, with well-moistened electrodes placed one by the outside of each breast for twenty minutes, resulted in the re-establishment of the secretion in five days. In the second case, after eight days suppression, three *stances* of twenty minutes resulted in re-establishment of the secretion. A third case is also referred to where the same result was obtained in a woman seven months after her confinement, where the suppression had been immediate. Pierron also has treated by faradization a number of cases of suppression and diminution of the flow of milk. His method is the following: "The positive electrode, having the form of a spherical cup, is placed over the nipple, while the negative electrode, terminating in a ball, is placed below the breast." Afterwards the positive electrode is moved over the entire surface of the gland, while at the same time the negative electrode is displaced in such a way that the former will converge towards the latter. The current should not be strong enough to excite pain. Each application should last ten minutes and be renewed every twenty-four hours until milk is obtained, which is rarely later than four days.

JAMIESON'S METHOD OF PROPHYLAXIS OF SCARLET FEVER.—Dr. Jamieson and Mr. Alexander Edington have carried out a series of experiments leading to the identification and localization of the germ of scarlatina, to which germ they give the provisional name of bacillus scarlatinæ. The results, which are published *in extenso* with colored illustrations in the *Brit. Med. Jour.* of June 11th, lead to confirmation of the views of Dr. Jamieson regarding the methods of dissemination of the contagium, and the prevention of the spread of the disease. " The two sources of infection are probably the exhalation from the mouth and throat in the early stage, certainly the particles of dry cuticle cast off in the later. The method [of disinfection] recommended was to disinfect the throat with a strong solution of boracic acid in glycerine (a saturated solution of boro-glyceride in glycerine). In dealing with the skin more exact methods were available. Those consisted in the employment of warm baths every night from the very first, and in the application to the entire surface of the body, including the head, of an ointment composed of carbolic acid thirty grains, thymol ten grains, vaseline one dram, simple ointment one ounce, night and morning." A number of cases are reported in which the efficacy of the above-described procedure was demonstrated. This method was first published three years ago, and since then it has not once failed.

TREATMENT OF UTERINE FIBROIDS BY ELECTRICITY.—Dr. Woodham Webb gives, in the *Brit. Med. Jour.* of June 4th, an account of the apparatus for electrical treatment of uterine fibroids as carried out by Dr. Apostoli, of Paris. He uses a battery capable of giving a continuous, uninterrupted current, rising from ten to two or three hundred milliampères in strength, and provided with a rheostat, rheotome and galvinometer, the graduation of which last extends to at least 250 milliampères. The positive electrode is a platinum sound or trocar, of a length sufficient to reach the fundus of an enlarged uterus, and provided with an insulating canula in which it may be fixed by a screw so as to provide for the proper amount of penetration of the uninsulated point. "By having one end of the electrode sharpened it is enabled to penetrate the presenting part of the tumor if necessary. In the negative pole lies the special feature of the arrangement. Wet modelling clay is spread in a uniform layer about half an inch thick, and large enough to cover the lower part of the abdomen. The form, which is best made in a mould, is preserved by its being enveloped in folds of a large-meshed tarltan. A small plate of metal connects with the negative pole. This cutaneous electrode keeps the skin moist, and presents a large surface, so preventing cauterization of the skin even after the passage of a current of a strength of 200 milliampères for eight or ten minutes.

ACROMEGALIA.—Under the name of acromegalia, P. Marie, in 1886, had described a peculiar affection of which he had seen two cases in Charcot's wards in the Salpêtrière, and which appeared to have certain well-defined characteristics. The disease develops in the latter period of life and consists essentially of hypertrophy of the extremities and head, with certain other, generally nervous, symptoms. Another case is reported by Minkowski, of Königsberg. The patient, a man of healthy ancestry, noticed, at the age of twenty-eight, that his fingers were becoming thicker; within two years he had become the subject of headaches that gradually increased in intensity and continuance, and now he noticed that his feet were becoming larger, his boots getting too small, and instead of number nine rubbers he had to wear tens, then elevens, and finally twelves. The hands kept increasing in size so that he could no longer play the violin; he took up the cornet and soon found that he needed a larger mouthpiece as the lips had become greatly increased in size. Both ears and the nose showed marked thickening. The hands are described as colossal. The disease has been mistaken for myxœdema, but it differs from the latter by the existence of bony hypertrophy, by the absence of characteristic changes in the skin, and by the physiognomy, which in acromegalia shows a lengthened oval instead of the "full moon" face of myxœdema.—*Berl. Klin. Wochens.*, No. 21, 1887.

THE RELATION BETWEEN KIDNEY AFFECTIONS AND EYE DISEASES.—Dr. Fürst, of Berlin, in a communication on this subject to the *Berliner Klinische Wochenschrift*, says that although so much careful work has been done within the domain included in the title given that it would seem that nothing remains to be done, yet the general practitioner has an advantage over the oculist in being able to watch his cases for a longer time, and during the critical period when the patient is confined to bed. As is well known the visual disturbances resulting from kidney affection are of two forms : chronic, as retinitis albuminurica, more rarely, optic neuritis, or even choked disk ; and acute, as total sudden blindness from uræmia. In retinitis albuminurica there occurs only a progressive impairment of vision, that indeed is often the first clue to the discovery of the existence of kidney affection because in these cases dropsy is for the most part absent, and other symptoms such as headache, nausea, dyspnœa, etc., are of doubtful meaning. Retinitis, as found in different forms of nephritis chronica, is by far most frequent in contracting kidney, while in chronic parenchymatous nephritis, with large amount of albumen in the urine and moderate dropsy (even after years, or until the fatal ending), visual impairment and retinal affections are seldom observed ; and still more rarely, secondary amyloid kidney. Hence, in most cases, retinitis albuminurica offers a bad prognosis as indicating contracting kidney which goes on progressively to the fatal end ; yet it does occur that the visual disturbance and kidney affection both disappear, and the fundus, as seen by aid of the ophthalmoscope, returns to a normal appearance. Thus the occurrence of retinitis albuminurica will not determine an absolutely fatal prognosis.

THE TREATMENT OF PULMONARY TUBERCULOSIS WITH KREOSOTE.— Under this title Prof. Sommerbrodt, of Breslau, contributes to *Berl. Klin. Wochenschrift*, No. 15, 1887, an article. He has for nine years treated all his cases of the disease, amounting to about 5,000, with kreosote. From 1878 until 1880 he used in all tubercular cases, whether of the lungs or larynx, Bouchard's solution of kreosote, but since 1880 he has employed gelatine capsules, each containing 5 centigrams (¾ gr.) of kreosote, and 2 decigrams (3 gr.) of balsam of tolu, the preference for this method being that it is more agreeable and cheaper. In the dosage he gives : on the first day, one capsule; on the second, two, and then for eight days, three. The dose being given after meals with a tablespoonful of water. During the second week he gives, in three times, four capsules per day; in the third, five, and in the fourth six. The method has to be modified according to the circumstances of the case, and to avoid the patient's becoming habituated to the use of the drug, it is withheld at times for a day or two, or the dose is lessened. When he desires to be especially careful he uses only half the above dose. When the remedy is well borne, and this is the rule, for in many hundreds of cases there is often only one which revolts at the further exhibition of the remedy on account of violent eructations, retching, vomiting, etc., he permits the use of six capsules per day for two months, increasing until nine per day are given. Then he often withdraws the remedy for four weeks and afterward continues it for a year if necessary. He considers that in very many cases of tuberculosis the employment of kreosote as a remedy is of extraordinary service and that the greater the dose that can be borne the better its action.

DIAGNOSIS OF HYSTERICAL HEMIPLEGIA, by Dr. Oserez Kowski, Russia:

1. Hysterical hemiplegia develops itself frequently after a mental irritation.
2. They often appear as monoplegiæ, sharply differing from organic paralysis by grave disturbances of sensibility, absence of contractures, etc.
3. In hysterical hemiplegia the peripheral parts of the extremities are less palsied than the central ones ; the larger joints less movable than the small ones.
4. The mobility of the extremities returns at first on the peripheral parts and on the small joints; whereas the reverse takes place in organic hemiplegia.
5. The facialis and the hypoglossus are hardly ever affected in hysterical hemiplegia (Charcot only observed a spasm of the facialis on the other side).
6. Anæsthesia runs here parallel to the paralysis.
7. The participation of the anæsthesia may be peculiar in hysterical hemiplegia, with a full hemianæsthesia; hand and foot may remain intact.
8. Aphasia is rare, but mutism may be present. Hemiopia is also rare.
9. The diagnosis of hysterical hemiplegia is strenghened by the presence of other hysterical manifestations : anæsthesia faucium, polyopia, transfert, hysterogenous zones.

—*Centralblatt für Neroenkunda*, 6, 1887.—S. L.

IODOFORM AS AN ANTISEPTIC.—*Der Fortschritt*, No. 8, April 20th, 1887, reproduces from the *Deutch. Amerikanische Apotheker Zeitung* the abridgment of a paper entitled "Is Iodoform an Antiseptic?" in which the authors, Messrs. Ch. Heyn and Th. Roosing, deny the antiseptic properties of iodoform. They instituted a series of experiments in order to verify the generally alleged germ-destroying power of this drug. They tested the action of sterilized solutions of iodoform in olive oil and in serum, and of iodoform powder on cultures of different kinds of microbes. They also inoculated rabbits with these cultures mixed with iodoform, and found that the presence of iodoform never prevented the development of bacteria, and therefore refuted its antiseptic value in surgery. They further maintain that it is not only inefficacious, but that it may itself, if not disinfected before its use, become the means of conveying germs of different maladies to the patient. They therefore suggest having the iodoform previously disinfected with solutions of sublimate, if it is employed from other reasons for dressing wounds, etc. It has, therefore, to be borne out by other unbiased investigations, how far this verdict, which is contrary to the general experience, is justified, or whether the authors have not been misled by having used an adulterated substitute of iodoform, or by errors of optical observation or otherwise. Their opinion, however, is supported and confirmed by Dr. Tricomei, of Naples, who, in the meeting of the Surgical Congress at Geneva (April 4-7, 1887), reported that he had tested the action of iodol and of iodoform, in powder and in solution, on different kinds of micro-organisms, and had convinced himself, by numerous careful experiments and observations, that both these drugs are inefficacious and destitute of any antiseptic property.—*Lond. Med. Rec.*, June, 1887.

THE ETIOLOGY OF PROSTATIC HYPERTROPHY.—The view of Guyon that prostatic hypertrophy and its consequences are distinctly different clinically from other affections of the genito-urinary apparatus, and that the morbid phenomena are not wholly dependent upon a purely mechanical disturbance from obstruction to the outflow of urine have received strong support by the investigations of Launois upon the urinary apparatus of the aged. These show that in the aged the whole urinary tract, even up to the kidneys, has undergone specific changes that may be embraced under the term sclerotic—changes which affect the whole organism and which, in the tunics of the blood vessels, result in atheroma or arteriosclerosis ; the changes affect also the connective tissue of the mucous membranes and glands, and in the kidneys induce the well known although insignificant senile contraction; in the bladder lead to *vessie à colonnes*, and in the prostate to new formation of connective tissue, or so-called hypertrophy. This sclerotic process is accompanied by impaired circulation in the affected organs, producing lessened nutrition as well as—and this is specially important—a venous stasis or congestion. It is thus plain that the bladder of an old man is to be considered a weakened organ. It appears, indeed, often to be hypertrophied, as in a young patient suffering from stricture, but in fact it is only a pseudo-hypertrophy; the musculature is lessened and is not able to exercise powerful contraction, and thus arises the frequently observed diverticula and the so usually observed, although slight in the beginning, insufficiency. If now, such a bladder has increased demand made upon it, there comes in play an additional but mechanical factor due to the interference with the outflow of urine by the enlarged prostate. First comes incomplete, later complete retention, and finally, through the united influence of the above-named factors, vesical ectasia with dribbling of urine, but without voluntary power of evacuation. Cystitis need not be combined with this state, but may at any time break out, whether from cold or from the use of alcoholic drinks; or, and this is the most frequent cause, from the use of the catheter. The influence of the latter is far less through the introduction into the bladder by it of germs than by the sudden lowering of the internal pressure within the viscus, as the result of which an action equivalent to suction is set up in the over-filled veins, and hæmaturia and vesical catarrh follow.—*Berl. Klin. Wochens.*, No. 18, 1887.

ON THE VALUE OF CUNDURANGO BARK AS A REMEDY IN CARCINOMA OF THE STOMACH.—Under this title Dr. L. Riess contributes to *Berl. Klin. Wochenschrift*, No. 10, 1887, a long article based upon several years' experience. After giving a history of the introduction of the drug into medicine and some considerations of the contradictory and in many cases doubtful reports from earlier observers, he gives first the negative results of his experience. He does not believe that it holds any place as a stomachic. In about fifty cases, during the course of some years, of dyspepsia from acute and chronic catarrh of the stomach or from simple ulceration he found that the remedy, while free from any injurious influence, was of no greater value and indeed often of less than the old and well-known bitters and aromatics. Similarly, he saw rarely any striking result from the drug as a remedy for carcinoma when this was not connected with the stomach or was not limited in great part to that viscus. Of such he had about thirty cases in mind, embracing carcinoma of the peritoneum, primary cancer of the gall bladder, or large hepatic tumors (metastatic) extending to the stomach, and here the cundurango, while temporarily helpful in the loss of appetite, as well as for the pains, had no influence worth mentioning upon the other symptoms and the general condition. He had also eight cases of cancer of the œsophagus which, under the long continued use of cundurango, were much improved in their most annoying symptoms (dysphagia, cachexia), but there is doubt whether or not this result was not attributable to dietetic treatment and the use of the bougie. But it was quite otherwise in cases of pure, frank cancer of the stomach. Of such he had from 1878 till 1886, in the General Hospital at Berlin, about 105 cases, besides other cases. With 800 clinical histories before him he sums up that in no case was the remedy without influence. Even in patients in the last stage of the disease, and, in fact, in some with whom the use of the remedy was begun only during the last few weeks of life, there was improvement of the appetite and a certain amount of sense of well-being ; of course, in such cases the results could not be considered convincing. But far more striking was the action of the remedy where it could be continued for a longer time, at least for three or four weeks. And here the physician had the unusual and agreeable experience that the cundurango, even in patients suffering from stomach affections, who so frequently are sensitive and prejudiced against every remedy, was almost without exception taken with pleasure, well borne and without any aversion, even after long continued use. The doses given were larger and more frequent than had been recommended by most other observers, a decoction of ten grams per day being taken in teaspoonful doses so that the doses were repeated every hour. As instances of the long continued use of the drug he mentioned two women who took 800 and 900 grams, and three men who took respectively 830, 870, and 1,000 grams in decoction. It should be remarked that the hospital patients were, before beginning the cundurango treatment, kept under other therapeutic measures for a certain time, at least from eight to fourteen days, in order to determine their exact condition and to exclude any favorable influence from change of regimen and residence. In the cases treated with cundurango there was, as a rule, after a few days, improvement in the appetite, disappearance of nausea, and if vomiting existed it ceased unless due to severe stenosis of the pylorus and ectasia of the stomach. After the action was continued from eight to fourteen days there followed, almost without exception, a favorable change in the stomach pains ; where these had been continual there occurred now periods of freedom from them. Attacks of cardialgia, if present, became fewer and finally the pains ceased almost entirely. At the same time with improved diet there was an increase in the assimilative power, shown soon in a subjective sensation of well-being and increased body-strength. These improvements were conclusively established by weighing the patients, and it may be remarked that in a case of carcinoma of the stomach it is to be looked upon as a favorable sign when the body-weight in the last stages, in contradistinction to the usual rapid loss, remains tolerably constant or only slowly decreases. There occurred, too, in not a small number of cases a considerable increase of body-weight, and in many this continued until within a short time of the fatal ending. The writer holds that treatment by cundurango lengthens life in cases of cancer of the stomach and considers it worthy of recommendation in all cases where the diagnosis can be surely established or even with probability.—O'C.

NEWS.

CORNS.—Dr. R. T. Cooper, of the London Homœopathic Hospital, advises the use of *ferrum piericum* for corns on the feet.

APPOINTMENT.—Dr. Philip Porter has recently been appointed Professor of Gynecology in the Pulte Medical College, in place of Prof. Eaton, resigned.

WANTED.—An ambulance surgeon is wanted at the Brooklyn Homœopathic Hospital, 109 Cumberland Street. Candidates should apply at once, stating references, time and place of graduation. Address Charles L. Bonnell, M.D., Chief of Staff.

ANOTHER ERROR.—The *Record* is slightly mistaken when it states that the *Hospital Gazette and Students' Journal* is the only successful students' medical journal in existence. The *Chironian*, published and edited by the students of the New York Homœopathic Medical College, was a marked success from the start; has now an extended circulation, and is established on a permanent basis.

A SIGNIFICANT VERDICT.—A suit was recently tried in Brooklyn which shows that it is not always safe to speak lightly of a physician. Dr. W. J. Cruikshank secured a $1,600 verdict in his suit for $50,000 against William Gordon, the trial of which was brought in the Supreme Court. The doctor asserted that Mr. Gordon went to the mother of a child he was attending and urged her to secure another physician without delay, as, in his opinion, Dr. Cruikshank had not the skill necessary to attend a sick dog.

HOMŒOPATHY IN INDIA.—An account is given in the *Homœopathic World* of the celebration in Calcutta, India, of the 132d anniversary of Hahnemann's birth. There was a crowded audience and the hall became so full that many had to go away for want of seats. Dr. Sircar delivered the address of the evening. But a short time previous to this meeting the Calcutta Hahnemann Club was organized. The inaugural meeting was held on the twenty-second of March, at seven P.M. Homœopathy is evidently dying out in India in its usual fashion.

A HANDSOME CATALOGUE.—The Twenty-eighth Annual Announcement of the New York Homœopathic Medial College, just received, is exceptionally neat and tasteful.   A ground plan of the new college and hospital buildings is given, and, also, an excellent cut of the Laura Franklin Free Hospital for children, recently opened, and which affords additional clinical advantages to the students.   The college has, undoubtedly, acted wisely in deciding to make the three years' course obligatory in the future.   The announcement states : "The optional plan will be entertained for one year longer, but with the opening of the session of 1888, the graded course of study, extending over a period of three collegiate years, will be made obligatory."   There are no changes in the Faculty.   The laboratory course will be extended and improved.   The college library is growing rapidly and promises to be of great value in the near future. There seems to be no doubt but that the college has entered upon a new era of prosperity.

TOXIC EFFECTS OF LEAD.—Mr. Wynter Blyth has had an opportunity of examining portions of the bodies of two out of five persons who have, at different times, died more or less suddenly, from, as it is believed, the effects of lead poisoning.   In one case he separated about a third of a grain of sulphate of lead from the liver, and about the thirteenth of a grain from one kidney, besides finding lead qualitatively in the brain.   In the other he was enabled to examine the brain with more minuteness, and estimated that here the cerebrum contained about a grain and a half and the cerebellum about a quarter of a grain of sulphate of lead.   Mr. Blyth went on to remark in the paper he read to the Chemical Society of London on these investigations : "There has hitherto been no reasonable hypothesis to explain the profound nervous effects of the assimilation of minute quantities of lead, but if it is allowed that lead forms definite compounds with essential portions of the nervous system, it may then be assumed that in effects it withdraws such portions from the body ; in other words, the symptoms are produced, not by poisoning in the ordinary sense of the term, but rather by destruction—a destruction, it may be, of important nerve centers."—*London Lancet.*

IOWA SOCIETY.—The eighteenth annual meeting of the Hahnemann Medical Association of Iowa, was held at Des Moines, May 24-26.   From reports received the society seems to be in a flourishing condition.   The attendance was the best the association ever had.   Better still, the papers were excellent and the discussions animated, free and very instructive. All branches of the profession received attention, including the pharmacies, for whose benefit the following resolution was unanimously adopted : *Resolved*, " That this association deprecates the action of our homœopathic pharmacists in turning their pharmacies into general manufactures of all classes of drugs and combinations of the same ; also, in causing a lack of confidence in their preparations, by palming off upon the profession tinctures and dilutions made from the dry plant, as being made from recent importations of the green plant ; and that we resent, as an insult, the attempt to teach the profession Materia Medica by sending out circulars assuming to give us the action and use of drugs for specific purposes." The following officers were chosen : President, C. H. Cogswell, M.D., Cedar Rapids ; Vice-President, A. P. Hanchell, M.D., Council Bluffs ; Secretary, Geo. Royal, M.D., Des Moines ; Treasurer, S. E. Nixon, Burlington.   University Committee : Drs. J. E. King, B. Banton and F. Becker.

SWEET SUMACH.—The fluid extract of the root bark of the sweet sumach, *rhus aromatica*, an anacardiacea indigenous to the States, has lately been successfully employed in nocturnal enuresis of children.   It acts as an excitant in the non-striped muscles of the bladder, the uterus, and of the inferior portion of the digestive canal; and beneficial results have likewise been obtained from it in hemorrhage of the bladder, the uterus and the rectum, as well as in atonic diarrhœa. Dr. Unna recommends, from three years' experience, this extract in enuresis of children, for which it acts as a specific. He prescribes to infants and children, up to two years of age, five-minim doses in the morning and at bed-time; to children from two to six years of age, ten minims twice daily; and to older children, fifteen minims twice daily. He never observed any injurious concomitant effects, even after its uninterrupted use during several months. Its tonic effects, however, are not permanent, the paresis of the sphincter muscles of the bladder returning soon after discontinuing the remedy. It ought, therefore, to be given daily, as a rapidly-acting palliative, until the weakness has been gradually overcome by other adequate measures (training to the habit of regularly emptying the bladder, cold baths, douches, cool beddings, etc.), and only these to be gradually withdrawn.—*Homœopathic Journal of Obstetrics.*

ALLOPATHS ON ALLOPATHY.—Dr. Adams, the erudite translator of Hypocrates, says : "We cannot think of the changes in professional opinions since the days of John Hunter, without the most painful feelings of distrust in all modes of treatment." Claude Bernard, the eminent physiologist, candidly confesses : "Scientific medicine does not exist." Bichat, the illustrious physiologist, physician and author, makes this humiliating confession: "The Materia Medica is nought but a monstrous conglomeration of erroneous ideas. An incoherent assemblage of opinions, that are themselves incoherent, it is, perhaps, of all physical sciences, that which best illustrates the vagaries of the human mind. It is not a science fit for a methodic mind; it is a misshapen mass of observations, often puerile, of illusory methods, of formulas that are as grotesquely conceived as they are arbitrarily combined. Medical practice is said to be contradictory. I say more—it is not, in any respect, a profession worthy to be followed by sensible men." Sir Gilbert Blane wrote: "When it is further considered what a mass of credulity and error has actually accumulated in medicine; when we cast our eyes upon our shelves loaded with volumes, few of them containing any genuine profitable knowledge, the greater part of them composed chiefly of statements, either nugatory, erroneous, inapplicable, or mischievous, in which the dear-bought grain is to be sought in bushels of chaff, may it not be . questioned whether such researches have not tended more to retard and corrupt than to advance and improve practical medicine?" The great Boerhaare says : "If we weigh the good that has been done to mankind by a handful of true disciples of Æsculapius against the evil wrought to the human race by the great number of doctors since the origin of the art of medicine to our own times, we shall doubtless come to think that it would have been better had there never been any doctor in the world." Dr. Lauder Brunton says : "Our ideas are often hazy and indefinite. We give medicine at random, with no definite idea of what it should do, and trusting to chance for good results. When a remedy fails in its work we can give no reason for its failure. We do not even seek out a reason." Sir Astley Cooper said : "The art of medicine is founded on conjecture and improved by murder." Cullen wrote: "Our Materia Medicas are filled with innumerable false deductions, which are, nevertheless, said to be derived from experience." Sir John Forbes makes some damning admissions in respect to his new school : "Things," he says, "have arrived at such a pitch that they cannot be worse. They must mend or end." He asserts, "That in a large proportion of the cases treated by allopathic physicians, the disease is cured by nature and not by them. That in a lesser, but still not small proportion, the disease is cured by nature in spite of them." Kreuger Hamen says: "Medicine, as now practiced, is a pestilence to mankind; it has carried off a greater number of victims than all the murderous wars have ever done."—*Hom. League Tract.* This is the system offered in place of homœopathy.

BURMESE MIDWIFERY.—At a meeting of the Obstetrical Society of London held recently, an interesting paper was read which described the occupation, dress and physique of Burman women. The knowledge of the native doctors is handed down by tradition, and takes origin from fable, horology, astrology, etc. The midwives are of the poorest and lowest class, their chief qualifications being age and being the mothers of large families. The more decrepit, the more they are respected. All new methods are resisted. Nature is kind, as a rule, to the mother, and carries her safely through. A large store of firewood is laid in for the event. A room is set apart where the mother remains till convalescent. Regardless of all sanitary laws, every effort is made to keep out air, and especially the smell of cooking, which is supposed to be particularly injurious. A fire is made of wood, no chimney being provided, and the smoke renders the air stifling. The patient, when in labor, is surrounded by female friends, and a crowd of men and women squat behind the curtain which divides the apartment, and smoke or chew belel. When the pains become severe the patient squats upon the floor, supported by a woman sitting behind her. The midwife assists in front by pushing with her hands upon the abdomen, using more and more violence as the pains increase. A cloth is tied tightly around the body above the umbilicus, which is drawn tighter as the case proceeds, not with any idea of restraining hemorrhage, or supporting the uterus, but to prevent its rising in the chest. As the head progresses the woman is laid on her back, with her knees drawn up. Her attendants press on the abdomen with all their might. When the head presses on the perineum the midwife leaves the pushing to others, and in all first cases, tears the perineum, either with her thumb-nail, which has grown sharp and long for the purpose, or with her great toe-nail. In other cases the perineum is retracted, and as soon as the head is born the child is rapidly extracted. If the placenta does not follow quickly the cord is dragged on, and this failing, it is removed by the hand or torn away piece by piece. The mother is washed and the whole body rubbed with tumeris. The fire is kept up and hot bricks wrapped in rags, or bags of hot sand, are placed on the abdomen, and twice a day the patient has to squat over smoldering embers upon which tumeris has been thrown. The skin is often blistered by the application of heat, but heat is supposed to permeate the parts and heal them. The food is hot water, hot broth, with fish and rice. On the seventh day a hot "pack" is used for some hours, which produces free perspiration. When the blankets are removed the patient is bathed freely in cold water. When delivery is not rapid, various barbarous methods are followed, such as standing on the patient's abdomen and pressing or kneading it with the feet, or a bamboo or plank is placed across the abdomen, while the attendants endeavor to expel the child by using all their force at the two ends. This method is very usually fatal to mother and child, and often causes rupture of the liver or bladder. In cross births the part presented is torn or cut off, and the child removed piece by piece, the head being extracted by means of a large fish-hook. In all cases the object is to remove the child as quickly as possible, and regardless of risk to the mother, owing to the superstition that if a woman dies undelivered, the spirit of the mother and child haunt and bring misfortune to the relatives ever after.—*London Lancet.*

VOL. XXXV.   *AUGUST, 1887.*   (VOLUME II,)   No. 8.
                                   (Third Series.)

NORTH AMERICAN
JOURNAL OF HOMŒOPATHY.

ORIGINAL ARTICLES IN MEDICINE.

CYSTITIS.

By JOHN L. MOFFAT, M.D.,

Brooklyn, N. Y.

NAMES.—INFLAMMATION OF THE BLADDER—CATARRH OF THE BLADDER—
VESICAL CATARRH—STRANGURY—CYSTITIS—INTERSTITIAL CYSTITIS—
PARENCHYMATOUS CYSTITIS—CYSTITIS MUCOSA—C. SUBMUCOSA—C.
SUBSEROSA—C. PARENCHYMATOSA—C. URICA—CATARRHUS VESICÆ—
DYSURIA MUCOSA—INFLAMMATIO VESICÆ.

THE urinary bladder is subject to inflammation varying in degree
and kind according to the tissues affected, causes and duration
of the attack.

The catarrhal form is by far the most common, on account of the
exposure to morbid influences of the mucous membrane; but the inflammation may involve the submucous tissues, constituting interstitial
or parenchymatous cystitis, which is a more serious trouble and is
accompanied by marked constitutional disturbance.

ÆTIOLOGY.—The mechanical causes of cystitis are: Fracture of the
pelvis, more especially of the symphysis pubis; contusion in the
hypogastric or perineal region; bruising by obstetric forceps, or the
head of the child in labor; malposition of the uterus; extrophia
vesicæ; prolapse of the bladder; rude catheterism or the bung-
ling use of the sound; operations on the bladder; foreign bodies introduced per urethram; calculi, or crystals (most commonly of uric acid
or of the triple-phosphate) in the urine; sudden relief of pressure by
emptying the long over-distended bladder, and prolonged muscular
spasm, as in cases of neuralgia of the neck of the bladder, or in cases
of obstruction to the free exit of urine by polypus, enlarged prostate,
urethral stricture, etc.

The bladder may also become inflamed from the presence of too strong injections, whether intentionally or accidentally introduced.

The urine itself is irritating when highly concentrated, very acid or alkaline, and will often serve as a predisposing cause, or to heighten and prolong an already existing inflammation.

One of the most common causes of vesical catarrh is *retention* of the urine, whether from habit, obstruction, paralysis or anæsthesia, one of the latter two conditions being the most common factor in cases where cystitis supervenes upon spinal complaints—as posterior spinal sclerosis, typhus, coma, etc.

Retention of urine is a dangerous condition, because if not relieved, the urine will decompose. The carbonate of ammonia thus formed from the urea is very irritant to the vesical mucous membrane, besides, when absorbed, giving rise to constitutional symptoms simulating uræmia; in addition to which, one may have septicæmia, caused by the putrescent animal matter.

Next in frequency to irritation of the mucous membrane as a cause of cystitis comes *extension* of the inflammatory process from the prostate gland, urethra, ureters, or the pericystic tissues, as in neighboring abscess or pelvic cellulitis. And also poisoning by the contagion of pus corpuscles, of gonorrhœa, suppurative pyelitis, etc., as well as from the use of unclean instruments.

Cantharis, turpentine, oil of copaïba, and a few other drugs are generally recognized as having a specific action on the bladder, even when introduced into the system at some other point; and the old school explains the fact by saying that the kidneys excrete the irritating principle, whose presence in the urine causes the cystitis.

Homœopaths know that many drugs have a specific effect upon the bladder, even when administered in doses so minute as to preclude the theory of chemical irritation just alluded to. This, however, is opening up the question of drug-action, the discussion of which would be quite out of place in these pages; suffice it to state that the writer believes this dynamic power of the drug to be such as to influence the reception of life by, and consequently the growth and function of, the bioplastic cells of the bladder.

Under the head of Medicinal Causes, then, the reader is referred to the homœopathic therapeutics of cystitis, making note of the fact, however, that a transient, acute, vesical catarrh is frequently occasioned by the ingestion of poor new beer, or any other imperfectly fermented drink.

Sudden checking of perspiration on the abdomen or feet by exposure to cold or wet is also a fertile cause of the malady in question.

In brief, then, the causes serving to inflame the bladder may be summarily stated as mechanical, irritative (physical, chemical or medicinal) extension, local poisoning, metastasis (?) and exposure.

SEMIOLOGY.—The symptoms characteristic of cystitis are: frequent, urging calls to micturate, preceded or accompanied by more or less pain and straining, a sense of fullness, pressure, heat, and throbbing deep in the hypogastrium, and also in the perineum, when the trigonum vesicæ is affected, as is generally the case.

The pains are often burning, and radiate down the legs and to the scrotum, penis, loins and sacrum. The hypogastrium and perineum are more or less sensitive to pressure, and, in some cases, we recognize the bladder as a sensitive tumor behind or just above the pubis, or by rectal exploration. When the posterior aspect of the bladder is inflamed the rectum will be involved to the extent of a troublesome tenesmus.

Acute cystitis is generally accompanied by fever, malaise, more or less mental distress, and restlessness, and gastric disturbances, as anorexia and tendency to constipation, from which the chronic catarrh is comparatively free.

The urine in the acute form is generally heightened in color, with an increased amount of mucus, except in the first stage. In gouty subjects we are very apt to observe the presence of uric acid crystals, while the croupy and diphtheritic forms are characterized by shreds of false membrane, which are apt to plug up the urethra and give rise to agonizing attacks of strangury, until they are forced out of the meatus.

In the *later stages of vesical catarrh* the urine is found to be alkaline, with sometimes an ammoniacal odor, or even a putrescent smell in cases of long retention or gangrene. There is always a heavy sediment, consisting of mucus or pus (often rendered glairy by the carbonate of ammonia), and also crystals of ammonio-magnesian- commonly called " triple "-phosphate, as well as an amorphous deposit of phosphate of lime, urate of ammonia, and bacteria.

But the most characteristic element of the sediment, and that which is the most to be relied upon for our diagnosis in obscure cases, is the presence of epithelial cells from the mucous membrane of the bladder. These are of varied appearance, according to their location in the bladder—columnar, if from the mucous follicles; large round cells, twice the size of pus corpuscles, from the deeper layers of the mucous membrane, and larger, irregularly oval or polygonal, squamous cells from the free surface, characterized by a thickening towards the middle, and often by the imprint on their under surface of the round or columnar epithelium of the deeper layer.

According to L. S. Beale, we might infer the part of the bladder affected by the character of the cells, as he says that the squamous cells are more characteristic of the trigonum, while the large, columnar or rounded cells predominate at the fundus. The principal feature of bladder-cells, however, may be said to be irregularity, or rather diversity of shape, so much so that some experience is requisite to diagnose them readily under the microscope.

The phosphates may be distinguished from the urates of sodium and ammonium by the fact that they are dissolved upon the addition of nitric acid, while the latter are dissipated by heat.

A low, debilitating fever, with streaks of blood intermingled with the pus, indicates ulceration, a serious complication, endangering the patient's life from diffuse suppuration, septicæmia, or malignant peritonitis.

Diffuse suppuration and gangrene are indicated by a quick, weak pulse, prostration, clammy sweat, hiccough, cold extremities—in the latter case a sudden subsidence of pain—and by a putrescent or gangrenous odor of the urine, which is grumous in appearance, containing decomposed blood and pus and shreds of mucous membrane.

PROGNOSIS.—Cystitis may terminate in resolution, suppuration, gangrene or hypertrophy. The first-mentioned result is, of course, indicated by a gradual subsidence of all the signs and symptoms of the disease. The second by rigors, an abatement of the fever, and the appearance of pus in the urine. By suppuration, we mean to say that either a chronic catarrh is induced; diffuse suppuration supervenes (as alluded to above), or an abscess forms in the sub-mucous tissues, which may break into the cavity of the viscus and heal, or may pierce the outer coat of the bladder.

Perhaps the most favorable location for the abscess to point would be through the skin, just above the pubis, avoiding the peritoneum; for should this membrane be involved, great danger would ensue to the patient through peritonitis.

The abscess might break into the rectum or vagina and discharge safely; but if its contents were emptied into the cellular tissue of the pelvis, the patient must expect pelvic cellulitis and septicæmia.

When the abscess perforates all the coats of the bladder, a urinary fistula is established, producing infiltration of the cellular tissue, peritonitis, or a false passage, according to its location and direction.

Gangrene, which in the majority of instances appears within seven days after the invasion of the disease, is indicated by the symptoms of collapse mentioned above.

In old persons even simple vesical catarrh may prove dangerous to life by inducing complete retention.

PATHOLOGICAL ANATOMY.—In acute vesical catarrh the mucous membrane is hyperæmic, reddened, tumified and relaxed. The first stage is one of diminished secretion, while the reaction of the second stage is characterized by a profuse secretion of mucus on its free surface. When suppuration ensues, the epithelial cells proliferate too rapidly and degenerate into pus corpuscles, which, if the urine be strongly alkaline, will break down into a glairy, viscid mass.

In chronic catarrh the mucous membrane is thickened, of an ashy gray color, and covered with a layer of pus.

Diffuse suppuration is that condition in which the vesical wall undergoes purulent infiltration, with disorganization of its tissues. This most frequently follows ulceration, and is almost as grave a complication as gangrene.

In croupous cystitis the false membrane is merely a fibrinous exudation upon the free epithelial surface, which, when it is thrown off, leaves the mucous membrane intact; whereas in diphtheria there is infiltration and necrosis of the epithelial tissue, disorganizing it to such an extent as to leave an ulcer upon the removal of the diphtheritic membrane.

Interstitial cystitis may terminate in abscess, as above mentioned; but, when chronic, it is most apt to result in hyperplasia, causing hypertrophy of the bladder, eccentric or concentric.

In eccentric hypertrophy the cavity of the viscus remains unaltered, but the whole organ is enlarged, so as to be felt in the hypogastrium as a hard, inelastic tumor.

In concentric hypertrophy, on the other hand, the walls are contracted as well as thickened, so that, although the general size of the bladder may appear to be almost or quite normal, its capacity is reduced to two ounces, or even to half a fluid ounce.

This so-called hypertrophy is due to a deposit of connective tissue in the parenchyma of the organ, and it is not to be confounded with a *true* hypertrophy of the *muscular tissue*, resulting from prolonged and undue muscular exertion.

This is caused by any constant obstruction to the free discharge of urine, be it structural or functional.

This enlargement of the fasciculi of the detrusor muscle gives a reticulated appearance to the interior of the bladder, often resembling the columnæ carneæ in the heart.

If the obstruction be not removed, the mucous coat will eventually protrude between the muscular bundles, forming diverticuli or pouches varying in capacity from a few drops to several ounces. As these can never be emptied, the urine in them will decompose and deposit crystals, setting up an inflammation which is very apt to terminate in perforation, and consequently urinary infiltration.

An abscess protruding into the cavity of the bladder might, according to its location, obstruct the ureters or urethra, and so cause retention and much suffering.

DIFFERENTIAL DIAGNOSIS.—*Acute nephritis* sometimes arises from the same causes and has symptoms similar to acute cystitis, but the latter may be distinguished by the strangury, the locality of the pain and the quality of the urine; in *nephritis* the urine being more scanty, albuminous, with less mucus, and containing smaller epithelium cells. The presence of renal epithelia and casts of the uriniferous tubules is pathognomonic of inflammation of the kidney. In both diseases it is not uncommon to find the urine bloody; but the blood from the bladder is very apt to be coagulated, while that from the kidney is more intimately mixed with the urine, and if present in sufficient quantity, will appear as a brownish red powder; this, however, is by no means a certain rule.

Acute metritis is often very difficult to distinguish from acute cystitis, except by the character of the urine and physical vaginal exploration.

The practitioner must bear in mind that the detection of vaginal epithelium by the microscope is of no assistance in forming the diagnosis, because there is always more or less of it in the urine of females.

Chronic uterine troubles, characterized by a purulent discharge, as *endometritis* or *cervical leucorrhœa*, can be distinguished from chronic vesical catarrh only by ocular inspection and careful catheterization.

In *urethritis* there is less irritability of the bladder, and we do not encounter the deep-seated pain and fullness that characterize cystitis. There is also less pus discharged, and generally not so much constitutional disturbances. In urethritis the pus or mucus appears with the first urine passed, while, if the bladder be the seat of the trouble, it is voided at the end of micturition.

It is almost impossible to recognize *abscess* of the vesical wall, as there are no special signs to differentiate it from sub-mucous suppuration, they both having prolonged, intense fever and rigors. A sudden appearance of pus in the urine would naturally indicate the breaking of an abscess, provided the discharge were followed by a mitigation of the symptoms of the patient; but it is difficult to say whether the abscess originated in the bladder-wall or the surrounding tissues, and if there already existed a purulent discharge, the sudden accession of pus would probably escape notice.

Vesical spasm or *neuralgia of the neck* of the bladder, is as painful as acute cystitis; and, in fact, simulates it closely, but the urine is quite normal, and even may be profuse and watery.

A *dermoid cyst* might break into the bladder, but the presence of fat and dermal tissues would serve to distinguish it from ordinary tissues.

The following table from Van Buren & Keyes should render it an easy matter to distinguish between

Acute Cystitis of the Neck and	*Prostatitis.*
1. Characteristic vesical tenesmus; frequent uncontrollable calls to urinate.	1. Much less vesical tenesmus. Rectal tenesmus more marked.
2. Micturition particularly painful during the passage of the last drops of urine, when there is a convulsive contraction.	2. Nothing similar.
3. At the end of micturition, excretion of a thick fluid, a mixture of pus and blood; often a flow of pure blood.	3. Nothing similar. Urine normal.
4. Simple perineal sensibility; pains radiating towards the anus much less violent than in prostatitis.	4. Perineal pains deep; very violent; increased by motion, defecation, etc.
5. Prostate normal.	5. Rectal exploration reveals a prostatic tumor, hard, very painful, etc.
6. No retention of urine.	6. Dysuria; retention of urine.
7. Slight, or no general symptoms.	7. General symptoms well marked; fever, anorexia, etc.

TREATMENT.—The first and cardinal point of treatment, is to remove the cause, if possible.

In the acute affection, rest on the back, with the hips elevated, to relieve the bladder of the pressure of the abdominal viscera and uterus is strongly insisted upon.

In all cases the patient should enjoy dry, pure air and surroundings, and be warmly clothed; while in chronic vesical catarrh he is much benefited by gentle exercise, sea-bathing, change of scene, and avoidance of exposure to inclement or suddenly-changing weather.

When there is retention of urine, the diligent use of the catheter is necessary, and if its introduction is extremely difficult and painful, a pure rubber flexible one may be tied in, provided—and only so long as—the neck of the bladder will tolerate its presence.

All catheters should be kept scrupulously clean, for which purpose a two per cent. solution of carbolic acid is perhaps the most effectual. In cases of profuse discharge or of decomposing urine, the bladder may be washed out twice a day, if the patient can bear the introduction of the catheter.

In eccentric hypertrophy systematic catheterization alone may suffice to restore the contractibility of the bladder walls, a result much facilitated by the aid of an elastic abdominal bandage.

In concentric hypertrophy, on the contrary, the indication is for the patient to retain the urine as long as possible, provided it is in a normal condition; and it is even recommended to use large injections of warm water to try and dilate the viscus.

The diet should be simple, nutritious and readily digestible, there being nothing better than pure milk in abundance, fruit, oysters and other animal food.

The physician should interdict all coffee, tea, beer, asparagus, salt and lemon juice; but grated lemon *peel* may be allowed as a flavoring.

Alcohol is not permissible in acute cystitis, but in the atonic chronic vesical catarrh, Lebert recommends the moderate use, at meals, of the following light, red wines as astringent tonics (an effect attributed partially to the tannin they contain): Bordeaux, Burgundy, Rhone, Assmanshäuser, Erlauer, and the red Rhine and Hungarian wines.

Much benefit is found in the judicious use of hydro-therapeutics.

In acute inflammation nothing is more comforting to the patient than hip or general baths of luke-warm water at a temperature of 80° or 90° F. At first, the bath should be of about half an hour's duration, but this may be gradually increased to two hours, and even repeated in the course of the day.

Tieman makes a flat hot-water bag with a tubular prolongation that fits the perineum, at the same time applying the heat to that locality and the hypogastrium. This is a valuable adjunct, as it is readily applied and obviates all danger of a chill from wet clothing.

Cold applications occasionally relieve the pain of acute cystitis, but are of not so universal efficiency, and require close watching.

Enemata of hot water often soothe the inflamed bladder, more especially when the posterior aspect of that viscus is involved.

In chronic vesical catarrh, cold water is more efficacious than hot. The patient should be sponged daily, and as soon as practicable take river, or preferably, sea baths, or even sulphur baths, according to the recommendation of some authorities.

Various mineral waters are strongly recommended as alkaline diluents, the favorite ones being Seltzer, Vichy, Wildung, Ems and Karlsbad, as well as the chalybeate springs of Pyrmont Schwalback and St. Moritz. Several of our American springs seem to have an analogous composition to the above-mentioned waters, and should have a similar effect, but of these we cannot speak authoritatively, as their reputation is not yet sufficiently established.

The physician should bear in mind, when prescribing or permitting the use of strongly-carbonated artificial waters, that they are very apt to prove irritating to the bladder.

Counter-irritation is much relied upon in the old school as a valuable adjuvant. The abdomen is kept reddened by a thin poultice sprinkled with mustard; or, the same effect may be obtained more neatly and with less trouble by applying moistened mustard-paper under a hot-water bag.

Van Buren & Keyes hold that there is never any necessity for blood-letting.

The systematic introduction of soft wax bougies has proven efficacious in the obstinate congestion and hyperæsthesia which so frequently follow an attack of gonorrhœa. This same method of treatment has also relieved retention and incontinence of urine dependent upon irritable neck of the bladder.

Soothing injections of warm water have been often recommended, but it is doubtful whether their quieting effect is not over-balanced by the irritation caused by the introduction of the catheter. Niemeyer directs—when they are used—that the temperature of the water should be gradually lowered to 65° F., more especially if the patient be a woman.

In cases with an obstinate chronic discharge a mildly-stimulant injection is often necessary to excite a reaction sufficient to enable the medicine to make an impression.

A good rule is, that the injection, unless very strong, should be retained for five minutes or thereabouts, and then should be partially withdrawn so as to leave a little in the bladder.

Medicated injections should be made immediately after emptying

and washing out the bladder, and be sufficient in quantity to distend
the viscus and reach all parts of the mucous surface.

All astringents should be used with caution.

The following are the principal injecting fluids now in use:

>*Tannin,* 5–15 grs. to 1½ ozs. of water; then gradually in-
>crease the strength to three per cent. or more, and inject
>at intervals of two or three days, and later every day.
>"There is nothing better than this, especially in obstinate
>cases."

℞ Sodæ bibor., ℨj.
  Aquæ,
  Glycer., āā ℨij.

>Mix.—S. One tablespoonful to a 4 oz. injection.   Is soothing
>and checks the formation of pus.
>
>*Silicate of soda,* one per cent. solution is claimed by the
>French to check suppuration.
>*Acetate of lead,* ⅙–⅓ gr. to 1 oz. of water.
>*Dilute nitric acid,* 1–2 min.   "   "
>*Chlorate of potash,* 5–15 grs.   "   "
>*Nitrate of silver* is not in so great favor as of old; Van Buren
>& Keyes hold that it is rarely of service.   It requires
>more caution than any other agent.   When used it is
>best to begin with a solution of about 1 gr. to ℨiv. of
>water, or weaker, and gradually to increase the strength
>and size of the injection, if necessary.
>*Carbolic acid* does not meet the approval of any of the authori-
>ties consulted by the writer.
>*Salicylic acid,* 1 to 500, is much used now, although many
>prefer *salicylate of soda,* in a somewhat stronger solution.
>*Quinine* and *zinc* are also sometimes used.

The diluents are innumerable and should be imbibed profusely
and persistently in order to accomplish their purpose—that of diluting
the urine and so rendering it less irritating to the vesical mucous membrane.   They all are mutually interchangeable, according to the taste
of the patient, as none have specific virtues.

The urine is almost always acid on entering the bladder, its alkaline reaction being developed there by the decomposition of urea into
carbonate of ammonia; hence *alkalies,* and not acids, are indicated in
order to neutralize the urine and render it innocuous on its entrance
into the bladder; they should be taken frequently and in small doses,
alone or in carbonated water or some diluent.

Aside from the *alkaline mineral waters,* the following are often resorted to, and may be alternated with each other:

Citrate of potash in 20-30 gr. doses three times a day, according to the concentration and alkalinity of the urine; also, *bicarbonate of soda, acetate of potash* and *liquor potassæ,* etc.

HOMŒOPATHIC TREATMENT. —The law *similia similibus curantur* holds good in this disease — as in all others—our failures to cure being attributable to the carelessness or ignorance of the prescriber, and not to any limitation in the application of the law itself. But it must be borne in mind that this grand principle is a therapeutic law, governing only the selection of the remedy; and, as true physicians, we are bound by the best interests of our patients to neglect no hygienic, dietetic or surgical precaution that may aid the medicine in eradicating the disease.

As the limits and purpose of this paper forbid a detailed picture of each drug mentioned, only the bladder symptoms are given (with a few clinical hints) as an aid to the choice of the remedy, according to Hahnemann's prime rule of "covering the *totality* of the symptoms."

The most prominent of the remedies discussed are : (1) *Benz. ac., berb., cann. sat., canth., caust., dulc., equiset., pareira b., prunus* and *puls;* or, (2) *Acon., bell., arg. n., arn., ars., bals. peru., camph., cann. ind., chimaph., copaiva, digit., lyc., merc.* and *sulph. ;* and (3) *Apis, aloe, am. c., aur. mur., ant. c., aur. met., bry., calc., capsic., carbo an., carbo. veg., a. cepa, colch., coloc., con., erigeron, eupat. purp., euphorb., hyos., kali. c., kreos., lach., mez., natr. mur., nitr. ac., nux v., phos., polyg., ruta* and *sars.*

Aconite.—† *Anxious, urgent desire,* almost constant, accompanied by a sight sense of swashing in the bladder. †Tenesmus of the neck of the bladder, and burning in that locality when not urinating. Retention, with pressure in the bladder, °especially in babies, with much crying and restlessness. When walking, pain in the bladder, or pains in the loins like labor pains.

Emission painful, may be *guttatim* or involuntary from momentary paralysis of the sphincter.

Urine scalding, scanty, deep red, bloody or brown, with brick-red precipitate, or deposit of coagula of blood.

°*Acon.* is most frequently indicated at the onset of the attack, especially if caused by exposure to dry cold, by suppressed perspiration or fright, accompanied by fear and anger.

Is well followed by *cann. sat.* It may be indicated after *arn., coff., sulph., verat.*

Agar.—Urgent desire, with but scanty secretion. Weakness of the sphincter, with dribbling. Urine reddish, scanty or profuse, clear and lemon-colored.

°Apt to be of use in typhoid cases, with a tendency to collapse, gangrene, or convulsions.

Aloe.—Frequent urging, worse at night, or in the afternoon. Burning micturition. Urine bloody. Yellowish, bran-like or slimy sediment.

°Bad effects from sedentary habits. Lymphatic or hypochondriac temperament.

Alum.—Can only pass water while straining at stool. Frequent ineffectual desire.

†*Feeling of weakness in bladder and genitals;* fears he will wet the bed. Spasmodic sensation in the neck of the bladder; violent urging, with difficult and delayed discharge.

° To be considered in chronic cases, characterized by great weakness and excessive irritability, as in hysteria and hypochondriosis.

Ambr. gris.—Strong desire; frequent urination at night. Urine passed in small quantities, of a pungent, sour smell. Turbid, reddish-brown, with a profuse sediment of acid urates.

°More particularly adapted for lean or aged persons.

Amm. carb.—Frequent urgency, with continued pressure on the bladder, and cutting pain. Nocturnal aggravation. Discharge scanty and painful. Urine turbid, reddish.

°Tendency to gangrene. °The patient is of a feeble constitution, uncommonly irritable, with excitement of the nervous system.

°Inimical to *lach.*

Amm. mur.—Urging, yet only a few drops pass, until the next stool, when it flows freely.

Frequent painful urging, pressure and tenesmus in the bladder, especially at the neck. Urine hot, concentrated, of a deep yellow color, cloudy, with a clay-like sediment.

°Suitable to fat, sluggish people with fat body and thin legs.

°Compare *K. B., mag. mur.* and *sep.*

Ant. cr.—Tenesmus arouses him from sleep at night. During micturition, cutting pain; frequent urination, with intense burning in the urethra and backache, and much mucus; or discharge *guttatim,* with burning.

Involuntary discharge after attacks of coughing. Urine dark, concentrated, with a deposit of acid urates.

°Compare *amm. mur.*

Ant. tart.—Burning in urethra during and after urination. Spasm of the sphincter. Violent urging, with burning, painful and difficult discharge; sometimes *guttatim*; the last drops bloody. Urine scanty, dark brown, turbid, very pungent, with a violet-colored sediment (excess of *indican*); or profuse, watery, clear, with a deposit of lime salts and triple-phosphates.

Apis.—Great irritation at neck of the bladder, with frequent burning urination—may be *guttatim*—preceded and followed by burning and smarting, and accompanied by a stitching pain in the urethra. Urine scanty, hot, red ; may be bloody.

°If caused by *canth.* Recommended by Hering in the bilious, nervous temperament, strumous diathesis, women and children.

°Antidotes, *canth. Rhus.* given after it has often disagreed. Concordances, *canth., tereb.*

Arg. n.—Frequent desire, vesical atony, spasm and tenesmus at neck of the bladder. Discharge painful, with burning and sticking in the urethra and soreness in the kidneys. Urine scanty, concentrated; profuse discharge of pus.

°Herpetic patients. °Antidoted by *natr. mur.* (chemically and dynamically).

Arn.—Constant urging, while urine passes in drops. Bladder feels overfilled; ineffectual urging. †Has to wait a long time for urine to pass. *Cystospasmus.* †Tenesmus from spasm of the sphincter. †Enuresis while asleep. Urine scanty, red, very offensive, stains napkin yellow-brown. †Hæmaturia.

°RESULT OF MECHANICAL INJURIES. °*Retention from exertion.* °To be considered in septic states, or when there is a typhoid tendency. °Hydrogenoid constitution of Grauvogl.

Ars.—Burning pain, especially at the commencement of urination. Bladder feels paralyzed, greatly distended, with no desire to urinate.

Dysuria or involuntary emission.

Urine scanty, dark, turbid, with pus, blood and deposit of red sand.

°In *typhoid* and *septic* states; *collapse* and *gangrene.*

Asa f.—Spasm in the bladder during and after micturition. Urine very hot, dark, acrid, smells pungent or ammoniacal.

°In hypochondriacal and hysterical persons. The venous hæmorrhoidal constitution.

Asar.—Constant urging, with sensation of pressure in the bladder; drawing pain in the urethra and glans.

°Nervous temperament; excitable or melancholic mood.

°Compare *cupr., nux, phos.*

Aur. met.—Constant urging. Painful retention, with pressure in the bladder.

Urine turbid, like buttermilk, with much mucus; is ammoniacal; decomposes rapidly.

°Scrofula. Sanguine temperament; light hair and ruddy complexion.

Bals. Peru.—Sticking in the urethra. Cutting on urinating. More frequent micturition than usual during the night (sixth and seventh days). Urine more scanty and darker (eleventh day). Red coating on the urinal (fifth day).

Bar. c.—Great desire; cannot retain the urine. Constant urging; frequent emissions every other day. Discharge scanty, painful, of dark brown urine.

Painful drawing in the hypogastrium, with vesical tenesmus.

°Scrofulous children. Old people, especially when fat.

Bell.—Sensation of turning and twisting in the bladder, like a large worm, without desire to urinate. Vesical region very sensitive to touch or jar. Urging and tenesmus; painful dysuria. Vesical spasm, or weakness of the sphincter. Retention. *Urine* scanty, high-colored, turbid on standing; excess of phosphates.

°Plethoric people.

Benz. ac.—Irritable bladder. Fleeting pains in bladder when not urinating. Dysuria, urging and tenesmus.

Urine very hot and dark red, or brown, with a strong, penetrating odor. Hippuric acid is present after the ingestion of large doses. Deposit of granular mucus, mixed with phosphates and lime salts. Muco-purulent sediment.

°Vesical catarrh from suppressed gonorrhœa, gout or calculi. Enlarged prostate. Dysuria senilis. Urate of ammonia concretions. Gouty or rheumatic diathesis. °Useful in gout after *colch.* fails. Bad effects from *cop.*

Berberis.—*With all the urinary symptoms the back is lame and sore,* with pains in the loins and hips. Urinary difficulties aggravated by movement. Burning pains in the bladder, whether it be *full or empty ;* or aching, or frequently recurring crampy pain in the bladder, increased by pressing upon it.

Violent cutting pain from the bladder to the urethra. Painful dysuria, worse when lying or sitting, better while standing.

Before urination, frequent urging, pain and tenesmus. *During* urination, burning in urethra and pressure upon the bladder. *After* micturition, *violent urging ;* cutting, burning in the urethra, and burning and pressure in the bladder.

Urine always *turbid* yellowish, greenish, bloody, or brown-red.

Sediment, light, gelatinous mucus, clay-like or blood-red ; mealy or bran-like deposit of urates and lime salts.

Borax.—Ineffectual, severe, urgent desire, worse at night. Infant passes water every ten or twelve minutes, and frequently cries and screams before the passage. Urine hot, of a pungent odor.

°Inimical to *borax, acetum, vinum.*

Bovista.—Frequent desire, even immediately following urination.

Urine bright red, with violet sediment ; or yellowish-green, with a reddish deposit.

Bry.—Frequent urging, even when the bladder is but scantily filled. Must urinate quickly. Irritable bladder. Cystospasmus.

°Often follows *acon., nux, op., rhus.*

Cactus.—Constant desire. Dysuria. Urine passes in drops, with much burning. Spasm of the sphincter. Retention. Hæmaturia. Urination prevented by clots.

Calad.—Bladder is sore on pressure. Stinging pain deep in the hypogastrium.

Bladder feels full, without desire to urinate. Slight vesical spasm.

°Lax phlegmatic temperament. °Antidotes mercury. °Followed well by *acon., canth., sep., puls.*

Calc. o.—Frequent urging, worse after walking. Dysuria. Unable to empty the bladder. Polyuria. Dripping after micturition. *Urine* very offensive, putrid, brown, with white sediment. Or clear and ammoniacal. Hæmaturia.

°Polypus in the bladder.

°Leuco-phlegmatic temperament.

°Follows *china, cupr., nitr. ac., sulph.*

May be followed by *lyc., nitr. ac., phos., sil.*

Calc. phos.—Frequent urging. Shooting pain in the mouth of the bladder. Violent pain in bladder and neighboring parts.

°Sulphur follows well.

Compare with *calc. o., sil., fluor. ac., berb.*

Camph.—Frequent urging, sometimes ineffectual. Dysuria. Strangury, discharge *guttatim*, burning and tenesmus of the neck. Retention, with pressure on the bladder, and desire to urinate. Complete retention, or *slow emission in a slender stream*, with burning in bladder and urethra. *Urine* red, reddish-brown, or *yellowish-green*, with a musty odor.

°Inflammation or spasm of bladder. *Caused by canth., bals. pop., tereb.*, etc.

°Blondes most affected, as are scrofulous children.

°Aggravates the effects of *nitrum*, and seems to be injurious if given after it.

Cann. sat.—Ineffectual urging. Pressure to urinate in fore part of urethra, when not urinating.

Complete retention, or constant urging, especially at night, with burning pain; passes only a few drops of bloody urine. Urethra feels very *sore*. Strangury.

°In typhoid fever.

°Gonorrhœal cystitis.

Follows *canth.* and *acon.*

Cann. ind.—Urging ineffectual. Emission frequent, scanty, with burning pain, in the evening. Has to wait some time before the urine flows. Has to force out the last few drops with the hand.

The urine dribbles out after the stream ceases. Urine loaded with slimy mucus, °after exposure to damp cold.

°Affects most persons of nervous and sanguine temperament; the bilous nearly as much; the lymphatic but slightly.

CANTH.—Strangury. Violent but ineffectual urging, with discharge *guttatim* of concentrated bloody urine. Violent *agonising* tenesmus, and *burning in the bladder*. Stinging, shooting, burning pains in the region of the bladder and urethra before and after urinating. Or cutting, pressing pain along ureters to bladder, relieved by pressing upon the glans. Spasmodic pains in the perineum, along the urethra, and down into the testes, which are drawn up. Cutting pains through the abdomen. Abdomen distended and painful to touch, especially in the region of the bladder. Great thirst, but drinking and even the sight of water increases the pain.

Painful retention. Hæmaturia. Urging worse when standing, still more upon walking, better when sitting.

Urine turbid, scanty, bloody.

Sediment white; clots of blood, or bloody mucus.

°From suppressed gonorrhœa.

°Inimical, *coff.*; antidotes, *acon., camph., lauroc., puls.*

Capsic.—Strangury. Cystospasmus.

Frequent, unsuccessful urging and tenesmus. Stitches in neck of the bladder on coughing. Burning in the bladder. Painful drawing in testes and spermatic cord when urinating. *Shuddering on urinating.* Burning, smarting, after micturition.

°Less frequently indicated in persons of tense fibre. Light hair, blue eyes.

Carbo. an.—Frequent, ineffectual urging, with painful pressure in loins, groins, and thighs. Stitches and lancinating pains in the abdomen, relieved by urinating.

Urine increased, fetid, more frequent at night, sometimes interrupted.

°Elderly, venous, plethoric persons.

°Young scrofulous subjects.

(*To be continued.*)

THE TEMPTATIONS OF A HOMŒOPATHIC PHYSICIAN.

By M. DESCHERE, M.D.,

New York.

ON the tenth day of last February, about 2 P.M., I was called to see Mrs. K., twenty-five years of age, married five years ; had never conceived. She had suffered from ovarian neuralgia during menstruation since her first period, for which she had been treated by various physicians of the old school, mostly with morphine injections.

I had succeeded in much relieving her troubles with bromide of potash and *lac. can.*, in higher potencies, about a year ago, after which time she left for Europe, and I had lost sight of her until I was called that day. She was in great distress. Excessive dysuria, with constant urging, and passing only a few drops, with burning and cutting pains; much nausea; great tenderness to touch in hypogastric region ; much thirst; pulse tense—about 110. She could not keep quiet long enough to have her temperature taken, on account of the constant urging to urinate ; urine dark, but clear. ℞ *Cantharis* 3, every fifteen minutes until relief should set in.

At 10 P.M., the urinary difficulty had much diminished, but the nausea had increased, and very painful vomiting of green fluid had set in, accompanied with violent empty retching. The pains were of a crampy nature and felt mostly in the hypogastric region. There were great anxiety and restlessness, with constant craving for ice-water. which was, however, immediately thrown up. The tenderness of the hypogastrium had increased since morning. Temperature in

---

*Read before the New York Homœopathic County Society, March 10th, 1887.

vagina, 104.8. Face looked pinched; voice very weak—just above a whisper; great general prostration; pulse 120; tense. After as careful an examination as I could make under the circumstances, I concluded that I had to deal with a pretty severe case of pelvic cellulitis, with circumscribed peritonitis. My prescription was : *Cuprum arsen.* 3, and the application of dry heat to the abdomen.

February 11th, at 8 A. M., the condition appeared unchanged—worse if anything. The patient had not slept all night, which made two sleepless nights passed in agony, and I was urgently requested to give an injection of morphine. *I positively refused.* Mrs. K., otherwise a most amiable lady, said with her weak voice, but indignantly : "Doctor, you are brutal ; you would not give me morphine if I had to die from these pains." And the husband added : "Well, if you will not use morphine, I must get some one who will." *There was the temptation.* I explained the condition to them, I told them that I could do better with a drug accurately suiting the patient's condition. I reminded them of their former treatment, and that they had preferred homœopathy at that time because of the injurious effects of the opiates received. But all was in vain. I now reflected in this manner : If I do not administer a "hypodermic," I should first lose the case; homœopathy would be ridiculed, and the poor victim fall back into the infernal tortures of the morphine habit. So I made the following compromise and said : " I can tell you before, that you will be worse after the action of the morphine has passed away. For the drug will only benumb your sensation for a short while, as it has no curative effect on the inflammation of the parts, and your nerves will be more highly sensitive from the after effect. But as you insist, I shall now inject one-half grain of morphine, if you will let me have my way afterwards if things shall be as I foretold you. I sent for Magendie's solution and a syringe, injected fifteen minims into the arm, and after a few minutes left Mrs. K. feeling comfortable.

At my next visit, 8 P.M., when I was sent for, I heard that until 1 P.M. the patient had not slept, but felt no pain nor retching; then, however, the symptoms gradually reappeared and increased in severity, so that the condition was unbearable. She was much exhausted; the vomiting as before, the least fluid being immediately rejected by her stomach; excessive lancinating pains in the uterine region, drawing left leg up forcibly, so that the thigh is firmly flexed upon the abdomen, and the leg upon the thigh ; the least attempt to extend it caused screaming from pain.

Now I was master of the field; morphine was no more asked for, but I should try my best for relief. Under the circumstances I could not do any better than prescribe *colocynth* every fifteen minutes. It was the similimum of the case at that time.

The next morning the picture had changed. The retching and vomiting much better; after the third dose she had fallen into a slumber for about half an hour, then had several short naps of sleep with intermediate suffering, but much less than during the day. The skin was moist, the pulse 100; temperature in vagina, 101½.

My patient was as well as she possibly could be, beside her exhausted condition, by the evening of that day, under the continuation of *colocynth* every two hours. Two days afterwards she was up. Everybody felt happy.

From this case I drew the following conclusions.

1. It is wise policy to follow the urgent desire of a patient *in an exceptional case to convince him of his error* and *to strengthen his confidence in pure homœopathy.*

2. I consider such circumstances very *dangerous for a young physician*, who, after the *apparent* relief he gave to his patient *momentarily*, may be tempted to continue his morphine injections out of *want of confidence in his homœopathic remedies* and *he will be lost in the abyss of palliative treatment after that.*

3. It needs constant, *life-long study of materia medica* in reference to our case, to get that firm conviction in the correctness of a prescription which is necessary to prescribe at all.

4. We can only gain this point by *always using a single remedy;* for as long as we alternate, we can never know what remedy has done the work.

5. We must not be weakened in our conviction by the lamenting of the patient; but if they need constant dosing, let us feed them with placeboes to their hearts' content, while we *critically watch the action of our remedy.*

6. The greatest difficulty in prescribing homœopathically lies in the *examination of the patient.* If we have every point of interest, if ever so insignificant, drawn out of him, it is easy to find the remedy afterwards.

8. I therefore brought this case before you to show where the danger of temptation lies, and that we must use our strongest degree of will power, based upon the firm conviction of the undoubted superiority of the correct homœopathic selection, to avoid its dangers. Let us be true to ourselves, and truth will conquer.

CONCERNING THE EARLY DIAGNOSIS AND PREDISPOSING CAUSES OF MYOPATHIC SPINAL CURVATURE.*

By ALFRED WANSTALL, M.D.,

Batimore, Md.

"The earliest indication of spinal curvature is generally seen in increased projection of the right scapula, and in most cases the dressmaker is the first to call attention to this condition."

THE above quotation from Hamilton illustrates sufficiently the insidious nature of this affection, by which I mean its supposed almost universal development without special symptoms other than the established deformity itself. It pictures the affection after it has become habitual, and at a time when it is only partially, or not at all amendable by treatment, owing to the secondary changes of compression and rotation of the vertebræ themselves. No stronger argument could be used to demonstrate the importance of an early recognition of this trouble, and at a stage when it can be completely arrested.

By way of introduction, I will briefly relate the following case in which my attention was first called to neuralgia or myalgia, as an early symptom of myopathic scoliosis.

About three years ago I was summoned in haste, during the evening, to see a girl ten years of age, who was suffering greatly with pain in the left side. The pain had set in suddenly, and the sufferings of the little patient were so severe as to alarm the parents, who had telephoned for several physicians. I was the first to arrive and found the patient suffering, as already stated. The pain was located in the left side and front of the chest, in the region of the sixth, seventh and eighth ribs. Nothing definite could be learned from the child as to the character of the pain, partly owing to her youth and partly to her severe suffering, nor could any cause be assigned for it. The most searching examination failed to reveal anything wrong—no fever, nor thirst, no indications of general disturbance, and the functions all normal. The pain gradually subsided in the course of an hour or more, and on the following day the child was in her ordinary good health and attending school, as usual.

I was summoned in haste again during the following evening. The pain had returned as on the preceding day, beginning suddenly

---

*Read before the Maryland State Homœopathic Medical Society.

about her usual bed-time. To be brief: the pain occurred daily, with more or less regularity and severity, for upwards of two weeks, always coming on during the evening, and during the day the child would be in good health. The neuralgic character of the trouble was apparent, and the cause seemed undiscoverable until I noticed that the child, while sitting unoccupied, assumed the *oblique position* (to be more particularly dwelt upon). This symptom, already familiar to me, led me to have the child stripped to the waist and examine her back for curvature. A moderate lateral curvature, convex to the right, was found. Appropriate treatment, comprehended in removal from school, massage, and judicious exercise on the horizontal and vertical bars, was followed by speedy recovery from the neuralgia and curvature.

Later experience has taught me that neuralgic pain in the trunk is by no means an uncommon, early symptom in spinal scoliosis, and as it is the symptom that frequently drives these patients to the physician, it is all important that its significance should be recognized.

Since the above, two girls, both approaching puberty, were brought to me for pain in the right side, in the region of the liver. The history in both cases was alike; the pain occurred at irregular intervals, and had existed for a long time, and was markedly alike from its indefinite character and the absence of any apparent cause. In both cases the oblique sitting posture led me to look for and find spinal curvature.

In another instance my attention was asked to a child who complained greatly of pain over the left scapula, above the spinous process. No cause could be given for it, and all the mother could say about it was that it occurred at irregular intervals, and at times was very severe, and that rubbing and the use of liniments seemed to relieve it temporarily.

After some inquiry, directed to the patient herself, it transpired that the pain appeared during or after lessons or practice at the piano. This circumstance led me to suspect asthenia of the dorsal muscles, but the examination failed to furnish any decisive evidence of spinal curvature. However, after the child was seated a short time, she assumed the oblique position, which led me to assure the mother that there was a loss of equilibrium of the dorsal muscles, which, uncorrected, would lead to lateral curvature. The child was only temporarily under my care, her home being in Richmond. I have since learned from her aunt that she is under the care of a prominent surgeon in that city for scoliosis.

Before considering these symptoms further I will glance briefly at the predisposing causes of this trouble, and without discussing the several theories, I will simply state that I hold to the view that myopathic curvature is primarily due to a loss of functional energy of one set of the great erector muscles or the spine; and that the other changes, as increased energy of their antagonists, the curved column, with compression and rotation of the vertebræ, etc., are secondary.

According to Alex. Shaw, Esq. (Holme's Surgery, Vol. III.), the lumbar curve is the primary one, and the dorsal the secondary or compensatory curve. He bases this view on the fact that fatigued persons instinctively seek the position known in military parlance as "standing at ease." That the frequent assumption of this position has ever anything to do with the development of scoliosis, I do not think the facts confirm, though it is, perhaps, frequently due to it.

Lateral curvature is essentially a disease of the early school years; it is rarely seen prior to the sixth or seventh year. If this affection tended to develop from an attitude assumed from fatigue of the lower extremities, we would expect to find it more frequent in the earlier years, when we have all the conditions in the way of soft and yielding tissues to favor it, combined with the fact that the growing child, from the time it learns to walk, until it is compelled *to learn to sit* when it begins school, is almost incessantly upon its feet.

The attitude so graphically described by Alex. Shaw, Esq., as "standing as ease," is essentially one of adult life, when the bones and fibrous tissues have sufficiently hardened to permit the body to hang, as it were, upon them.

The spinal column may be said to be maintained in a state of unstable equilibrium, and is poised upon the pelvis, in the erect position, only by the constant and harmonious action of the muscles of the trunk, acting in concert with each other and with those of the lower extremities; and as the pelvis, its point of fixation, is being constantly elevated and depressed, the muscles of the trunk are necessarily rhythmically and insensibly contracting and relaxing— pulsating, if I may use the phrase.

When the school years begin, new relations are at once developed. The child who has previously spent the greater part of its waking hours on its feet, with unrestricted use of all its muscles, has now *to learn* to pass them in the sitting posture, with more or less restriction of the muscles. The pelvis, as the base of the spine, instead of constantly altering its level, as before, now becomes fixed, and the erector muscles of the spine are suddenly called upon for more continuous exertion, for a more tonic contraction, in order to maintain the trunk erect.

It is a common fact that a muscle works longer when its action is interrupted than when continuous. Therefore, it is obvious that more nervous energy is required to maintain the trunk erect in the sitting posture than when standing and walking.

Nor is this all. A disturbing element has also been introduced. The associated nervous relation of the muscles of the trunk with those of the lower extremities, so intimate in the upright attitude, is interrupted, and the habitual impulse of the nerve centers is altered, as now the muscles of the trunk are called on for uninterrupted and, therefore, greater energy, while those of the lower extremities are almost inert.

In this connection these additional factors are also potent. The system generally is undergoing the changes incident to the approaching puberty; and the mental faculties are being called upon, by study, to yet further exhaust the nervous energy, and the affection under discussion prevails among girls who have primarily deficient nerve force.

The position at the desk, the greater use of one arm, etc., abundantly explain the greater loss of functional energy of one set of erector muscles; the hanging of the spine upon its ligaments for support of the tired muscles, the stretching of these yet unhardened ligaments, compression of the soft vertebræ, their later rotation, altered position of the ribs, scapulæ, etc., which are mainly secondary and mechanical, complete the picture of habitual scoliosis.

It is a noteworthy fact that this affection is incomparably greater among the children of the affluent than those of the poor, and ten times greater among girls than boys; and it is among the girls of the wealthier classes that the factors I have been discussing are found to prevail.

Cervico-brachial and dorso-lumbar neuralgia or myalgia are, no doubt, familiar to you as not uncommon symptoms of habitual scoliosis, and these neuralgias are explained by the distortion of the spine, ribs, etc., occasioning compression or tension of the nerves and muscles. If this is true of habitual scoliosis, it is also true of the incipient affection, which, like its analogue, strabismus, intermits before it becomes habitual.

The symptom I have designated as the oblique position is simply a certain awkward attitude *unconsciously assumed while sitting unoccupied* by persons suffering from dorsal muscular asthenia and scoliosis, which, once intelligently observed, will not be forgotten, and is, perhaps, the sitting equivalent of the position already referred to as "standing at ease." The secret of the position is that the back of a chair does not furnish support in the proper place to aid the weak set of muscles in keeping the spine erect in comfort, so that the patients seek additional support to another part by unconsciously and instinctively drooping to one side and resting as well against the arm as the back of the chair, *sitting obliquely.* The position is less obvious if they sit to a desk or table, as they attain the same end by using an arm as a support. It is an unconscious and instinctive attitude and is to be sought objectively, and without the knowledge of the patient.

This symptom is probably always present and fixed in habitual spinal scoliosis, and is probably the earliest and most constant (though perhaps intermittent) symptom when this affection is impending.

Patients with myopathic kyphosis or lordosis tend to sit, either with the elbows resting on the knees, or when leaning back they sit on the sacrum, or, to use an exaggerated comparison, on the shoulder-blades, with the feet elevated. Parents largely attribute a squint to imitation, or speak of these awkward sitting attitudes as slovenly, and attribute them to habit, but the careful physician will always look deeper for the cause of the so-called "habits" of children.

There is another class of cases deserving a word in this connection, namely, persons who have past puberty, and who have one or both of these symptoms, and whose spines have not undergone the secondary changes. They are variously suspected to suffer from nervous exhaustion, spinal irritation, uterine displacement, etc., but whose real compliant is dorsal muscular asthenia. I call to mind the case of a man with an exaggerated lumbar curve (lordosis) who suffered terribly for years with sacral pain after any unaccustomed exertion, who was completely relieved by exercise directed especially toward strengthening the lumbar muscles.

The diagnosis of incipient curvature is not always a simple matter, as the patient is generally examined under the most favorable conditions for concealing the trouble. In assuming the standing posture, and having their attention concentrated, unless the secondary changes (compression and rotation) have already taken place, these patients are frequently able to straighten the column and keep it so during the time consumed in an ordinary examination. The unsupported sitting posture will more thoroughly and quickly betray the weak muscles, as in this position the nerve impulse is less.

To sum up. The tendency of children to assume the oblique position when sitting, and the presence of dorso-lumbar, or cervico-brachial pain of an obscure character, should always lead us to look for spinal curvature. In the absence of positive objective signs of a curved spine, the presence of these symptoms is assumed to be absolutely indicative of a weak back, or dorsal muscular asthenia; or, in other words, of impending spinal scoliosis.

HISTOLOGY IN ITS RELATIONS TO THE PATHOLOGY OF DISEASE.

By J. W. DOWLING, Jr., M.D.,

New York.

HISTOLOGY, the science of minute anatomy, is one of the new-comers among those branches of study considered necessary for the education of the student of medicine, and though almost last, yet it is by no means least in importance. Not only as an aid to our knowledge of the body in a healthy state, but as a guide to the elucidation of difficult points in diagnosis and a sure basis for all speculations on disputed points of pathology, the histology of disease. This it is which makes its study so imperative, a knowledge of its minutest points so important; and it is to the advances made in this branch of learning during recent years that are due the many facts now known and accepted by all, which only recently would have been laughed to scorn as the wildest creations of fancy.

Histology itself has a beginning in the discovery of the first of the principles of the microscope, which has accomplished so much in adding to the world's stock of knowledge. When this instrument, in the crude and imperfect form in which it first appeared, was given to the scientific world, it seemed as if a new era had been entered upon—an era of boundless discovery, of unlimited research, and of an unending series of revelations of the secrets of nature, so long held to be beyond the reach of man. New worlds were revealed in a single drop of water; thousands of new forms of life were added to those already known, and it was predicted by enthusiasts that the very *first cause*, life itself, would be discovered. Unfortunately, the limits of this method of research were soon reached; and though it has fallen short of what was hoped, yet in what it has accomplished in the one direction of medicine alone, it has been of incalculable benefit to science, and through the practical application of knowledge thus obtained, to the lasting benefit and continual improvement of the human race.

Histology is the science which has done all this, and histologists have been the means—and do we not justly feel proud and honored that such men as Wagner, Virchow, Cornil, Ranvier and others of equal celebrity, have devoted their lives to its pursuit, and that we can call them brothers in a profession which is honored the world over?

It was not many years after the first beginnings had been made by the discovery of the elements of the blood, the cell as the ultimate anatomical structure, and other of the more simple facts of the science, that an approximate and fairly accurate knowledge of the structure and arrangement of all the tissues of the body was acquired, and when this had been accomplishd, the natural result was that the question "Of what practical use is all this knowledge of cells, fibres, tissues and the like?" began to be answered in the new ideas which were formed as to the changes, great and small, taking place, as the results of disease in these very tissues, whose normal structure had but just been ascertained. That wonderful discovery, the microscope, was again put to work, and every morbid process that could be found to have occurred was subjected to its scrutiny, and results, wonderful and valuable, were brought to light. With the normal structure on the one hand and the diseased tissues on the other, it was possible to demonstrate to the dullest mind the workings of the disease process, which had hitherto been but a sealed book to the wise and learned. By studying the successive phases of disease, it could be shown with positive accuracy that every step in the process was distinct, and that in similar cases the changes were constant, thus giving, for the first time, a solid foundation on which to build theories of disease or pathology, and towards which to direct practicable means of relief; in other words, preventive and curative medicine.

Consider what a gain this was upon the old and now obsolete methods of determining the nature of a sickness. Then the most skilled physician was limited in his knowledge to those facts, gross and coarse, which could be distinguished by the sense of touch, of sight, of hearing, and even these, from a lack of knowledge of what should be the normal conditions, were more often wrong than right. Microscopical examinations were all that could be given, and in a *post mortem*, how bare and almost useless were the facts that could be gleaned by the sight and touch, without a knowledge of the minute structure of tissues, the microscopic anatomy which is so essential. For instance, we can gain no idea of the structure of the normal liver by merely looking at it and handling it, and still less can we obtain any clear idea of a diseased liver by the same means. But, knowing as we now do, the normal histological structure of that organ, we cannot fail in arriving, after proper investigation, at the departures from its normal condition, the results of disease, and thus at the nature of the disease itself.

Pathology is the study of diseases not only in their manifestations and results, but in their very nature. Morbid conditions induce the individual to believe that he is not in his usual state of health or well-being; in other words, that he is sick, and these conditions may bring about certain changes in his general appearance and bodily condition which can be seen and appreciated by the physician. These phenomena, subjective and objective, are merely indications of the presence of something which we designate by the name disease. The disease itself is the cause of these signs, and the disease is really some change in the condition of one or more of the organs of the body, due to interference with the performance of its natural functions or to failure of the organ or organs to perform their functions, from inherent weakness and not from obstruction.

This being the nature of disease, how great and detailed our knowledge of histology must be, for it is this which gives us the standard normal conditions and structure of the organs of the body that is the healthy state, and enables us to appreciate and understand all changes from this standard; in other words, disease.

There is another and important way in which histology has a bearing on pathology. As a rule, all disease is divided into two classes—organic and functional—the former, of course, embracing all those in which structural change of any kind can be found in the organ involved; and the latter, the functional, those forms in which no such changes exist. Owing to the steady increase in our histological knowledge of normal structures, we are with more and more certainty able to detect changes in tissues hitherto undiscovered, and thus to transfer one condition after another from the class of functional to that of organic diseases, thus simplifying and making much more certain our ideas as to the nature and treatment of morbid conditions. It is possible that in time, with continued diligence in histological research, that the class of functional diseases will be no longer in existence.

Again, histology has accomplished another result in pathology. Owing to the increased stimulus given by it to minute investigation and to accurate description, it has made us much more careful and particular in our use of pathological terms, and in our descriptions of pathological processes to be much more exact. What more general, for instance, in the early days of the recognition of condition, than the confounding, both in name and description, the condition known as fatty infiltration of the heart with that of fatty degeneration of the heart, roughly grouping them both under the name of "fatty heart." It is true that in both cases the heart is "fatty," but it is also true that the former condition is one in which fat is deposited in globules and droplets upon and between the muscle fibres of the heart, and that its effect is mechanical—an obstruction to the free action of the muscle; in the latter case, owing to disease process or aberration of nutrition, the very substance of the fibre itself breaks down and *becomes fat*, the muscle structure being lost. Histology, by demonstrating that the normal heart muscle fibre does not contain fat, has enabled us to recognize the condition of fatty degeneration of the heart, and its gravity with reference to a prognosis; and it has also taught us to realize the comparative benignness of the fatty infiltration, and has put it in our power to give hope and comfort to unfortunate patients who have been nearly frightened into a decline by the statement from some physician, careless as to his histological and pathological knowledge, that there was a condition present—a grave condition—known as fatty heart, upon which the poor patient must forever look as the name of the torture which is to put him to death.

The proper explanation of those processes to which we give the name "inflammation," would be but poorly formulated, were it not for the light thrown upon them by the results of histological research. The old definition that inflammation is a process characterized by heat, swelling, redness and pain would have to be sufficient to answer all questions, were it not for what histology has proven. We know that leucocytes exist in the blood; we know that these leucocytes possess an amœboid motion; we know that the capillaries are tubes formed of cells; we know that the leucocytes, as a result of an irritant action from without, tend to stagnate in the capillaries; finally do come to a condition of stasis; and then, by means of this very amœboid motion, pass directly out of the vessels into the surrounding tissues, and once here, we know that if they live they become newly formed elements, and that if they die they become pus corpuscles. This is the process of inflammation as shown by the results of the study of the histology of the blood and vessels and their changes during inflammatory action.

This very matter—the histological structure of the blood—has been of the first importance in giving us a knowledge of the pathology of that condition known as *chlorosis*. How would we have been able to know that patients suffering from the signs and symptoms of this disease were susceptible to proper treatment and certain to attain recovery had not our histologists first given us the normal conditions of the blood, and then, branching out into pathology, hit upon the idea of examining the blood of such patients, and then, finding in the departures from the known state of that vital fluid, the root of the whole difficulty.

A patient presents herself for examination. The skin is blanched; lips and mucous membrane pale, with great loss of strength, and dyspnœa on the slightest exertion, and with more or less derangement of every function of the body. We examine the heart. Its area is normal, its apex in the normal position, its sounds pure, though feeble. The lungs yield the same negative results. What is there to indicate the root of the trouble? Place a single drop of the blood of such an one on the slide of the microscope and the whole matter is explained. Histologists have demonstrated that normal blood contains two elements, red and white corpuscles, which always bear a certain relative proportion in number to each other and to the quantity of serum. In the blood from a chlorotic person we readily see that this definite standard is no longer maintained; that there are far too few blood discs and corpuscles for the quantity of fluid. How would this be known but for histology; and in its very diagnostic function histology, aided by chemistry, here points out the way of cure—the therapeutic guide. Again, in the condition known as leucæmia, histology is our guide, both as to the pathology and diagnosis. Differing from chlorosis, we have a great decrease in the ratio of the blood discs to the white corpuscles, due to very marked increase in the number of the latter, this going on to such an extent that the proportion of one white to two red is not uncommon, when the normal proportion is one of the former to 350 of the latter. Thus again, with unfailing exactness, histology has shown us the nature of this otherwise obscure disease. The subject of disease of the kidney—this all-important and yet imperfectly understood question—is one of the departments in which histology, as applied to pathology, is still at work and with great results yet to be achieved. Formerly the histology of the kidney was considered settled, and from this, arbitrary rules were laid down as to its pathological condition in various diseases; notably that combination of lesions known as *Bright's disease*. It was assumed that there would henceforth be not the slightest difficulty in the diagnosis of this malady. Was it not discovered that albumin appeared in the urine; that this was the result of disease, and that, therefore, albumin being found, there could be no doubt as to the existence of the malady? There arose two theories in regard to this albumin. One, that it only percolated through the walls of the glomerulus when the disease existed. Another, that at all times it might be found in the urine in the tubules, but that it was reabsorbed through the agency of the epithelial cells lining them, and that albuminuria was due to failure of these cells to perform their function. This is still an open question, awaiting a satisfactory solution.

Pathology, acting on the knowledge given by histology, has also divided this disease into a glomerulo-nephritis, a parenchymatous nephritis, and an interstitial nephritis. This division has been accomplished; but in the practical application of it to the diagnosis during life and the treatment, much yet remains. Formerly it was albuminuria which was the universal guide; now it is announced that specific gravity is of the greatest importance. When casts were discovered, to these were assigned the duty of acting as guiding points in diagnosis. Lately their importance has decreased, and now they are, in some cases, almost without significance. Heretofore, the various cells found in the urine were considered almost as important as casts; now, owing to the multiplicity of cells and the uncertainty as to the location from whence they come, these, too, have lost credit in influencing our opinion.

Who shall predict what will next be announced as the true solution to all these problems. Let us only hope that in the years to come, pathologists, first making sure of their histology, will, by its aid, so all-important, be able to find an answer to all these difficult questions, and then let due credit be given, in the study of pathology, to the histologists who have pointed out the straight road to correct ideas as to the nature of pathological lesions.

ORIGINAL ARTICLES IN SURGERY.

APPARATUS IN POTTS' DISEASE WHERE THE PLASTER-JACKET IS NOT APPLICABLE.*

By FRED S. FULTON, A.M., M.D.,
New York.

IN presenting this paper, I shall not attempt any systematic treatise of Potts' disease, but merely speak of some of the methods of treatment which I have found useful, particularly where that faithful old stand-by of Dr. Sayre's, the ordinary plaster-jacket, for one reason or another does not fulfill all the necessary requirements. We know that the causes of Potts' disease are constitutional and traumatic. The

---

* Read before the New York County Homœopathic Medical Society.

most rational view to be taken of its etiology is that the disease is produced by some traumatism acting upon an individual who is the
heir of some constitutional vice, such as scrofula, tuberculosis,
syphilis, etc.

The symptoms are marked even before any structural alteration in
the vertebræ can be detected. Intestinal disturbances of a flatulent
character, impairment of the function of the bowel and bladder, either
as lack of sensibility, or irritation and inability to retain their contents;
gradual loss of that easy and unstudied action of the muscles throughout the body, and fixation of various parts, such as the head thrown
back, shoulders elevated, spine held rigid, pelvis and limbs under constant watch lest an unguarded movement or jar should disturb the diseased surfaces and start up the pain, against which the child is always
involuntarily upon the guard; the peculiar method of stooping, constantly keeping the spine erect, the effort, always exerted, to relieve
the spine of its incumbent weight by means of chairs, tables, its own
arms, etc.; the relief of symptoms by forcibly stretching the spine between the knees or in an apparatus, and the spasmodic action of
muscles and the reappearance of suffering on compressing the two
extremities of the column ; all, or a large part of these will warn
the watchful physician of the approach of structural disease of the
vertebræ. Later on, the deformity in some portion of the column
manifests itself either as kyphosis or lordosis.

The pathology—thanks to Percival Pott—is known to all, namely:
structural alteration and absorption of the bodies of the vertebræ in
kyphosis, or of the spinous and transverse processes in lordosis,
accompanied by evident deformity of the spinal column and chest.

It is regarding certain methods of treatment about which I particularly desire to speak. The first object to be attained is to arrest
the destruction of the vertebræ; and the second, which in the
ultimate sense is the first, is to reduce as much as possible the
deformity.

The older method of entire rest in the prone position upon a hard
bed, without rising, tended to prevent further destruction, but could
have but little effect upon the reduction of existing deformity. The
plaster-jacket, introduced by Dr. Sayre, offers a very cheap—and if
well borne and properly managed—a most excellent means of treatment. The method of its application is perfectly known. It is in
constant use in the Laura Franklin Hospital and in our clinic in the
dispensary. It gives most excellent results. In order to secure its
greatest good, it should be well arched up over the back and chest.
If this is not done, the necessary depression to prevent rubbing in the

axillas renders it so low that it does not give the needed support. The jacket should also be taken off about once in four or five weeks and a new one applied. If a child does well in one of them, it will outgrow it in about that time, so that it will either be uncomfortable, or, what is more important, no longer conform accurately to the altered shape of the child's body, and thus it fails to give the necessary support. This observation is true regarding all the apparatus used in this disease.

But there are certain cases to which this mode of treatment with the orthodox jacket is not applicable. It may prove too heavy, too hot, or may, in sensitive children, cause excoriation, and even deep ulceration of the apex of the curvature. In anterior curvature of the lumbar and sacral vertebræ the ordinary jacket is not applicable, because the pressure of the base of the jacket comes at the small of the back and would tend to aggravate the lordosis rather than relieve it. Also in posterior curvature of the same locality the jacket cannot be made to exercise sufficient pressure at this point with support of the spine below the angle. In these cases we must resort to other methods of treatment.

To overcome the objection of weight or heat, a felt or leather perforated jacket can be substituted. Dr. Wilcox, in an admirable paper upon "Lateral Curvature," read before this Society in November, described the method of its application. It needs no further description. The perforated leather jacket is expensive and can be made only by a certain process, which is not convenient for the ordinary physician to employ. They are made by S. A. Darrach, of Newark, who has also his wheeled contrivance for the additional treatment. These are very light, fit the body and can be altered in shape to meet the requirements of the case. The felt jacket has the advantage that it can be applied and readjusted by the surgeon himself without being placed to the trouble of submitting it to a third party. If the skin be very sensitive or the patient object to a jacket or corset, Taylor's brace can be substituted. This is a most excellent apparatus.

It is made with two padded strips which are shaped to fit over the prominence of the spine. At the back, the two long arms, which reach to the shoulders and to the hips, are hinged and so adjusted with screws acting upon the iron brace which fits over the curvature, that the pressure upon the shoulders, lump, and hips can be adjusted to meet the varying demands of the case. In this way the shoulders can be subjected to pressure acting upon the curvature in the back as a fulcrum to prevent the natural drooping forward and so to materially lessen the deformity.

The following case illustrates the usefulness of the brace :

Lillie Hatfield, æt. 4 years, admitted to the Laura Franklin Hospital November 24th, 1886. History is rather indefinite; all that could be obtained was that nine months before admission the little patient suffered with pains in the back and legs. Upon admission only a very slight curvature was noticable; the child could bend over and pick up articles from the floor without much trouble. No treatment was given aside from entire rest in bed until December 29th, when she began to complain of pains in the back and of being very tired. She frequently cried out at night. On the 11th of January, 1887, I applied a plaster-jacket. At this time the curvature was pronounced and was getting rapidly worse. Three days after the child began to complain of still greater pain in the back and was very averse to sitting up. This condition becoming more pronounced on the 20th of January, the jacket was removed, when quite a deep and wide ulceration of the skin and underlying parts was observed. This ulcer extended over the prominence of curvature. Other slight abrasions were present.

This was a case in which, either from the sensitiveness of the child's skin or probably from the excessive pressure in one spot of the prominence, the jacket could not be tolerated. For this case I had an ordinary Taylor's brace made, such as I have mentioned. It worked admirably. Since its application the curvature has not increased any and a very slight reduction of its size has taken place. Since this paper was written the reduction has gone on rapidly and the child grown so in height that the deformity is scarcely noticeable.

In cases where the curvature, posterior, is so low down in the lumbar or lumbo-sacral region that a plaster-jacket would not exert the proper pressure, a modified Taylor's brace can be made with the short arm below and extending down well to the end of the coccyx. The upper arm can be held in place by the shoulder-straps and abdominal bands, while the short arm for the support of the vertebræ below the curvature can be held firmly by perineal bands, such as are used in the splints for hip-joint disease, united over the lower hypogastric region by a short abdominal band.

Another case, for which I found no instrument made, was for a very pronounced case of anterior curvature of the lumbo-sacral portion of the spine, sent to the hospital by Dr. T. F. Allen. Every apparatus I could find was inapplicable because it brought the pressure upon that very portion of the spine which would tend directly to increase the curvature. What was needed was to bring an anterior pressure on the spine, using the dorsal or lower sacral coccygeal region for points of posterior pressure. It was a slight device of my own, but it answered the requirements so fully, I feel justified in calling your attention to it. The child's history was as follows:

Marcus Monyea, æt. 6 years. No history of a fall. One year ago noticed that the right shoulder was higher than the left. Dr. Knight, of this city, treated him with one of his braces, which I honestly believe doom more children in the city to irremediable suffering and deformity than any other one agency we possess. He became steadily worse until sent to Dr. Allen, who referred the case to me for admission into the hospital, providing I thought anything could be done to help the child. At this time he could neither stand nor sit up without the brace, and with it on, the anterior curvature or saddle-back would have taken in a good-sized loaf of bread, while the protuberance of the abdomen would have done credit to a boodle alderman in his fourth term.

I had a brace of steel bands 10 inches by 3 inches fashioned in rectangular shape. I then slung the child in a plaster-jacket swing, and with a piece of lead obtained the exact curvature of that portion of his spine. The steel brace was then made to conform very nearly to this curve, the only difference being that the curve was a little less than the one in the child's spine. A few days later, when it had been shaped, the child was again suspended and a jacket applied. After circling the child's body about twice the brace was laid upon the bandage with the lower border of the brace extending down until it rested upon the posterior prominence of the sacrum. The bandage was then gradually applied downward over that, being careful not to carry it laterally over the crests of the ilia. It made a jacket of ordinary appearance in front, but with a long, narrow posterior projection which, when on, made the whole resemble a fashionable coat of the swallow-tailed variety. This jacket was borne easily and with apparent benefit. On February 12th it was removed, the curve of the steel brace approximated more nearly to a straight line and re-applied as before. On March 26th the jacket was re-applied with still less curve in the brace. On May 4th I took off the jacket the fourth time and had the steel brace made perfectly straight. The improvement in the child's condition is remarkable.

When removed this last time the child could stand perfectly straight without difficulty; the large protuberance of the stomach and the extreme lordosis have almost completely disappeared, so that as he stands with his jacket on one would not notice that there was the least deformity. I am aware that in probably the majority of cases, saddle-back is secondary to some other trouble; but in this case I could find neither luxation or deformity of the femurs or of the pelvis, nor could I find that it resulted from any disparity of action of the dorsal muscles, and on that account attributed the deformity to incipient structural changes of the spinal vertebræ. In this case this device was of the greatest service.

RECENT ADVANCES IN RECTAL SURGERY.*

By SIDNEY F. WILCOX, M.D.,

New York.

IN SURGERY, as in other branches of art and science, the results most difficult of attainment are the ones most sought after. Those easy operations which have been performed for years, with little or no variation in the method of procedure, and which are followed by a pretty definite proportion of good and bad results, soon obtain an established status, and here rest, apparently having reached the limit of improvement. This *status*—if I may use such a term— may exist *for years* or decades, and no progress be made until some radical and restless mind, not satisfied with what has been done, and longing for an improvement, suddenly breaks in upon the still quiet of established custom and opinion, and with an innovation opens wide an unknown gate and makes a great step forward in methods and results.

Thus it has been with regard to the surgery of the rectum. To be sure, cures have been effected, but the processes by which they have been obtained have been tedious and oftentimes extremely painful. Take, for instance, the treatment of fistula in ano, as laid down in almost all the works on surgery. The treatment advised is of two sorts—that by the knife and that by the ligature. This is, of course, leaving out of the question the probability of effecting a cure by medicine or by local applications. For, while it is admitted that occasionally, under very favorable circumstances, a cure of fistula may thus be obtained, such a result is so improbable and of such infrequent occurrence, as to leave these methods practically out of consideration. With regard to the knife, the method is good as far as it goes, but in the past it has not gone far enough. The treatment by the knife has consisted simply of slitting up the fistula in such a manner that the entire tract is laid open and the sphincter divided. Then the gap has been packed and stimulated to granulate from the bottom. But this process is a slow one and requires a great deal of after-treatment.

Speaking of the results by this method, Dr. Stephen Smith says, (*Medical Record*, Vol. XXIX., p. 669): "The Immediate Closure and Rapid Cure of Fistula in Ano." "Even when those (fistulæ) having a large abscess cavity finally healed after free incision, there was often a deep cicatrix, which was a constant source of irritation from the

---

*Read before the N. Y. Homœopathic County Med. Society.

tendency to accumulation of filth in the deep sulcus.   Occasionally there was a certain troublesome defect in the action of the sphincter, which remained as a permanent disability."

With regard to the ligature, the solid rubber elastic is the one most frequently used.   Probably no greater delusion was ever offered the victim than what he is led to expect from this innocent bit of rubber. He is assured that there will be no danger from hemorrhage, and is led to expect that he will have little or no pain, and can go about his business as usual after its application, and so, from dread of the knife, and a natural desire for ease, comfort and safety, he accepts the ligature.   Now for the result.   From my experience with the ligature, I am led to wonder whether or not the surgeon, in advocating its use, is not speaking two words for himself and one for the patient.   He— the surgeon—certainly feels no pain, and he is in a comfortable state of mind regarding hemorrhage ; but the patient,—he has no fear of bleeding to death, but none of the patients whom I have seen had any particular desire to go to business while wearing an elastic ligature.   The most of them, after trying to get into an easy position, have spent the most of their time in bed, calling for morphine to ease the pain.   It takes from one to two weeks for this ligature to cut through, and then the end is not yet.   There is generally quite a deep cleft, which must be left to heal by granulation, with the attendant daily treatment necessary to the attainment of this result.

So much for the old methods of treating fistula.   We will consider the more modern and more satisfactory treatment further on.

The treatment of internal hemorrhoids has always had in view the removal, or obliteration of the tumor and the avoidance of hemorrhage.

The surgical treatment has been by means of the ligature to strangulate the mass, the cautery and clamp to burn off the mass and at the same time seal up the mouths of the vessels, and the injection of carbolic acid, combined in varying proportions either with oil or glycerine, into the substance of the pile, thus producing sloughing or shrinkage of the growth.

All of these methods are successful, but have certain objectionable attendant features.

The ligature is, as a rule, extremely painful for the first two or three days, and after the mass has sloughed an ulcerated surface is left to heal by granulation, and if this surface is very extensive there is danger from too great cicatrical contraction.   The use of the cautery and clamp, by Henry Smith's and Kelsey's methods, are much less painful than the ligature, but there is more danger from hemorrhage in inexperienced hands, and the same liability to cicatrical contraction as from the preceding method.

Speaking of the method by injection of carbolic acid, Dr. Chas. B. Kelsey, (*Medical Record*, Aug. 7th, 1886), says, in comparing this method with that by the clamp and cautery, which he greatly favors : "The method of carbolic injections can only accomplish, by repeated operations, what the clamp and cautery does by a single one. Each injection is a surgical operation, and may cause greater pain and longer confinement by its effect upon a single hemorrhoid than the operation with the clamp will entail in effecting a radical cure of the disease. I do not mean to say that this will be the case, only it may be, and the operator must be prepared for it. This is, in itself, a great objection. It prevents the surgeon from giving any positive prognosis as to the time necessary for a cure, or as to the amount of trouble, pain and confinement the patient will have to endure. All he can promise is a cure in the end, and one which, if things go well, will be very satisfactory, in that it involves nothing that the patient considers a surgical operation, and no confinement to the house. He cannot, however, promise that things will go well."

On a preceding page, in comparing the results of the clamp and cautery with the carbolic injections, he says : "The cure will be equally satisfactory to the patient for a time in either case, but more satisfactory to the operator in the former (clamp and cautery), because he is sure the disease cannot return, as it may, in a measure, after the treatment by injections."

Out of many hundred cases treated by injection he gives two in which serious trouble ensued. In one there was scantiness of and difficulty in voiding the urine, enlarged glands in the groin, and a small abscess at the verge of the anus. In the other case the injection "was followed by a severe ischio-rectal abscess, lymphangitis running up the rectum, and enlarged glands in both groins. After the rather diffuse phlegmon had limited itself, the usual operation for large abscess in this region was performed, but the incision had to be carried into the bowel and the patient only recovered after weeks of treatment."

I have given this much on the injection method in order to show that it is not, as ordinarily supposed, entirely free from danger.

Now, having discussed the old methods, we will turn to the new.

For information on the subject of the treatment of fistula, I turn to the article by Dr. Stephen Smith, already referred to. He lays down the following as the three principles which should be borne in mind in the operation for the immediate closure and rapid cure of fistula in

ano : " 1. Complete removal of the lining membrane of the fistula and
of the abscess cavity which may exist. 2. Accurate and permanent
adjustment of the opposing surfaces. 3. Thorough antiseptic treatment of the wound."

He gives the details of the operation, which I will condense as
much as possible. The patient is prepared by having the bowels
emptied by doses of castor oil for two days before the operation.
The parts about the anus are washed, shaved and irrigated with a
corrosive sublimate solution. The rectum is also irrigated with the
latter solution and a large sponge pushed up in order to prevent any
fæces coming down during the operation. The fistulous passage is
incised in the usual manner, and then the lining membrane of the
passage and the abscess cavity thoroughly dissected out with the
knife or scissors. The ragged and thin margins of the wound must
also be cut away. All bleeding vessels are ligated. The assistant
then, with his forefinger introduced well into the rectum and bent like
a hook, extrudes the bowel, thus bringing the whole track of the fistula into view. Then with a long piece of chromic gut, with needles
at both ends, he sews down the length of the mucous membrane with
a saddler's stitch, which everts the edges of the membrane and brings
the deeper structures into apposition. The margins are afterward
more closely approximated by a continuous suture. A drainage tube
is inserted at the external extremity of the wound, and the operation
completed by introducing several deep carbolized silk ligatures,
which pass completely under the wound and which are tied over an
iodoform gauze pad laid along the wound. The parts are then irrigated, the sponge withdrawn, a suppository inserted, and the patient
put to bed. The diet is milk and the bowels are kept quiet for about
six days.

My own experience with the operation is confined thus far to two
cases, one of which was unique.

CASE 1.—Mrs. G——, mother of one child, was sent to me last
October by Dr. Griswold, of Elizabeth, N. J., for examination. She
stated that she had had an abscess some time previously which had
opened in two places. I made a careful examination, but could find
but one opening externally. She entered the Hahnemann Hospital
a few days later and I operated, following essentially the method laid
down by Dr. Smith. The fistula, apparently a simple complete one,
had a track about an inch and one-half in length, opening into the
rectum about three-quarters of an inch above the margin of the anus.
The track was about the size and shape of a piece of clay pipe stem,
and was easily dissected out and the wound closed up with catgut for
the mucous membrane, and three or four wire sutures for the deep
portions. All went well for a couple of days when she complained

that the fæces passed through into the vagina. I told her that could hardly be possible, as I certainly had not made a recto-vaginal fistula. But she insisted that she was right and I made an examination and found that the abscess had opened into the vagina as well as the rectum, and externally on the buttock. The passage to the vagina being very small I did not suspect its existence, having made no vaginal examination. The removal of the tissue and the presence of the sutures had caused the opening to enlarge to the size of a slate pencil, thus admitting of the passage of gas and fecal matter. The sutures were removed on the eighth day with the result of findˆing the external passage completely healed. But the recto-vaginal fistula still remained, passing just above the external sphincter, and a few weeks later I operated on this. Introducing one blade of a large pair of scissors *per vaginam* through the fistula into the rectum, with the other blade placed externally on the perineum, I split the perineal body with one stroke. Then after dissecting out the inˆdurated tissue, the wound was closed with catgut sutures along the vaginal and rectal margins of the mucous membranes, and deep wire sutures externally. Everything progressed favorably, the wire sutures were removed about the tenth day, with the result of a complete cure.

CASE II.—Mr. F——, age twenty-four, single. Had had a fistula for eight years. It had been cut three times and had once healed up, but only remained so for six weeks. When I saw him there was an internal opening low down, an external opening about an inch from the anus, but a long sinus had burrowed for about four inches under the integument on the buttock. This was slit up and the wound treated as before. The wound healed rapidly with the exception of a small portion near the anus, which had to be sewed once more. I account for the imperfect result by the fact that the patient took ether badly, and I was obliged to hurry the latter part of the operation.

With regard to operating upon phthisical subjects or those inˆclined to phthisis, the preponderance of authority is in favor of operˆating, if the lung disease is not far advanced. I cite as authorities: Allingham (1), Henry Smith (2), Hamilton (3), Morton and Wetherill (4), Pollock (5), Fagge (6), Erichsen (7), and Kelsey (8).

Most of these gentlemen consider the operation beneficial, and Dr. Hamilton says if an issue appears necessary it would be much better to establish it on the arm.

Time will admit of only a brief reference to the new and brilliant operation for internal hemorrohoids. This operation was introduced

1. International Encyclopædia of Surgery. Vol. VI. P. 108.
2. Holmes' System of Surgery. Vol. II. P. 648.
3. Hamilton's Principles and Practice of Surgery. P. 783.
4. Pepper's System of Medicine. Vol. II. P. 898.
5. Fagge's Practice of Medicine. Vol. I. P. 986.
6. Fagge's Practice of Medicine. Vol. I. P. 986.
7. Erichsen's Surgery. P. 832.
8. Kelsey's Diseases of the Rectum and Anus. Pp. 81, 82.

by Mr. Walter Whitehead, of Manchester, Eng., and a full account of it may be found in the *British Medical Journal* for February 26th, 1887, as well as an editorial in the *Medical News* (Phila.) for March 26th, 1887, and a report by Dr. Lange in the same journal, for February 12th, 1887. The results in Mr. Whitehead's hands have been "three hundred consecutive cases of internal hemorrhoids cured by excision, without a death, a single instance of secondary bleeding and not followed by such complications as ulceration, abscess, stricture or fecal incontinence," (*Med. News*, March 26th, 1887.)

The operation is based upon the frequency of relapse following other operations by which single loops of enlarged vessels are removed, and not the entire amount of diseased veins which completely surround the gut. This new operation removes the entire plexus of diseased veins up to healthy structure, and is described in brief as follows :

The patient, having been previously prepared, is anæsthetized and placed in the lithotomy position; the sphincter thoroughly stretched, and an incision made at the margin of the anus, following accurately the junction of the mucous membrane with the skin. Then the entire ring of gut, including the plexus of vessels, is dissected up from off the sphincter, with a blunt-pointed instrument until healthy tissue is reached. This is pulled down and the diseased mass removed by cutting transversely, a little at a time ; as this is done the margin of the healthy membrane is stitched to the skin with carbolized silk, or or silk-worm gut. All bleeding vessels are either tied with catgut or twisted.

The advantages of this operation are : 1. All the diseased tissue is entirely removed. 2. All bleeding is as perfectly controlled as after an amputation of a limb. 3. There are no sloughing portions to come away, or ulcerated surfaces left to heal by granulation. 4. There is much less pain following the operation, especially where the ligature is used; and 5. The patient gets well much more rapidly and completely than by other methods. Of course antiseptic details are employed.

My experience with this operation is limited to one case.

CASE. Mrs. J——, about thirty years of age, was sent to the Hahnemann Hospital by Dr. Dowling, who asked me to operate on her, which I did on April 9th, 1887.

The case was a very aggravated one, the tumors which came during pregnancy were very large, and the patient said that she "suffered untold misery for from three to twenty-four hours after each movement of the bowels.

The operation was quite long, a large amount ot tissue being removed, and the bleeding about as much as would attend a secondary operation for lacerated perineum. Thorough antisepsis was observed, and at the close the wound was covered with iodoform and an antiseptic pad.

Rapid recovery ensued. The highest temperature was 100 deg., Fah. She had comparatively little pain, and most of the sutures were removed about the tenth day. The first movement of the bowels was on about the sixth day, and being brought on through a mistake of the nurse in giving too large doses of Hunyadi water, was very fluid, and the patient not having regained entire contractile power of the paralyzed sphincter, was unable to control it. This difficulty, however, soon disappeared, and she had natural movements with little or no pain, and was able to go out of doors and take a drive at the end of two weeks. The urine had to be drawn for the first two or three days.

With regard to irritable ulcers of the rectum, I can recommend an application which was introduced by Dr. Fulton. This consists of a thick paste of pure carbolic acid and iodoform, which is applied to the surface of the ulcer after thoroughly stretching the sphincter. I have had excellent results from its use.

INTOXICATION BY SMALL DOSES FOR QUININE.—Rizu reports case of a woman, twenty-two years of age, who had contracted malarial fever four years previously. She was given a two-grain pill of sulphate of quinine, and an hour later she began to feel a sort of itching round the eyes and upper lip, accompanied by violent and continued sneezing ; the patient cried out that she had taken quinine and was poisoned. She then related that some time previously, at Bucharest, she had taken ten grains of quinine, and had almost died in consequence ; that, just as then, the symptoms had commenced with itching and sneezing, followed by œdema and congestion of the face, with lachrymation and disturbances of vision and hearing. While she was telling Dr. Rizu this, her face gradually changed form and color, and the whole of the above symptoms recurred. The pulse was feeble—ninety-five per minute ; the temperature was above normal, and the muscular system was in a state of marked relaxation ; respiration much hindered. She was given hot, strong coffee, and in about an hour the symptoms passed off. The patient called Dr. Rizu's attention to the fact that, under the influence of quinine, cold water applied to any part of the body provoked an erythematous eruption. The symptoms were reproduced on several subsequent occasions when quinine was given.—ALFRED S. GUBB, in *Lond. Med. Rec.*, June, 1887.

EDITORIAL DEPARTMENT.

EDITORS.

GEORGE M. DILLOW, M.D., ...	Editor-in-Chief, Editorial and Book Reviews
CLARENCE E. BEEBE, M.D., ...	Original Papers in Medicine.
SIDNEY F. WILCOX, M.D., ...	Original Papers in Surgery.
MALCOLM LEAL, M.D., ...	Progress of Medicine.
EUGENE H. PORTER, M.D., ...	Comments and News.
HENRY M. DEARBORN, M.D., ...	Correspondence.
FRED S. FULTON, M.D., ...	Reports of Societies and Hospitals.

A B. NORTON, M.D., ... Business Manager.

The Editors individually assume full responsibility for and are to be credited with all connected with the collection and presentation of matter in their respective departments, but are not responsible for the opinions of contributors.

It is understood that manuscripts sent for consideration have not been previously published, and that after notice of acceptance has been given, will not appear elsewhere except in abstract and with credit to THE NORTH AMERICAN. All rejected manuscripts will be returned to writers. No anonymous or discourteous communications will be printed.

Contributors are respectfully requested to send manuscripts and communicate respecting them directly with the Editors, according to subject, as follows: *Concerning Medicine, 21 West 37th Street; concerning Surgery, 256 West 57th Street; concerning Societies and Hospitals, 121 East 70th Street; concerning News, Personals and Original Miscellany, 461 West 71st Street; concerning Correspondence, 152 West 57th Street.*

Communications to the Editor-in-Chief, *Exchanges* and *New Books* for notice should be addressed to *102 West 43d Street.*

HOMŒOPATHIC—HOMŒOPATHIST.

HOMŒOPATHIC—"pertaining to homœopathy!" Homœopathist—"a believer in homœopathy!" It is interesting at the present time to note how much misunderstood these two words have been and still are, and to consider the varied shades of their definitions (especially among our old school friends) that have taken place within the past twenty-five or thirty years. A quarter of a century ago, in the estimation of the so-called "orthodox" body, "homœopathic" was synonymous with everything appertaining to the worst forms of quackery.

The medical journals of that period—especially do we remember the *London Lancet*—abounded in articles, editorial and contributed, regarding "the silly heresy," the "scandalous and nefarious trade." When, in spite of prophesies of downfall and maledictions showered mercilessly, not only upon the homœopathic practitioner, but even upon the laity who employed him, the system still gained ground; then the efforts were redoubled and the "earnest appeals" to the profession and to the public to suppress the "quackery rampant" which was threatening the temple of Æsculapius with destruction, and the profession of medicine with dissolution, were pathetic in the extreme.

When Henderson, for thirty years the accepted and honored professor of pathology in the University of Edinburgh, boldly declared himself a homœopathist, his teachings were declared pernicious, and the editorial cry resounded throughout Great Britian, "What kind of pathology *can* this man teach ?" So monstrous was considered this homœopathic heresy, that those who dared to avow their belief in it were stigmatized as "knaves or fools;" were debarred not only from professional, but from social intercourse; they were deemed unworthy to consult with medical men; they were driven out of the medical societies, and tabooed from the medical periodicals.

These are all matters of history, and humiliating must be the remembrance of them to the honest and upright members of the allopathic school, as they dispassionately review the history of homœopathy throughout the world.

The true and stanch men—who, having the courage of their convictions, were thus driven out from the great body of medical men, given the "sectarian" name "homœopathists" and shunned by the medical profession, walked steadily on by the light of scientific truth, proving day by day the efficacy of their law, confident of its ultimate triumph. *Tempora mutantur.* Behold the signs of the times ! Behold the change in the definition of the word homœopathic ! Behold the liberal and learned men of the old school, splitting it in twain and burying Percival and his ethics, by the recognition of homœopathy, not now quackery, but *one* of the methods of curing disease! We can read in the advanced text-books and periodicals how pneumonias are treated with aconite ; how belladonna is given for angina ; how castor oil in drops (shade of Paracelcus !) is recommended for enteritis in children ; how the second and third triturations ot bichloride of mercury, and colocynth are to be prescribed for the bloody flux, and calcium sulphide (hepar sulph.) for the suppurative process. Repetition is unnecessary. The more advanced allopathists of to-day only object to homœopathists on the ground that we are known by the name with which their medical ancestors, with cursing and bitterness, christened us. There are also some recalcitrant followers of the Hahnemannic law who consider that this distinctive title should be dropped ; they are so pseudo-scientific in their notions of liberality, and hyperæmic in their ideas of universality in medicine, that they consider "sectarian" proclivities prejudicial to the welfare of science—whereas the history of the world shows the entirely opposite condition. The arguments adduced to uphold this position are at first sight plausible ; it is affirmed that the advanced homœopathists, do not adhere exclusively to the law of similars in the treatment of disease ; that those who do so rigidly follow the law must relinquish great and valued auxilliaries, which, if the homœopathist adopts, he is sailing under false colors, and is necessarily a fraud. This is very specious pleading and strikes home to those who do not bestow much thought upon the matter.

It is high time, however, that the word "homœopathic" be understood by the public ; it is high time that the true definition of the term "homœopathist" be given. It means "one who believes in homœopathy"—nothing more, nothing less—and why a believer in homœopathy does not have just as much right as a believer in allopathy to use all the adjuvantic treatment that he may think necessary for the welfare of his patient we are at a loss to determine.

Because a physician is a believer in homœopathy is he to believe nothing else ? Is he to be debarred from using any other treatment which he may consider best for his patient? Can he not administer morphine hypodermically for the mechanical pressure of gall stones or of a kidney calculus ? Shall he allow a patient to die in torment from cancer, or in the excruciating pain incident to mutilating accidents or surgical operations ? Shall the agonies of phthisis and other incurable disorders inflict themselves upon a human being—and a physician—because he believes in homœopathy—stand passively by without attempting to offer his euthanasia to the suffering and the dying ? The interrogatories are so preposterous that they need no reply.

The truth is this: the homœpathic physician believes in the law *similia similibus curantur* to such a degree that it moulds and directs his practice in the majority of his cases ; he believes it to be the best, and, indeed, the only scientific law upon which therapeutics are based, and endeavors to follow it as conscientiously as he can in the practice of his profession. But because he does this, and so announces, is he to treat cases of poisoning without antidotes? Is he to trifle with pains incident to incurable diseases? Is he to forswear the influence of chemical action? Is he, in other words, to make a fool of himself to the detriment of his patient because he is a believer in homœopathy?

There is still another consideration which evolves itself in the consideration of the subject. It is this : strive as we may to possess the similar to certain presenting symptoms, it may happen either from the lack of knowledge of the materia medica (few men being able to master it completely in a life time) or from the imperfectness of provings, or indeed from the absence from the materia medica of certain drugs, that it is impossible to enunciate the law in prescribing; then, surely, though it is less scientific in every way, the humane physician must fall back to the next best resource, which is the medicine of experience.

It must also be remembered that men now practicing, for the most part, homœopathy, hold a diploma which gives them most emphatic power to practice as they please. The document first states that they are not only " doctors of medicine," *with all the rights and privileges thereunto belonging*, but are in addition created " doctors of homœopathic medicine."

That the time will come when distinctive titles regarding systems of medicine will be dropped, and educated and conscientious practitioners be allowed, without let or hinderance, to practice their profession without regard to "pathies," there can be no doubt.

That the demand of our sponsors in baptism to forget the name which, not so long ago, they rubbed into our foreheads with cruelty and persecution is now being made ;—is a fact.

That *magna est veritas et prevalebit* is as true to-day as when the early christians were slaughtered for their belief, is past contradiction, and therefore those who believe that the law *similia similibus curantur* is the best formula to follow in the treatment of disease need not be ashamed of their title, and may, without scruple or hinderance, employ any other means they desire for the relief of suffering humanity.

COMMENTS.

EXCELLENT ADVICE.—President Orme not only presided with dignity at Saratoga, but he also delivered an address, which added much to the interest of the session. Presenting a brief account of the recent progress of homœopathy, describing in detail the changes of front of the so-called "regulars," as successive defeats compelled them to shift their grounds, he finally passes, toward the conclusion of his address, to the "duty of making suggestions." While he asserts that this duty shall rest lightly upon him, nevertheless he succeeds in making some recommendations of the greatest practical value. The homœopathic materia medica has grown during recent years with a rapidity almost incredible. The increase in bulk has been so excessive that the center of gravity comes near to falling without the base. A huge, cumbersome, unwieldy mass, of great value, it is true, yet ill-digested; the terror of the student, a constant torment to the physician, it still rears its shapeless bulk aloft and casts a deepening shadow athwart the homœopathic system of medicine. The attempt to master it, or even a comparatively small portion of it in its present condition, would be quite as hopeless as was the task Sisyphos was condemned to perform. The earlier materia medica comprised few drugs, but they were well proven. The symptomatology was authentic and undoubted. A thorough study of one drug was justly considered of much greater importance than the imperfect and uncertain trial of an hundred. It was remembered then that homœopathy is *par excellence* the science of therapeutics. But in later years scientific methods of investigation gave place to crude conjecture and unwarrantable generalizations. A mad frenzy for sudden therapeutical riches seized upon too many of the profession. New drugs of every sort and description were pressed hurriedly into service, labeled distractedly, only to be buried in turn by fresh arrivals and rivals. To improve and perfect our knowledge of drugs already shown to be valuable seemed to be desired but by few. And so our materia is now a great heap of ore from which each one may extract, as he is able, some of the pure gold and silver it contains in such abundance. But the coming materia medica must be made of the refined and purified gold and not of the ore. It is gratifying to observe that a reaction has begun and the process of purification is at hand. It is a process imperatively demanded. In his address President Orme says: "We, as a school claiming to have a more definite and accurate method in prescribing, should aim at the utmost degree of precision as regards our materia medica and therapeutic appliances. On this account we should proceed carefully, repeatedly, scientifically—under test conditions—and hold fast to that which is good. We have many articles that we know to be good, and we should learn further of their qualities, avoiding a waste of time upon questionable substances. Hahnemann's words should be well considered when he says (*Organon*, § 122): 'No other medicines should be employed (in provings) except such as are perfectly well known, and of whose purity, genuineness and energy we are thoroughly assured.' Let us build further and more securely upon foundations already laid, and not allow ourselves to be enticed too far into the proving of new and, perhaps, valueless or unneeded materials. Unless an article promises to be useful in spheres in which we require new remedies, let us give what time we have to spare in improving our knowledge of the full value of, say fifty or one hundred of our test remedies. Already the gardens, the fields, the mountains, the plains, the seas and even the bowels of the earth have been explored with a view to discover drugs to prove, until we have listed over 1,000 substances, which are called medicines. Some of these are of such a character that to name them would be indelicate, to think of them disagreeable, to administer or to take them revolting. The profession suffers from a knowledge that such materials are included in our medical *armamentarium.* Let us cease researches in these directions and rather apply ourselves to the work of expurgation. We are all aware that there is a limit to human capability, and that it is beyond the capacity of the most comprehensive intellect to compass a knowledge of the full value of one-tenth the number of medicines advertised by our pharmacies. I am moved, therefore, to suggest to our Bureau of Materia Medica that it might be well to take up the subject of determining, by such methods as may be devised, upon a certain number of the most valuable remedies we have, in order that study may be chiefly confined to them. We suffer now from an embarrassment of wealth; the student is confused. We have scattered too much and we should now combine and concentrate. Our State and other societies should co-operate with our Bureau of Materia Medica and our Standing Committee upon Drug Provings. We may then expect good and trustworthy results—such as we may point to with pride."

A Choice Morsel.—*The Record,* in its issue of July 9th, offers a choice bit of news for the delectation of the "regular" palate. This pilule of information does credit to the laboratory from whence it came. The sugar-coating is as thick as can be applied, but it is a bitter pill for the allopaths to swallow. The heading is "Homœopathic Troubles." "The visiting physicians to the London Infirmary for Consumption have all resigned, because the Governors have voted that homœopaths may be allowed on the staff." This may be a sweet morsel to roll under the tongue, but we doubt it. It is widely known that in the struggle at the Margaret Street Infirmary the allopaths were completely routed. Discovering that some of the staff used medicines in accordance with the homœopathic law, the "regulars," with characteristic bigotry, sought to have them removed. Foiled and beaten at every turn, smarting with defeat, the allopaths resigned. There was nothing else for them to do. Their places have already been filled by capable and more liberal men. To the disinterested reader it would seem that the "trouble" in the matter was almost and altogether lodged in the old school camp. *The Record's* way of putting the tale brings to mind the story of the unlucky pugilist who, belligerently inclined by nature, one day picked a quarrel with a gentlemen of mild and inoffensive aspect. When the battle was over the pugilist, banged and battered beyond recognition, eying his recent opponent, who stood almost without mark, naively remarked : " Well, I made him a great deal of trouble, any-how." In that sense there is no doubt about the "Homœopathic Troubles."

ALLOPATHIC TROUBLES.—The waters are troubled again in the old school camp. This time it is the New York County Medical Society. The brethren do not appear to dwell together in peace and harmony. A lack of interest is manifest, the attendance is limited, and the membership is growing, by degrees, beautifully less. The worthy president of the society, noting these things, cast about for a remedy. After much and presumably weary cogitation, he prepared a little prescription which he deemed a certain cure for the trouble. But the dose, unfortunately, produced the opposite effect from that which was expected (a thing that happens now and then with "regular" physic), and the last state of the society is infinitely worse than the first. The plan adopted to reclaim wandering members was a specially brilliant one. A directory of all physicians in New York was published. First came a list of the members of the County Society (strikingly brief), and then under a heading, which intimated that the society was not aware that any of the physicians whose names followed were legally qualified, came a list of the remaining physicians in the city—homœopaths, allopaths (those not members of the society), eclectics, etc. This by no means poured oil upon the troubled waters. In fact, it added fuel to the flames. We wish our " friends, the enemy," joy of their family quarrel.

DEAD MEN.—Some men would die of inertia were it not for the fact that respiration is involuntary. Every profession numbers in its ranks a certain proportion of men dead to every ambition, deaf to all appeals—Rip Van Winkles, dreamers, dozers, men who vegetate. They gravitate naturally to the bottom. Nobody disturbs them. Nobody ever goes out of his way to kick a dead man. They are submerged. Their identity is lost. The still waters of oblivion cover them. It is doubtful if they will be resurrected. They are too dead. No one ever hears of them. They belong to no societies. They never contribute anything to journals. They make no discussions. They pursue no given line of study. They are buried even while alive. They exert no influence. They disappear and are not missed. The homœopathic profession has no use for dead men.

BOOK REVIEWS.

A PRACTICAL TREATISE ON DISEASES OF THE EYE, by DR. EDOUARD MEYER. Translated by FREELAND FERGUS, M.D. Pp. 647. Philadelphia : P. Blakiston & Co., 1887.

It has become quite a fashion of late years for young men fresh from their studies and with limited experience to write—no, compile— a text book on the eye. It is, therefore, with pleasure that we review a work by one so well qualified by reputation and experience to write a book as Prof. Meyer, of Paris. The work now under review is the English translation by Dr. Freeland Fergus, of Glasgow. That it is no new aspirant for favor, and that it possesses merit is evidenced by the fact of its having gone through three French and four German editions, besides having been translated into the Italian, Spanish, Polish, Russian and Japanese languages.

The author in the first chapter describes very concisely and clearly the different methods of examination of the eye, and also gives general indications in treatment. After which he considers in succession, diseases of the conjunctiva, cornea, sclera, iris, ciliary body, and choroid; glaucoma, diseases of the optic nerve and retina, amblyopia and amaurosis; diseases of the vitreous body and lens; refraction and accommodation; muscles of the eye; and diseases of the lids, lachrymal passages and orbit.

Preceding the description of each disease the anatomy of the part is very briefly yet clearly set forth; a much better plan than placing the anatomy all in one section, as is so often done. In the description of the various diseases, the diagnostic symptoms are first given, then follow the progress and termination, prognosis, ætiology and most approved old school treatment; all of which is stated in such terse, concise language, that though brief it is still full, so that the reader can without difficulty readily understand the author's meaning and obtain a lucid picture of the disease.

His classification varies occasionally from that most commonly adopted, which, though it may not improve, does not materially injure the work. Some omissions have also been noticed here and there, as for example : Under the head "choroiditis with suppuration," we miss the familiar term "panophthalmitis," which most fully describes this affection, since, though the inflammation may begin in the choroid, yet it almost invariably involves the whole eye. Here also we find no consideration given to irido-choroiditis metastatica, only a passing reference to it in the ætiology of suppurative choroiditis. Among the various forms of inflammation of the retina, no mention is made of retinitis diabetica, though rarer forms of retinitis receive full attention. It is possible that these diseases are more rare in France than in this country, and so explain the author's omission. Again, no reference is made to keratoscopy, which of late has become a very popular method of examination of the refraction. Though the reviewer does not believe it should be relied upon in prescribing glasses to the extent that it is by some ophthalmologists, yet it surely should receive some mention in a text book upon the eye.

Whenever it has been necessary in explanation of certain points in ætiology to give theories, the doctor has been careful to give *all* those most generally accepted, thus rendering apparent to the reader the various opinions upon a disputed subject. Another feature which increases very materially the value of the book is the copious manner in which it is illustrated ; there being 267 excellent illustrations, besides three colored plates from Liebreich's Atlas.

It may truly be said that no book has yet been written, in which some faults could not be found, but all authors appreciate honest criticism; we have, therefore, in reviewing this book, pointed out some of its most glaring defects which, as may be seen, are not very serious. Take it as a whole we consider it one of the most concise and most comprehensive works on diseases of the eye now found in the

English language, and as such we most heartily recommend it as a text book for the student, and as a practical treatise for the guide of the general practitioner in the diagnosis and surgical treatment of ophthalmic diseases.

Dr. Fergus deserves credit for his excellent translation, and nothing but praise can be given the publishers for the able manner in which they have done their work, both in the text and in the illustrations.   G. S. N.

A PRACTICAL TREATISE ON OBSTETRICS, Vol. IV., by A. CHARPENTIER, M.D., Paris. Illustrated with 191 wood engravings and one colored plate. This is also a volume of the "Cyclopedia of Obstetrics and Gynæcology" (12 vols.), issued monthly during 1887. New York : William Wood & Co. Vol. IV. contains 388 pages, and treats, under "OBSTETRIC OPERATIONS," of *version*, the *forceps*, the *lever*, the *induction of artificial labor*, *induced miscarriage*, the *Cæsarean section*, *Porro's operation*, *post mortem Cæsarean section*, *embryotomy*, etc. A concluding part of one hundred pages is devoted to "THE PATHOLOGY OF THE PUERPERIUM," or to a consideration of the various forms of *puerperal fever*.

Much space is given, very properly, to a discussion of *the forceps*, and throughout the author insists on the need of wise delay before, and intelligent care in, the use of this valuable instrument. He says (p. 86) : " How many labors would have ended happily, and yet have terminated in the death of the mother and child, because inexperienced or hurried physicians have used the forceps prematurely * * * ! " And again in reference to the locking of the forceps (p 98) : "Either the head is well grasped and locking is easy, or else the head is badly grasped and locking impossible ; and then the rule should be to begin over, a hundred times, if need be, rather than to use any force."

The author naturally advocates the French method of applying the forceps—parallel or as nearly parallel as may be to the sides of the head (bi-parietal), without regard to whether the forceps are *parallel* or *oblique* to the sides of the pelvis. In doubtful cases, at least, we believe it better to follow the German method of applying the forceps—parallel to the pelvis—and re-apply them as the head rotates and descends. The American (and preferable) mode of inducing anterior rotation in occiput posterior positions, is well described by the editor on page 119.

This volume fills the expectations formed from an examination of the three preceding volumes. To the practitioner this work will be valuable for reference, and to the student it will afford additional information on matters which are less fully treated in other works on obstetrics.   D——n.

SEXUAL HEALTH, companion to "Modern Domestic Medicine, HENRY G. HANCHETT, M.D. Revised and issued by A. H. LAIDLAW, A.M., M.D. Charles T. Hurlburt, 3 East Nineteenth Street, New York.

This little work treats of sexual hygiene from infancy ; the proper management of the child and youth in order to aid in escaping the many dangers which naturally surround the sexual development ; and the treatment of the more common diseases of these organs. The suggestions are sensible in the main. We should not be able, however, to agree with the author in the statement that a true gonorrhœa is at times the product of a benign non-specific vaginal or cervical catarrh. This might produce a urethritis ; but a simple urethritis is quite a different disease from a specific gonorrhœa. Also in his directions as to taking a hot douche, he directs the patient to take it in the sitting posture. Practical experience has shown that a douche taken in this way is little better than none. In order to obtain the good effects of hot water the patient should lie upon her back with hips elevated over a capacious bed pan. Also, he recommends that the douche be used very warm at first, and then the temperature of the water gradually reduced to 85 deg. This would fail entirely of securing the very effect for which the douche is given, namely a tonic, astringent, anæsthetic action. The douche to be of service should be given as above, and the water should be as hot as the patient can comfortably endure.   F.

MODERN DOMESTIC MEDICINE, by HENRY G. HANCHETT, M.D. Revised and issued by A. H. LAIDLAW, A.M., M.D. Chas. T. Hurlburt, 3 East Nineteenth Street.

We are glad to see this volume of domestic practice, and believe that Dr. Hanchett has added materially to the popular knowledge of disease and treatment, and placed a book in the hands of the laity which, while not intended to supplant the physician or in any way to dispense with his services when needed, gives very plain, definite instructions regarding the management of disease when slight or until a physician can be summoned.

The suggestions regarding *treatment* and *prophylaxis* are reliable and are the best that we have ever seen in this variety of book. It does not transcend, in its recommendations, the ability of the patient to follow and execute them, nor does it use the practical ignorance of the laity as a screen behind which to hide its own lack of scientific knowledge, or upon which it can safely foist worthless suggestions and useless expedients. We regard the ideas upon hygiene and treatment as sensible and reliable and believe it to be the best book for the family that we have yet seen.   F.

SIXTH ANNUAL REPORT CF THE STATE BOARD OF HEALTH OF NEW YORK. Transmitted to the Legislature March 19th, 1886. Weed, Parsons & Co., Albany, N. Y.

This volume covers much ground, being composed of special reports upon the analysis of water, in which Croton water appears to advantage, having only 0.3 per cent. of chlorine, 0.001 of free ammonia, and 0.012 of albuminoid ammonia, no nitrogen, and 7.38 per cent. of solids ; special reports from the Sanitary and Darinage Committee ; of the food, drug and beer laws ; registration and vital statistics ; effluvium nuisances, and school hygiene. The analyses of beer, ales, and porter shows that there is scarcely any substitution for hops or malt; and drugs, such as iron, citric acid, iodide of potash, ether, chloroform, etc., were found of fair or good quality. Much instruction regarding drainage, sewer contamination, paludal influences, etc., can be gained from the reports.   F.

REPORTS OF SOCIETIES AND HOSPITALS.

HOMŒOPATHIC MEDICAL SOCIETY, COUNTY OF NEW YORK

THE regular monthly meeting of the Homœopathic Medical Society of the County of New York was held May 12th, 1887. President Beebe in the chair.

There were present fifty-seven.

Minutes of previous meeting were read and approved.

The Executive Committee presented a report recommending that an assessment of two dollars be levied. Upon motion of Drs. S. Strong and Houghton it was so ordered.

The Committee on Surgery, Dr. Wm. Tod Helmuth, Chairman, reported the following list of papers, which were duly read by their authors:

"Tumors of the Bladder," F. E. Doughty, M.D.; "Recent Advances in Rectal Surgery," Sidney F. Wilcox, M.D.; "A Case of Fibro-cystic Tumor of the Uterus—Abdominal Section, with Specimen," H. I. Ostrom, M.D.; "Apparatus in Pott's Disease, where the Ordinary Plaster-jacket is not Applicable," Fred S. Fulton, M.D.; "A Case of Sarcoma of the Fibula," Wm. Tod Helmuth, M.D.

Dr. Helmuth:—I was greatly interested in the paper read by Dr. Doughty. It is only recently that this subject has attracted attention and been brought within the field of surgery. In the last three years there occurred three cases of tumor of the bladder in my practice which I watched with great care. The symptoms presented by these patients resembled those enumerated by Dr. Doughty.

Persistent hæmaturia, which rest and the usual medicines did not relieve, and the presence of blood, glairy on account of the mucus which it contained, are pathognomonic of tumor of the bladder. In those conditions of the kidney which were accompanied by frequent and prolonged hæmaturia, the kidney would, in the majority of cases, be enlarged. This could be ascertained by employing renal ballottement, which he considered an important test in the diagnosis of such cases. The kidney could be percussed on the outside of the loin and its area found by the extent of the dullness. Renal ballottement is performed by placing one hand over the abdomino-parietal region and with the other giving the loin a sharp thrust.

The origin of this blood containing glairy mucus, especially if the odor is bad, generally is the bladder.

After a malignant tumor of the bladder has existed for some time the characteristic infiltration may be detected by an examination per rectum.   ·

I consider explorations of the bladder very necessary. Among the various operations for this purpose, the supra-pubic was the only one by which ocular evidence could be obtained. The examination by the catheter amounted to nothing, but, in the female, either forcible or gradual dilatation of the urethra, even to the extent of admitting the finger, was feasible and should always be tried, although in some cases the procedure might be followed by paralysis of the sphincter or incontinence of the urine.

By extending the operation over two or three sittings, the female urethra can be dilated to a surprising extent. Cocaine may be applied beforehand, to make the operation painless. Through the dilated urethra the growth can be felt with the finger, and if the location of the neoplasm is favorable it may even be seen by the electric light.

All my cases were papillomas. The hemorrhage in many cases is so severe as to endanger life. They can be scraped with Simon's spoon or cut off with Thompson's forceps, the operation being followed by washing out the bladder, as after lithotrity, I used Bigelow's straight tube and his original aspirator.

Malignant tumors are apt to recur. Medicinal treatment in my experience was unsuccessful.

A complication to be expected in these cases is an extension of the disease up through the ureters to the kidneys, accompanied by the presence of a very large amount of albumen in the urine, even to two or three per cent. in the advanced stage.

Dr. Dillow:—In reference to the albuminuria occurring in the course of tumors of the bladder, alluded to by Dr. Helmuth, I would call attention to the facts that, excluding the albumen to be accounted for by blood often present, it may arise either from (1) transudation of albumen through the capillary walls of the vessels of villous tissue; or (2) from a co-existing cystitis; or (3) from a consecutive pyelitis, with its associated nephritis; or (4) from some one of the forms of consecutive nephritis. I believe that only rarely does the albumen transude from the villous vessels themselves. I have never observed such a case myself, but it needs to be borne in mind, as it may be attributed wrongly to the kidneys. Excluding villous albuminuria as rare, the albumen must usually be traced to inflammation of the mucous membrane and kidneys, resulting from the cystitis developed by the tumor.

It is very unusual for villous tissue to extend up the ureters into the pelvis of the kidney, although a very few cases are recorded where the kidneys, ureters and bladder were invaded by such a growth. But there is nearly always a time in the course of a vesical tumor when cystitis develops and the inflammatory process extends secondarily up the urinary tract.

Usually there is secondary pyelitis, with involvement of the kidney. But even without pyelitis there may be a resulting nephritis; and this nephritis, principally interstitial in type, may be either acute, chronic, or subacute, and sometimes develops into the suppurative form. The tendency to death is generally through this consecutive nephritis. I would call attention to the frequent, even usual, absence of casts in this variety.

Before operating it is important to determine whether nephritis exists, on account of the dangerous effect of ether on existing renal inflammation, and also of interference with the bladder. Probably the French method of epi-cystotomy is preferable, because there is then less interference with the trigone of the bladder, between which and the kidneys the reflex nervous connection is peculiarly intimate.

I believe that it is more practicable to make a diagnosis of villous tumors by urinary examination alone than is usually supposed. It is not necessary that characteristic villous tufts, with well marked capillary loops, should be present. Profuse recurring hemorrhage from the bladder is in practice almost always to be attributed to tumor. If, in addition to the blood, we find numerous blood-stained bladder epithelia, some with large and sometimes double nuclei, in connection with shreds of newly-formed, delicate connective tissue, the diagnosis is pretty well established.

From these signs alone I have made a positive diagnosis of villous tumors where I had nothing to judge from except the specimens of urine, all other information being withheld. The diagnostic importance of connective tissue in urine is not sufficiently realized. Of course, it may come from other causes than villous growths—from erosions of the mucous membrane, with granulating connective tissue, from abscess, etc.   But a fairly trained microscopist, taking into consideration the special epithelia and other microscopic elements present, and differentiating between the newly-formed variety of connective tissue and that coming from broken-down normal tissue, can exclude one condition after another, and come to a satisfactory conclusion as to its origin.

The appearance of connective tissue from villi is more easily shown than described ; once seen, it can be usually recognized subsequently.

In one case of mine the shreds closely resembled hyaline casts, though their contours were not so regular, their thickness was very much less—being more flat—and they showed very faint, delicate striations.

Dr. S. F. Wilcox then read his paper on " Recent Advances in Rectal Surgery" (*vide* page 483).

Dr. B. G. Clark:—Mr. Whitehead has the reputation of being a good observer, and I am sure that an operation suggested by him, and performed by our friend, Dr. Wilcox, would be successful.   Rectal surgery has been much neglected in the past, and any improvement in the modes of operating should be hailed with satisfaction.   I have seen (by invitation) the operation as suggested by Mr. Whitehead, performed by Dr. James B. Hunter, at the Woman's Hospital in this city. Dr. Hunter used silk sutures in closing the wound, and the ice-bag locally after the reaction from the ether.   I think it is a good operation.

Dr. Doughty :—I am surprised at the statistics of Whitehead's operation ; that so large a number of cases were treated without any alarming hemorrhage.

On more than one occasion I have seen extensive primary hemorrhage following the old operation.

In one aggravated case of hemorrhoids, complicated with prolapsus of the rectum, in which I stretched the sphincter, pulled down the tumors one at a time, transfixed with a Peaslee's needle and ligated, there occurred an extensive hemorrhage.   I endeavored to stop it with ligatures, but as they were applied it commenced to bleed somewhere else.

The actual cautery was applied, but still it kept on.   A solution of persulphate of iron met with the same result.   It was finally stopped by introducing a tampon in the rectum.

In such a case he thought Whitehead's operation would have been followed by more alarming hemorrhage still.   It is strange that not more bad cases of hemorrhage follow.   The blood usually oozes, but after transfixion with Peaslee's needle it may spurt.

Dr. Helmuth:—Although these operations are all new and brilliant in results, I should not recommend a too hasty withdrawal of the old methods until they are well tried.   The amount of pain caused by the elastic ligature can be regulated by the tightness with which it is drawn.   I have found that when it is put upon extreme tension it caused great pain, but when gradually tightened every few days a very satisfactory operation can be made.   When the fistula can be reached this operation of Dr. Wilcox is one of the best.

Hæmorrhoids are often diverticula.   Certain phlegmatic people have profuse bleeding from hemorrhoidal tumors at times, while during the interval they do very well.   It is a question whether the sudden suppression, or rather prevention of the hemorrhoidal flux, is not followed by disastrous consequences.   Some years ago two patients of mine, both of them plethoric in habit, were operated upon by a quack with injections of carbolic acid and sweet oil. They were cured very rapidly, but three years later one died of apoplexy and the other became paralyzed.

In one case of my own, where there were six tumors, the mass closely resembling a big tomato, I injected them all with carbolic acid and sweet oil. It caused great pain, but they shrivelled and soon disappeared. Two years later the gentleman died of apoplexy.

It is a question whether it is safe to stop off this diverticulum in patients who are well advanced in life and of a plethoric habit. It is now my custom to operate on one hemorrhoid at a time, with an interval of six weeks between.

Dr. Wilcox:—I used the silk suture in sewing up the fistulæ and always stretched the sphincter because of the great pain which followed if this is not done.

With regard to the distance up the bowel, Dr. Smith has operated on cases where the wound extended for three inches from the anus.

Dr. H. I. Ostrom presented his paper, " A Case of Fibro-cystic Tumor of the Uterus."

Dr. J. H. Thompson:—Ether should be administered without the inhalation of air after the first few respirations. I have had better results in its use when two or three ounces of brandy were given beforehand. Nausea is best prevented by giving a hypodermic of atropine 1-200 of a grain; morphine ⅛ to ¼ grain.

Assistants who do not understand the proper method of administration are apt to leave the inhaler away from the nose when renewing the ether, thus allowing the patient to take one or more inhalations of air. On account of this, it requires a much longer time to get the patient under the influence of the anæsthetic and a larger quantity of ether. The system becomes saturated with it and the recovery to consciousness is longer delayed.

Dr. Fulton:—I was rather surprised at Dr. Ostrom's statement that chloroform was a safer general anæsthetic than ether. The general sentiment of surgeons and the statistics are quite opposed to this statement. Statistics of European hospitals give a mortality of about five for chloroform to one of ether. In the large hospitals of this city, chloroform is discarded, unless a speedy narcosis is required, or the condition of the kidneys contra-indicate ether, or the patient is not susceptible to the influence of the latter drug. While resident surgeon of Hahnemann Hospital I gave ether over 200 times without the slightest bad result. Since then, in connection with hospitals and in private practice, I have never seen any bad results follow its use. The success of its administration depends, to a very great degree, upon the person giving it. I always thoroughly saturate the cone and hold it about three or four inches from the patient's nose. As the patient becomes accustomed to the pungent odor, the cone is gradually approximated to the face, bringing it a little nearer with each inspiration. By the time it reaches the face the inhaler has become accustomed to it and rarely offers any resistance, the primary anæsthesia having been induced. By this method the patient may be entirely saved the nervous shock and distressing pulmonary spasm which so often seriously embarrasses the administration of the anæsthetic. When the cone is once over the nose and mouth it should be held so as to exclude all air, unless the heavy, stertorous breathing indicates a too profound condition of anæsthesia. If evidences of vomiting appear, fresh ether, vigorously applied, will generally check it.

Dr. Doughty:—Statistics are not always reliable, as fatal results are apt to be withheld. I have met with alarming effects from chloroform, and prefer ether, except when the condition contra-indicates it, or in operations about the mouth.

Should a coroner's jury inquire of me which was the least dangerous, I should unhesitatingly say ether, and I would feel guilty, indeed, should I have a fatal result following the use of chloroform when given for no other reason than to produce narcosis quickly for my own convenience.

I am in favor of giving ether rapidly, as it saves shock and avoids vomiting.

Dr. Helmuth:—According to my experience, anæsthesia produced rapidly is the safest. Twenty minutes before giving the anæsthetic it is my custom to administer, hypodermatically, ten minims of a solution representing 1-6 grain morphine, and 1-100 grain atropine. By this means the circulation in the surface capillaries is preserved and coldness and shocks are not so likely to supervene. This method is known as "*the mixed anæsthesia*," and to me has been very satisfactory. Lately I have been using the metallic cone, invented by Dr. Packer, in the administration of ether, together with the polyclinic ether bottle. In the last five days I have performed three supra-vaginal hysterectomies, all of which are doing well. I attribute my success in the operations for fibro-cystic tumors to three things:

1st. The use of the elastic ligature in preference to any variety of clamps.

2d. The application of Dr. Wilcox's pins with the ligature; and

3d. The extra-peritoneal method of treating the stump, thus allowing the sloughing process to proceed outside of the abdomen.

When fibro-cystic tumors are interstitial, they are always well supplied with blood and the tissue is very dense. I have broken Tait's, Thomas's and Wells's clamps in endeavoring to sufficiently compress the fibrous pedicle to prevent bleeding; and as the pedicle shrinks, it is necessary from time to time to screw up most of these instruments to preserve a sufficient amount of constriction.

With the elastic ligature, however, the contraction is constantly maintained and the danger from hemorrhage is *nil*.

Dr. Helmuth then exhibited a number of very interesting specimens of fibro-cystic tumors which had recently been removed by him. One of these was of especial interest. The uterus developed into a large myfibromatous mass; at one point contained large calcareous formations, rendering it as hard as stone, to the left tube an ovarian cystoma was attached.

Dr. Wilcox:—From some recent experience, I have become afraid of all anæsthetics, though I think it is more the person giving it and the manner in which it is given, than the anæsthetic used.

Dr. Fred S. Fulton read his paper on "Apparatus Useful in Potts' Disease where the Ordinary Plaster-jacket is Inapplicable." (*Vide* page 478.)

Dr. Wilcox:—I do not think the felt jacket is applicable in a case of Potts' disease, as it is not rigid enough, especially during the hot weather. I have seen the patient mentioned by Dr. Fulton. The child is much better and walks well.

Dr. Wm. Tod Helmuth read his paper on "A Case of Sarcoma of the Fibula."

The Society then adjourned.

RECORD OF MEDICAL PROGRESS.

ANTIFEBRIN IN EPILEPSY.—Dr. Adolf Salm, of Strasburg, gives, in *Neurologische Centralblatt*, June 1, 1887, a series of investigations upon the value of antifebrin as an anti-epileptic. His conclusions are summed up as follows: In the eleven cases of epilepsy treated with this drug no noteworthy result was attained. In no case did the attacks cease or show any notable lessening, and even when in single cases an insignificant decrease in the number of the attacks occurred, in others there was a considerable increase. And these differences were well within the usual variations so common in epilepsy, and give no reason for supposing antifebrin to have any favorable influence on the disease. Under the action of the drug almost all the cases showed a more or less evident cyanosis as well as dark color of the urine. According to received views, the cyanosis is due to the formation of methæmoglobin in the blood, but in these cases tests of the blood made by Dr. Kahn, gave no evidence of methæmoglobin. The subjective state of these patients under antifebrin was influenced only very slightly, and even when the blue coloration of the lips was considerable no serious symptoms were observable.—O'C.

PARALYTIC PHENOMENA IN SIMPLE PSYCHOSES.—Dr. Theodore Ziehen, of Jena, says (*Berliner Klinische Wochenschrift*, No. 26, 1887), that the occurrence of paralytic phenomena during melancholia or maniacal exaltation, usually leads to the opinion that a fatal ending will result from progressive paresis. In opposition to this view, Seifert, in 1853, had described cases, in part at least, of pure mania and melancholia, accompanied by disturbances of iris-innervation, two cases showing dilatation of the pupil on one side, which disappeared with recovery. Bailarger also showed, in 1858, that *manie ambiteuse*, with slight motor disturbances, did not always lead to dementia paralytica. Nasse supported Seifert's observations and maintained that a symmetric innervation of the facial, hypoglossal and fifth, whether continuous or transitory, might be of no special importance and could occur in functional psychoses. Later, Tigges has described similar paralytic phenomena, especially one-sided facial paresis, in simple melancholia, mania and dementia. In contradistinction to these older publications, the later treatise and text-books are silent concerning such partial hemipareses. Ziehen has observed three cases of functional psychoses accompanied by one-sided facial paresis, not dependent on organic affection of the nervous system, or hysteria, or trauma, etc., but simply the accompanying phenomena of severe melancholia. Brissaud and Marie have lately described cases of hysterical hemiplegia in which the facial and hypoglossal were both implicated. In the clinic at Jena, there is a case of hysterical paranœa in which the left half of the body, including the facial innervation to the mouth, is paretic; the tongue does not deviate, but there is dilatation of the left pupil, the intensity varying with that of the hemiplegia. The pupillary reactions are retained. In a case of imperative conceptions, a man aged sixty, there is a difference in the size of the pupils lasting for days, and sometimes for weeks ; at one time the right pupil is larger, and after a while the left will be more dilated. At times there is equality of the pupils. Theoretically such paralytic phenomena as mere accompaniments of simple psychoses may be attributed to congenital low innervation, exhaustion and circulatory disturbances of the cortical and subcortical centers.—O'C.

TWO CASES OF POISONING BY CANNABIS INDICA.—Dr. Graeffner, of Breslau, reports, (*Berliner Klinische Wochenschrift*, No. 23, 1887): Case I. A woman aged twenty-three, had taken one and a half grains of *balsamum cannabis ind.* and half an hour after, about 10 P.M., went to bed and immediately was the victim of the most frightful dreams. She had the feeling that although in the presence of the most threatening danger, she was neither able to escape or to call for help. Soon there was a nameless anxiousness, in which she thought she was dead and buried, and that she was able to follow every phase of the dying process. Suddenly she recovered power over her limbs, sprang out of bed and ran to the kitchen, giving such a frightful cry that the servant, thinking there were robbers in the house, shut the door between her mistress and herself and would not open it till she had summoned help. Dr. G. found her in a state of frightful bodily excitement, in a continual to-and-fro motion, with the fingers in motion, now searching on the bed for something, and again seeing visionary objects, and with a flood of ideas expressed in a ceaseless, rapid monologue. In spite of this the patient saw and recognized all that was going on about her. The pupils were moderately dilated and sluggish, the pulse was increased in frequency, and the arteries were moderately compressible; the temperature in the axilla, 37.9 deg. C. The treatment consisted in stimulants and cold compresses to the head. Case II. Was a man aged forty, cabinet-maker. He lay down on a sofa after taking the drug; soon fell asleep and after an hour was awakened by a customer who wanted a receipt signed. He found it impossible to make even a stroke with the pen, and partly astonished and partly vexed, he endeavored to overcome the disagreeable condition by going to work in the shop; but a mist before his eyes, and the feeling of the whole body being asleep, compelled him to return to his room. Then he passed into a state of apparent death, in which he heard everything, but was incapable of any motion or even of calling for medical help. The ideas that swept through his brain during this time were mostly concerning religious matters. The patient was treated in the same way as No. 1, and by the next morning he was free from trouble and his mind was clear.—O'C.

PHYSOSTIGMIN IN THE TREATMENT OF CHOLERA AND OTHER HYPERKINETIC DISORDERS.—L. Riess gives, in *Berliner Klinische Wochenschrift*, No. 22, 1887, under this title a study on the action of physostigmin. From 1879 to 1885, he treated all the cases coming in the general hospital in Berlin by this means. Thirty-four of them were children and young people, most of them being fresh attacks, though a few had existed for months. Six other cases were in older people, two being acute and four chronic. Of the young cases, four were of a severe, fatal type, not rare in Berlin, and in these, owing to the rapid course of the disease, the eserin was of as little service as other remedies; the four cases in older people were of the "habitual" form and naturally could only be improved somewhat, but the improvement was manifested after a relatively short time of the treatment. The other cases were completely cured, two of them, indeed, slowly, after a number of weeks, but they were especially unfavorable, one being accompanied by a severe psychosis, and the other having existed nine months. In all the other cases the cure was accomplished in a remarkably short time, the very first dose showing its influence on the disease; in some cases the disease disappeared within five or six days from beginning the treatment. The treatment was not begun until the patients had been in the hospital for about eight days so as to exclude any favorable influence that might result from the influence of hospital regimen. The observer noticed in a series of cases, less in number, of nervous affections having, in common with chorea, a determinate type of muscular contraction and body motion, favorable result from this treatment; the cause for such hyperkinetic phenomena being considered an irritative condition of the ganglionic portions of the brain or cord or both. Among these forms tetanus seemed less amenable to the treatment; in two severe cases other remedies, such as chloral, curare, permanent baths, etc., being employed at the same time, and in three light cases it is difficult to say whether or not the method was of any value. In some other hyperkineses the results were very favorable, as in twelve cases of tremor, of which four were senile, four alcoholic, two hysterical, one following after typhus, and the last probably being symptomatic of brain tumor. In eight of these cases, after treatment with injections of physostigmin, continued from fourteen days to three weeks, there was essential improvement; in the other four, the post-typhus case, one sentile and both hysterical cases, complete cure followed very shortly. The post-typhus tremor, said to have existed two years, disappeared in about fourteen days; one of the hysterical cases, which had lasted many years, after six injections, and the senile case, in a women aged sixty-eight, after the second injection. Further, there were four cases of paralysis agitans treated by this means, the injections being given in a series of fourteen days, and repeated in some; every time there resulted a rapid improvement in the tremor lasting even after withdrawal of the remedy for a number of weeks. Marked good effects were shown in two clear cases of multiple sclerosis of the brain and cord, especially in one case where, after several series of injections of two to three weeks duration were used, there was noticed at the same time with the lessening of the intentional tremor, a marked bettering of the speech and locomotor ability, with increase of the general well-being. Also in three cases of Charcot's post-hemiplegic chorea (tremor), a several weeks' treatment with physostigmin injection brought about a marked improvement, as well as in two cases of athetoid spasmodic movements apparently symptomatic of brain tumor. Finally is to be mentioned a peculiar case of an hysterical man in which all reflex movements were enormously increased; the symptoms disappeared after a two weeks' treatment with eserin after other nervines had been employed in vain. The preparation used was Merck's sulphate of physostigmin, the solution being made up in the smallest amounts, and when the slightest sign of decomposition was evident by the reddish color of it, it was discarded. The dose was generally one milligram (1–60 grain), injected subcutaneously once a day during the first day, and then twice a day. In small children the dose was one-half the above.—O'C.

A NEW OPERATION FOR HEPATIC ABSCESS.—Dr. George Zancarol, surgeon to the Greek Hospital, Alexandria, has performed a new operation for hepatic abscess in a large number of cases during the last two years, with excellent results. This consists in making an opening sufficiently large to expose the whole cavity of the abscess, and in thoroughly cleansing it of all pus and *débris* of sloughing hepatic tissue. The operation may be divided into three stages: (1) Exploration of the liver; (2) opening the abscess; (3) cleansing the abscess-cavity.

(1) *Exploration of the Liver.*—The skin having been washed with a brush and soap and water and a two per cent. solution of carbolic acid, an exploring trocar is plunged into the liver to find the abscess. The puncture may have to be repeated several times, so that a good idea may be formed of the size and direction of the abscess.

(2) *Opening of the Abscess.*—An opening is made with the thermo-cautery into the lower third of the abscess, two or three inches long, according to the size of the abscess, and as much as possible in the direction of its greatest diameter. The opening must be sufficiently large to enable the surgeon to see the whole cavity with ease when the edges of the opening are held well apart by retractors. To obtain this result in abscesses of the left lobe an opening in the soft parts will suffice; but if the abscess is in the right lobe, resection of one or two ribs will be necessary. This resection is also performed with the thermo-cautery, using an elevator to detach the periosteum, and Liston's bone-forceps. Care must be taken not to wound the intercostal artery; should this happen, the hemorrhage will cease as soon as the abscess is opened. The abscess is then opened with the thermo-cautery, keeping always in the direction of the resected rib. With the aid of two strong retractors held by an assistant, the margins of

the incision, whilst they are kept open, are pressed against the liver, in close contact with the abdominal and thoracic walls, so as to prevent either pus, or the liquids used for washing out the abscess, from finding their way into the abdominal or pleural cavities. If this precaution be observed no harm will result, even should there be no adhesion between the wall of the abscess and the parietal peritoneum ; for once the abscess has been thoroughly cleansed, adhesions will be established before fresh pus can accumulate. In fifty such operations performed by Dr. Zancarol no pus has ever escaped into the cavities.

(3) *Cleansing the Abscess-Cavity.*—The retractors being still held by an assistant in the position described, a strong current of warm distilled water is allowed to play within the abscess-cavity by means of a siphon. Every particle of adherent pus and necrosed tissue is removed with the fingers, or with sponges fitted to holders ; and the washing out is continued until the walls of the cavity look perfectly clean, often granulating, and the water returns clear. The retractors are then withdrawn ; two drainage tubes of large caliber are inserted in the cavity ; and the dressings applied, which are left undisturbed for twenty-four hours. At the end of this time the cavity is again washed out with warm distilled water, and the current kept on until the water returns perfectly clear.

As a rule, the temperature becomes normal immediately after the first washing. If fever should reappear, or if the pus is abundant, washing out should be repeated every twelve hours. If, in spite of all this, the fever persist, or diarrhœa set in, this would indicate that other abscesses exist in the liver, and such cases are invariably fatal.—(*Brit. Med. Jour.*, June 11th, 1887).

THE VALUE OF TURKISH BATHS IN DISEASES OF THE CIRCULATION.— In a recent paper Frey records his experience as to the value of Turkish baths in patients suffering from disturbances in the circulation. He first of all determined the normal effects of such baths by observations on himself with special reference to their influence on the pulse, arterial tension, respiratory capacity, renal excretion and body weight generally. According to these observations, the quantity of blood in the body is lessened by the free excretion which takes place through the skin and lungs; the body weight is reduced ; and the work of the heart is in this way lightened, at the same time that its substance is better nourished by the improved quality of the blood supplied to it. The peripheral arterioles of the body, too, become dilated and filled with blood, thus effecting a corresponding emptying of the vessels of the internal organs. At the same time, albuminous bodies, and still more fat, become more rapidly broken up, the loss in weight being thus explained. Lastly, as the result of the alternate warm and cold douching, the vaso-motor energy of the vessels is increased, thus rendering them more capable of resisting any strain thrown upon them. The good effects of the Turkish baths in disease find their explanation in these physiological considerations. Thus the diminution in weight is well illustrated in cases of *obesity*. By such patients the baths are extremely well borne. The only precaution necessary is, that the cold douche ought not to be used in such cases, as the sudden shock produced, acting on a heart overloaded with fat, or the fibers of which may already have become fatty, may readily prove dangerous. In all cases it is important to have regard to this rule—that the sweating stage ought never to be continued after the pulse rises above 100. The diastole of the heart then becomes too short to allow sufficient time for the heart to nourish itself ; and under such circumstances, the effect of the bath is to weaken rather than to strengthen the cardiac action. In cases of *aortic and mitral disease* dependent upon rheumatic affection, and not the result of atheroma, the baths are also well borne. This effect is most marked in cases in which compensation is disturbed, with anasarca of limbs, failure in secretion of urine, and a dilated right heart. So far from the pulse gaining in frequency under the influence of the bath, after the first ten to fifteen minutes it generally falls, remaining between 90 and 100 as soon as perspiration commences; it becomes softer, less tense, more dicrotic in character; visible arteries, *e. g.* the temporal, are seen to distend, and respiration becomes freer, deeper, and sometimes even more slow. In the after treatment the cold douche is in the first instance to be avoided, a douche at the temperature of the body being used instead. The bath can be repeated daily, or on alternate days, according to the strength of the patient. As improvement goes on, recourse is gradually had to colder douches, then, finally, the coldest of all may be freely used. The tone of the heart and vessels is in this way greatly improved. In cases of *chronic Bright's disease*, where there is hypertrophy of the left ventricle, œdema of the legs, increase in albumen, and some failure in the secretion of urine, the baths also prove useful. It is necessary to have care in the use of the cold douche. By *emphysematous* patients, on the other hand, the Turkish bath is not well borne. In their case the use of the vapor baths proves far more efficacious, and is often extremely beneficial. Lastly, in all conditions characterized by disturbances in the circulation dependent upon weakness, local or general, *e. g.* œdema of the lower limbs or around joints, the result of general weakness, paralysis, rheumatic affections, etc., the Turkish bath proves of great value. It is, indeed, under such circumstances, that the full effects of the baths in improving nutrition, and raising the general vaso-motor tone, are best observed.— (*D. Archiv f. klin. Med.*, April, 1887).

OIL OF WINTER-GREEN IN GONORRHŒAL RHEUMATISM.—Dr. R. W. Taylor read a paper on this subject at the meeting of the Association of Genito-Urinary Surgeons. He tried it in all varieties, both acute and chronic; and without speaking enthusiastically of his results, he is well satisfied with them. He thinks this remedy will be found of most benefit in recent cases, where the fibrous structures of joints and muscles are involved, and in which there is a large amount of serous effusion. In cases complicated with hydrarthrosis, the results were sometimes disappointing, whilst in the very chronic cases it did not prove itself a very trustworthy remedy. It is powerless to remove structural changes when they have once taken place, but is of service in relieving and curing the accompanying cachexia. A trial of it should not be allowed to supersede the methods by counter-irritation and other means.—(*N. Y. Med. Jour.*, June 4th, 1887.)

THE DESTRUCTIVE EFFECTS OF ETHER INJECTIONS.—MM. Pitres and Vaillard have published some notes on the effects which the subcutaneous injection of ether has produced on the nerves in its neighborhood. They find that when the injection has been so directed as to reach near to the main nervous trunks, it has set up, after a few hours, a neuritis, in which the myeline first blends with the cylinder-axis, and then the whole nerve-structure becomes indistinct, in a state of acute inflammation. The subsequent degeneration spreads downwards, never upwards, and regeneration begins in a special fashion. In short, ether under these conditions produces an immediate necrosis of nerve-fibers; and it is just possible it may be of use in those cases where nerve-stretching is at present employed.—(*Progrès Méd.*, May 21st, 1887).

NEWS.

ONE MORE.—*The Record* states that the use of gaseous enemata has been entirely abandoned in the fourth division, Bellevue Hospital, where they have been earliest and longest tried.

APPOINTMENTS.—Drs. J. O. Reed and D. H. Arthur were recently appointed internes at the Homœopathic Insane Asylum, at Middletown. A competitive examination determined the selection of the successful candidates for the positions. Both of the gentlemen appointed are graduates of the New York Homœopathic Medical College.

A REMINDER.—The Committee on High Potencies, A. R. Wright, M.D., Chairman, has sent out a supplementary circular, reminding physicians of their former "appeal for the collection of the results of reliable clinical experience in the treatment of cases by the thirtieth or higher attenuations." The committee has in view not "the discussion of the relative merits of high and low attenuations," but desires "simply to ascertain if there is any efficacy in the thirtieth or higher attenuations."

SIGNIFICANT.—Coming college classes, like coming events, cast their shadows before them. It is probable the entering class at the New York Homœopathic College this fall will be the largest in its history. An unusual number of letters of inquiry have been received by the secretary of the Faculty, and there is every reason to believe that the session of '87-'88 will be a most prosperous one. After this year the three years' graded course is obligatory upon all students, and the college fees are slightly increased to cover the longer period.

NOT READY TO SURRENDER.—"We are not yet ready to surrender the heritage that Hahnemann conferred upon us. It is not our friends but our enemies that are freely advising and suggesting that we drop the word 'homœopath' from our vocabulary. If we follow their advice what do we get in return? It offers tradition and fashion in therapeutics; uncertainty for certainty. To every conscientious practitioner of our system of medicine the word 'homœopathy' means a positive science in therapeutics. It means that when under this law the action of a drug is once established it remains the same during all time."—DR. CLAYPOOL, *Med. Era.*

WHAT THEY THINK OF THEMSELVES.—Here is the opinion pronounced on his own school by the responsible editor of the chief medical periodical of Germany, the *Wiener Med. Wochenblatt*, which has often distinguished itself by its virulent attacks on homœopathy: "What is praised by one is ridiculed by another. What one doctor dare not give in small doses is given by another in large doses, and what is praised by one as something new is considered by another as not worthy of being rescued from oblivion. The favorite remedy of one is morphine; another treats three-fourths of his patients with quinine; a third expects favorable results from purgatives; a fourth, from the healing power of nature; a fifth, from water. One blesses, another curses mercury. Within a short period of time the treatment by mercurial inunction flourished, was set aside, and then came into repute again; it was looked upon as buried; funeral orations were pronounced over it, and then it was disinterred, and lately its praises have been sung by enthusiastic admirers. And such things happen within a few decades in the self-same "school," under the sway of the same infallible despot, girded with the sword of triumphant science."

A few years later this same organ of allopathic opinion says : " We must here allude to that gross fraud which the high-priests of medical science impose on their disciples, although neither they themseves nor the majority of medical men believe it. I mean the fables of the so-called pharmacodynamics of the materia medica. * * * * * This modern pharmacology, which is taught at the colleges and about which large volumes are written, which students are obliged to learn almost by heart, belongs, in virtue, at least, of nine-tenths of its contents, to the domain of fable and fairy tales, and is a survival of the old belief in magic. The numerous announcements of newly-discovered remedies, which in all the journals are recommended by the apothecaries, and provided with testimonials as to their infallibility by physicians, show that efforts are being made to extend the empire of magic and superstition.—*League Tract.*

INFLUENCE OF TEA AND COFFEE ON DIGESTION.—Dr. James W. Frazer, in the recent number of the *Journal of Anatomy and Physiology*, has recorded the results of an interesting series of experiments on the action of our common beverages on stomachic and intestinal digestion. The experiments have been most carefully arranged from a physical standpoint and give us some valuable hints on the digestion of the chief alimentary principles, but they have no bearing,it should be mentioned,in individual variation in human digestion, or on the influence of the various glands in preparing the gastric or intestinal juices. A summary of dietetic advice is added to Dr. Frazer's observations which will, in the main, agree with that which is now given by our best authorities in cases of dyspepsia ; and we are glad that experimental inquiries afford so strong a basis of support to empirical clinical observations. (1) That it is better not to eat most albuminous food stuffs at the same time that infused beverages are taken, for it has been shown that their digestion will in most cases be retarded, though there are possibly exceptions. Absorption may be rendered more rapid, but there is a loss of nutritive substance. On the other hand the digestion of starchy food appears to be arrested by tea and coffee; and gluten, the albumenoid of flour, has been seen to be the principle least retarded in digestion by tea, and it only comes third with cocoa, while coffee has apparently a much greater retarding action on it. From this it appears that bread is the natural accompaniment of coffee and cocoa when used as beverages at a meal. Perhaps the action of coffee is the reason why, in this country, it is usually drunk alone or at breakfast, a meal which consists much of meats, and of meats (eggs and salt meats) which are much retarded in digestion by coffee. (2) That eggs are the best form of animal food to be taken along with the infused beverages, and that apparently they are best lightly boiled if tea, hard boiled if coffee or cocoa is the beverage. (3) That the casein of the milk and cream taken with the beverage is probably absorbed in a large degree from the stomach. (4) That the butter used with bread undergoes digestion more slowly in presence of tea, but more quickly in the presence of coffee or cocoa; that is, the fats of butter are influenced in a similar way to oleine. (5) That the use of coffee or cocoa as excipients for cod liver oil etc., appears not only to depend on their pronounced tastes, but also on their reaction in assisting the digestion of fats.—*London Lancet.*

STRANGE MEDICINES.—The *Living Age* for July 9th, contains an interesting article describing some curious medicines in use in Japan, and incidentally throwing no little light on the medicine lore of our own immediate ancestors. The writer, C. F. Gordon Cumming, says : " The quaint old man, whose legal adherence to the customs of his ancestors afforded me such an interesting illustration both of old Japan and old Britain, was a seller of *curoyakie, i. e.*, carbonized animals; in other words, animals reduced to charcoal and potted in small covered jars of earthenware, to be sold as medicine for the sick and suffering. Formerly all these animals were kept alive in the back premises, and customers selected the creature for themselves, and stood by to see it killed and burnt on the spot. Now the zöological back yard has vanished, and only the strange chemist's shop remains, like a well-stored museum, wherein are ranged portions of the well-dried carcasses of dogs and deer, foxes and badgers, rats and mice, toads and frogs, tigers and elephants. The rarer the animal and the farther it has traveled, the more precious, apparently, are its virtues. From the roof hung festoons of gigantic snake skins, * * *. So lizards and dried scorpions (imported as medicines) also found a place in this strange druggist's shop— an "interior" so unlike anything I have ever seen elsewhere that the recollection of it remains vividly stamped on my memory —the multitude of earthenware jars containing the calcined animals, all neatly ranged on shelves, the general litter of oddities of various sorts strongly resembling an old curiosity shop, and, in the midst of all, the eccentric old man who might have passed for a Japanese wizard, rather than a great physician. It was a strangely vivid illustration of what must have been the general appearance of the laboratory of the learned teachers of Britain in the days of our forefathers. Before glancing at these, however, it may be interesting to note a few details of kindred medical lore in China, on which subject a member of the French Catholic mission says : "May Heaven preserve us from falling ill here. It is impossible to conceive who can have devised remedies so horrible as those in use in the Chinese pharmacopœia. Such as drugs compounded of toads' paws, wolves' eyes, vultures' claws, human skin and fat, and other medicaments still more horrible, of which I spare you the recital. Never did witch's den contain a collection of similar horrors." But England was given over to the same superstitions. "In the official pharmacopœia of the College of Physicians of London. A. D. 1678, *the skull of a man who had died a violent death,* and the horn of a unicorn, appear as highly approved medicines ; again in 1724, the same pharmacopœia mentions unicorn's horn, human fat, and human skulls, dogs' dung, toads, vipers and worms among the really valuable medical stores." Here are some prescriptions of the early part of the eighteenth century. "For quinsy, take old swallows, burn them in a pot, take the powder thereof, mix it with honey and annoint the throat therewith. For falling of the hair, make a tea of the ashes of cows' dung, wherewith wash the head. The blood of a shell crab anointed breeds much hair. The ankle-bones of a swine or the hoofs of a cow burnt and drunk cures the colic. To stop bleeding, take a toad, dry it very well before the sun, put it in a linen cloth and hang it with a string about the party that bleedeth; let it touch the breast of the left side near the heart." The *Living Age* for 1887 has contained an unusual amount of interesting reading matter. It is one of the most valuable of our exchanges.

VOL. XXXV.   *SEPTEMBER, 1887.*   (Volume II, Third Series.)   No. 9.

North American

JOURNAL OF HOMŒOPATHY.

ORIGINAL ARTICLES IN MEDICINE.

OUTLINES OF A SYSTEMATIC STUDY OF THE MATERIA MEDICA.

By T. F. ALLEN, M.D.,

New York.

(*Continued from Page 325.*)

BEFORE entering upon the examination of the acids and their compounds, it will be well to turn our attention to a few drugs derived from the vegetable kingdom, whose action is very like that of *amyl nitrite* and *glonoine*. The plants from which these substances are obtained possess, usually, flowers of a strong odor, or have active principles of a similarly powerful perfume, and our preparations are made either from the flowers alone or from portions of the plant which contain this perfume. Among these substances we find *cactus, melilotus, magnolia, anthoxanthum*, and plants which contain coumarine (an active principle similar to melilotol, and readily convertible into it: coumarine $C_9 H_8 O_2 + H_2 O = C_9 H_{10} O_3 =$ melilotol, the change being due to the simple additions of a molecule of water). The coumarine plants, principally *dipterix odorata* (the Tonka bean), *asperula odorata, liatris odorata, angroecum, ruta, aceras*, and other heavily perfumed orchids, produced disturbances of the circulation similar to those caused by *cactus* and *amyl nit.;* and when fully proved will certainly cause vertigo, nausea and vomiting, violent headache, flushing of the face, oppression of breathing, disturbances of the action of the heart and kidneys. These plants are, in their physiological action, allied to the whole carminative group, all of which produce a dilatation of the arterioles of the intestinal tract, with a feeling of heat, which relax spasm and relieve accumulated gases, but whose action, it may be said in passing, is too little understood and too much assumed.

The night-blooming cereus (called *cactus*) expends nearly its whole energy upon the circulation, causing at once flushing of the face and head, intense, throbbing headache, with a feeling as if the head would burst; it also causes symptoms of a rush of blood to the chest, to abdomen, fullness of extremities, all more or less associated with a disturbed action of the heart. The most characteristic feature of these congestions of *cactus* is the *sensation of stricture;* this is particularly violent about the heart and chest, but it is felt about the head, throat, abdomen and extremities, as if they were grasped by a tight, un-yielding hand. This sensation seems to be as generally pathogno-monic of *cactus* as the throbbing is of *glonoine.* Other noteworthy effects of *cactus* are the intense pressure on the vertex, the constric-tion at the neck of the bladder, and the excessive pressure and full-ness in the rectum, with hemorrhage, or a feeling as if bleeding would relieve the symptoms. Mad. Rubini speaks of the daily recur-rence of the chilliness, heat and sweat at one P.M., and this observa-tion has been verified in a few appropriate cases. Our own experi-ence is that *cactus* is indicated in a form of congestive marsh ma-laria, characterized by an incomplete resolution and by hemorrhages of dark blood, the paroxysm coming on at about the same hour each day. It promptly (instantly) cured for me an ague in a child who had two "congestive" chills on successive days; the first attack con-sisted of a prolonged cold stage, followed by a profuse hemorrhage of dark blood from the rectum and some perspiration; the second attack came on at the same hour (in the afternoon), the child continued cold, became unconscious, and finally had convulsions and involun-tary bloody stools. *Cactus* (a low potency—the third, I think—in water), brought about a resolution, and the paroxysm never returned. The family lived in one of the unhealthiest districts near New York, and were all frequently attacked. I did not see the patient, but was guided in my choice by the twenty-four-hour recurrence of the paroxysm and by the hemorrhage, considering the convulsion of minor significance.

The provings of the allied species, *cereus bonplandii* and *cereus serpentinus* correspond closely enough to those of *c. grandiflorus,* to show that the same active principles exist in other species of cereus.

The provings of *cereus bonplandii* especially, seem to have elicited almost identical symptoms in many regions, but the *bon-plandii* is only a variety of the *grandiflorus* and might be expected to produce similar results; the provings, however, were made with a tincture prepared from the stems when the plant was not in flower. The provings of *c. serpentinus* are more meager and exhibit nothing characteristic. It is probable that very little, if anything, will be gained by retaining either of these varieties of *cereus* in our symptomatology.

Melilotus.—Dr. Bowen's provings of *melilotus* exhibit the same features of disturbed circulation found in *cactus*—the very red face, vertigo and nausea, terrible headache, oppression of chest, fullness in chest and head, fullness in abdomen, frequent micturition, pressure in the rectum, and feeling as if he would have an internal hemorrhage.

These symptoms are produced by a tincture of the dried root, but Mrs. Bowen and her mother are powerfully affected by the odor of the flowers, which causes a violent, congestive headache. This effect of the odor of the flowers has been noticed from other similar flowers, such as magnolia, tuberose, orchids and others, and some persons are so sensitive to these exhalations that they cannot remain in a room with the flowers without experiencing flushing face, headache, vertigo and nausea. Clinical experience confirms the provings, and *melilotus* has been found of great service in violent, neuralgic headache, with intense flushing of the face, nose-bleed, and other symptoms. As yet no characteristic symptoms have been found ; it may, however, be remarked that the headaches are apt to be one-sided, either right or left, and are always violent, driving the patient to desperation.

Magnolia.—I had for many years known the fact that some persons could not tolerate the perfume of these flowers on account of the oppression of breathing caused by them (the observation is recorded in the encyclopedia), but the plant has never been proved. No analysis has been made of the species and no experiments recorded. Two species are highly prized in China, where they have been used for a long time—one, *magnolia hyposteum*, of which the bark is used; another, *m. yulan*, the flowers of which have a very strong and agreeable odor; of this a tea is prepared and highly prized for *pulmonary trouble*. It was, therefore, with peculiar interest that I read the provings of *yolotxochill* (magnolia grandiflora), by Dr. Talavera of Mexico, in the *Hahnemannian Monthly* of September, 1882. I turned at once to the chest symptoms and there found most wonderful corroborations of previous observations, meager though they were concerning other species of *magnolia*, and a confirmation of the clinical value of these species in pulmonary engorgements, as recorded by the Chinese.

These provings of *magnolia grandiflora* exhibit a wonderful analogy to those of *cactus*. The Aztecs used it in the treatment of heart troubles, and its use has been handed down to the Spanish inhabitants. *Pain in the heart,* with *suffocation* and *constriction of the throat;* with fear, suffocation by paroxysms, congestive, throbbing headache, lancinating pains in left side of head, nausea, with vertigo, hemorrhage between menses, congestion of left ovary, shifting pains, startings from sleep from pain in the heart, chill in afternoon, followed by fever, etc.

These provings are, without doubt, extremely valuable. The features of the drug which arrest our attention are the suffocation and pain about the heart and the left-sided character of the head, chest and ovary symptoms. Many features remind one of the nervous phenomena of *lachesis,* but the essential characters are those of *amyl nitrite* and *cactus.* I have heard travelers say that the native Chinese doctors had knowledge of a great number of simple infusions which gave marked and prompt relief, and that, as a rule, one's health would be better cared for in their hands than in those of the more pathological, but less practical, foreign doctors; certain it is, that domestic medicine the world over has been repeatedly justified by investigations into the nature of the herbs used, and these provings of *magnolia* add to the list already large.

Tongo.—The provings of the Tonka bean, by Neuning, are not wholly satisfactory, partly, perhaps, on account of the limited range of action of the drug. The principal effects are shown in the head (confusion, throbbing headache, weight, pressure and throbbing on the vertex; the sides of the head feel as if in a vise). We find, also, nausea and vomiting, burning in abdomen, burning in the chest, with a lot of indifferent symptoms of no decided character. *Coumarine,* the active principle in this bean, causes nausea, vomiting, vertigo, stupefaction and violent headache, and, in a general way, resembles the effects of *turpentine.* *Turpentine* (with the vegetable substances yielding the different sorts of *turpentine*), produces dilatation of the arterioles over the surface (even when inhaled), in the head, chest, abdomen, and, particularly, in the kidneys, where the action is very persistent (due in part, perhaps, to its elimination by the kidneys), resulting in violent hemorrhage from that organ. It also produces vertigo, stupor, nausea and vomiting, and violent stupefying headache and nose-bleed; its action on the heart is very marked and, in a way, similar to that of *cactus,* causing violent oppression and pain; taken altogether, it belongs to this same field of symptomatology, and should be studied in this connection. At the same time *turpentine* marks a transition from the group now under consideration to the one next in order, typified by *ergot,* namely, a group characterized by *contraction* of the arterioles and engorgement of the veins, resulting in hemorrhages.

To return to *coumarine*—we have found its action similar to *melilotus*, *cactus*, and other members of our group, and we may briefly look at some of the substances which contain it as their active principle. It may be remarked in passing that, in addition to the general vaso-motor paralysis caused by it, there is a decided stimulating action on the muscle of the heart, and, to some extent, feebly, I believe, it antagonizes the action of *agaricus* (muscarine). The heavy perfume of *asperula* produces the familiar symptoms above noted, and to these nothing is to be added from what is known of the effects of the other coumarine-bearing plants. It would be interesting to examine chemically the tuberoses and the allied members of the lily family—*agapanthus, funkia, phormium* and others, which possess a heavy perfume so distressing to many persons. The effects of these are similar in kind to those we have noted, but may possibly have individual peculiarities, which might prove very valuable. The effects even of *asafœtida* could almost be classed with this group, characterized, as they are, by violent, pressing, frontal headaches, burning in the eyes, great heat of the face, constriction of the throat, distention and pulsation in the abdomen, chest symptoms, which might almost be exchanged with those of *magnolia grandiflora*, and palpitation. Surely the hysterical phenomena, so marked in *asafœtida* clinically, are not more developed pathogenetically ; indeed, not as much so as in *cactus*, *magnolia*, and other similar drugs. The globus hystericus in the throat is almost the only distinguishing feature ; like *magnolia*, the left side is chiefly affected, and it is found very useful in spasmodic asthma and in functional troubles of the heart. But if we open up the *asafœtida* group, we shall be led off in a different direction again ; it is spoken of rather to show how from the field we have entered upon pathways of research opened up in the most natural and inviting manner. The study of materia medica cannot be followed along a single line of inquiry, but its groups rather resemble the halls and labyrinths of the minute structure of bone, a lacuna here, with canaliculi leading in every direction, up and down, hither and thither, to other lacunæ, all of which are variously connected with their neighbors. In this study we may imagine ourselves in a well-arranged botanical garden, with plants grouped according to their pathogenetic affinities, growing upon and related to their proper inorganic congeners, fertilized and attended by members of the animal kingdom—a garden full of interest on every side and at every step.

We will now retrace our course and take up the study of the nitrous compounds, beginning with the *nitric acid* series. These we have seen produce a fall of blood pressure, dilatation of arterioles, flushed face, fullness of head and pulsating headache, diuresis, palpitation, etc.

(*To be continued.*)

SPINAL DISEASES AND THEIR TREATMENT.
By SAMUEL LILIENTHAL, M.D.,
San Francisco, Cal.

IN the July, 1887, number of *l'Art Médical*, its editor, Dr. P. Jousset, gives some cursory remarks, which are of some interest.

1. *Congestion of the spinal cord* he considers more frequently symptomatic of severe fevers; of variola, and especially of typhoid fever. In asphyxia and in tetanus it plays the part of a lesion; it is an effect and not a cause. Congestion of the cord has a more independent existence, in consequence of a fall, from excessive coitus; from sudden suppression of menses; from poisoning with *strychnine, carbon dioxyde* and *nitrite of amyl.* A congestion of the meninges always accompanies that of the cord, and it may be even the product of a neuritis. Its symptoms are, more or less severe pains all along the vertebral column, contractures, or more often, incomplete paralysis. Remedies: *Belladonna, arnica* and *tobacco*, and perhaps also *strychnine* and *nitrite of amyl.*

Remarks.—We could have desired that the learned clinician would have given us the indications, for his remedies do not fill up the gap. In cases of concussion or congestion from a fall, we prefer *hypericum perforatum* to *arnica*; in congestion from excessive coition (and we doubt here the congestion), the salts of lime, our *calcarea ostrearum*, loom up as of great importance. *Belladonna* might serve well in sudden menstrual suppression, though in such congested states our own *gelsemium* and our old standard-bearer, *aconite*, must not be neglected. Especially where such a congested state of the cord is the product of an ascending neuritis, we would not neglect *gelsemium*, and especially think of *cuprum*, should the totality indicate this metal.

2. *Anæmia of the spinal cord.*—Arterial obliterations cause a sudden anæmia of the cord, and if complete, the symptoms show a paralysis in proportion to the extent of the anæmic region; if incomplete, pains and contractures precede the paralysis. Large hemorrhages, especially uterine flooding, cause paralysis from medullary anæmia, which may last for a long time. *Secale cornutum* is the remedy most often indicated in the treatment of these palsies.

Remarks.—The physiological action of *secale cornutum* is contraction of the arterioles; and it may be indicated in the incomplete paralysis of this anæmia as long as there are contractures and increased reflex irritability, or in the complete one, with its tendency to dry gangrene and rapid emaciation. Still, our choice in anæmia of the cord from flooding would lead us to *cinchona*, from which we realized some splendid effects, and often removed the last traces of such anæmia by the steady use of the *phosphide of sinc.*

3. *Hemorrhages of the spinal cord.*—Charcot and Hayem deny the existence of a hemorrhage in the spinal cord, as they consider such hemorrhages always in connection with a myelitis; but Grasset reports autopsies which discovered hemorrhage in the cord without myelitis. Chief symptom is the suddenness of the attack, an extremely acute pain at the moment when the hemorrhage takes place; radiating like a girdle sensation, followed by motory and sensory paralysis, and death in a few days or months. It is still questionable whether a cure is possible. Cases were observed in young girls, in consequence of the suppression of the monthlies. *Arnica* and *belladonna* ought to be alternated during the acute stage, followed by the remedies suitable to the consecutive myelitis and paraplegia.

4. Hemorrhage of the meninges of the cord is symptomatic of traumatism, of poisoning by *strychnine* of fevers; it is sometimes seen in new-born infants, and may be preceded by a pachymeningitis. It may also arise spontaneously, and the symptoms are nearly the same as in hemorrhage of the cord; an extreme pain, forcing the patient to scream; formication; slight convulsive twitchings, paralysis less perfect; sphincters paralyzed or not; rapid death. Grasset recommends *ergotine.* *Arnica* and *belladonna* may also find indications. Clinical experience is still wanting.

Remarks.—For the hemorrhage very little can be done, and the great absorbent, *arnica*, may be as good as anything else; we would rely, in such cases, more on *phosphorus;* small wounds bleed much, profuse hemorrhages pouring out freely, followed by anæmia and great debility; great irritability and nervousness; thrombosis and emboly also belong to the symptomatology of this drug. *Carbo. veg.* and *lachesis* may be thought of. Will *ledum* do anything, which has ascending paralysis and copious discharge of bright-red blood? *Ergotinum* has more passive bleeding, with sensation of pressure in chest and anguish and faintness.

5. *Myelitis.*—In relation to treatment, we differentiate between diffuse acute myelitis or diffuse and chronic polymyelitis of infants and of adults, tabes spasmodica and amyotrophic lateral myelitis. In the former number of this journal we treated of *sclérose en plaques*, pro-

gressive muscular atrophy and locomotor ataxia. It is still impossible to give indications of drugs for each of these diseases. We can only study the effects of different drugs on the cord; and we might mention the *solanea, strychnine, secale,* the snake poisons, *plumbum, argentum, phosphorus, cicuta, chelidonium, veratrum, acidum oxalicum, arsenicum, mercur.*

Belladonna.—We have seen that *belladonna* is the remedy at the beginning of locomotor ataxia, and that it is also the principal remedy in the beginning of acute diffuse myelitis. It is indicated for sudden, incomplete paraplegia, for paralytic numbness of the extremities, the tottering gait, impossibility to stand firmly. The paralysis of the eye muscles, the dilatation of the pupil, the paralysis of the bladder and of its sphincter, especially indicate *belladonna.* (We may have in the myelitic state tonic and clonic convulsions, but the weight of the disease soon falls on the posterior column, and we find then loss of coördination of the muscles, though motor weakness of the lower extremities is easily observed. May not the origin of this myelitis be originally higher up, as symptoms of affection of the oculomotorius and of the optic nerve show themselves at an early stage. It is a myelitis descendens, for which *belladonna* finds its best indications).

Stramonium finds particular indications by the presence of convulsive phenomena, trembling and contracture. The convulsions are excited by the least touch. Dose of *belladonna* and *stramonium,* tincture to third dilution. (Hyperæsthesia of mind and body characterize *stramonium* more than they do *belladonna,* and prevail even in the paralytic state, hence we find it valuable in paralysis dolorosa, where we may even have an alternation of convulsive and paralytic symptoms. Though consciousness may be undisturbed, a perfect mania for light and company characterizes the *stramonium* patient).

Nux vomica and strychnine are indicated for tetanus and for the fulgurant pains of locomotor ataxia. *Strychnine* in toxic doses produces a genuine myelitis, and we might therefore prescribe it with some chance of success in diffuse acute myelitis where the following symptoms exist: cramps, contractures, tonic convulsions excited by motion, noise, light, even touch. The convulsions are accompanied by excessive pains, with tingling. Dose, second trituration of *strychnine sulf.* (of *nux vomica* we might well say), cerebro-spinal system secondarily affected, the primary source of irritation occurring in the alimentary canal, and this very thing shows us that the alkaloid may often widely differ in its action from the mother plant, for *strychnine* affects primarily the spinal cord, leaving the brain most frequently undisturbed. According to Jousset *strychnine* suits the inflammatory stage, before the neuralgia become sclerosed and paralytic symptoms follow, hence when there are still the fulgurating pains, the premonitory stage of locomotor ataxia, but the mother plant, the *nux vomica*, acts beautifully in all paralyses, originating in a neurasthenia from loss of vital power, and we see it therefore sometimes recommended in alternation with *china*. Venous stasis causing a weakened heart, and thus illy sustained nerve-force, is the keynote for the use of *nux vomica*, but not for the tetanic *strychnine*.

Secale cornutum* produces myelitis, and Jousset cured a case of subacute diffuse myelitis, setting in suddenly, with *ergot*. A sensation of tingling and of torpor in the extremities ; a progressive ascending paralysis and decubitus indicate this drug. Dose, first trituration (though we cannot always agree with Jousset in his use of the lower potencies, we think he is right in *secale* and *ergotin*. There is paralysis of the vaso-motors, dilatation of the arterioles, languid circulation, the distant parts fail to be supplied with their quantity of circulating fluids, the distant and superficial nerves are starved, and necessarily ascending paralysis and dry gangrene follow. The intermittent pulse, the weak palpitation, only felt at night, in the horizontal position, show the waning powers of life, for which *secale* and in other cases *carbo vegetabilis* remain our sheet anchor. What then, if any, are the indications for the higher potencies of *secale?*) ·

The snake poisons. Lachesis, crotalus and *naja* are recommended in the treatment of myelitis. *Crotalus* has Elb of Dresden, for its sponsor ; hardly any sensitiveness to pressure on the vertebral region; general debility; weakness of all the extremities, especially the lower ones; sensation of numbness and of coldness ; decrease 'of mental power; difficulty of speech ; periodical fits of dyspnœa—it may be therefore of benefit in chronic myelitis, and especially in *sclerose en plaque. Lachesis* suits better, paraplegia with permanent contracture, sensation and painful tingling of the parts paralyzed. *Naja* acted well in several light cases of amyostheny and anæsthesia. Dose, third to sixth dilution. (If we keep in mind that *crotalus* has for its primary effect, dissolution of the blood and death of the red blood-corpuscles, and only secondary symptoms in the nervous system, while *lachesis* paralyzes primarily the nervous system, and that *naja tripudians* just stand in its action between the two former, we get a keynote which explains all the other symptoms of these valuable drugs, for which we have to thank especially Hering, Dunham and Hayward.)

Plumbum produces paralysis, with muscular atrophy. It is the medicine for limited fascicular myelitis of the gray anterior horn, whether acute or chronic; for infantile paralysis, for acute spinal paralysis and for progressive muscular atrophy. *Plumbum* in the thirtieth dilution cured for me a case of acute spinal paralysis in a rheumatic patient.

Argentum nitricum in toxic doses causes myelitis, and it is one of the most important drugs in locomotor ataxia, but acts well also in spasmodic myelitis, a fasciculated myelitis of the lateral columns. It was employed in low and high dilution successfully. (The earlier this drug is prescribed, the more beneficial will be the result. The old school has used and abused it for years in cerebral diseases, especially epilepsy, and as a cerebro-spinal irritant they used it on homœopathic reasons without knowing it. We ought to use it only in the higher potencies to get its full effect, just as Jousset uses *lead* in the thirtieth.)

Phosphorus produces, in toxic doses, lesions of the spinal cord (Danillo), so far very poorly described. It causes and cures paraplegia, and according to Gallaoardia, it is more indicated in ascending paraplegia with tingling. (It is a curious fact that in several autopsies on lunatics, the normal quantity of *phosphorus* in the brain was found diminished, and it is equally well known that phosphorus produces venous stasis, thrombosis or emboly, with consequent fatty degeneration; may we not therefore conclude that it must be indicated in progressive cerebral and spinal affections, leading to mental and bodily paralysis, and that we found in *phosphorus* just the drug to inhibit the furthur progress of the disease?)

Conium maculatum produces an ascending paraplegia, which finally becomes bulbar, causes dysphagia, loss of speech, dyspnœa, asphyxia and syncope, it may be indicated in acute myelitis and in acute spinal paralysis. Dose? (Let us keep in mind that *conium* is our great remedy for excessive sexual indulgence, natural or unnatural, as well as for the consequences of suppressed sexual desire, paralyzing first the peripheral nerves and finally the cord and the bulbas; a motor palsy without the least spasm, though tremors might prevail, as it is also, with *lycopodium* a great aid in the treatment of old women (*Barium* more for old men).

Chelidonium majus may, according to its pathogensis, be indicated in tabes dorsalis spasmodica and in disseminated sclerosis; paresis of inferior extremities with stiffness of the muscles and trembling during motion, pain in the cord increased by pressure. (Is here the liver the *fons et origo malis?* We never used it so far in spinal diseases, except where the cerebral or spinal symptoms were reflex of abdominal pressure.)

Veratrum album also suits tabes dorsalis spasmodica, as it produces a muscular rigidity which prevents the muscle for a long time from returning to its normal state. (We meet the same tension in the mental sphere where the *white hellebore* is indicated, and we would beg our readers not to neglect the study of that old pamphlet, by Hahnemann, on "Helleborism," and we may learn therefrom its beneficial use in nervous diseases, if steadily given for a long time. In painful paralysis with its constant jerks in the limbs, and the icy coldness, so characteristic of the drug, it has not received the full attention, which it deserves.)

Acidum oxalicum. Richard Hughes recommends it for ascending paraplega, with pains in extremities, from a chronic meningo-myelitis. (The keynote is: pains occupy small spaces, limbs stiff, muscular twitchings, extremities heavy, powerless, numb, weak. Whether it is a remedy for sclerosis of the posterior root zone, may be doubted, but who ever expects a clear-cut pathological state, in this disease? When *oxalic acid* suits, we expect the cerebellar and lateral tract drawn into the inflammatory zone. All our remedies need reproving in relation to spinal affections.)

Arsenicum produces paraplegia, and according to Hughes, myelitis, especially chronic. The paraplegia of *arsenic* is accompanied by loss of sensibility, muscular atrophy, tingling, cramps, muscular shocks and œdema. It may be therefore indicated in locomotor ataxia and tabes spasmodica. (Cases are on record where it was necessary to give Fowler's solution after meals in the doses of the old school to get the desired effect, and therefore it may be more considered as a palliative than a real curative remedy in these organic nervous disorders, but where we find burning, tearing, lancinating pains, especially at night and during sleep, nearly driving the patient crazy ; greatly oppressed breathing and anxiety ; constriction and tightness of chest as if bound with a hoop (girdle sensation); bruised sensation all along the spine, with violent startings and weariness of all the limbs, and especially where also œdema and emaciation make their appearance, we may prescribe the metal or the iodide with confidence.)

Mercurius. Baehr reports a case of acute myelitis (?) cured by *mercur.* and it may also be indicated in locomotor ataxia and tabes dorsalis spasmodica, when we meet weakness of the lower extremities, accompanied by cramps and contractures, a vacillating gait, and the legs are involuntarily jerked forwards. Baehr used the sixth. (According to high authorities locomotor ataxia finds very often its cause in syphilis, and thus we easily understand the action of the mercurials in these final syphilitic affections. It has in its pathogenesy the lightning-like, shooting pains of this sensory progressive paralysis, the nocturnal aggravations so characteristic of syphilis, the stiffness in the limbs, the tremors; and we can see therefore no reason why Jousset should doubt a cure of myelitis or meningo-myelitis, made by such an excellent prescriber as Baehr was known to be.

Some of our best remedies Jousset has not touched yet, as *onosmodium* in that sclerosis of the posterior root zone with co-affection of the lower portion of the lateral column. He leaves out *cuprum* and *zincum*, so often indicated in diseases of the cerebro-spinal system, *calabar bean* and *piric acid*, and many more. Here we have a theme which was never worked out and we need not wonder at it, for the diagnosis of spinal and bulbar diseases, hardly dates back a few decades. We thank the Bureau of Materia Medica of the American Institute, that they took up the study of *zincum*, and let us trust that the provings will be made with all the lights which recent studies have shed on this interesting branch of medical science.

CYSTITIS.

By JOHN L. MOFFAT, M.D.,

Brooklyn, N. Y.

(*Continued from page* 465.)

Carbo veg.—Blennorrhœa vesicæ. Urine reddish, turbid, bloody, with red sediment.

°In chronic cases, when the acute inflammation has subsided, leaving a blennorrhœa. Vesical catarrh of old people ; accompanied by varices of the anus and bladder.

°Low vitality. Venous system predominant.

°Ailments from quinine or mercury.

Caust.—*Cannot tell when he is urinating unless he looks, or feels with his hand. After he thinks he is through and lies down, more passes involuntarily. Urging, and he waits long for the urine to come.* Intermitting flow. *Involuntary discharge upon coughing,* etc. Retention, with frequent, urgent desire ; a few drops occasionally dribble away. Retention, with difficult expulsion of the urine.

Paralysis of the bladder. Anæsthesia of the urethra. *Urine* dark brown, turbid, and cloudy on standing.

°Dark hair and rigid fibre most affected.

Children with delicate skin.

°Inimicals, acids, *coff.*, *phos.*

A. cepa.—†Frequent micturition, with burning in the urethra. Fullness and pressure in the bladder, with urgency to urinate. Violent pains in the bladder and left side of the abdomen. Region of bladder very sensitive to touch.

Sensation of weakness or of warmth in bladder and urethra. Irritable bladder. Urine very red. Iridescent film.

°Spasmodic strangury from getting the feet and bowels cold.

°Old age—gangrene.

°*All. sat., scilla, aloes,* do not follow well or antidote it.

Cham.—Very frequent urging, with dragging down the ureters, like labor pains.

Burning in the neck of the bladder when urinating.

Urine scanty, turbid, clay-colored, thick soon after passing ; or yellow, with flaky or yellow sediment.

°Nervous, excitable temperament.

Chelid.—Frequent urging, with scanty, painful discharge. Violent pain in the ureters preceding discharge of turbid urine. The urine has vesical mucus, biliverdin, and profuse urates. The chlorides are diminished.

°Spare people. Blondes.

°Follows *led.* well. *Ars.* will often be useful after it.

Chimaph.—Awakened repeatedly by constant desire to micturate. Urging immediately after urination. Pressing fullness in the region of the bladder.

Urine frequent, thick, ropy, brick red, throwing down a copious bloody, or muco-purulent sediment, accompanied by hectic fever and night sweats. (E. M. Hale.)

°Dysuria in plethoric, hysterical women.

China.—Frequent discharge of turbid, scanty urine. Sediment white, loose, dingy yellow; scanty, greenish yellow, brick dust, or pinkish.

°Swarthy persons. Debility from exhausting discharges.

°Inimical to *selen.*

Clemat.—Urine frequent, but scanty. Flow jerking, interrupted. Burning during urination, worse at the beginning of the flow, or during the interruptions. Involuntary discharge of drops at the close of micturition. Purulent sediment.

°Vesical neuralgia, the urethra or seminal cord most affected.

°Light hair, torpid, cachectic condition.

°Follows *sil.* well.

Coccus c.—Tension and heaviness in the bladder, spasmodic pain in the neck. Frequent desire. Urine scanty, watery; falls from the end of the penis. Cystospasmus.

Colch.—Cystospasmus. Tenesmus and burning in the urethra.

Urine acid; concentrated; sour; dark; turbid; bloody, almost inky; scanty; flowing drop by drop; whitish sediment, much urate of ammonia.

°Often indicated with old people.

○Follows well where *nux v.* or *lyc.* has relieved.

Coloc.—Freqent tenesmus, with scanty emission.

Urine turbid at first, but on standing throws down a tough mucus, which may be drawn into strings; or which becomes jelly-like. Urine fetid; viscid; like brown beer.

Con.—Strangury, with vertigo, especially on lying down. Spasmodic feeling of pressure in the bladder. Painful dysuria. Cutting pains during, and burning or smarting after, urination. Flow intermits. Frequent micturition at night. *Urine* pale, with gray or white sediment.

°Old men ; old maids. Light-haired persons. Marasmic children.

Copaiva.—(Tincture of the balsam.)

†*Burning in the neck of the bladder and urethra.*

Dull pain in the bladder. Pressure on the bladder, with frequent ineffectual urging, and passage of urine *guttatim.*

Hæmaturia; strangury; ischuria. Painful discharge by drops.

The urine is more abundant, more acid, and has a very strong smell of violets.

Frothy, dark yellow urine.

Cyclam.—Urine dark red, with much flocculent matter. Scanty, with urging; frequent, or seldom.

Digit.—Constant urging, ineffectual, or with scanty discharge. Increased desire after a few drops have passed, causing the patient to walk about in distress, although motion aggravates the desire. Feeling of fullness in the bladder, persisting after micturition. Throbbing pain, during the tenesmus, in the region of the neck of the bladder. The neck of the bladder is principally affected. Retention, with a constrictive pain in the bladder. Cystospasmus.

Urine scanty, thick, very dark, turbid, with brick dust sediment (*uric acid* or urates). The chlorides are diminished.

Dros.—Frequent, scanty urination, often *guttatim.* Urine dark and of a strong odor.

Dulc.—Constant desire felt deep in the abdomen. Painful pressing down in the bladder and urethra ; discharge of a few drops, with a mucus sediment. Retention. Strangury. Enuresis. Urine fetid, scanty, turbid ; upon standing becomes oily and deposits a white, tough, jelly-like mucus, mixed with particles of blood.

Muco-purulent sediment.

Paralysis of the bladder.

°If caused by a cool change in the weather, or exposure to *damp cold*.

°Chronic cases.

°Is followed well by *kali* or *phos*.

°Incompatible, *bell.*, *lach*.

Etat.—Pains upon urinating so violent as to induce spasms. Constant heat at the neck of the bladder.

Equiset.—Urine *very scanty; syrupy* from the abundant transparent mucus. Constant desire.

†*Constant feeling of fullness and severe and dull pain in the bladder, as if micturition failed to empty it.* Aching pain in the back and down either sciatic nerve.

Constant desire to urinate. †*Pain in the bladder, as from distension.* †*Tenderness in the region of the bladder and lower abdomen, extending upward from the groin, worse on right side. Pain in bladder, with tenderness and soreness.* †*On standing the urine showed great excess of mucus,* but was otherwise normal.

Erigeron.—Frequent painful urination ; dysuria ; ischuria. Urine copious, of a strong odor, very acrid.

°*Dysuria of teething children.* °Vesical irritation from *calculi.*

Eup. purp. —Constant desire; even after frequent passages of urine the bladder still feels full. Desire, accompanied by a cutting, aching pain in the bladder; soreness and pain in the bladder; deep aching; uneasiness. Very frequent emission of a few drops at a time.

Euphorb.—Strangury. Frequent desire, with scanty discharge. Urging to urinate—the urine was passed by drops, with sticking in the glans penis, followed by a natural discharge. An itching stitch in the forepart of the urethra when not urinating. Much white sediment in the urine.

Fagop.—Frequent desire. "Difficulty in voiding the last few drops; think I am done, then several drops pass away." Urine light and clear.

Fluoric ac.—Burning before and after micturition, with aching in the bladder. Dysuria. *Urine* dark, scanty; alkaline, with whitish or purplish sediment. Or, urine bright colored, very frequent, with thirst

°Old age. Weakly constitution.

°After abuse of *mercury*.

Gambogia.—*Micturition seldom.* Frequent, but scanty. Emission of one or three drops at a time, then intermitting, then finally returning, then burning at the orifice.

:℥ *Gels.*—Alternate dysuria and enuresis. Paralysis of the sphincter. Spasm of the bladder.

°Nervous persons; excitable.

Graph.—*Before* emission, cutting and downward pressure in both kidneys. *During*, pain in the sacrum. Burning in the urethra between the acts. Very frequent micturition at night. Urging, with scanty discharge.

Urine sour, dark brown; becomes turbid, and deposits a white or reddish sediment.

°Follows well after *lyc.*

Guaiac.—Continuous urging, even after the discharge of profuse fetid urine.

Stitches in the vesical neck, after ineffectual pressure to urinate.

°Dark hair and eyes. Old women.

°After abuse of *mercury* in gout or rheumatism.

Guarea.—Cystitis. Frequent urging in the evening. Involuntary micturition. Clay-colored urine.

Hamam.—Frequent or continual desire.

Profuse urination, but only little at a time; seems that the bladder fills up very quickly; light-colored urine.

"A greasy deposit, which sinks to the bottom of the vessel, rising to the top when shaken; looks like laudable pus."

Hedeoma.—(No bladder symptoms in Allen's Encyclopedia. Hale attributes to it): Tenesmus; painful urination; scanty emission, with frequent urging desire.

Urine very dark, like black tea.

Helleb.—Frequent spasmodic urging, causes convulsions. After great pressure he passed, with much pain, a few drops of blood. Passes blood and slime, with burning and stinging. Bladder overdistended and paralyzed. Retention from atony.

Urine scanty; dark, with a coffee-ground sediment.

°In bad cases, where the irritation at the neck of the bladder threatens to run into inflammation.

Helon.—Strangury. Involuntary discharge after the bladder seems to be emptied.

oMental depression from *kali brom.*

°Climaxis. Nervous atonicity.

More especially for women.

Hepar.—Urine passed slowly, from atonicity of the bladder. Feels as if the bladder could not be emptied thoroughly.

Urine dark, bloody; acrid, corroding the prepuce. Greasy, opalescent pellicle.

°Against abuse of *kali. iod.* Antidotes, *mercury* and *iodine.*

Hydr.—Vesical catarrh; sediment of thick, ropy mucus. Urine smells decomposed:

°Old people. Bad effects from *mercury.*

Hyos.—"Has no will to urinate." Retention, bladder largely distended. Spasm or inflammation of the neck of the bladder. Dysuria. *Urine* frequent, scanty, turbid, with muco-purulent, or red, sandy sediment.

°Sanguine temperament. Hysterical subjects.

°Complaints from inhaling *ether*, or abuse of *bellad.*

Hyper.—Nightly urging, with vertigo. Urine scanty, bloody, turbid, and of a peculiar odor.

°Hyper. is the "Arnica of the nerves."

Ign.—Sudden irresistible desire. Pressure to urinate from drinking coffee.

°After grief. In nervous persons.

°Ailments from coffee, brandy, tobacco.

Iod.—†*Copious frequent micturition.*

Constant desire, attended by dribbling.

Urine dark, thick, ammoniacal; dark, yellowish-green; milky; acrid; covered with a variegated pellicle.

°Dark hair and eyes. Scrofula.

°Frequently suitable in ailments from *mercury* or *nitrate of silver.*

Ipec.—Unsuccessful urging. Frequent, scanty micturition. Great burning and urging before the discharge, not followed by tenesmus. Hæmaturia.

†Urine red, scanty.

Kali bich.—Continuous desire during the day. †After micturition burning in back part of urethra, with sensation as if one drop had remained behind, with unsuccessful effort to void it. †Frequent discharge of watery, strong-smelling urine, awakening him at night. *Urine* scanty, with a white film and mucus sediment. Painful drawing from perineum into urethra.

°Fat, light-haired persons.

Kali carb.—Frequent desire. Pressure in bladder for some time before the urine passes. Violent cutting and tearing in the neck of the bladder and urethra. After long waiting the urine flows slowly, with soreness and burning. Interrupted stream without any pain. Urination, immediately followed by painful desire to micturate.

Urine hot, scanty, frequeut, with red slimy or purulent sediment.

°Old people. Lax fibre, dark hair.

Anæmic persons.

°Frequently suitable after *bry. lyc., natr. mur., nitr. ac.*

After *k. c.* are frequently indicated *carbo. veg., phos.*

Kali iod.—Irritable bladder. Congestion and heaviness in the neck of the bladder, with priapism. Frequent painful urging. Contraction of the sphincter just as urination begins and during its continuance. The bladder is full and swollen, but cannot be emptied. *Urine* smells very badly, and decomposes almost immediately. *Sediment* of triple phosphate ; yellow or gray deposit sticking to the sides of the vessel like calcareous concretions.

°Scrofula. Syphilis.

°After abuse of *mercury.*

Kobalt.—Frequent, scanty emission of urine, with a greasy pellicle, and strong, pungent smell. Frequent urination in the morning, after drinking coffee.

Kreos.—Strangury and *burning.* †*Frequent, profuse.* †*Excessive urging to urinate; she cannot get out of bed quickly enough.* †*Urinates with great haste and profusely.* The urine spurts from her during each cough.

Urine †*offensive;* chestnut-brown ; reddish or colorless ; cloudy ; with a red or white sediment, triple phosphates, lime and urates.

°After *carbo. veg.* it may disagree.

Lach.—Ineffectual urging. Burning when the urine passes. Dull pain in the bladder. Sensation as of a ball rolling in the bladder or abdomen when turning over. Vesical catarrh. *Urine* foamy, almost black; offensive mucus. *Pressure upon the bladder.*

°Climaxis. Cyanosis, venous stasis. Septicæmia.

Lactic ac.—Bladder feels sore, as though strained or over-taxed; must keep bent forward to take off the pressure, in which position he feels much more comfortable.

†*Frequent urination; the attempt to retain the urine causes pain.* *Urine* profuse; clear, white and thick; scanty, high colored; normal, with the exception of a greasy film.

Lactuca v.—Increased desire; urine profuse, and of a violet odor. A constant sensation while sitting still as though a drop were running through the urethra.

Lamium.—Frequent *urging*, with very *scanty* discharge. Crawling sensation in the urethra. Sensation as though a drop of water were running through the urethra, though no moisture was noticed at the orifice.

Lauroc.—During urination pain in stomach; or often spells of palpitation of the heart and gasping for breath. Retention or slow emission as if the bladder were paralyzed. Enuresis. *Urine* acrid, corroding the labia; *sediment* thick, reddish, with floating jelly-like flakes.

Led.—Urgent desire; almost constant; desire in day time, not at night. Frequent micturition. Stream often intermits. Discharge of pus.

°From abuse of alcoholic drinks.

Lil. tigr.—Frequent or constant urging, with scanty discharge, followed by acrid smarting in urethra, and tenesmus. The urging is worse towards morning. Continuous pressure in the bladder. A congested sensation in the chest if the desire to urinate is not complied with. Urine milky; scanty; dark and increased; hot like boiling oil.

Lith. c.—Before urinating, flashes of pain in the bladder, extending towards the right side; after the act, the pain extends into the spermatic cord. Quick, strong tenesmus, with sensitive pain in the middle of the urethra; worse in the evening; on walking. In the morning on rising to urinate, a pressure in the cardiac region, not ceasing until after micturition.

Urine scanty, acrid, dark; *emission* painful, difficult. Sediment dark-reddish brown; uric acid; mucus.

Lyc.—Strangury. Frequent urging, forcing the patient to retain the urine, and to support the abdomen with both hands. Heaviness and dull pressure in the bladder. Urging, but must wait long for the urine to pass. Emission delayed, with pain in the back, which is relieved soon after the flow begins. Micturition *preceded* by much pain in the back, eliciting screams; *accompanied* by itching in the urethra and burning; and *followed* some time after by itching and violent shooting, tearing or cutting pains in the urethra. Stitches simultaneously in anus and neck of the bladder.

Pains worse on lying down, especially at night; relieved by horseback riding.

Urine foamy; turbid; milky, with an offensive, purulent sediment; scanty, dark-red, clear, with deposit of uric acid or "red sand." Hæmaturia.

° Chronic cases, with disposition to calculi.

° Follows well *calc. or lach.*

Followed often indications for *graph., lach., led., phos., sil.*

Magn. mur.—Urine can only be voided by bearing down with the abdominal muscles. Frequent desire, with scanty emission.

° Women; especially if hysterical. Children, during dentition.

Mang. acet.—Frequent desire, profuse urine. Cutting in the urethra between the acts. Earthy, violet colored sediment.

Mephitis.—Frequent emission of clear urine. Difficulty in voiding water during the day. Stream interrupted. Urine turbid in the morning, and after the evening fever.

Merc.—Sudden irresistible urging, with copious flow. Hæmaturia, with frequent violent urging. Constant desire not relieved by micturition. Violent urging, with thin stream, or discharge by drops, containing mucus, blood, or pus.

Perspires during urination. Enuresis. Region of the bladder very sore to the touch.

Urine burning; dark-red and turbid; sour, or pungent odor; contains white flakes, pus or flesh-like shreds of mucus.

°*Merc.* and *sil.* do not follow each other well.

Merc. bin.—Frequent desire; she cannot hold her water for a moment. Ulcers in the bladder. *Urine* red, thick, and dark when passing.

Merc. cor.—Great tenesmus. Retention. *Urine* scanty, hot, bloody; flows drop by drop, with great pain; brown, with brick-dust sediment. Mucus in filaments, flakes, or dark flesh-like pieces. Strangury.

Mez.—Very urgent, frequent desire; immediately after urinating. †*After micturition a few drops of blood are passed.* A pinching sensation in the bladder.

†*Urine hot, with a reddish sediment.* Urine scanty, flaky.

Hæmaturia, preceded by a crampy pain in the bladder.

°Phlegmatic temperament.

°Frequently indicated against bad effects of mercury.

Millef.—*Hæmaturia;* the blood forms a cake in the vessel.

°Purulent discharge after lithotomy.

°Calculus, with retention. Vesical catarrh from atony.

Mitchella.—Uneasiness at the neck of the bladder and urging to urinate. *Urine* high colored, with a white sediment.

°Vesical catarrh especially in women.

°Dysuria accompanying uterine complaints.

Mur. ac.—Frequent micturition. Slow emission; atonic bladder. Must wait long for the urine to pass; has to press so that the anus protrudes. *Urine* red, violet, milky. Enuresis.

°Follows well after *rhus.* and *bry.*

Natr. c.—Frequent urgent micturition. *Urine* smells like that of the horse; sour; fetid; dark yellow; mucus sediment.

°Follows *sep.* well.

Natr. mur.—Frequent, sudden, irresistible desire, with copious emission. Enuresis when walking, laughing, coughing. Has to wait long for urine to pass; especially if there are others near him. Intermitting flow. *During* urination stitches in bladder; smarting, burning in urethra; smarting and soreness in vulva. *After* micturition, burning and cutting in urethra. In the pauses (intermitting flow) stitches in the urethra. Hæmaturia.

With violent tenesmus, passes large quantities of mucus.

Mucus like boiled starch (Schüssler).

Urine dark, like coffee, with brick-dust sediment.

°It antidotes *arg; nitr.; quinine*, bee stings.

Followed by *sep.*

Natr. sulf.—Piercing pain in the groins, with urging to urinate, in the afternoon, while walking out of doors.

Pinching around the umbilicus while sitting, with urging to urinate, the pain going into the groin.

Urine scanty, burning, with yellowish red sediment; in the morning yellowish white.

°Hydrogenoid constitution.

Nitr. ac.—Urging *after*, and shuddering along the spine *during* micturition. *During* urination, burning in the urethra increased by the act, and stitching in the abdomen. Painful retention. Hæmaturia.

Urine smells like that of the horse; smells strong; scanty; dark brown; intolerable odor; looks like the dregs of a cider barrel.

Urine cold when it passes; small stream. Incontinence.

°*Inimical, lach.*

Nitrum.—Dysuria; frequent urination, with pain and heat.

Urine profuse, pale, with reddish sediment; cloudy, mucus sediment; salts increased; *sp. gr.*, 1030–1040.

°After *canth.*, turpentine, condiments, stimulating injections, cold, gonorrhœal extension, onanism.

Nux. mosch.—Tenesmus. Dysuria, with urging to stool; worse after dinner or supper, or bodily exertion.

Urine scanty, high colored, of a violet odor.

°Strangury from beer or wine. Pain from calculi. Complicated with uterine troubles, or hysteria.

Nux. vom.—Painful, ineffectual urging. Desire, with violent pains *during* and *after* scanty or *guttatim* emission; may be accompanied by tearing or burning pains in urethra, bladder, kidneys, or loins. Spasmodic strangury. Micturition *preceded* by pressure on the bladder, *accompanied* and *followed* by contractive pain in the urethra.

Urine pale; later thick, purulent; reddish, with brick-dust sediment. Hæmaturia. Paralysis of the bladder; urine dribbles.

°After drugging; indulgence in liquor; suppressed hæmorrhoidal flow, menses, or gonorrhœa.

Follows well after *ars., ipec., phos., sulph.*

Is followed by *bry., puls., sulph.*

Op.—Slow, difficult emission in a thin stream. Stream interrupted (spasm of the sphincter). Paralysis of the bladder, especially of the fundus. Enuresis. Retention.

°Retention in nursing child after passion of the nurse.

Urine seldom, scanty, dark brown, with brick-dust sediment.

Oxal. ac.—Thinking of micturition causes a necessity to urinate. Frequent profuse emission of clear, straw-colored urine.

°Sugar, coffee and wine disagree.

PAREIRA BRAVA.—*Constant urging* and tenesmus, with violent pain in the glans, extorting screams. Left testis drawn up tightly. Pain in the thighs. Paroxysms from three to six A. M.; or midnight until morning; comparative ease the rest of the day.

Has to get upon the hands and knees to urinate. Rectal with the vesical tenesmus. Emission *guttatim*, with a sensation as if much were coming. Drawing, cutting pains down the legs to the heels.

Urine turbid; *abundant mucus*, transparent, thick, tough, sticks to the sides of the vessel. Sediment of red sand. Strong ammoniacal smell to the urine.

Paris q.—Frequent passage of acrid urine, dark red, with a reddish sediment and a greasy pellicle.

° Is followed well by *led., lyc.,* and *rhus.*

Petrol.—Itching in the (female) meatus urinarius during micturition, preceded by an urgent desire to urinate. Discharge frequent and scanty, of a brown fetid urine. Enuresis. Constant dripping of urine.

°Light hair.

Phos.—Frequent urging, with rectal tenesmus. Frequent desire, with twitching and burning in the urethra. Emission prevented by a dull pain in the hypogastrium; in the morning. *Urine* profuse, pale and watery; or frequent, scanty, turbid, like curdled milk, with a red sediment.

°Tall, slim, woman; disposed to stoop.

°Inimical, *caust.*

Ph. ac.—Constant urging. Involuntary emission at night; profuse discharge of a clear, watery urine. Creeping in the urethra, between the acts.

Urine †*milky*, with bloody jelly-like pieces of mucus. Decomposes rapidly.

Phytol.—Urgent desire. Pain in bladder before and during micturition.

Plat.—Frequent urination, with slow emission. *Urine,* pale, watery, red, with white clouds; turbid, with red sediment.

°Females. Dark hair, rigid fibre. Haughty disposition.

Plumb.—Strangury. Retention, as from atony of the bladder. Discharge *guttatim.*

Urine dribbles; is high colored and fetid.

Necrotic cystitis, from decomposed urea.

Polyg.—Painful cutting and feeling of strangulation at the neck of the bladder when urinating, lasting a long time. Constant desire. Pain in sacrum and bladder, with desire to micturate, not relieved by voiding large quantities of urine. •

Populus.—Urine scanty, with large quantities of mucus or pus, and severe tenesmus as soon as the last drops are voided, or a little before.

°Vesical catarrh in elderly persons, with ardor urinæ, or perfect retention.

PRUNUS.—Has the tearing, cutting pains of Pareira b., but not the sediment.

Terrific *burning* in the urethra and bladder, which always feels full, and is more comfortable when containing urine.

Urine scanty; the patient cannot void it beyond the fossa navicularis.

PULSAT.—Continued pressure on the bladder, without any desire to urinate.

Frequent, almost ineffectual urging, with cutting pains. Desire to urinate, with drawing in the abdomen. *After* micturition a spasmodic pain in the neck of the bladder extending into the thighs. Tenesmus, and stinging in the neck of the bladder. Dropping of blood at the end of micturition. Hæmaturia, with burning at the orifice of the urethra and constriction around the umbilicus.

Retention, with redness, soreness and heat in the region of the bladder. Cannot retain the urine; it passes in drops when sitting or walking. Enuresis on coughing or passing wind.

Urine scanty, red brown. Sediment tough, slimy; bloody or reddish; mucus, jelly-like and sticking to the vessel; purulent, with the bloody urine.

°From exposure. Women and children. Light hair, blue eyes, pale face. Easily moved to tears.

Ranunc. sc.—Frequent desire, with scanty emission of light yellow urine. Drops escape some time after urinating. A short time after micturition, a burning pain in the fore part of the urethra. A tickling, crawling sensation at the orifice of the urethra.

Raphanus.—Frequent desire. Urging to urinate causes suffering, as if from retention, and does not cease, except while she is passing water; returns immediately after, and is always accompanied by pain in the sides and loins. Desire to urinate, with pain in the region of the *mons veneris* like a pressure in the fundus of the bladder.

Ratanhia.—Frequent ¡pressure to urinate, always with the evacuation of only a few drops. *Urine* scanty, becomes turbid after a time.

Rheum.—Bladder weak, must press hard to urinate. Burning in the kidneys before and during micturition.

· °Children. After abuse of *canth.* or *magnes. carb.* Follows *ipec.* well.

†*Rhod.*—Frequent urging with drawing in the region of the bladder.

Urine greenish, profuse, very offensive.

Rhus.—Tenesmus, with discharge of a few drops of blood-red urine. Frequent urging. Belching of wind during micturition.

Retention. Emission slow, stream divided. Enuresis worse while at rest.

°Incompatible with *apis.*

Rumex.—Sudden urging. Enuresis on coughing. Urine less copious, red and turbid, with a flaky deposit, and oily surface ; next day a heavy brick-dust sediment.

Ruta.—Constant urging, could hardly retain the urine. If forcibly retained it could not be voided. Pressure in the bladder, as though it were constantly full ; at every step, after urination, she feels as if the bladder were full, and moving up and down. Frequent pressure to urinate, and scanty emission of green urine.

Spasm of the sphincter vesicæ.

Enuresis at night, and in the day while walking.

Sabad.—Urging, especially in the evening. After voiding a few drops only, violent urging, with a drawing in the urethra from before backwards, and violent burning in the urethra.

Urine dark, muddy, like clay water.

°Light hair, muscles lax.

Sabina.—†Irritable bladder, °depending on the gouty diathesis. Strangury.

Frequent violent urging, with profuse discharge.

Retention. Hæmaturia.

°Chronic ailments of women.

Sant.—Fullness and sensitiveness in the bladder. Frequent, painful desire, with scanty discharge.

Urine greenish ; turbid when voided ; stains the clothes yellow.

Strangury. Dysuria. Hæmaturia.

Sars.—Ineffectual urging. Tenderness and distention over the region of the bladder.

Vesical tenesmus, with discharge of white acrid pus or mucus. Painful retention.

During micturition air passes from the bladder.

Flow in drops without pain, or in a thin, feeble stream. Severe pain at the end of micturition.

Sand in the urine, the child screams before and while passing it.

Urine copious, passed without sensation.

Urine, irritating, bright and clear; or scanty, slimy, flaky, with deposit of sand.

°Dark hair. Sycosis.

°*Sars.* and *sep.* follow each other well.

°Vinegar appears at first to increase the effects of *sars.*

Sec.—Unsuccessful urging. Discharge of thick black blood from the bladder.

White cheesy sediment.

Ischuria paralytica.

°In old people, thin and crawny.

°*Cinchona* follows well after *sec.*

Senecio.—†*Vesical tenesmus* in the morning.

†*Urging to urinate followed the chilliness ; urine tinged with blood.* Urine scanty, high colored ; of increased specific gravity.

Sep.—Urging with violent itching in the region of the bladder. †*Urging, from* †*pressure on the bladder,* urine passes only after waiting some minutes.

Frequent micturition.

A feeling as if drops were passing out of the bladder when it is not the case.

During and after urination, heat in the head.

Mucus discharge, periodical, not at each micturition ; sometimes pieces of coagulated mucus clog up the urethra.

Violent burning in the bladder.

†*Feeling as if the bladder were full, and its contents would fall out over the pubes, with constant desire to press them back ;* this feeling of distension of the bladder is different from the pressure downwards, as if everything would be pressed out through the vulva.

†*Urine thick, slimy, and very offensive, depositing a yellowish pasty sedi-*

ment the next morning. †*Urine fetid with much white sediment.* †*The urine when passed is frequently cloudy and dark as though mixed with mucus.* †*Turbid, clay colored urine with red sediment. A brick-dust sediment, and the glass was coated white.*

A white adherent film ; sediment slightly pinkish ; easily dissolved on slight heat, *not* by a few drops of nitric acid (*urates*).

The white film adherent to the glass was removed by *caustic potash, ammonia,* or *nitric acid,* not by water alone, or acetic acid.

Urine, of increased specific gravity, leaves a pink stain on the vessel which is very hard to remove.

°Frequently indicated after *puls., sil., sulph.*

Dark hair. Women.

Sil.—Continuous urging, with scanty discharge.

Urine turbid with red or yellow sand (*uric ac.*) Ischuria.

°*Sil.* is frequently indicated after *bell., bry., calc., cina. graph., hep., ign., nitr. ac., phos.*

°Scrofula. Rachitic anæmic persons ; over sensitive. Mal assimilation.

Spig.—Frequent urging, mostly at night.

Urine drips involuntarily. Whitish sediment.

Spong.—Frequent urging. Enuresis.

Urine scanty, frothy, with thick grayish, white or yellow sediment.

°Women and children. Light hair ; skin and muscles lax.

Squilla.—Fæces escape during micturition.

Frequent urging, with scanty emission.

Continuous painful pressure on the bladder.

Urine red or bloody.

°Useful after *bry.*

Stann.—Deficient urging, as from insensibility of the bladder, which feels full, yet the secretion is scanty. After urination, continued urging.

Urine brown ; milky.

°Follows well after *caust.*

Staph.—Urging after micturition, as if the bladder were not emptied. Frequent urging, with discharge either scanty, in a thin stream ; by drops, of a dark urine ; or profuse, of pale watery urine.

°*Coloc.* and *staph.* act well after each other. Incompatible, *ran. b.*

Stram.—Unusual straining required to empty the bladder, the stream stops before it is emptied, and the ejection has to be completed by several successive efforts, the flow stopping as soon as the bearing down effort is discontinued, *e. g.,* to take breath.

Micturition, dribbling or *guttatim* ; may be accompanied by rigors and rumbling in the abdomen. He cannot hasten the emission or press out the last drops ; no pain, but sensation as if a cylinder were pushed through the urethra.

Could retain the urine, but still felt always as though he had not the power to do so and to close the neck of the bladder; sometimes a sensation as if the urethra were too narrow, and unable to expand.

Urine, dark, pungent, thick and turbid.

Ineffectual urging. *Bladder empty*.

°Young plethoric persons.

Sulph.—Constant painful desire, with discharge of bloody urine— requires great effort to avoid it. Retention. Cutting in the abdomen before urinating.

Urine fetid, with greasy pellicle.

°Intercurrent, or if other remedies have failed. °Followed well by *calc.*, *ars.*, or *carbo. veg.* °Suppressed skin eruptions, gonorrhœa, or hæmorrhoids.

°Lean, stooping persons.

Sulph. ac.—Pain in the bladder if the call to urinate is not acceded to.

Cuticle on the urine. Sediment, blood-like.

°Light hair. Old people ; women.

Follows *arn.* well ; antidotes bad effects of lead water.

Sumbul.—Constant desire, amounting to pressure.

Desire immediately after urinating.

Frequent, ineffectual efforts, with a sensation as if a stool would soon pass; cutting in the arms, and coldness in the back. Frequent desire, sensation as if the bladder were empty, or nearly so.

Urine scanty, ammoniacal.

Sediment, reddish brown, thick, muddy, with an oily pellicle on the urine ; cloudy mucus, with white shreds in it ; rosy pink, clinging to vessel when shaken about; white, tenacious.

Tabac.—Constant desire. Paralysis of the bladder.

Urine, red, offensive, ammoniacal; deposits, urates and mucus.

Tanacet.—Constant desire, not amounting to strangury. Constant desire, with dull heavy pains in the small of the back (secondary). Urine very fetid, high colored (primary).

Tarant.—Cystitis with high fever, gastric derangement, excruciating pains, and ischuria; the bladder is swollen and hard.

Great tenesmus, debilitating the patient, with passage only by drops of a dark red, brown urine, fetid, which deposits a gravel-like sediment.

Tereb.—Strangury. Sensitiveness of the hypogastrium. Tenesmus.

Urine smells sweet, of violets; deposits a slimy, black, muddy sediment.

Thuja.—Frequent urging, with profuse discharge, more towards, and in the evening; with stitches in the urethra.

Stitches from the rectum to the bladder.

Wants to urinate, but feels as if a tape prevented.

Bladder feels paralyzed, has no power to expel the urine.

Continued urging, passes a few drops of blood.

After urinating feels as though a drop were running down the urethra.

Brown mucus sediment.

°Follows well after *merc.*, *nitr. ac.*

°Sycosis.

Uva Ursi.—Strangury. Dysuria. Frequent urging with little discharge, followed by burning cutting pains.

Has to lie on his back to pass urine.

Profuse mucus sediment, very tenacious; pus or blood; passed with great straining.

Valer.—During micturition much straining and prolapsus recti. Red or white sediment.

°Nervous, irritable, hysterical patients.

Verat. a.—Continuous urging. Frequent urination with violent thirst and hunger.

Involuntary discharge on coughing.

°Typhoid. °Anæmia. °Lean, choleric or melancholy persons, children.

Violatric or *Jacea.*—Constant urging and tenesmus, with profuse discharge.

Urine turbid, offensive; smells like that of a cat.

Zinc.—Can only pass urine while sitting bent backwards.

Violent pressure on the bladder; sits with legs crossed; although the bladder feels full, none passes. Enuresis while walking, coughing, sneezing.

Urine turbid; loam colored in the morning.

Frequent emission of a pale yellow urine, which on standing deposits a white flaky sediment; much "sand" in the urine.

°Followed well by *ign.*

Incompatible, *cham.*, *nux. v.*

Zingiber.—Complete retention °in typhus.

Frequent desire, with aching in the kidneys.

Urine thick, dark brown, of a strong smell.

ᵖSchüssler recommends:

Ferr. phos.—Inflammation of the bladder with violent fever. Irritability of the neck of the bladder. Enuresis from weakness of the sphincter. First stage of inflammation, so long as there is no exudation or suppuration.

Kali. mur.—Cystitis, after the fever.

Greenish yellow, or white mucus, like "milk glass."

Kali. phos.—Cystitis, with vomiting; pale face; prostration; dry tongue.

Kali. sulf.—Yellow mucus, especially in chronic cases.

Magn. phos.—Spasmodic retention.

Natr. mur.—Mucus like boiled starch.

(*To be continued.*)

POPULUS IN CYSTITIS.

By JAMES A. FREER, M.D.,

Washington, D. C.

SO AVERSE is the mind of the profession at this day to resurrections from that comprehensive category of our medical armamentarium, which is popularly denominated "trash," that it is not without some trepidity that I approach this subject, but convinced as I am that nine-tenths of what would be passed off as honest conviction by those who cry "trash" is evidence of laziness and lack of investigation, I will pay this small tribute to *populus*—it is a comparatively new drug and has not been thoroughly proven, and so far as records show, but very little used by the homœopathic profession.

I have recently administered it in a few cases of cystitis of different types and in different stages, and with such excellent results that I feel justified in trying to elevate it to a more prominent position as a remedy for this painful and not infrequent affection.

Hale, in his "New Remedies," gives the following concerning the physiological and therapeutical action of this drug, gleaned from the record of the experiments of eclectic and old school practitioners:

"TOXICAL EFFECTS. In doses of five or ten grains in a healthy person it produces a warm, pungent sensation in the stomach, followed by a glow of heat on its entire surface, and a copious discharge of urine, and if the dose is repeated every two hours until forty or fifty grains are taken, it causes nausea, vomiting, and slight purging of bilious matter, with fierce, burning sensation in the stomach, fiery, copious discharge of urine, irritation of bladder and urethra, with slight fullness about the head and general nervous excitement."

"Suppression and retention of urine are readily relieved by *populus*. Paramount to all the rest is its property of relieving painful micturition, heat and scalding of the urine. Did it possess no other curative value, we should consider it an indispensable constituent of our materia medica. Its value in this respect is more apparent when the symptoms above named occur during pregnancy."

"In diseases of the bladder, urethra and prostate, I have found the greatest benefit from this article. In several most inveterate cases of catarrh of the bladder, I have found that two or three grains administered four or five times a day produced a most favorable impression. In the case of an old gentleman who had been troubled with this affection, together with *ardor urinæ* and chronic enlargement of the prostate for many years, and who was not able to obtain benefit from any of the ordinary remedies, relief was promptly given by the use of two grains of *populus* three times a day. The medicine was continued in this case for four or five months."

"In large doses *populus* causes *ardor urinæ*, irritation of the bladder and urethra, with copious discharge of urine."

"In cases cured by me there was little pain during urination, but as soon as the last drops were voided, or a little before, a severe cramplike pain set in just behind and above the pubes; this pain often lasted ten or fifteen minutes."

My attention was first directed to the remedy by an old homœopathic practitioner, who had used it in the case of an old gentleman suffering from irritation at the neck of the bladder, caused by enlargement of the prostate; he suffered intensely from *ardor urinæ*, which lasted for some time after the act of urination. The voided fluid contained a large proportion of pus, which was of vesical origin. *Populus*, two grains, was administered, with the result of producing a decided amelioration of the pain, and at the same time diminishing the amount of pus secreted.

CASE I.—Miss W., æt. 22 years. This was a somewhat complicated and very aggravated case of cystitis. The trouble commenced in an inflammation of the right labium majus, which finally terminated in an abscess. The whole labium was involved and was the seat of most excruciating pain at the time when we first saw it. From the above origin the inflammation extended to the vagina, setting up an intense vaginitis, and adding much to the misery of the patient.

Swelling of the labia now obtained to such an extent that it encroached on the orifice of the urethra, rendering urination progressively more and more difficult, until, in spite of all treatment, this act became impossible without mechanical aid. A catheter was now employed, though with great difficulty, owing to the distortion of the parts caused by the swelling ; the sensibility was allayed by the application of cocaine hydrochlorate, 4% solution.

As the catheter was introduced some of the products of inflammation were carried with it along the urethra, notwithstanding a vaginal douche had been previously used, the result was violent inflammation of the urethra and bladder. The employment of the catheter was obligatory from this time until the abscess was lanced two or three days later, after which the urinary function was re-established.

Cystitis of a high grade now obtained, giving rise to frequent desire for urination, which was accompanied by burning, which increased during the act, reaching its greatest intensity some time after, when the burning and tenesmus at the neck of the bladder were intense. The urine was very scanty, high colored, and contained a large proportion of mucus. The usual remedies were employed as called for by indications, *nux vomica, cantharis, cannabis indica,* etc., being administered, but the condition grew worse, urination became more frequent, and was followed by excruciating burning and tenesmus at the bladder's neck, compelling the patient to cry out. This pain lasted from the end of one act of urination until the beginning of the next, continuing day and night, with a slight aggravation in the early evening, which was followed by some amelioration during the early morning hours, assuming vigor again as the morning advanced to day. The sediment of a specimen of her urine was now examined microscopically and found to contain mucous and pus cells in great abundance, together with some bladder epithelium. Vesical irrigation was now deemed advisable and preparations made for its accomplishment, but owing to the difficulty in introducing the catheter, caused by the nervousness of the patient and the swollen and sensitive condition of the parts, it was postponed. A final search of the therapeutics of cystitis in the meantime led to the selection of *populus,* which was administered in the second decimal potency, a powder every two hours. At the time appointed for irrigating the bladder some abatement in the intensity of the symptoms had taken place ; observing this the local treatment was postponed indefinitely and the *populus* continued at lengthened intervals. Convalescence progressed from this time, and in a few days the urine had cleared up and every symptom of cystitis disappeared.

CASE II.—A young married female, who was a chronic sufferer from uterine displacement, attended with its usual local and reflex symptoms, the latter being of an unusually aggravated type. She was taken with mild symptoms of cystitis, for which she applied promptly for treatment. The local symptoms present were some burning during micturition, which increased after the urine had ceased to flow, when the burning and tenesmus would be intense ; when this was at its height a few drops of blood would be voided, after which the pain would gradually subside.

Several remedies were administered successively during four or five days, but, notwithstanding all, she grew gradually worse.

It was at this juncture that she came under my care. Her urine was very scanty and high colored and the call for micturition, frequent (about once an hour). Urination was accompanied by considerable burning, but the chief part of the pain, as above stated, followed the act and lingered until urging to urinate commenced again. Examination of the urine revealed the presence of a small percentage of albumin, and microscopically, large quantities of vesical epithelium, and mucus which had begun to assume the characteristics of pus.

Populus in the second decimal trituration, was administered, a powder being given once in two hours. The first dose was followed by relief, but the powders being continued, according to directions, in six or eight hours aggravation resulted. The medicine was now interrupted and convalescence progressed satisfactorily, a few powders more being given at long intervals.

On the third day following the beginning of the administration of the *populus* the urine was again examined, and scarcely a vestige of the evidence of her previous trouble remained. Subsequently the trouble returned and was again relieved by *populus*. The tendency to recur led to a vaginal examination, when the uterus was discovered to be anteflexed. This being remedied, no further trouble was experienced from cystitis.

ORIGINAL ARTICLES IN SURGERY.

ABDOMINAL SECTIONS.

By S. H. KNIGHT, M.D.,

House Surgeon, Helmuth House, New York.

THE method of treatment detailed in this article is based upon a series of forty cases, which, since April, 1886, has come under the writer's care as House Surgeon of the Hahnemann Hospital, afterwards at the Diakonissen, and more recently at the Helmuth House. The operations were done mostly by Dr. Helmuth, some few by Drs. F. E. Doughty, and S. F. Wilcox. They include abdominal sections of every description, from a simple exploratory incision to ovariotomies, hysterectomies, laparotomy for volvulus, etc.

When a patient comes to the Helmuth House for a laparotomy, a certain systematic course of preparatory treatment is always carried out. An easily assimilated diet is prescribed, the bowels are regulated, a record of the morning and evening temperature and pulse taken, and the abdomen rubbed daily with vaseline. On the evening before the operation the patient is given a laxative or a cathartic, in order to insure a full movement the next day. On the day of the operation the patient's breakfast consists of coffee, eggs and toast, and, four hours before the operation, she receives a cup of strong beef tea. During the forenoon she has a warm bath, a full enema, a vaginal douche. The abdomen is then shaved. Just before receiving the anæsthetic she passes her water, her abdomen is scrubbed with soap and water, and covered with a solution of iodoform in ether. The ether evaporates, leaving an antiseptic layer, which penetrates even into the pores of the skin. At twenty minutes before the time set for the operation, an hypodermic, consisting of ten (10) mins. of a solution containing *morphiæ sulph.* eight (8) grains, *atropiæ sulph.* one-half (½) grain to the ounce, is administered. This solution quiets the patient, stimulates the heart's action, and, very often, after the operation, secures for her a refreshing nap for an hour or two. The anæsthetic is always ether or the mixed method.

The operation is done in one of the operating rooms on the same floor with the patient. The room is thoroughly cleaned, disinfected with sulphurous oxide, and then shut up for eighteen (18) hours with carbolic vapor. Before the spray is set going, all the linens, towels, etc., to be used, are brought into the room. The instruments are picked out the night before and polished. One-half (½) hour before the operation they are immersed in a 1–4 carbolic acid solution.

As little of the anæsthetic as possible is given the patient. She is kept quiet simply, and once or twice allowed to partially recover consciousness. When the anæsthesia is complete, the chest and legs are covered with a rubber cloth, leaving exposed only that portion of the abdomen which has been covered with the iodoform solution. The incision is made in the median line, through fat and other tissue, down to the peritoneum. All bleeding is now thoroughly stopped, and the peritoneum carefully opened upon a director.

If the condition of affairs be such as not to be readily determined by inspection or by the forefinger, an exploration is now made by the hand. If the tumor comes into view when the peritoneum is opened, a sound is passed about it to determine the amount of adhesions. If there be no adhesions and the tumor be cystic, then the operation is easily finished.

Antiseptic flannels are placed about the incision, the tumor itself drawn closely up to the opening and the trocar plunged in. Smaller cysts within the larger can be broken with the hand and pulled through the wound without enlarging the incision. During all these manipulations, by careful attention to the flannels packed about the incision, not a drop of fluid need enter the abdominal cavity. After the sac has been drawn through the wound, the pedicle is usually secured with Tait's knot. Pure antiseptic silk should be used for the ligature, neither silver wire nor catgut being adapted to the purpose. After searing with the Pacquelin, the pedicle is ready to be replaced within the abdominal cavity.

If the tumor be a fibro-myoma of the uterus and is to be removed by a supra-pubic hysterectomy, the tumor is raised from its bed and brought outside the abdominal cavity—an operation sometimes of great difficulty. If necessary, there should be no hesitancy about lengthening the abdominal incisions. Two (2) Wilcox pins are now thrust through the base of the tumor at right angles, and a stout rubber ligature wound as tightly as possible around the pedicle, below them. Great care must be taken not to include the intestines or bladder. Such a mishap may bring about a fatal result.

The tumor may now be severed from its pedicle, and no matter how vascular it may be, there is absolutely no bleeding from the stump.

The surface of the pedicle should now be seared with the Pacquelin, and the abdominal wall sown up around it. As a rule no drainage tube is necessary, but a small space may be left below the pedicle which will allow the escape of any fluid that may unexpectedly gather in the cavity. The wound is dressed with iodoform and a thick layer of bichloride cotton, all held in place by a muslin body bandage.

Dr. Helmuth attributes his success in the operation of super vaginal hysterectomy—ten (10) pure cases with two (2) deaths—principally to two things : the extra-peritoneal method of treating the stump, and the use of the rubber ligature. In all operations in the abdominal cavity, of first importance are the experience and skill of the operator, but of scarcely less importance is the rapidity of the operation. To this end the assistants should be trained, and should understand what is expected of them. Advantage should be taken of every device to shorten the time necessary for the removal of the tumor.

There is much questioning as to the best method of sewing up the abdominal wound. Interrupted silver stitches passed through the recti muscles and tightly twisted serve every purpose. They can be quickly introduced and are strong enough to resist any vomiting. Even better than silver wire, in that the stitches are rapidly put in and give little pain when taken out, is horse hair.

Unless the operation has been exceptionally long, the patient comes from the table with a flushed face, a good pulse, and regular breathing. She is hurried into a bed previously warmed, and left in quiet with her nurse.

Her pulse and temperature are taken every two hours; plenty of cracked ice is given her, or sips of hot water. Her diet for thirty-six to forty-eight hours consists of a tablespoonful or two of rice or barley water every two (2) hours. Gradually the patient is given a small quantity of peptonized milk, or milk diluted one-half (½) or two-thirds (⅔) with rice water, but no animal food for seven (7) days. Beef tea may then be alternated as a change with the milk or the juice of a steak, or some of the prepared foods, as Murdock's or Liebig's. Patients who say they cannot take milk, will take it if peptonized, diluted with lime water, or flavored with tea. There are some who crave tea and beg for it even on the second day. I always allow them to have it, weak, with no milk or sugar. I have seen it stop vomiting and give the patient more relief than any remedy. Attempts to vary the diet before the seventh day have always been regretted, and are never attempted no matter how well the case progresses. Simple gruels, as oatmeal, rice, arrowroot, etc., can be interchanged with the milk if the patient tires of it. After the seventh day the diet is cautiously increased to the full hospital fare, so that in three (3) weeks the patient eats almost anything.

The shock of the operation may last some thirty-six to forty-eight hours, and needs every effort to combat it. *Camphor, veratrum alb., aconite,* hypodermics of brandy, aromatic spirits of ammonia, all have their use.

The particular symptoms of *camphor* are well known, also *ars.* and *veratrum ; aconite* will be found a good remedy when restlessness, anxiety, wakefulness, high temperature and excitement combine. As a rule, when on the third or fourth day the temperature begins to go up a little, if no other remedy is particularly called for, *aconite* is the one to give. If the patient cannot be quieted in any other way, rather than cause harm by the tossing about, give her a hypodermic of morphine. Unless the patient has used it previously, it is rarely necessary.

For pain from the operation, give *hypericum.* Give it the first night.

Another symptom that will tax the ingenuity of the physician is the vomiting. It comes on, as a rule, as soon as the patient wakes from the ether, partly from the anæsthetic and partly from shock. It may occur only two or three times, or last for three days.

Ice, sips of hot water or tea, long deep breaths, some effervescing water, all help quiet the stomach. For remedies, small doses of *soda bicarb., soda bromide, verat alb., arsenicum, ipecac, nux vom., ant. tart., oxalite of cerium, lacto-pepsine, pepsine wine,* all of these the writer has found useful at some time or other. I have more confidence in *ars.* and

veratrum than any of the others, yet I have seen *lacto-pepsine* check
it when everything else failed.

For a secondary vomiting which accompanies a rise of temperature, and denotes septic peritonitis, Dr. Gil Wylie recommends the use
of an enema, and something as a sedlitz powder to move the bowels.
The writer has seen this tried but once, and though the results were
not so brilliant as in Dr. Wylie's hands, still the patient was relieved.

Septic symptoms may be combatted with *ars., sulpho. carbolat.,
soda, muriatic acid, rhus., lachesis, carbo veg., baptisia, quinine,* etc.
Sulpho carb. of soda and *muriactic acid* are especially useful; sometimes also *quinine.*

There is a condition of flatulent distension with eructation, that almost always follows an abdominal section. The three remedies for
it are, par excellence, *carbo veg., chlorate of potash* and *lycop.* Gas will
escape per rectum, generally in from forty-eight hours to three days.
It may be encouraged by use of the rectal tube and gently turning
the patient slightly on one side. Distention of the abdomen, and failure
of the gas to pass are often disagreeable and obstinate symptoms. The
patient becomes uneasy; eructations and bringing up of food
distress her, and bitter liquids are often vomited. Sometimes the
condition is almost one of stoppage.

Lycop. is the remedy for such conditions. I have never found it
to fail. The fifteenth trituration seems to work better than any other
form.

For two or three days the patient must be kept perfectly still on her
back; after that the nurse may gently turn her a little, and prop her
with pillows.

Unless the patient's bowels give her unusual trouble, nothing need
be done with them until about the seventh day. An enema sometimes fails to secure a good movement, but if one of oil be given, ten
or twelve hours before the water and oxgall, success will be the rule.
After the first movement, with the help of *nux* or *bell.,* they will generally take care of themselves; if not, and repeated enemas are distasteful,
a gluten suppository morning and night, or a preparation of *cascara*
and *maltine* will be very useful.

On the tenth or twelfth day the stitches may be removed. If there
be any stitch hole abscesses, pack them with iodoform. If there be a
pedicle to dress, tighten the rubber ligature every other day, sprinkle
with iodoform, and when it comes off dress with balsam of Peru.

On the fourteenth (14) day the patient sits up, and if all goes well,
in four (4) weeks goes home. Visitors are prohibited until the ninth

or tenth day, when one may be seen for five (5) minutes if deemed advisable, but it is always best for the patient to see as few as possible before leaving the institution.

The following are two of the many cases operated upon at the Helmuth House this winter, and are selected because they show some of the many difficulties which sometimes arise after all seems well.

CASE I.—Cystic tumor of the right ovary. The previous history has no bearing upon the after happening, and the tumor was treated in the way described, except that there were many adhesions, particularly of the pedicle, making it impossible to remove it. Accordingly a small portion of the tumor was included in the ligature. Patient recovered nicely from the shock. Very little vomiting. The patient had been accustomed to the use of morphine, and it was found necessary to administer it for a few days after the operation. At the end of a week the temperature, instead of falling to normal as it ought, rose to 102°–103° at night, with 100° in morning. The pulse stayed between 112–128. She passed a great deal of gas, and her bowels moved several times a day. On the fourteenth day evidences of deep fluctuation could be detected in the median line of the abdomen. Poultices and *hepar sulph.* were ordered, and on the third day an opening was made which let out a pint of the foulest, darkest and rottenest pus. No bottom to the abcess cavity could be felt with the probe. In a day or two the abcess burst of itself in another place, and all in all some gallon of the same foul pus escaped from the cavity. The temperature immediately fell to near normal on letting out the discharge. Poultices were kept up for a week, then the cavity was washed out with a solution of *calendula* and afterwards of per oxide of hydrogen. Her recovery was only a question of time, and she went away in three weeks.

CASE II.—The previous history was of no particular interest. The operation was a simple removal of a small cyst of the right ovary and was completed in thirty (30) minutes. For two days the patient did fairly well, vomiting occasionally. On the third night the patient commenced to vomit fecal matter. This vomiting lasted all night, occurring at very short intervals. Two large enemas of soap suds and oxgall were given with no effect ; also *nux vom.* 3x, every half hour. Her temperature continued about 99⅘ and pulse 88–96. In the morning the patient was very weak and had but little life left. Dr. Helmuth decided that her only chance was to open the wound and see what caused the obstruction in the bowels. This was accordingly done, and the small intestines were found twisted twice around the pedicle. The gut was very much congested and purple, but not black or gray. The twists were straightened out, then returned into the cavity and the wound sewed up. During the operation the patient sank very rapidly, but was kept alive by hypodermics of brandy.

In an hour after the operation her temperature was normal, and pulse 112. The patient vomited once or twice during the day. In about six (6) hours she passed about four (4) ounces of liquid feces through the rectal tube, and in four (4) hours more gas escaped freely without any tube. For a few days her bowels moved five or six times a day, and for two weeks there were pain and tenderness in the right iliac region. Her recovery was rapid.

OPERATION FOR THE ADVANCEMENT OF THE INTERNAL RECTUS MUSCLE OF THE EYE.

By CHARLES C. BOYLE, M.D.,

Surgeon of the New York Ophthalmic Hospital.

WHEN the operation for strabismus was first performed years ago, the eye was as apt to turn in the opposite direction as much as it did in the other.

This was due to the surgeon's loosening the muscle from its attachment to the sclera too much, allowing it to retract and attaching itself so far back as to diminish its power to such an extent as to have the eye turn the other way, that is, if it were originally an internal strabismus, it became an external.

You do not come across a great many of these cases now, as the trouble has been corrected by the eye surgeons of the present day; but occasionally you will meet them, and it is not always that the operation dates very far back, but has been performed by some unskillful hand.

I came across lately a case of this kind; a young woman, who had been operated upon for an internal squint of both eyes, by some traveling quack, with the result that after the operation the eyes turned in the opposite direction, with inability to turn them inwards. I advised an operation; but as she was married, she did not consider it necessary at present.

The only remedy for this result is the advancement of the internal rectus, which has been set back too far, and separating the attachment of the external rectus, allowing that to re-attach itself further back, thus offering less resistance to the other.

This is considered a difficult operation to perform successfully on account of the nice calculation required as to how far forward to bring the muscle. If brought too far forward, you will have the original condition existing, and if not enough, you have not corrected the difficulty.

Not long ago I operated a lady for this deformity, which had resulted from an operation for internal strabismus fifteen years before.

Cocaine was used instead of ether, which is much more satisfactory in this operation, as your patient remains conscious and you can direct her to move her eyes as you wish. I first divided the attachment of the internal rectus, together with the episcleral tissue, as far back as the equator of the eyeball, and then made a cut with my scissors above and below, on a line with the upper and lower margins of the cornea, extending inwards as far as the tissue was loosened from its attachment, thus forming a tongue-shape piece of conjunctiva, which included on its under surface the tendon of the internal rectus, which was to be brought forward for re-attachment.

This was drawn forward and five sutures passed through it near its free end as far back as considered necessary; the needles of the sutures were then passed through the corresponding part of edge of conjunctiva, which had been left for that purpose on inner border of cornea.

The threads were now drawn together; but before tying, it is necessary to see if you are bringing the muscle too far forward or not enough; it appeared sufficient; then the portion of the tongue in front of suture was cut off and the edges of the wound brought together by tying the sutures. After this the attachment of the external rectus was divided and a double thread was passed through a fold of conjunctiva in front of the attachment of external rectus; this thread, which was to draw the eyeball inwards, thus relieving the strain on the five sutures, was fastened by plaster to the bridge of the nose.

After the operation was finished, patient was placed in bed and ice bags kept on eye to keep down the subsequent inflammation which necessarily follows.

On removing sutures the third day, I discovered that I had overcorrected the difficulty slightly, causing a slight internal strabismus; but when the eye had recovered from the first operation, I corrected this by loosening the new attachment of the internal rectus slightly, just enough to make the correction, with the result that the eyes were straight and remained so.

A CRITIQUE.

By HENRY SHERRY, M.D.,

Chicago, Ill.

BEFORE me lies the March number of the *Polyclinic*. Turning over its leaves, the first article is a clinical lecture by John Ashurst, Jr., M.D., Professor of Clinical Surgery in the University of Pennsylvania. The author has not only a national, but an international reputation. I expect, therefore, to find here something worth the reading ; and as I read down the page, here is what he says :

"The first patient that I bring before you this morning is suffering from a compound fracture of the right leg. * * * Dr. Wharton * * * * finding a small wound of the integument and no apparent injury of the great vessels, made the attempt, as should always be done, to convert the fracture into a simple one by covering the wound with a little lint soaked in compound tincture of benzoin. I saw the case the day following and continued the same treatment. Yesterday, however, I found the limb swollen, and it was evident that suppuration was taking place. I therefore removed the pledget of lint and enlarged the opening. I also made an incision upon the inner side of the limb where the skin was very tense and where sloughing was imminent. * * * * * In addition to making the incisions before referred to, I applied over the entire leg a poultice."

That a great surgeon should advocate such primitive methods of treating such a solution of continuity in this year of our Lord one thousand eight hundred and eighty-seven, hardly seems possible. Instead of being content to wait for developments, which was virtually the course followed, the wound in the integument should have been enlarged, and all broken down tissue, clotted blood and splinters of bone removed, a counter opening at the point of greatest bagging made and a drainage tube inserted ; the leg, from the toes to above the knee, encased in a thoroughly antiseptic dressing ; over this a fixed dressing of plaster, reinforced by strips of tin or zinc.

Again, by what process of reasoning a man arrives at the conclusion that a poultice is the proper thing for tissue rapidly going to destruction, is another pathologico-surgical puzzle.

Further down the page I read as follows:

"After a time we shall apply some simple dressing, such as alcohol or a simple unguent."

In answer to such teaching, I do not hesitate to say that salves, cerates, ointments, etc., are an abomination and a direct prevention of the pathological reparative process, as we understand it to-day.

Should any so-called irregular practitioner follow out the teachings herein described by Professor Ashurst and the result prove disastrous, I have no doubt but that surgeons of the dominant school would accuse him of criminal malpractice.

EDITORIAL DEPARTMENT.

The Editors individually assume full responsibility for and are to be credited with all connected with the collection and presentation of matter in their respective departments, but are not responsible for the opinions of contributors.

It is understood that manuscripts sent for consideration have not been previously published, and that after notice of acceptance has been given, will not appear elsewhere except in abstract and with credit to THE NORTH AMERICAN. All rejected manuscripts will be returned to writers. No anonymous or discourteous communications will be printed.

Contributors are respectfully requested to send manuscripts and communicate respecting them directly with the Editors, according to subject, as follows: *Concerning Medicine, 21 West 37th Street; concerning Surgery, 256 West 57th Street; concerning Societies and Hospitals, 111 East 70th Street; concerning News, Personals and Original Miscellany, 461 West 71st Street; concerning Correspondence, 152 West 57th Street.*

Communications to the Editor-in-Chief, *Exchanges* and *New Books* for notice should be addressed to *102 West 43d Street.*

BOOK REVIEWING.

IN very many cases the reviewer of a book seems to be totally at fault in his views as to his province and the proper execution of his task. We find some conscientious workers whose review of a book is of practical value to the readers, but the great majority appear to be in league with all parties concerned, including themselves, against the medical public, to whom alone they should hold themselves directly responsible. Many seem to be under the impression that the total significance of a review is either to flatter it as much as an exceedingly plastic conscience will admit, in order to cajole the publisher and author into good humor, or to be able to add another volume to their library with as little personal effort as a most cursory glance between the covers renders possible.

Neither of these considerations should in the least influence a conscientious reviewer. Readers look to this department of journalistic literature for a reliable and honest estimate by one capable of forming such an opinion of a book of which they may stand in need. It must be remembered that the majority of readers are not fortunate enough to reside where medical literature is published or kept in large stock. They must form their opinion largely from reviews. If a book be worthy it should by all means be praised; but if it be of a different nature, the reviewer who, for selfish and unworthy reasons, either applauds it, knowing its deficiencies, or without any proper examination of its subject matter, dismisses it with a reproduction of its table of contents, is not only guilty of a gross abuse of duty and privilege, but also lowers the authoritativeness of his journal and voluntarily throws away the respect and confidence of his readers.

A thorough and trustworthy review of a book is no easy task, and there is a very strong temptation for those whose dominant characteristic is a love of personal ease, to shamelessly shirk. Honesty in work is always a matter of prime importance in all departments, but it is especially essential now in this field of literary labor. Books, good, bad, and indifferent, are fairly deluging the market; many are published with no other thought than personal display and advertising. There appears to be no *raison d'être* for such works; the authors have no new information to impart, nor even a good classification of what has already appeared. And yet such books receive from some derelect reviewer a favorable criticism, which is eagerly seized by the publishers, and the book is boomed, and foisted on a deceived profession. The various journals should see that books are reviewed not only by one who is willing to give a fair opinion, but also by one who is thoroughly qualified to criticise the subject matter itself from a more than ordinary amount of learning in that particular branch of which the book treats. Books on special subjects should be reviewed by specialists in that department. It is eminently absurd for one who knows only the rudiments of a subject to attempt to guide one who is deeply versed, in the selection of his special library. Many of the books now published are almost worthless, and the journals owe it to the profession to expose the true inwardness of such publications. It is only by fair, honest, fearless criticism that medical literature can be kept upon the high plane of its best publications and the profession prevented from being constantly duped into purchasing books which are not only unworthy of the subject of which they treat, and of the valuable time of the physician, but tend directly to the degeneration of medical literature.

ONE of the most lasting impressions made on our minds by the National Conventions of Homœopathists held this year is the marked tendency to rely upon clinical and empirical experience rather than upon the pure provings of drugs. To our mind this is most lamentable, for there is nothing more sure than that success in the treatment of disease is in direct ratio to the practice of homœopathy. The causes of this departure are not far to seek. It is so easy to copy others, to try a remedy because some one has had good results after using it, and it is not so easy to study and remember our symptomatology. The decadence of homœopathy will begin just at this point, and will involve a resort to more medicine of the wrong sort to produce an impression which one fails to get from small doses of the improperly selected remedy, to all sorts of expedients, and finally to allopathic methods in general. Empiricism cannot be covered up by fluxion potencies, and while it was rampant at the American Institute of Homœopathy, it was also rife at the meeting of the Internationals. It seems a double crime to select a remedy which has never been proved and then to administer it in a potency which is purely mythical, so the note of warning must be sounded. Let us adhere to our law, and excuse cannot now be made that our materia medica is too fragmentary or too inaccessible; the trouble really is, doctors are too much disinclined to study it.

Excuse can be made that nearly all of our physicians are overworked. There seems to be no doubt that the average homœopathic physician does the work of about two average allopathic physicians, and the homœopathist has too little time to study. Some good advice was given to medical students by a professor of materia medica, when they were told to study their first cases with the greatest care *while they had time*, and so gradually accumulate an accurate knowledge of indications for the use of remedies, which would serve them well when they became busy and were often obliged to prescribe rapidly. One of the most accurate prescribers in our school is said to be one of the most rapid prescribers; a few telling questions bring out the exact information required and the remedy is decided upon. This facility—the knowing how to put the questions—has slowly grown with the increasing experience of the prescriber, who, in his earlier days, when patients were few and far between, labored with his symptoms till the key was found.

It has elsewhere been urged that a materia medica, simplified and condensed, was needed to make better homœopathists of us. It is also needed to purify the materia medica we now have—but that is an old theme and well worn; it only occurred to us by seeing a copy of "Hering's Guiding Symptoms," which is a great work, but not one for homœopathy. Such guides lead surely to empiricism and allopathy.

The *Medical Record* of this city is in a "state of mind." Poor *Record!* Some months ago when the Laura Franklin Hospital was opened it cried that to place such a splendid endowment under the charge of homœopathic physicians and surgeons was a crime against civilization, a blot on the nineteenth century, and all that sort of thing. We wonder if it will eat its words when it receives the first annual report of the Institution and compares the results with those of other similar institutions? But just now it is the Cook County Hospital of Chicago. Here is what it says in its issue for September 3d, 1887 :

"MIXED HOSPITAL BOARDS AND THE MORTALITY RATE.

"The annual reports of the Cook County Hospital reveal some facts in which the profession should feel some interest. On the opening pages we find a list of the members of the 'regular medical board,' and below of the 'homœopathic medical board.' Such juxtaposition seems a little at variance with conventional ethics, but in this we may be mistaken.

"The point that is of real importance is, that both in its totals and in the medical and surgical departments the mortality of patients treated by the homœopathic medical board is less than that of the regular board. And this is true not for one year, but apparently for a series of years. For example, in 1884, the mortality on the regular medical side was about $\frac{1}{11}$ of the total treated (406 to 4,692), that on the homœopathic side about $\frac{1}{12}$ (103 to 1,242).

"In 1885-86 the figures were for the regular school $\frac{1}{13}$ (448 to 5,909) to $\frac{1}{15}$ (105 to 1,532), and a similar excess of mortality rate is carried through the medical and surgical departments.

"It is possible that the cases sent to the homœopathic side are of the less severe and acute character. Unless some such explanation as this exists, the reproach upon the skill of the regular medical staff is a severe one. Hospital statistics are extremely fallacious things, to be sure, and no inferences should be drawn from them without careful examination. But in the Cook County Hospital such examination seems demanded."

We should think that some examination was demanded! and not only an examination of the methods by which in Cook County Hospital the homœopathists come out ahead, but an inquiry into the meaning of the superior results reported from the Middletown Asylum for the Insane and from every hospital where homœopathy is practiced. We can enlighten the *Medical Record*, or rather we believe that the *Medical Record* knows already perfectly well that homœopathy is a superior method of therapeutics. Why not say so? Why not advocate it? Is there any earthly reason why every physician should not do the best for his patients? Are you afraid?

THE fact is, that before long the homœopathic law will have to be taught in all medical schools. "Regular" physicians want to know about it, and the fear of the "Knights of Labor" of the American Medical Association is dying out.

THE records of the Cook County Hospital are not so remarkable as we might expect. Frequently the comparisons have been much more favorable to homœopathy; often a difference of fifty per cent. in the mortality rates. We are driven to the conclusion that the allopathic practice in that hospital is remarkably good; that mild measures and good nursing is the rule. The difference between eight per cent. for the allopaths and seven per cent. for the homœopaths is not enough. Cannot the homœopaths give still less medicine?

WE were quite impressed this summer by the remark of a wise and far-seeing president of one of our celebrated universities, that non-sectarian institutions did not, as a rule, flourish well; that a "*sect,*" both in theology and medicine, was a good thing to develop power and evolve truth. "While I do not employ a homœopathic physician, I believe the founding of that school has been of inestimable benefit to humanity, and I hope it will stick to its colors and not seek to be absorbed by the regulars, falsely so called." There seems to be a decided and increasing respect for the homœopathic school as a school of medicine. It is no longer looked at askance, nor are its members considered half educated, box-and-a-book men. We are winning our place in the community, and also in the profession at large, by a steadfast adherence to our principles, while those who try to ride the fence and "practice both ways," lose all respect. Illustrations of this are multiplying about us daily.

COMMENTS.

SAVING THE GOLD.—The student of the eighteenth century no longer hopes or expects to compress within the narrow limits of his cranium the knowledge he longs to possess, and although he may grow in learning so that he rivals Goldsmith's schoolmaster, and the wonder may be how one small head can carry so vast a load of erudition, yet the greater and sometimes the better part of his learning and wisdom is to be found arrayed on his book-shelves, ready to hand. properly arranged and classified. For it is not what a man holds by sheer force of memory that is always most valuable or sensible, but a skill in knowing just what information is wanted, where to find it, and how to use it to the best advantage when found. As the knight of old, laying aside his cumbersome and oppressive armor, retained, perhaps, the graceful Damascus blade for the ordinary combats of the day, but when serious battle threatened, sought his armor and more ponderous weapons, so the scholar of to-day, well-equipped for common strife, when more serious warfare comes, retires to his study and there finds the weapons that he needs. But only those can arm themselves who possess an armory kept in careful order. Physicians are too apt to allow their weapons to rust for want of use. A want of method is the worse enemy some physicians have. They seem to have no idea of classified knowledge, either as carried by the brain or as stored in a library. Books are purchased, magazines are received, yet but little benefit is derived from them all. They may be read and some suggestion at once acted upon, made the reader's own, but the greater part of information lies forgotten and buried beneath fresh arrivals. And so the doctor's weapons, which should be kept bright by frequent inspection, are allowed to rust in confusion on the floor. When some especial information is wanted in haste, how does then the medical man hie him to 'his study and view, with rueful countenance, the wilderness of disorder before him. How often failure follows attempt to find, and even if successful, how tedious the search. A little system would change all this. A habit of noting valuable articles or suggestions in the various journals, and recording in a reference book, kept specially for the purpose, the date and name of the magazine and title of the selection or article, would afford a ready means of reference in future time. This simple index could, of course, be enlarged upon in many ways. But by its use alone the gold in the books and journals would be saved for each one to use when wanted. Then the journals, instead of being a nuisance and littering up the room, would be welcomed as aids in the warfare with disease.

MEDICAL JOURNALISM.—If we assert that the secular press mirrors forth each day society as it really exists—its wants, its aspirations, its attainments, its blunders and crimes;—if we agree that the religious papers reflect, with tolerable accuracy, the condition of affairs in the religious and theological world, then we are prepared to admit that the medical journals of to-day paint for us, weekly and monthly, a truthful and unflattering picture of the medical world as it is at the present moment. Medical journalism is controlled by the same inexorable laws that rule supreme in the management of ordinary journals. The daily paper has been said to be the history of the world for a day. In a certain limited sense this is true. And because this is true it follows that the paper cannot, and does not (with rare exceptions), rise above the people whose deeds and words it reproduces. It caters to the masses. It seeks patronage. It tries every method by which the list of subscribers may be increased. In other words, it prints to live, and by no means lives to print. It cannot rise above its source. It must print what its readers want and bend to their wishes, or lose ground rapidly. This is not a description of an ideal paper. By no means. It is a description of the newspaper of to-day—the practical paper. It knows what the people want and prints it. No market has ever been found for the paper no one wanted. If too many of our papers are vulgar, sensational and coarse, it is not primarily the fault of the press. The people demand it and the demand is supplied. The remedy obviously is to educate the readers of papers, and so elevate their minds and morals that a demand shall arise for something better. The multiplicity of medical journals is undoubtedly an evil. But it is an evil whose roots are embedded in the profession itself. An over-supply of medical journals inevitably brings cheapness and mediocrity. And if a certain number of imperfectly edited and inferior journals attain a sufficient circulation to sustain life, are we to blame them for their continued existence? The profession supports them and is responsible for their continuance. The medical press will become whatever the profession requires whenever the demand is made. The question of the elevation of the medical press resolves itself into the question of the elevation of the profession. So it is that while the journals may do much to elevate and quicken, the profession owes a similar duty to the press. Consideration does not necessarily improve a paper, nor is a high price always an index of worth. As is the doctor, so is his journal.

MIXED HOSPITAL BOARDS AND THE MORTALITY RATE.—Under the above caption the editor of the *Medical Record* (September 3d, 1887), writes: "The annual reports of the Cook County Hospital reveal some facts in which the profession should feel some interest. On the opening pages we find a list of the members of the 'regular medical board,' and below of the 'homœopathic medical board.' Such juxtaposition seems a little at variance with conventional ethics; but in this we may be mistaken. The point that is of real importance is, that both in its totals and in the medical and surgical departments, the mortality of patients treated by the homœopathic medical board is less than that of the regular board. And this is true not for one year, but apparently for a series of years. For example, in 1884 the mortality on the regular medical side was about $\frac{1}{11}$ of the total treated (406 to 4,692), that on the homœopathic side about $\frac{1}{12}$ (103 to 1,242). In 1885–6 the figures were: for the regular school $\frac{1}{13}$ (448 to 5,909) to $\frac{1}{15}$ (105 to 1,532), and a similar excess of mortality rate is carried through the medical and surgical departments. It is possible that the cases sent to the homœopathic side are of the less severe and acute character. Unless some such explanation as this exists, the reproach upon the skill of the regular staff is a severe one. Hospital statistics are extremely fallacious things, to be sure, and no inferences should be drawn from them without careful examination. But in the Cook County Hospital such examination seems demanded." Comment is unnecessary.

TWO POPULAR DELUSIONS.—Among the beliefs widely prevalent with the laity these two stand prominently forward—that fish is a brain food of great value and an exceedingly good diet for invalids, and that ice is always pure, no matter how filthy the water from which it was formed. Nor is it at all certain but that the profession has held, at different times, these same sadly erroneous beliefs; indeed, it is feared that some even yet cling to the fish as an article of diet especially created for the sick room. The truth is that fish, as a brain food, is worth no more, nor as much, as many other foods, and as an article of diet for sick rooms, in the majority of cases, is absolutely injurious. Relapses have been caused frequently by fish when given after fevers and nervous complaints. Loss of weight followed a fish diet and very promptly. It should be stricken from the diet card for sick rooms. To convince the average man that ice is or can be filthy is a hard task. But it can be done, and the people should be taught that ice may be as unfit for use as water, and for the same reason, that freezing does not remove all impurities, nor kill disease germs. It is true that some of the frozen matter is eliminated in congelation, but not all. The fact should be proclaimed that ice from stagnant pools or water that contains refuse of any kind, is not fit for use—that it may breed disease and death.

BOOK REVIEWS.

A PRACTICAL TREATISE ON THE DISEASES OF THE HAIR AND SCALP, by Geo. Thomas Jackson, M.D., Instructor in Dermatology in the New York Polyclinic; Assistant Visiting Physician to the New York Skin and Cancer Hospital, etc. 356 pages. E. B. Treat, 771 Broadway, New York. 1887.

Before considering the diseases of the hair and scalp, the author gives three valuable chapters on the anatomy and physiology of the hair, and hygiene of the scalp and hair. The latter chapter is particularly interesting and contains many sensible suggestions. The diseases are classified and treated of under the following heads: Essential Diseases of the Hair, Parasitic Diseases of the Hair, and Diseases of the]Hair secondary to Diseases of the Skin. The ordinary and many very unusual diseases are described under their appropriate heads. The diagnosis, including the symptoms and differentiation from allied disorders and treatment is particularly full. The illustrations add but very little to the book, as they are indistinct and would be of no service in assisting one to recognise a disease. Great numbers of citations from different authors are made, and, as illustrating their individual views of disease and treatment, are valuable. We believe they should be incorporated. What the author has failed in doing, however, and which is of great importance, is to make any satisfactory deductions from the many conflicting and dissimilar quotations. An author is supposed to have had a certain amount of experience with the remedies suggested by others and to have been able to form some definite ideas regarding the correctness of their hypothesis in the question of etiology and pathology. If he has not such information, the writing of the book had best be deferred till he has gathered it. If he possesses the knowledge, he should give the reader the benefit of his longer experience and not compel him to experiment with a mass of empirical remedies till he has found the one which is of service. In this respect the book is not as valuable as it should have been made. The chapter on parasitic diseases is not so open to criticism on this ground, the author here giving the treatment which his own experience has found valuable. The new remedies in most cases are, no doubt, good; but we should like to know which is the best.   F.

HASCHISCH. A Novel. By Charles Galchell, M.D. (Thorold King). Chicago: A. C. McClurg & Co. 1886. 314 pages.

As might be expected from its title, this work of fiction deals with certain problems in the domain of medicine not yet wholly solved. In fact, the turning point of the story hangs upon what may be termed "unconscious cerebration." It is, as an old lady once remarked of another work, "a medicated novel." The plot is strong, the characters well defined, and the action is brisk. The style is vigorous and carries the reader easily on to the conclusion. If at times somewhat of the machinery is visible and the tale drags slightly, these are faults that may be excused, for they are not grave. For summer reading, Dr. Galchell's book is to be recommended. It will pass away some leisure hours very pleasantly and afford food for reflection after the book is completed and the covers closed. The book is well bound and excellently printed.

CORRESPONDENCE.

To the Editors of the NORTH AMERICAN JOURNAL OF HOMŒOPATHY :

About the first subject of a medical nature which engages the attention of a practitioner who has started on a European journey, is that very usual affliction to those who travel by sea—"sea-sickness." If he experiences personally the *mal de mer*, he is forced to be interested, and gets a pretty fixed idea of its symptoms and their sequence ; on the other hand, if he is fortunate enough to escape this reversal in the onward course of matter, the affection still remains one of great interest to the profession, from the fact that most measures taken to prevent it have heretofore generally failed to insure immunity from attacks of less or greater severity.

It may be assumed, I think, without here stating the reasons for the assumption, that sea-sickness (as a certain writer said of poverty) "is an unmitigated curse;" to reason otherwise—that an attack is beneficial—is to forget the causes which led to it, and that ordinary health after an attack seems in comparison like the most perfect type of well-being, therefore, all proper means to prevent or relieve an affection which robs ocean travel of much of its pleasure, both anticipated and real, and also causes much individual suffering—may well interest the mind and duty of physicians.

Like many another illness, the *causes* of *mal de mer* are probably not of a nature to be prevented wholly, if at all. Of the various theories of the causation of sea-sickness, two only, it appears to me, are worthy of consideration. 1st. The continuous moving acts through the optic nerve to set up disturbance in the nervous centers, which is reflected through the nerves which supply the stomach and other parts engaged in vomiting. 2d. The *up* and *down* motion of the vessel so gravitates the blood in the larger venous trunks as to produce more or less cerebral anæmia, and leads to reflex nausea and vomiting. The former theory is weak. Continuous and even more rapid movement of objects before the eyes in land travel, does not cause symptoms similiar to sea-sickness, except with comparatively few individuals. The second and latter explanation is supported by the fact that the smallest per cent. of cases occur amid-ships where there is the least up and down motion, and that taking the recumbent position, with the head low—sometimes lower than the feet, ameliorates the symptoms to some degree.

If the causes (known or unknown) cannot be removed so as to prevent sea-sickness, we may try to anticipate or relieve its most annoying effects; here the law of "similiars" undoubtedly is of great service, not by selecting *our* remedy on general principles, but by carefully choosing one adapted to the needs of *each individual.* I am quite aware of the skepticism in regard to this matter among the profession, but from my experience during the past four years in giving remedies to prevent sea-sickness, I believe the doubt arises more from the results obtained from too general prescribing rather than from any failure of the law. Remembering my personal acquaintance with sea-sickness twenty years ago, and having this time taken a homœopathic preventative (successfully, as it proved), I was glad of an opportunity to observe the attacks in others, and to watch the effects of drugs given to afford relief. In the dozen cases under observation, in no instance did the medicine fail to relieve the annoying symptoms in a few hours, and led to speedy recovery when the indications were clear for the remedy used; while other cases, not under close attention, but known, and treated, if at all, empirically, were in many instances ill for days. The drugs found most useful were *tobaccum, petrolĕum, cocculus* and *nux vomica.* In exceptional instances, when clear indications were wanting, *cocoaine tablets,* used empirically, were efficacious.

Dr. Doughty, with whom I spent a day at Interlacken, had also found them useful in the nausea and vomiting of sea-sickness.

In my cases no effort was made to regulate the diet beyond the avoidance of soups of all kinds. Iced champagne, as heretefore, was found the most refreshing of drinks as soon as the stomach permitted the indulgence, even the over scrupulous might say in their cases *venia necesitati datur.*

Regarding the many Alpine health resorts for which Switzerland is deservedly known, little need be said; our own country is probably equally endowed by nature, but in many places yet remains less accessible than those distant places. Of those I have visited, Lucerne and its vicinity appears to afford the most advantages; the lake is ever present to charm the eye, and the surrounding mountains speak of rest and strength. Mt. Rigi is so accessible by boat and rail, that one may reach almost any altitude with ease, and find accomodations for comfort. Even the climate varies on different sides of the mountain, from mild on the southern slopes, to the more stimulating atmosphere on the northern. If invalids are in doubt as to the locality best suited to their needs, it is wise to consult some local medical practitioner, who is familiar with the various situations. At whatever altitude chosen, mountain climbing, which has (properly regulated) proved so beneficial in cardiac and other troubles, may be indulged in to any extent desired.

After a day or two at Geneva, I hope to see something of the hospitals of Paris during the balance of time remaining, and to meet some of the prominent members of our school, and especially to secure the promise of regular material for the JOURNAL.

H. M. DEARBORN.

Lausanne, Aug. 1887.

To the Editor of the NORTH AMERICAN JOURNAL OF HOMŒOPATHY:

DEAR SIR—One is surprised on visiting the different hospitals and clinics of Paris to find so great a number of medical students in attendance, and there is much more activity in medical study than one would imagine.

My principal object in visiting Paris was to study Dr. Apostoli's method of treating uterine fibroids, and other diseases peculiar to woman, by electrolysis, and it is to this I wish to call your attention. Dr. Apostoli's clinic is held in a very poor part of the city three times a week. Patients come to it as they do to any out-patient clinic in New York—some coming on the recommendation of those who have been benefited, while others are sent by their medical advisers.

The number of cases in attendance at each clinic is from twenty to thirty. More than half of these are cases of uterine fibroids, the remainder being various diseases peculiar to women, but principally chronic metritis and sub-involution.

Dr. Apostoli's clinics are open to the profession for inspection—every clinic being witnessed by physicians from various parts of the world. English physicians have made it a special study and are applying the same methods in their country with success.

Dr. Apostoli and his assistants not only extend a cordial welcome to all visitors, but insist upon their making examinations to satisfy themselves as to the correctness of the diagnosis. I also examined a few cases that were treated from one to three years ago and who are as well to-day as when discharged cured by Dr. Apostoli, thus proving the completeness and permanency of the cure.

All cases of uterine fibroids are amenable to treatment, but the hemorrhagic and non-hemorrhagic require the application of different poles. With the former the positive electrode is used internally; with the latter, the negative.

Very powerful currents are used ranging from 100 to 250 milli-ampères.

To illustrate its prompt action in checking hemorrhage, I can do no better than to give the history of a case that came under my observation : One evening about the 1st of August, one of Dr. Apostoli's assistants was sent for by a physician to try and ·check a hemorrhage due to a sub-mucous fibroid, which had been treated by him without effect, until the patient had become so anæmic that it was apparent, unless something was done to check the flow, the patient would die. He inserted a positive electrode and let on a current of 250 milli-ampères. The hemorrhage was decreased almost instantly.

The next day the hemorrhage was scarcely perceptible.

The third day she was treated in the same way as before, when the hemorrhage entirely ceased and has not yet showed any signs of returning.

The cases of sub-involution and chronic metritis are treated with the Faradic current. A double electrode is inserted in the uterine cavity and a strong Faradic current allowed to pass. The muscular fibres of the uterus are made to contract so that the cavity of the uterus will measure from one-eighth to one-half inch less at the end of the treatment than it did at the beginning, thus cutting off the supply of extra nutrition and causing the uterus to come back to its normal size.

In conclusion, I wish to say one could not witness the great care taken in making a diagnosis, the complete clinical record kept, and the thorough antiseptic precautions used, without feeling the sincerity of Dr. Apostoli and his assistants.   W. H. KING, M. D.

PARIS, August 10th, 1887.

REPORTS OF SOCIETIES AND HOSPITALS.

HOMŒOPATHIC MEDICAL SOCIETY OF THE COUNTY OF NEW YORK.

THE regular monthly meeting of the New York Homœopathic County Medical Society was held in the Reception Room of the New York Opthalmic Hospital, corner of Twenty-third Street and Third Avenue, Thursday evening, June 9th, 1887.

President Beebe in the chair.

Dr. W. Storm White, Chairman of the Committee of Pathology and Preventive Medicine, presented the following papers :

"Difficulty of Diagnosing Tumors of the Thorax and Abdomen, with Specimens," J. M. Schley, M.D.; "Histology in its Relations to the Pathology of Diseases," J. W. Dowling, Jr., M.D.; "Carcinoma, Pathologically Considered," W. Storm White, M.D; "Specimen of Bronchial Cast, from a Case of Croupous Bronchitis," C. E. Beebe, M.D.

Dr. J. M. Schley presented the first paper.

Dr. Knight :—I should simply like to say, in confirmation, that the question of diagnosis of tumors of the abdomen is very difficult. It reminds me of the old saying that seeing is believing, for it is only by seeing them that one can be positive. My experience at the Helmuth House leads me to believe that very few understand diseases of the abdomen. Those who see cases only occasionally are apt to make mistakes. Many cases are sent to us for operation where the diagnosis is wrong. One case diagnosed as an abscess of the spleen turned out to be simply fatty abdominal wall. Another case diagnosed as an ovarian tumor turned out to be pregnancy, with the fœtal heart sounds to be plainly heard over the abdominal walls. Another case diagnosed as cancer of the omentum, in which the symptoms were very similar to this disease, proved to be, on *post-mortem* examination, an intestinal obstruction located just where the large and small intestines join. Again, patients are sent where the tumors, although existing two or three years with circumscribed dullness, etc., promptly disappear on the administration of ether. Other cases, really ovarian tumors, come to us diagnosed as ascites, Bright's disease, disease of the liver, etc.

Experts, however, can make pretty definite conclusions.

When it is possible it is better to make an exploratory incision ; it can be done without much danger if the proper precautions are applied. I have seen a number of them performed with no bad results.

It is advised by such men as Thomas, Emmet, Tait and Helmuth.

Tait says he now commences with an exploratory incision and ends with an ovariotomy, where he used to commence with an ovariotomy and end with an exploratory incision.

It ought to be made if the patient has a chance to get through it.

Dr. Fulton : — Before reaching a positive diagnosis in abdominal tumors it is necessary, in many cases, to see that the bowels are thoroughly opened by a strong cathartic.   Many such tumors will disappear under its influence.   In one case of mine diagnosed as abdominal tumor, in which the dullness was circumscribed and the tumor had a boggy feeling, I gave a strong cathartic as a diagnostic measure, and in a few days the tumor and the symptoms had entirely disappeared.

Dr. J. W. Dowling, Jr., then presented his paper.   As there was no discussion, Dr. W. Storm White read his paper on "Carcinoma, Pathologically Considered."

Dr. Knight :—I should like to ask Dr. White if in his investigation he has found, or is there claimed to be, a distinctive pathognomonic cancer cell.

Dr. White :—In answer to Dr. Knight's question, I would say that there is no such cell.   None has ever been discovered.   The cells are not true epithelial cells, but are epithelioid elements.   The microscopic diagnosis of carcinoma does not lie in the character of the cell, but rather in the peculiar alveolar arrangement of the fibrous net-work which incloses the cells.

Dr. Fulton :—In classifying cancers as connective tissue growths, Dr. White is at variance with nearly all of the best authorities upon malignant growths.   With scarcely an exception, they agree that the sarcomata belong to that group, but that the carcinomata should be classified as epithelial in nature and origin.   In this, Virchow, Billroth, Ashurst, Holmes, and all American authorities agree.   They base the epithelial nature of cancer upon the following grounds: that true carcinoma (and the alveolar sarcoma must be distinguished from cancer), do not develop except in structures which are essentially epithelial in nature and origin.   Lately the researches of His and Waldeyer have shown that the peritoneum, pleura and pericardium, instead of being formed from the mesoblast, as was supposed, are diverticula from the gastro-intestinal tract, and are, therefore, epithelial in origin, and is first lined with true epithelium, which ultimately becomes flattened.   This removes almost the last objection to considering carcinoma epithelial in origin.

In bone and muscle, which are the two typical, connective tissue groups, true primary carcinoma do not exist.   Secondary deposits are another matter.   In older writers and in those at present who do not distinguish between the sarcomata and carcinomata, cancers of such structures are reported, but it is probable that all such neoplasms should be classified as sarcomata.   As the distinction is becoming recognized, cases of true primary carcinoma of the bones and muscles are becoming almost unknown, and it is probable that in cases which are put down as such, there has been a faulty diagnosis.

The cell contents of carcinoma do not in the least resemble connective tissue elements, but are exactly like the epithelial cells found in other parts of the body.   The similarity is so exact that it is an impossibility, with our present methods of investigation, to differentiate a malignant cell element from the epithelium lining the ducts of the kidney, lobules of the lungs, or the glandular portion of the active breast.

They all, in common with the malignant cell, have a round, oval, or caudate form, are more or less granular in appearance, and possess, in the great majority of cases, one nucleus, although sometimes two are detected.   As Dr. White says, there is no typical cancer cell, and this fine distinction between epithelioid elements and epithelium is merely a multiplication of terms, to the utter confusion of the student.   The diagnosis of cancer is made from the peculiar arrangement of the cells and their investing stroma.

Dr. White also excluded, in his classification, the epithelioma from the group of cancers.   Practical experience has shown that the epithelioma is as deadly in the long run as the scirrhus or encephaloid. The histological elements also are epithelial, precisely as are those of the latter growths. I assisted Dr. Thompson in the removal of a growth on the thumb, which had softened and destroyed the soft tissues and bone to such an extent that amputation at the wrist was necessary. The microscope showed it to be a pure epithelioma in an advanced stage. All the rational symptoms of cancer were present and the malignancy was certain. Another specimen which I have, taken from a breast which I twice excised, shows in the superficial granulations the characteristic pegs and pearls of the epithelioma, while below, in the deeper portion, the delicate and widely-meshed alveolar arrangement of the encephaloid is observed. We should scarcely expect to find growths in the same specimen which had no common relationship as to character and origin. Both on technical and pathological grounds I believe that the epithelioma should be classified among the cancers. The great work of pathologists at present is not analytical, but synthetical.

Dr. White :—My classification is taken directly from Cornil and Renvier, who are certainly good authority. In answer to Dr. Fulton's statement that they are found only in organs which are epithelial in origin, I would state that I recently found one located in the heart muscle, where there are no epithelial cells.

Dr. C. E. Beebe then presented a specimen of a bronchial cast, which was a perfect reproduction of the various ramifications of the tubes down to a very small size. It was the second or third one which had been extracted. After each one thrown off, the child perfectly recovered its health.

The Society then adjourned until September 8th, 1887.

THE LAURA FRANKLIN HOSPITAL.

The Laura Franklin Free Hospital for children, which has excited so much interest and attention not only in this city but in other places, is doing a magnificent work in its special department and well justifies the great outlay of money made by the Delano family for its erection and maintenance. It is one of the most cheery, comfortable and enjoyable hospitals in its domestic appointments that can be found in the country. The wards are fitted up with pictures, and many would do credit to the most elegant drawing-rooms ; with rolling-chairs and beds which, in point of comfort and convenience, are models. Mosquito netting entirely envelops the beds which contain children, who are especially attractive to flies, and in every way the comfort and happiness of the little ones, as well as their physical improvement, are made objects of constant watchfulness. The medical and surgical equipment is as fine as money, added to skill and hospital experience, can make it. If anything is found lacking at any time the deficiency is immediately supplied. Another great blessing, which will be more highly appreciated by those physicians who have had previous connections with other hospitals. lies in the fact that it is not controlled and hampered, its harmony entirely destroyed, and ultimately its usefulness and success as a hospital completely and absolutely destroyed, by a board of lady managers, or more properly, mismanagers. The homœopathic profession in New York does not need but one Hahnemann hospital to teach it the utter uselessness and stupidity of such administration.

The Laura Franklin is under the control of the Episcopal Sisterhood of St. Mary, and under the immediate supervision of Sister Gertrude, who embodies and centralizes in herself all authority and power over all the various departments of the hospital. It has one head, which is what most hospitals lack.

To say that the management is entirely satisfactory, would only half express the sentiments not only of the medical staff, but of all in any way connected with the institution.

The hospital received its first patient November 21st, 1886. Since then it has treated 127, of which number fifty-five have been discharged cured; twenty-four improved; nine unimproved; two not treated; one transferred; four have died, and thirty-two are at present in the hospital. It would surely be difficult to present a more favorable report.

Nearly every form of disease, excepting those which, by their nature, are either incurable or contagious, have been under treatment, and so far the results have justified the confidence we feel in homœopathic medication. A large proportion of the cases are surgical, and many are such as do not show immediate brilliant results. Very many are bone or articular diseases, the treatment of which is necessarily slow. From time to time, as interesting cases present themselves, we shall record them in this department

The following are a few of many instructive cases which have been treated at the hospital:

Service of Drs. B. G. Clark and Martin Deschere—Chronic eczema.— Eddie Knox, aged 18 months, admitted to the hospital January 20th, 1887, for chronic eczema of the face. When the child was four months old, a slight pustular eruption appeared on the face. Since then it had constantly grown worse. On admission to the hospital, the eruption completely covered both cheeks and was plentifully sprinkled over the brow, neck, hands and arms. It was worse about the chin and eyes, which were red, watery and inflamed. Previous to admission he had been under more or less constant treatment. The little patient was given *rhus.* 3. On the 27th he was worse, his eyes being inflamed and deeply injected. He was given *bell.* in alternation with *rhus.;* at the same time his face was rubbed with sweet oil. January 30th the face, hands and forehead were covered with thick scabs, and the patient was restless, peevish and fretful; did not sleep well. ℞ *graph.* 30. February 1st the face was red and inflamed, and there was considerable fever. *Clematis* 30 was prescribed, to be given three times a day. On February 5th the scabs were dryer and the face less red and inflamed, but the child continued restless, peevish and disturbed in its sleep. *Cham.* 30 was given for two days, when the nervous symptoms having subsided and sleep being restored, the *clematis* 30 was resumed. On February 11th a large scab formed on the forehead and much matter was secreted beneath it. On the 14th, as the child was worse, no medicine was given. On February 22d *mezerium* was prescribed, which a little later was followed by *dulc.* 30, and later by *bapt.* 30, as the glands were enlarged and the color was bad. On March 30th *psorinum* 30 was given for two days, when the *mezerium* 30 was resumed. There had been more or less constant improvement, but now it became very decided, and soon the face was perfectly clear.

The child subsequently came back to be treated for croup and pneumonia. The eruption slightly reappeared. Later Dr. Fulton circumcised him, and when he left the hospital on June 20th, his skin was as clear and white as any child of that age could desire.

Dr. Sidney F. Wilcox's service—Sequestrum of tibia.—Eddie Menger, aged 10, admitted May 23d, 1887, upon recommendation of Dr. E. M. Pettet. Two years ago a man had struck him on the leg with a stick, causing him much pain. Previously his health had always been excellent. After the blow the leg swelled, and ultimately a large abscess was formed, which broke, discharging a large amount of pus and some pieces of bone. The abscess had continued to discharge ever since. On examination with the probe the roughened surface of dead bone was plainly detected. On May 24th he was anæsthetized, and Dr. Wilcox made a long incision over the outer surface of the leg, cutting through the sinuses and down upon the bone. Small cloacæ were discovered leading into the tibia, which at this point was very greatly enlarged. The probe entered these and dead bone was discovered within. Nature had done her best to encyst it. With a bone chisel and gauge one of these openings into the bone was enlarged so as to admit the little finger, the great diameter of the opening being in the axis of the bone. As the opening was enlarged, a perfectly formed sequestrum was seen. By the aid of the sequestrum forceps this piece of dead bone, which was perfectly loose, was gradually withdrawn from its bony chamber. It proved to be about 4½ inches long and was very fragile. Its greatest diameter was about 3-16th of an inch. It was in a typical condition for removal. The interior of the bony chamber was then thoroughly scraped out; all degenerate tissue within and about the sinuses removed; the whole thoroughly cleansed with a 1 to 2,000 solution of corrosive sublimate, which in all surgical operations at the hospital is constantly used for irrigation; two rubber drainage tubes inserted; one going into the bony chamber; the deeper portion of the wound closed with sutures of silk-worm gut attached to lead buttons wtth superficial sutures of silk. The whole was then covered and dressed with borated cotton in corrosive sublimate gauze and secured by a roller. This dressing was removed June 5th and the stitches removed on the 12th; the ankle was swollen and inflamed. This broke and discharged a large amount of pus. On the 16th the leg again swelled and was poulticed. After it had discharged it was washed out with a solution of peroxide of hydrogen. The leg continued to swell and discharge until July 4th, when it celebrated its independence of diseased conditions and began steadily and rapidly to improve. At present the wound has entirely healed and the patient is awaiting his discharge.

Service of Dr. Fred. S. Fulton—Central abscess of the right metatarsal bone.—James Enwright, aged 5 years, admitted January 14th, 1887, upon the recommendation of Dr. J. W. Dowling, Jr. Three years ago he violently struck his toe against the bed. It caused him a great deal of pain for a time, but soon passed away and no more notice was taken of the injury until four months afterwards, when it was noticed that the boy walked on the inside of that foot. On examination no trouble was discovered, except that the metatarso-phalangeal joint was enlarged. This swelling increased slowly, until nine months ago the boy became feverish and the joint acutely inflamed. Last November the joint discharged pus and had continued to do so until his admission into the hospital. The discharge was not constant, but would cease for a number of days or weeks and then suddenly break out and flow quite freely for some time. On examination, the toe was found but little sensitive; the phalangeal end of the metatarsal bone of the foot was enlarged and reddened. The joint proper was not involved. A small opening led down to the bone. Upon inserting a probe, it would strike the healthy bone, covered with periosteum, but would go no further. No dead bone could be detected. Being confident that it was a central abscess of the bone, Dr. Fulton, after placing the child under the influence of an anæsthetic, cut down in the line of the sinus, making an incision about ⅓ of an inch in length. It was then found why the probe did not detect dead bone. On pushing the skin and subcutaneous tissue back and downward, the opening into the bone was found on the under side of the bone, while the external opening was on the side of the foot. The sinus thus covered on itself. The osseous opening was very small, merely admitting a probe, which, upon insertion, readily detected the roughened bone. This opening was enlarged so as to admit the little finger, which easily passed into a large, round cavity, large enough to readily admit the end of the index finger. This was filled with dead bone and *debris*. It was all cleaned out; the roughened bone removed by the gouge and scraper until the interior was healthy. This left a mere shell of bone covered with periosteum on the outside. The joint was not entered, though the plate between the abscess cavity and articulation must have been extremely thin. The cavity was packed with balsam of Peru and marine lint; the incision was stitched with silk at its extremities. The whole was covered with corrosive sublimate gauze. This dressing was reapplied every day or two. The cavity was large and it took a good while for it to fill up. Later the subnitrate of bismuth was substituted as a dry dressing. The case progressed slowly, and on May 14th, 1887, he was discharged, the bone having been filled and the external wound closed.

The following case is given, not to illustrate the marvelous effect of treatment, but to record a case of immense hypertrophy of the spleen. It is the largest we have ever seen or read about. She was a patient of Dr. B. G. Clark, who placed her in the hospital:

Bessie S., aged 11 years, born at New Brighton, Staten Island. For more than a year the patient has suffered with malarial fever and bronchitis. Her temperature has been high, pulse frequent; she has lost flesh, and looks pale and thin. Her spleen was enlarged. She complained of pain in her right side and sore throat. At times she would be feverish, thirsty, drowsy, and occasionally had diarrhœa. At various times she was given *phos., rhus., china, ars. ac., bry., hepar. sulph.*, etc., but without much effect. On January 9th, 1887, a long, exploring hypodermic was inserted into the tumor, but only a slight amount of blood was withdrawn. On examination by Dr. Fulton, it was found to contain only red and white blood corpuscles, the latter being in great abundance. The impossibility of differentiating between the latter and pus corpuscles when the latter are mixed in small quantities with blood, made it impossible to state definitely whether the corpuscles were due to leucocythæmic condition of the blood or to a general purulent infiltration of the spleen, thus giving rise to the fluctuation of temperature. The latter was considered more probable, as her looks and general condition were septicæmic. Her temperature during almost her entire stay at the hospital was about 98 3-5' degrees in the morning, and 100 2-5 degrees in the afternoon; at times the temperature rose to 101 2-5 degrees. Several careful examinations were made. From the last one, made by Drs. Clark and Fulton on May 6th, 1887, we extract the following from the case books of the hospital: "External veins over the entire body are very prominent and blue. The tumor occupying the left portion of the abdominal cavity extends upwards to the eighth interspace in the axillary line, forwards to a point in the median line, four inches below a line connecting the two nipples. From here it extended obliquely to the left, till at the level of the navel it extended 1½ inches to the right of the umbilicus. Two inches below this the tumor extended 2½ inches to the right of the median line. The tumor thus completely filled the hypogastric, left inguinal, lumbar and hypochondriac regions and the great portion of the umbilical. Posteriorly, the tumor extended from the crest of the ilium to the upper border of the tenth rib, close to the spine and for a space extending upwards 2½ inches from the crest of the ilium, and 2½ inches in width, in which there is tympanitic resonance." The pulse was 134 at the time of examination. The patient continued about the same; the tumor, which was regarded as an enormously enlarged spleen, did not apparently increase or diminish in size. She soon afterwards left the hospital and returned to her home on Staten Island. The tumor was hard and sharply defined and at times was slightly sensitive.

The case is most unusual on account of the tremendous and exceptional enlargement which the spleen had undergone, no doubt from the effect of long-continued malarial poisoning.

RECORD OF MEDICAL PROGRESS.

NASAL DISEASE AND OCULAR TROUBLES.—Dr. Bettman in the *Jour. of the Am. Med. Assoc'n,* gives detailed report of six cases in which epiphora, conjunctivitis, photophobia, and pain above the eyes, were due to nasal disease, and disappeared on treatment of the nose.

RHINITIS ULCERATIVA AS PRODUCED IN ARSENIC AND CHROME WORKERS.—Carlas writes in the *France Médicale,* May 12th, 1887, that the ulcerative rhinitis provoked by arsenical powder, is absolutely identical in its course and evolution with that observed among operatives in chrome. It is the same mechanism, the same process, with this difference, that the corrosion of the mucous membrane, and the necrosis of the cartilage advances much more rapidly with the chrome than with the arsenic workers. In arsenical rhinitis, when there is ulceration, it is always at the anterior extremity of the inferior tribinated bone, and the projecting fold formed by the extreme edge of the ala.—Joal, in the *Jour. of Laryngology and Rhinology,* August, 1887.

TREATMENT OF SCIATICA BY CUTANEOUS IRRITATION OF THE SOUND LIMB.—Dumontpallier, in 1879, read before the *Acad. de Medicine* a note on local therapeutic analgesia, determined by irritation of the similar region of the opposite side of the body, and now, at the meeting of the *Soc. de Biologie,* of July 23d, reported in the *Jour. des Soc. Scientif.,* August 3d, 1887, calls attention to the results obtained by M. Jacquet, as supporting his view. M. Jacquet, in using Debove's method of treating neuralgias by local refrigeration, by means of liquid methyl chloride, noted the fact that " if in a case of violent sciatica, we act with the methyl chloride on the healthy limb, we obtain an immediate cessation of the pain." His report of ten cases so treated will be found in the *Jour. des Soc. Scientif.,* July 27th, 1887.

EPIDEMIC HYSTERIA.—A curious outbreak of convulsionist mania, analogous to those which occurred from time to time during the middle ages, has shown itself in Agosta, in the province of Rome. For some weeks past the country people have been laboring under the delusion that the district is under the immediate government of the evil one, and before retiring to rest they carefully place on the threshold the broom and the salt, which are credited with the power of keeping off evil spirits. Many of the younger women have epileptiform attacks, during which they utter piercing shrieks, and are violently convulsed. A medical commission appointed to investigate the cause and nature of this outbreak, examined a number of the sufferers, mostly young women, some of whom were alleged to have vomited nails, horseshoes, and other equally indigestible substances, while others barked like dogs. Measures have been taken to prevent the spread of the mischief. In a milder degree, this contagious form of hysteria is not infrequent, especially in places where ignorance and superstition favor manifestations of nervous disorders. The worst excess of popular outbreaks, like the French Revolution, have been attributed to similar influences, and with every appearance of justice.—*Brit. Med. Jour.,* July 23d, 1887.

TREATMENT OF CONICAL CORNEA BY THE ACTUAL CAUTERY.—Mr. W. J. Cant, in the *Brit. Med. Jour.* for July 23d, gives a *résumé* of the operation, as proposed by the late Dr. Andrew, of Shrewsbury, for the correction of keratoconus. In brief, this operation consists in making a minute opening in the apex of the cone, with a very fine and highly heated cautery needle.

This opening permits a continuous escape of the aqueous humor for from seven to fourteen days, giving rest and time for the weakened cornea to contract to its normal curvature, the contractile power of the cicatrix helping. The pupil is first dilated. No speculum is used and no pressure put upon the eye. Directly the needle has penetrated the anterior chamber it must be removed, the eyelids closed and not opened again for three days. A little castor oil with atropine being gently rubbed along the lashes every morning, and the wool pad readjusted. The results obtained in two cases are given : in the first—operated by Dr. Andrew—the vision increased from 20-200 to 20-70, and in the second—by Mr. Cant—from 20-200 to 20-36. The advantages claimed for this operation over the removal of a portion of the cornea with knife or trephine are : " (1) it is easily performed ; (2) there is no risk of anterior synechia ; (3) the slow and continuous drainage of the anterior chamber allows rest and contraction of the cornea ; (4) the cauterized opening in the cornea leads to further contraction ; (5) the scar is a small one."

ATTEMPTED REMOVAL OF A NEEDLE FROM THE HEART.—At the seventeeth congress of the German Society of Surgery held in April, a report was made by Dr. Stelzner, of Dresden, of a case in which an operation had been performed for the removal of a needle from the right ventricle of the heart (*Beilage zum Centralblatt für Chirurgie*, No. 25, 1887). The patient, a young student, had attempted to kill himself by thrusting a sewing-needle into the heart. After an interval of twelve hours, during which there had not been any serious symptoms, the patient suffered from pain in the cardiac region, and from dyspnœa, and a loud pericardial rubbing sound was heard at the apex of the heart. Twenty-four hours later these symptoms had increased to such an extent, and the patient had become so seriously collapsed, that it was thought necessary to remove the needle by operation. No trace of this could be found just under the skin or in the intercostal space. After resection of a portion of the fifth rib, whereby the pleural cavity was opened, and subsequent opening of the pericardial sac, from which about a teaspoonful of turbid fluid was discharged, the needle could be felt in an oblique position, in the right ventricle. By the pressure of a finger passed under the heart, the eye of the needle was thrust through the anterior wall of the ventricle, and fixed by the operator's finger-nail. An attempt to seize the end of the needle with forceps failed in consequence of the very violent movements of the heart, and the foreign body suddenly slipped back into the heart, where it now occupied a vertical instead of an oblique position. Under these circumstances no further attempt was made to remove the needle. It now unfortunately happened that an iodoform tampon which protected the exposed pleural cavity, was, during a deep inspiration, drawn into this cavity, and could not be found again. Notwithstanding pneumothorax and extensive pleuritic effusion, the patient made a good recovery by the end of the fourth week, and, at the date of Dr. Stelzner's communication, was quite well, and free from any uneasiness. There was neither bruit nor abnormal condition of the pulse, nor any trace of pleuritic exudation. It remains uncertain whether the needle remains in the heart or has wandered into the mediastinum, and whether the patient will continue in his present state of good health, or at some future time be attacked by some fresh and sudden danger. In the course of the discussion on this case, Dr. Hahn showed a portion of a knitting-needle that had been removed, during life, by von Bergmann, from the heart of a girl, aged eleven. This had been accidently forced into the left side of the chest through a blow with a slipper. Below the third rib on the left side was observed a small black spot, formed by the point of the needle. A systolic bruit was distinctly heard over the apex of the heart. The needle was removed within a few hours after the accident. During its slowly effected extraction, it presented very distinct pendulum movements. The extraction was effected very slowly, in order to allow of coagulation along the course of the wound in the wall of the heart, and so to guard against hemorrhage into the pericardium, which is so often, in cases of punctured heart, the cause of death. Immediately after the removal of the needle, the pulse, which had been very rapid, sank to 90 to the minute.—*Lon. Med. Rec.*, July 15th, 1887.

BURNS AND SCALDS.—Prof. Mosetig during the past five years has treated forty-eight cases of severe burns and scalds with satisfactory results. He uses iodoform in very limited quantities. He either does not apply the powder at all ; or he sprinkles it in thin layers only on those places where the integument has been burnt in its whole thickness and has assumed a parchment-like appearance. As a rule he covers the injured parts directly with compresses of iodoform gauze, not prepared in the usual way, by thickly dusting the gauze with the powder, but by impregnating with an etheric solution of iodoform, the purified gauze which has previously been freed of grease. He proceeds in the following manner : After opening and excising the vesicles, and cleaning the burns with cotton-wool, which had been steeped in a half per cent. solution of table salt, and well pressed out, he covers the wounds with dry compresses consisting of several layers of iodoform gauze, prepared as stated above, of corresponding size, which are exactly and smoothly laid over the whole surface of the injury. Over this an equally large or somewhat smaller piece of gutta-percha tissue is placed, taking care that it does not form folds or creases. The whole is wrapped in a very thick layer of medicated absorbent cotton-wool which overlaps to a great extent the compresses, or, better, surrounds the whole limb or injured part of the body. This cotton-wool is finally fixed by several turns of bandages, which at the same time exert a gentle pressure. This simple dressing, which, moreover, has the advantage of taking up very little time, is allowed to remain, without being changed, as long as possible, *i. e.*, as long as cleanliness permits, and no rising of the temperature takes place. The secretions from the wound drain off beneath the gutta-percha tissue, and are taken up by the absorbent cotton-wool. Slight straining of the bandage is no sufficient indication for renewing the dressing, which ought to be permanent ; in case of real imbibition and offensive smell, only the external dressing has to be removed and changed ; the iodoform gauze and the gutta-percha covering, however, should not be interfered with. In case, in the meanwhile, fever should set in, which betrays by its character septic causes, generally the demarcation and separation of the mortified part having commenced, or a retention of the secretion of the wound having taken place, the dressing must be removed, the abscess opened, and free discharge of the pus secured ; the mortified shreds and the eschars must be removed by means of forceps and scissors. The new dressing is put on in the same manner as the first one. The impermeable covering of gutta-percha tissue is very essential, and ought never to be omitted, because the drying on and sticking to the wounds of the gauze, stiffened by the imbibed secretions, is always injurious, and may moreover cause, like a scab, retention of the secretion. The discharges may be allowed to dry in the external portion of the dressing, but never on the wound itself. By the permanent iodoform dressing, the infection, both by the air and by contact, is prevented, and burns of the second degree, as a rule, heal under a single dressing ; in burns of the third degree, aseptic separation of the eschar, with but slight secretion, frequently takes place, and even if the latter be not the case, the granulating surfaces heal in a far shorter time, and the cicatrization is smoother, more even, and altogether less disfiguring than in non-aseptic treatment. In burns and scalds of the face the mode of dressing described will, of course, be impossible; instead of it an iodoform-vaseline ointment (1 : 20) is employed, and covered with a mask of gutta-percha tissue. The ointment has to be daily renewed, and is always spread on the thickness of a knife-blade.—*Lon. Med. Rec.*, July, 1887, from *Centralbl. f. die gesamte Therapie*, March, 1887, and *Wiener Med. Presse*, Nos. 2 and 3, 1887.

NEWS.

THE Laura Franklin Free Hospital for Children is the most completely equipped of its kind in America.—*Ex.*

A PROPHYLACTIC.—Femplé recommends the placing in the mouth of a fragment of myrrh if one finds himslf in an infected atmosphere, and he has employed this means with happy results in several epidemics. Physicians in the east use this means constantly in visiting patients.—*Recorder.*

APPOINTMENTS.—Dr. J. G. Gilchrist has been appointed Professor of Surgery, and Dr. C. H. Cogswell Professor of Obstetrics and Diseases of Children, in the Homœopathic Department of the University of Iowa. Governor Beaver, of Pennsylvania, has appointed Mr. A. J. Tafel a member of the State Pharmaceutical Examining Board.

THE DETROIT HOSPITAL.—Work is being vigorously pushed on the new Homœopathic Hospital, or to speak more correctly, the McMillan and Newbury Free Hospital, in Detroit. It is expected to be ready for occupancy early next year. The greatest care is exercised in the building, and the appointments and various appliances will be of the very best. It is said that further bequests have been secured.

FIFTIETH ANNIVERSARY.—The fiftieth anniversary of the introduction of homœopathy west of the Alleghanies will be celebrated in connection with the twenty-third annual meeting of the Homœopathic Medical Society of Pennsylvania, at Pittsburgh, September 20th, 21st and 22d, 1887. Drs. W. Tod Helmuth, of New York; J. P. Dake, of Nashville, and R. Ludlam, of Chicago, are expected to be present and deliver addresses.

NOT UNUSUAL.—The town of Dedham is under prohibition law, apothecaries alone being permitted to sell alcoholic stimulants. The other day a son of the Emerald Isle entered a drug store there, and taking a bottle from his pocket, asked for a quart of whiskey. The salesman asked to what use it was to be put, and the reply was, "To soak roots in it." The order was filled and the clerk, after handing over the bottle and its contents, inquired in a conversational manner, "What kind of roots are you going to soak?" Pocketing the bottle the customer said, "The roots of my tongue, be jabers."

THE *Union Médicale* notes that when what is usually cleared out of the Seine is duly considered, it becomes evident the water of that river is not the impure and deleterious fluid it has hitherto been supposed to be, but a nourishing soup. The following were removed in Paris in 1886: 2,021 dogs, 977 cats, 2,257 rats, 507 fowls, 210 hares and rabbits, 10 sheep, 2 foals, 66 sucking pigs, 5 pigs, 27 geese, 27 turkeys, 2 calves, 2 monkeys, 8 goats, 1 snake, 2 squirrels, 3 porcupines, 1 parrot, 600 various birds, 5 foxes, 130 pigeons, 3 hedgehogs, 3 peacocks and 1 seal, besides 3,066 kilogrammes of offal. We should like to see the returns from the New York harbor.

NITRITE OF AMYL.—Mr. F. H. Kendle, of South Molten, reports the case of a lady who complained to him, the first day after delivery, of excruciating after-pains, which she declared were worse than any she had experienced during labor. The womb was found firmly contracted, lochia slight, and no clots larger than beans had been passed. As several hours must necessarily have elapsed before any medicine could have been sent her, Mr. Kendle broke a couple of amyl capsules (four grains in each) into a smelling-bottle, and directed the patient to take two or three deep inhalations when she felt a pain coming on. The effect was simply magical; the pains were immediately relieved and shortly ceased altogether, the patient being soon able to take some refreshing sleep. She made an excellent recovery. He has since tried the same remedy in two other cases of less severity, with similar results. He has also found the drug invaluable in the sickness of pregnancy and in obstinate cases of dysmenorrhea. Inhalation seems to be more certain and lasting than the internal exhalation of the drug. He strongly recommends this as a simple and efficacious plan of treatment.—*Lancet.*

THEISM.—Attention has recently been drawn to a new nervous disorder, said to be especially prevalent in England and America. It is called "Theism," or tea-drinkers' disease. It is said to exist in three stages—acute, sub-acute and chronic. At first the symptoms are congestion of the cephalic vessels, cerebral excitement and animation of the face. These physiological effects being constantly provoked, give rise, after a while, to reaction, marked by mental and bodily depression. The tea-drinker becomes impressionable and nervous, pale, subject to cardiac troubles, and seeks relief from these symptoms in a further indulgence in the favorite beverage, which for a time restores to a sense of well-being. These symptoms characterize the first two stages. In chronic cases theism is characterized by a grave alteration of the functions of the heart and of the vaso-motors, and by a disturbance of nutrition. The patient becomes subject to hallucinations, nightmares and nervous trembling. With those who take plenty of exercise, an habitual consumption often may be indulged in with impunity, but with women and young people who follow sedentary occupations, this is not the case. The best treatment for theism is said to be indulgence in free exercise, such as walking and open-air life.—*Lancet.*

AN EXCELLENT LECTURE.—In the *Homœopathic World* for June and July appears a lecture by Dr. J. H. Clark entitled, "The Treatment of the Sick." There are so many good things in this lecture that one hardly knows where or what to select for a specimen extract. In the course of the lecture Dr. Clark said: "In the face of all this wealth of material and the dearth of trustworthy guidance in the useful application of it, what is to be done? 'Let each man use his common sense,' is the counsel of some. But, unfortunately, the practice of medicine has very little to do with common sense. It needs sense of a very uncommon kind to choose and apply the right measures for the relief of the sick, and this sense is not acquired in a day. It is not even to be imparted in a course of lectures. It is partly a native gift and partly the outcome of patient and minute observation of the results of practice. So long as we are ignorant of the essential nature of therapeutic action of any kind, common sense rules and 'general principles' do not apply. Hence it follows that it is impossible to pooh-pooh any system of treatment as being *prima facie* absurd, for we have no fixed grounds, apart from experience, on which to presume any treatment either absurd or rational. There is only the ground of experience to go upon. Hence every kind of treatment must be judged by its results, and the facts must be fully recorded, and of such a nature as to preclude any other explanation of recovery than that afforded by the therapeutic measures. This we have not only a right, but a duty to ask before accepting any treatment that is urged on our attention. * * *

It is here the doctor must think of many other things besides his drugs. Success in life seldom depends on one thing alone, and the medical man must know many things besides the powers of drugs if he is to succeed in life. But the term 'accessory treatment' truly describes the relation that other remedial measures bear to the administration of drugs. In some cases 'accessory treatment' may be of more importance than the treatment by medicines, and among allopathists this is, doubtless, frequently the case. Those practitioners of eminence who openly confess their disbelief in drug powers, are usually great adepts in utilizing all the other means of assisting the sick that may be at command. Nor are they by any means to be defined as they are apt to be by the followers of Hahnemann. We give such an unusual amount of thought to our drugs that it is not to be wondered at that we should sometimes overlook minor matters that may yet be of great importance. This is a danger to be guarded against, for on these minor matters, in great measure, depends a man's success and reputation. * * * * Again there is the question of diet and regimen. These are two branches of treatment in which all must be experts. In many cases medicines act without any alteration of the ordinary diet and mode of life. In others all medicine is vain until some change is made. Thus diet and regimen may be actually curative when ordered on an intelligent plan, and this is a branch of practice which each one must learn for himself. Books and lectures may give many useful hints, but all must be checked by the facts of daily practice. * * * * There is no success in medicine possible without much careful attention to details. Personally, I abhor details. 'General principles' are my delight. For long I sought for 'general principles' for guidance in my practice until I found myself working my principles into my practice, instead of letting my practice form itself from my principles. My advice to you is, lay yourselves out for this from the beginning. Make each patient a study, and do not draw your conclusions too rapidly. Often you will only get at the real history of a case by slow degrees, and if you have not tact and patience you will never get to know it all. * * * * I have said above that the treatment of the sick is the sole end of the doctor's calling. It is strange that any other idea should have taken possession of the medical mind and found its way into print. Our position as curers of our patients is really our only excuse for the confidential relations we hold with them. What right have we to know the secret history of their lives, unless we can turn that knowledge to their own advantage? It can surely be no advantage to them that we make, by their assistance, a clever diagnosis, proving eminently satisfactory to our *amour propre*, if that is all we care to achieve. We may delude ourselves with the idea that if we do not accomplish anything for the individual patient, we are, at least, doing something great for posterity; but it is scarcely for that that our patient tells us his secrets, and it is not posterity that pays us our fees. Practicing on patients to-day for the good of posterity is not honest practice, ladies and gentlemen. And as soon as one of us finds that he can no longer do a patient any good, it is his duty to say so and give up the case. The man who does his best for his patients to-day is the man who is most likely to help posterity. His work is honest and his experience sound. If a man wants to leave behind him anything that posterity will find it worth while to look at, he must work for each individual patient, and have no grand ideas about abstract humanity. Such a man will find himself in possession of an abundance of shapely stones, cut with his own hands and brain from the granite of nature's quarry, when the time comes for him to build, whilst the experience of the abstract humanitarian—the posterity doctor, 'who works not for the one, but for the many;' not to cure patients, but to 'understand them'—will prove to be nothing better than a shapeless, incoherent mass of sand."

Vol. XXXV.   *OCTOBER, 1887.*   (Volume II, Third Series.) No. 10.

North American
JOURNAL OF HOMŒOPATHY.

ORIGINAL ARTICLES IN MEDICINE.
CONCERNING THE NECESSITY OF HOSPITALS IN GENERAL AND THE PROPOSED FREE HOMŒOPATHIC HOSPITAL IN PARTICULAR.*

By J. G. BALDWIN, M. D.,

New York.

WHOEVER has, by chance or design, taken a stroll through the parts of our city occupied by the people dwelling in tenements, especially of the lower class, must have been amazed at the rows of five and six story houses lining both sides of the several streets.

If he takes this stroll in the summer time, or on a Sunday, or on a holiday, or in the evening, he will be more astonished at the multitudes of men, women and children he will see.

The windows will be open, and at almost every one an occupant or two will be noticed trying to catch a breath of air a little different from the stifling fumes of the close rooms. At the same time the stoops and sidewalks are swarming with human beings in such numbers that he is at a loss to conceive where they can all be housed.

If the stroller should enter one of these houses, he would, after groping his way up a narrow, dark and dirty stairway, taking care that he does not run over, or trample upon, some of the numerous children who are constantly passing up and down, find a tenement of one living room and two or three small and dark bedrooms.

There are often four of these tenements or apartments on each floor of a twenty-five foot house.

If he were permitted to inquire into the condition of these rooms,

---

* Read before the New York County Homœopathic Medical Society, September 8th, 1887.

he would be horrified at the dark, dismal appearance, and the close, foul smelling and unhealthy air.

The large room is not only the living room, but the kitchen, dining-room and work-room. A sewing machine is frequently to be seen at each window. The operators on these machines, or the other workers, can scarcely spare the time to turn from their employments to the tables on which their meals, the cooking of which has filled the room with steaming odors, are spread. Owing to the pressure of work which must be done, or there will be nothing to eat, the vessels and dishes are frequently put by uncleaned, and with the decomposing garbage and refuse, for which no proper place is provided, unite in giving out their sickening odors and poisonous germs, never in the least ameliorated by the sunlight or the fresh air of heaven. The bed-rooms will be found to be small and dark, into which the sun never shines and the outside air never enters, except it be through a small window from the common hall, or through the living room, where it is robbed of all its life and freshness.

He will probably find this tenement occupied by a family large enough to furnish two or three persons to each room.

If he chance to enter a better tenement, he may find at the front of the house a small parlor room, and at the back of the house the living room, while the two or three bed-rooms are placed between them, without light or ventilation.

In each of the tenements of the better class and in the halls of the poorer class will be found a sink, with water faucet and an open waste pipe connecting with the common sewer. The water-closets are usually in a dark closet, without the least ventilation, and often without sufficient water to flush them properly.

The tenement population of New York City is enormous, almost surpassing belief.

In some quarters there are 298,000 inhabitants to a square mile, while in the densest parts of London there are only 170,000 to the square mile.

When to all this is added the fact, that the quality of the food used by this class is not, owing to their poverty, of the best or freshest kind, and the digestibility is not improved by the cooking, one wonders that there is not much more sickness among them than there is, and that so many do live, and year after year are able to labor and to maintain the struggle for existence.

This being the common and inevitable condition of so large a portion of the population when in health, what must it be when sickness comes upon them, or accident happens to them?

How can a patient with pneumonia, or peritonitis, or rheumatism, or any other serious disease, be cared for with even a slight chance of success? Who can be spared from among the bread-winners to do the required nursing or waiting?

What chance for quiet is there when every room is occupied by two or three persons? or when the incessant rattle of the sewing machine, or the swash of the wash-tub, or the clattering of the cooking, with the chattering of the operators, is almost at the bedside? Even when love and sympathy keep the immediate associates of the patient quiet, how is the noise of the surrounding tenements to be controlled?

When the rooms of families who are strangers to each other are separated only by the thinnest partitions, affording the merest impediment to the noise, the bustle, the quarreling, the merry-making, and even the ordinary conversation of the neighbors, how is quiet to be obtained?

If one of a family meets with an accident and has a broken limb, or a fractured skull, where are the conveniences for the patient or for the surgeon?

How can such an one be expected to recover without those necessities of life—fresh air, quiet and proper attention and nutriment?

If the conditions requisite for the proper treatment of the sick or disabled, with the necessary fresh air, quiet, and good, nutritious diet, cannot be had in their own homes, other places must be provided where they can be had. This other place is a hospital—a free hospital—to which the injured and the sick can be taken and properly cared for.

This is what renders such hospitals indispensable institutions wherever such a condition of the population exists, as it does in large cities. Such hospital accommodations should be somewhat proportioned to the population, and should be enlarged as the number of the poorer classes increases. There is no reason to fear there will be too many hospitals. It will hardly be possible for them to keep pace with the growth of the tenement classes. These hospitals should be so placed and endowed that they can fully offer to all needy applicants. such a home and such surroundings as shall afford them the best chance for recovery. They should be so located that they will be easy of access, both to the patient and to his or her friends whenever they wish to visit them.

Of such hospitals we have many, of which any people might justly be proud, and great good do they do, with their long lists of noble physicians, surgeons and nurses. But there is a class of the poor who are not satisfactorily cared for in the existing institutions. ·

I refer to that class who are believers in homœopathy and its methods of cure, as far as they understand them, and who earnestly desire to have themselves and their children treated in that way whenever they need medical treatment.

This is the reason for the effort to establish a new free homœopathic hospital which is now being made.

To do this a large amount of money will be required, and it can only be done by the liberality of those people of wealth who have themselves that confidence in and liking for homœopathic treatment, which begets in them the desire that the poor who wish it may have it also.

It is to be hoped that those who feel thus toward the worthy poor, and who have the means, will exercise such liberality that soon the Free Homœopathic Hospital will be so richly endowed that it can extend to all who need it the most generous, kind and skillful care.

Every member of this society should use whatever influence he or she can with his or her patrons in favor of this great and needed enterprise, so that it may speedily be placed on a firm foundation and be enabled to engage successfully in this glorious work.

RATIONAL TREATMENT OF UTERINE DISPLACEMENTS.*

By Mrs. M. A. BRINKMAN, M.D.,

New York.

UTERINE displacements with complicating tissue changes constitute the most common class of cases that meet the gynæcologist in daily practice. These cases often tax the skill of the physician, and in many instances they pass from one system of treatment to another, only to get steadily worse. If we consult the list of remedies for application to the vagina, cervix and endometrium, and the surgical and mechanical methods of treatment for displacements and their complications laid down in text books, we note how utterly inadequate and crude many of them are. Authors, while pointing out a line of experimental treatment, place guide boards all along the way, which point significantly to "counter indications" and "dangers." Almost every aspirant for gynæcological fame has invented a new pessary or modified one already known. Dilatation of the uterus and

---
* Read before the Homœopathic Medical Society, County of New York, Sept. 8th, 1887.

curetting its cavity have become a fashion. The young physician, often without any just reason for doing so, performs these surgical feats, fearing that if he fails to follow the " routine practice " he may fall short in his duty to his patient. There is also danger that oöphorectomy, so valuable in most carefully selected cases, may be so abused as to bring discredit upon us. The conscientious physician, finding many of the generally accepted methods of uterine treatment pernicious, seeks a more rational system.

Dr. Emmett, in his text book issued in 1880, sarcastically refers to physicians who '' have no faith in pessaries '' by hinting that they are unable to fit them. In a paper read before the British Medical Association in 1886 (*Brit. Med. Jour.*, Nov. 13) the doctor states that he *now* avoids as far as possible the introduction of any instrument or remedy within the uterus. He recalls cases treated years ago who were often under treatment year after year, and each relapse was then attributed to cold or imprudence, but never to the method of treatment. He makes a more judicious and limited use of pessaries, with the result, he tells us, of fewer instances of lighting up again an old "pelvic inflammation." The fact that in the hands of so skillful an operator as Dr. Emmett an old pelvic inflammation is occasionally rekindled, and inasmuch as pelvic peritonitis and cellulitis may cause a patient years of suffering, and not infrequently a condition of chronic invalidism, no further argument is needed for seeking safer methods. A thorough knowledge of diseases and their relations to distant organs is imperative to successful gynæcology. The testimony of the best authors tends to prove that much of the general suffering in displacements depends upon hyperæmia and hyperæsthesia of the pelvic organs, and that the sympathetic influences of the uterus are excited through the vaso-motor system. Prolapse of the uterus, with obstruction to the circulation, seems to be the prime factor in producing many of the symptoms. The nerve and blood supply being presided over by the same genito-spinal centre, accounts for many of the reflex symptoms accompanying displacements. These symptoms vary, according to constitution, temperament and complications. In every case of general nervousness, hysteria or chlorosis, as in all cases of sickness where uterine complications are suspected, the pelvic organs should be examined. Doubtless many women are sent to insane asylums for nervous and mental diseases through neglect of the physician to locate the cause of the trouble. Patients with displacements frequently suffer from melancholia, even to the extent of committing suicide. The fear of insanity is a common symptom, and many patients really show signs of mental disorder clearly due to the malposition. This is proved by the fact that when the uterus is brought into its normal position, and retained there, the disturbed thoughts almost at once disappear. Symptoms of uterine diseases being so varied and complicated, the local examination is particularly necessary in order to discriminate between surgical and non-surgical cases. It is not sufficient to recognize a displacement of the uterus ; we must also seek to learn the causes of the malposition, ascertaining as far as possible the primary and secondary conditions.

In the August number of the *American Journal of Obstetrics* is an article on Uterine Dyspepsia, in which the writer says : "While agreeing with Jaffe that there is a train of gastric symptoms due to uterine causes, and while subscribing in part to his views, that these will disappear when the complaining organ is relieved from suffering, he protests against a wholesale acceptance of this teaching—first, because in cases of long standing the symptoms become so pronounced and settled that they assume prominence as distinctive physiological conditions, which will not yield to pelvic therapeutics ; secondly, because the dyspepsia may be partly due to the hepatic derangement, to which also the constipation may be beholden. Both of these factors aggravate the chronic metritis, the old peri- or parametritis, and will not disappear coincidently with the uterine complaint." This writer has unconsciously pointed out the reason of so much failure in the treatment of uterine difficulties. It is a safe axiom that he who would become a successful gynæcologist must beware of "routine practice." There can be no exclusive system of "uterine therapeutics." In uterine difficulties, as in all other local expressions of abnormal action, there are not two cases alike, and the totality of the symptoms, *objective* and *subjective*, must decide the treatment to be pursued. This is true not only as regards the selection of the remedy homœopathic to the case, but as to measures which must be considered in a hygienic, physiological, chemical, mechanical and psychical sense. This last consideration may often be the most important in the case.

We have selected two cases from our note-book which will illustrate what seems to us a rational line of treatment in uterine displacements. We do not expect to advance anything original, but to emphasize anew what, it seems to us, there is danger of forgetting, that the homœopathic law of cure is here, as elsewhere, paramount to all auxiliaries, valuable and indispensable adjuvants as some of them undoubtedly are. We have chosen two cases of marked *Retroversion* in which the objective and the subjective symptoms differ entirely, as well as what appear to have been the primary causes. To sum up the history of these cases as briefly as possible, we find it necessary to enter somewhat into detail, as attention to details we believe to be the pivot upon which success depends.

Case I.—Is one of prolapse of the uterus with *retroversion* approaching the third degree, congestion and some leucorrhœa. The patient is of nervous temperament, with dark complexion; age, 32. She has been married five years, but has never been pregnant. At the time of marriage she enjoyed fair health, but family troubles then occurring, she suffered for many months grief, anxiety and mental strain, and for five years has been a constant sufferer. The husband was kind, considerate and exemplary in every way. The case is characterized by severe colic pains, aggravated by exertion and before the menses. The flow is scanty and light in color. The pains are intensified by attempted coition, which has never been satisfactorily performed. All such attempts are followed by vaginismus, spasmodic pains in the abdomen and spasm of the rectum, the latter followed by obstinate constipation for several days, although the bowels are otherwise regular. Vertex headaches, frequent and severe, often confined her to bed. Sleep is disturbed by distressing dreams. Frequent attacks of nervous chills with visible trembling, so that she requires to be held to assist her to composure. Severe attacks of hystero-epilepsy precede the menstrual periods and follow unusual worry or excitement. All the symptoms are worse in the morning. We first saw the patient in January, 1887. In May of the same year all the symptoms had disappeared, and all the functions were performed normally. The uterus had regained its normal position, and the patient was gaining in flesh and strength. There has been but one slight attack of hystero-epilepsy, and that occurred early in the treatment, brought about by worry from receiving bad news. Considering the temperament, and regarding the grief and mental strain as the cause of the trouble, *nux vom.* suggested itself as the remedy. "The pathogenetic action of *nux vom.*," we read (Hughes), "is to impress the sensory nerves, and the morbid impression is carried by them to the spinal cord, whence it is reflected upon the motor nerves and muscles. From this follow the phenomena of the motor sphere, which range from simple stiffness or twitching to complete tetanic rigidity and, finally, paralysis." "This influence extends to the involuntary muscles, as to those of the alimentary canal, the respiratory organs and the genito-urinary tract." In analyzing the case before us we notice that the symptoms are all spasmodic in character. We find under the characteristic symptoms of *nux vom.* "trembling," "spasms," "convulsions and epilepsy," "painful spasmodic stricture of the anus, and constriction and narrowing of the rectum, hindering expulsion of stool." Dr. Dunham has pointed out that the constipation of *nux vom.* is due to inharmonious and spasmodic action of the intestine, hence the "ineffectual desire for stool." We believe that the muscular spasm that caused the colic pains forced the uterus downward, while the uterine fibres, also partaking of the spasmodic action, superinduced by exertion and contact, further increased the displacement. *Nux vom.*, 30th dil., was administered at intervals during the period of treatment. The mechanical treatment consisted in replacing the organ at each visit and supporting it by a cotton tampon saturated with glycerine. When the congestion was removed, we simply lubricated the tampon with vaseline.

The method of replacing the organ and the adjustment of the tampon we believe to be very important. We must recognize what needs to be done, the object to be attained, and we must possess mechanical genius enough to accomplish our aim. This process is far more than stuffing a plug of cotton into the vagina. The tampon should not be so large as to stretch or exercise undue pressure on surrounding tissues, neither should the vaginal canal be packed, nor the uterus lifted too high. This point is especially important in cases of displacement with cellular infiltration and thickening. Properly adjusted, and not allowed to remain in position too long, this simple support places the uterus in a position favorable to free circulation, not so much by lifting the fundus, but by relieving the tension and dragging of the overstretched or relaxed pelvic fascia and connective tissue. Their blood-vessels are supported, thus diminishing their calibre and lessening the pelvic congestion. Many of the reflex symptoms are almost immediately relieved by the mechanical treatment alone, as we have often demonstrated. Judging from quite a large experience, we are led to think that in most of the cases of uterine displacements mechanical treatment is necessary. It certainly hastens the cure. We are opposed to the use of pessaries in all their forms. The element of danger cannot be eliminated even in the hands of the most skillful gynæcologist. Few have the mechanical faculty to fit them accurately, and even when well fitted, they exercise undue pressure and interfere with the mobility of the uterus. Postural treatment, the free exercise of the muscles of respiration, the weight of the clothing taken from the abdomen, are all valuable adjuvants, and are in the line of rational treatment. It is almost needless to add that in the case before us the proper hygienic conditions were prescribed with particular care. To encourage a healthy tone of mind, the patient was urged to go out of doors daily, to visit, to be amused, and to interest herself as much as possible in others. We mention these details because we think one portion of the prescribed treatment almost as important as the other.

CASE II.—While one of marked *retroversion* also, differs essentially from the first in history, symptoms and treatment. Mrs. L. had been out of health since the birth of her only child, now ten years old. She had been under the care of a homœopathic practitioner of good reputation, but the prescribed remedies failed to benefit her much. Her health continuing to fail, in spite of change of scene and air, she consulted us in October, 1886. There had been profuse yellowish green leucorrhœa for a year, of very fœtid odor, so profuse as to render the continued use of a napkin necessary. The menses were regular, but of late had become scanty and were preceded by intense colic pains. She suffered from dragging pains in the bowels. Exertion, ascending stairs, walking, etc., caused oppression of breathing. The patient was nervous and had frequent trembling spells. Severe pain in the epigastric region about two hours after eating. The skin was dry and harsh, with eruption like water blisters, appearing mostly upon the arms and in the bend of the elbow. They came in successive crops, and were itching and burning in character. The symptoms were aggravated in the morning and about five P. M. No pelvic examination had been made by the attending physician. We found complete *retroversion*, with extensive bi-lateral laceration of the cervix uteri and considerable thickening of surrounding cellular tissue.

Here, as in Case I., we had a case of retroversion, but the objective and subjective symptoms differed materially. The same mechanical treatment was instituted as in Case I., only the tampons were adjusted with regard to the infiltration and thickening of the tissues, care being exercised that no undue traction was made. The fundus was lifted as far as it would freely move and the tampon placed under it. The remedy chosen was *sepia 2*. The third day she reported that the leucorrhœa had ceased entirely, nor did it again return. We may note in passing that the patient could not use hot vaginal enemas. Whenever tried they had been followed by severe uterine colic, due perhaps to the open condition of the os. Trachellorophy was not indicated. In less than three months the symptoms had disappeared and the patient expressed herself as feeling well. The tissue changes and the position of the uterus were not *entirely* normal when I last saw her in the spring, but she wrote me last week that she remains perfectly well.

In all uterine cases we are impressed with the importance of discriminating as far as possible between the mechanical, the reflex and the constitutional symptoms. Displacements keep up the obstruction to the pelvic circulation, whatever may have caused the displacement primarily. Obstructed circulation gives rise to passive congestions, from which may result uterine catarrh and cellular infiltration. Oversecretion, according to Dr. Emmett, is due to obstructed circulation outside of the uterus, even when the discharge seems to be due to an injury, as from the surface of a lacerated cervix (*Brit. Med. Jour.*, Nov. 13). This seems to us highly probable. Passive congestion may cause menorrhagic or scanty flow. In selecting *sepia* for this case, we found that it acts "through the vegetative nervous system." It especially acts upon the vascular and lymphatic system of the genito-urinary tract. "It causes obstruction to the portal system." The uterine condition of which *sepia* is curative is one of "passive congestions." The characteristic symptoms, "pressing in the uterus, oppressing breathing," "profuse leucorrhœa having a fœtid smell," with "drawing pains in the abdomen," "violent colic before menses," "moist eruptions" and "cramp-like pain in the stomach," were present, these symptoms dif-

fering very widely from those of Case I., while the degree of retroversion was much the same in both. In the latter case the results of child-
birth were probably the primary cause of the congestion.   Particular
attention was paid to the diet, and the patient was persuaded to remain more quiet, to give the exhausted nervous system a chance to
recuperate.   We are more and more convinced of the necessity of
"individualizing the case" in uterine displacements of apparently the
same character as well as in cases of typhoid fever, etc.   The distinctive characters exist in every case, and the characteristic symptoms
will point to the constitutional remedy, as well as to the selection of
auxiliary means.

A REMEDY OF SOME VALUE IN THE RELIEF (CURE) OF ANGINA PECTORIS. IODIDE OF SODIUM.

By J. M. SCHLEY, M.D.,

New York.

THE remarks I have to make to-night deal with facts and clinical
observations made by myself during the past six years and nine
months. The use of this drug was not an original idea, and though
employed at first with much doubt, it has rapidly grown in my favor.
Those of us who read the leading journals must often notice how
many drugs are brought forward—sometimes by men who *should* be
able to speak with authority—as remarkable in their efficacy for
certain pathological states, and when put to the test by others in the profession, though they may be used in every detail as advised, are found
useless or nearly so. The frequency with which we see new medicines extolled, is a strong evidence of our inability to combat certain
morbid states; and again, if these praises of a fresh discovery or of
uses of an old remedy hitherto unfound or unsought were more carefully detailed, more accurately weighed, the length of time of its experimental application, the complicating maladies (beside the one it
is employed for), the correctness of the diagnosis of the disease for
which it is vaunted, the length of time during which the drug was
taken, the dose administered, and at what specified hour in the twenty-
four it was taken, fasting or otherwise, the objective symptoms noted ;
if all these items in each instance were looked into with care, the ex-
perimenter not permitting the result to bias his conclusions, many of
the profession would be more charitable in their therapeutic ideas,
many may enlarge their number of remedies employed, which might
redound to their comfort and that of the patient.

There is a wonderful sameness about the discovery, the sudden rise to popularity, the progress, the culmination, the decay and ultimate fall into oblivion of a new remedy.

At first most of the reports are decidedly favorable, then we read of a failure which is to be rapidly followed by others; and without the stimulus of continued success and faith in its merits, it falls to its true level, and is fortunate if the exalted hopes raised by its first exaggerated claims are not followed by a contempt which disregards its real worth.

To give lasting value to practical observations certain conditions should be fulfilled.

First and above all, a careful and accurate diagnosis of the disease we are treating, noting every and all complications of other organs, the possibility of their aggravating or so complicating the symptoms that some doubt about a final diagnosis is entertained. Next, a fair understanding should be had of the course of the disease when not influenced by any method of treatment. And finally, we should try and determine in what way medicines can benefit the condition : and we should in all such undertakings approach our subject with a broad, judicial spirit, with the desire to find out simply the truth, and not endeavor to prove or disprove anything.

In bringing this subject up to-night, I hope I may not be considered as acting too speedily, too hastily; and my excuse, if any be necessary, is the relief, absolute and continuous, that most of my patients have received as soon as they were under the effects of the medicine, and it is the CESSATION OF PAIN in one of the most agonizing of troubles, *vis.*, angina pectoris, that its greatest effect is shown.

The *iodide of sodium* was first prominently brought forward as a cardiac remedy of great value by Dr. Henri Huchard, in September, 1885, in the *Bulletin Général de Thérapeutique.*

In his first paper he treats of its undoubted merits in angina pectoris. In a second paper, read at Nancy, in August, 1886, before the French Association for the Advancement of Science, he dwelt upon its service in certain forms of organic heart disease, and has satisfied himself that murmurs, which were not functional, disappeared and had not returned after months and years of observation. In nine cases of angina pectoris, four were practically cured. In some of these there were valvular lesions, and disease of the coronary arteries. The *iodide* mitigated or stopped the angina and acted favorably upon the crippled valve.

Let us weigh these last two facts carefully, and if they are not disproved as true facts, what relief are we able to offer now to those sufferers, which was never thought of a few months ago! My experience has not been of sufficiently long duration to test the value of the *iodide* in valvular disease, or myocarditis, but I may state with some positiveness what I have seen it do in angina.

The *iodide* is more efficacious in the chronic contracting (sclerotic) inflammation of the endocardium.

Permit me to cite a case from my practice before Dr. Huchard read his papers.

Mr. W. B———, æt. 66, over six feet, weighing 220 to 240 pounds, retired minister; previous health always good. In the spring of 1883, I was hastily summoned to his house in the early morning, and on my arrival found him emerging from his first attack of angina pectoris. There was no apparent cause for it; on making a physical examination we found, an enlarged left ventricle, and an insufficient aortic valve, enlarged joints of his hands and a slight catarrhal nephritis, pulse moderate, full, hard, at times irregular. This patient was frequently seen by me during the following two years. His attacks of angina pectoris occurred at irregular intervals, and at all times of day or night. Their severity and duration were decidedly influenced by the inhalation of a few minims of *amyl nitrite*. He received *cactus, arsenic, phosphor., digitalis*, etc., persistently without any apparent relief. Finally he gave up taking medicines, as they seemed to avail him nothing, and relied entirely upon the *amyl nitrite*. He carried the capsules with him always. In the summer of 1885, he was seized with an attack while dressing, and died as he threw himself on the bed. An autopsy revealed an hypertrophied heart to the left, atheroma of the aorta, and aortic valve, with insufficient action, coronary artery atheromatous, myocarditis with some fatty degeneration.

This is about the history and course of the disease, as we are accustomed to follow it when medication is useless, or of little avail. In some instances the patient only survives one or two attacks at longer or shorter intervals. I have several cases of angina pectoris now under observation, where I have used the *iodide* with decided beneficial effect. I will, however, cite only three.

The first case that I would mention and one that has impressed me more than any other, is that of a Mrs. C. S——:

I was called to see this lady last winter, and found on examination a moderate bronchitis affecting the larger bronchial tubes, old pleuritic adhesions at both bases, an enlarged heart transversely, insufficiency of the mitral and aortic valves, pulse moderately full, at times irregular, atheromatous, slight enlargement of liver. She was the mother of five children, and æt 71. Her urine was normal, so I was informed; I never analyzed it myself. During my absence last summer, she was put on a solution of *iodide of sodium*, receiving about 3½ grains, thrice daily. Her attacks of angina prior to the administration of the *iodide* were terrible, occurring at all times, and lasting from a few moments to a half hour or longer. I have witnessed them myself, and all the symptoms of this disease were well portrayed. She has on some occasions had three and four in one day. Now six months have elapsed and there is not the faintest indication of their return. Her general health is improved, and she attends to her household duties notwithstanding her advanced age. In this case I can attribute this relief from pain, from an advancing disease, entirely to the *iodide*. She is not cured of her heart disease, but the constant fear of this returning agony has passed away and seems a thing of the past. Within a week from the time this drug was administered, comfort commenced. Her diet was restricted before its employment, and no other drug was taken, except for new symptoms foreign to her heart trouble. She, as some others for whom I prescribed this remedy, complained of nausea, heart-burn, dizziness, and a congested feeling towards the head. When any cerebral symptoms were mentioned the drug was diminished one-half, and if relief were not obtained then from them (the symptoms), it was discontinued for one week, and the dose gradually augmented when resumed. Only one of my eight cases could take 8 grains, three doses daily after meals, without complaining of sensations due to the drug, for, on its discontinuance these symptoms ceased, to reappear on its resumption. I claim that this Mrs. C. S——'s angina pectoris has been cured by the use of *iodide of sodium*. Her organic difficulty may eventually cause her death or be a complicating factor, not to be overlooked.

The next case is as interesting as the one just spoken of.

Mrs. J., æt. 48. History of no importance, beyond the fact of being always a great sufferer from migraine. The mother of six children. Aside from migraine, she suffers from fibroid phthisis of the right lung, following pleurisy with effusion; an hypertrophied liver; a floating right kidney and croupous nephritis, and has had repeated attacks of pelvic peritonitis. She also suffers from insufficiency of the mitral valve, with transverse hypertrophy. Patient is not of a neurotic habit. About one year ago she had her first attack of angina pectoris in the street car, and her daughter, who happened to be with her, thought she would die before she could get her home. She was prostrated in bed for four days following this brusque onset. Since that time until last October, patient had seven well marked attacks of different degrees of severity and duration. Since October, 1886, until the present writing, she has had one attack, and this was in November. I would say her valvular malady and other symptoms pertaining to her heart have rapidly grown worse until the administration of the *iodide*. Since then a decided improvement is noticeable to her whole family and myself. She takes 8 grs., three doses daily, with an occasional intermission.

I cannot see as yet any benefit to the chronic organic heart lesion, and in fact it would be too early to expect much of an alteration in such a short while. Huchard noticed the disappearance of murmurs only after eighteen months or two years of drugging. My last case is perhaps the most interesting of the three on account of the serious complications, and her having had, under my supervision, ether administered for one hour.

Miss A., æt. 49, of a neurotic family, rheumatic history, suffers from a large pyo-salpynx (which was once evacuated by aspirator), gravel in a marked degree, croupous nephritis and insufficiency and stenosis of the mitral valve with all their accompanying symptoms. When I sailed for Europe in June, I little expected to find her alive on my return, and strange though it may seem, this patient's general health is better at this moment than it has been in eighteen months. Her attacks of angina, which were severe, long and frequent, have disappeared. She has had none since October; her pulse is as full again; not so rapid; dyspnœa easier; cyanosis less, and the murmurs not so loud and rasping. This lady, though pampered for years on account of her many ailments, is more able to walk without fatigue and dyspnœa than for many months. She is still taking the *iodide.*

Whatever may be the final termination of the cardiac disease in these three cases, I am personally convinced that the *iodide of sodium* has relieved them of much suffering, and may so in time act that the danger of sudden and painful death will be done away with.

My total dissatisfaction in treating angina pectoris with all the known means, was the simple reason of my resorting to this familiar remedy. In all of these cases my diagnosis was affirmed by others more competent than myself to speak on such a subject. The complications were ferreted out by myself and were simply cited for fear that a suspicion may lurk in the minds of some that I may have been misled. In one instance only did I find marked spinal irritation with intercostal neuralgia, and this lady's case is not embodied in those cited. We all know of the line that this familiar disease follows, and our *only* remedy in no way wards off an attack; it simply relieves—palliates—and this drug is *amyl nitrite.* Some persons are affected by it unfavorably, or cannot use it at all.

I do not want to throw any discredit upon our own remedies, such as *aconite, spig., ars., cactus, calc. c., rhus. tox., digitalis, bell.,* and *verat. vir.,* for I have time and time convinced myself of their merits.

The *iodide of sodium* was chosen by Huchard instead of the *iod. of potas.* on account of its unirritating properties upon the kidney, its easy assimilation and pleasanter taste (?), and the less likelihood of its injuriously affecting the cardiac muscle by prolonged use.

The *iodide of sodium* may be prepared either by treating a solution of caustic soda with iodine or by double decomposition between iodide of iron and carbonate of sodium precisely as *iodide of potassium* is obtained by the corresponding processes for that salt.

Iodide of sodium seems to have the same therapeutic effects and is used in the same diseases as *iod. of potassium*, and when given in large doses, even, seems to produce none of the unpleasant effects of the latter.

The next thought that suggests itself to one after being convinced of the efficacy of the *iodide* in angina pectoris and organic valvular disease is, How does this drug bring about this change? how does it produce this curative result?

There are *two* ways alone in which it may be brought about: first, through the nervous system; secondly, in a purely dynamic (chemical?) manner.

As the action of the *iodide of sodium* has been found similar to that of the *potassium*, and as the latter has not been used for purely nervous affections, whether functional or of any other nature, unless it has a specific luetic base, it is evident that the *iodide* must perform its curative result by other channels.

The etiology of angina, its explosive and sudden onset, and mysterious, immediate or gradual subsidence, are still shrouded in some mystery.

The paroxysm has been tried to be explained as a purely neuralgic (and that such forms of angina exist without gross lesions of the coronary arteries, valves or myocardium, I have no doubt—and such cases are readily cured, as proven by a contemporary of Dr. H. Huchard, a Dr. Robin)—a vaso-motor spasm (witness the relief following the inhalation of a few minims of *amyl nitrite*); and again, by some unaccountable state brought about by a partial occlusion of either the anterior or posterior coronary artery or both, from atheromatous changes. If, then, the *iodide* be taken in sufficient doses for a sufficient length of time, it must so work upon the exciting cause (whatever that may be—a myocarditis—an enlarged and laboring ventricle, upon a valve crippled within itself, and replaced in part by a hard, dense fibrous tissue—or what is more probable—a constricted coronary artery), that it is removed, and the patient recovers.

It seems to me that the dynamo-homœopathic action is the only one that will explain the relief brought to those suffering from organic valvular disease in Dr. Huchard's cases. It is supposed—nay, it is strongly maintained—and I think with some justice, by syphilographers, that the action of the *iodide of potassium* in the tertiary form of syphilis (gummata, periostitis), is a purely chemical one. Its absorbing power, its abortive tendency is shown here to the greatest advantage.

RHEUMATIC ENDOCARDITIS (?): GLONOINE.

A CLINICAL CASE.

By ALFRED WANSTALL, M.D.,
Baltimore, Md.

MISS N. F., aged 16, a robust girl, called at my office on the 24th of April, 1882, complaining of severe pain in the right side of the chest, which came on suddenly while in school. No fever. *Bryonia* 6. On the following morning I was called to see her at her home, and found her confined to bed with moderate fever. During the evening of the preceding day she had had a slight chill. The pain had disappeared from the right side, and she now complains of severe pains in the neck, head and right shoulder. The pains are sharp and shooting, particularly in the head, and the scalp is extremely sensitive to touch. There is loss of appetite, with moderate thirst, and a heavily coated tongue. She shows great aversion to being moved, or interfered with in any way. *Aconite* 3 and *bryonia* 3 in alternation.

On the morning of the 26th I found that the patient had had a bad night, having been unable to sleep on account of pains in her head. Temperature 104.5, pulse 120, febrile, irregular and intermitting. Has had another moderately severe chill. Skin hot, and the scalp very sensitive. The pains in the head, neck and shoulder continue, but there is no redness or swelling. The action of the heart is tumultuous and irregular, with a marked systolic blowing sound over the right heart (tricuspid valves), masking and prolonging the first sound of the heart only over the fourth intercostal space and adjoining right side of the sternum, at all other points the sounds of the heart appear intact. Prescription of the preceding day continued. At my evening visit I found my patient worse. In addition to the severe scalp pains there are dreadful throbbings in the head, and there have been several spells of palpitation, and one sharp, but short, attack of dyspnœa ; respirations accelerated. The patient will not move nor be moved, neither will she talk nor be talked to, owing to her extreme sensitiveness to noise, and even the noise from filling the coal-hod in the cellar, although she is in the third story, is intolerable. She lies with her head and shoulders elevated, and desires to be fanned constantly. Substitute *spigelia* 3 for the *bryonia* in the prescription of the last thirty-six hours.

On the morning of the 27th, I found her much better, and tolerably free from pain. Pulse less rapid and more regular, but still intermitting occasionally. Tricuspid murmur present, but less loud. During the day she had another slight chill, and by night she was in about the same condition as on the evening of the previous day. *Aconite* and *spigelia* continued.

On the morning of the 28th, she was again easier as on the preceding forenoon, only to be in greater suffering by night than at any time previous. At my night visit, I found her in the following condition : Action of the heart violent and irregular, blowing sound over the right heart very marked ; pulse rapid and febrile, irregular and intermitting ;

violent pulsation of the carotids. Pains in the head (particularly the throbbing) agonizing. She complained especially of a sensation in the head as if a cog-wheel were turning there, the cogs of which, one after the other, were coming in contact with the brain. The sensations within the head were mostly on the left side, and compression of the corresponding carotid mitigated them to a great extent. *Glonoine* 3x dil., xii drops in xii teaspoonfuls of water, one teaspoonful every fifteen minutes. Before the medicine was gone the sufferings in the head were relieved, and disappeared entirely during the night, so that for the first time during the sickness she enjoyed a good sleep.

On the 29th I found her cheerful and comparatively comfortable, the pulse, for the first time, as low as 100, and soft and regular. She is almost free from pain, with the exception of some in the right shoulder. The blowing sound over the right heart is still present, but less marked. Continue *glonoine* every two hours.

April 30th.—There was no aggravation on the preceding night, and the patient is comfortable and continues to improve. Pain in the right shoulder continues. *Aconite* 3.

May 6th.—The patient is slowly convalescing, and is only able to sit up two hours of the twenty-four. She has little appetite, and gains strength slowly. An examination of the heart made on this day reveals the blowing sound as just distinguishable. Frequent examinations of the heart made later failed to reveal any abnormal sounds.

It is noteworthy that the convalescence was very protracted, and out of all relation to the length of the active trouble itself, if not to its gravity. At the beginning I was sure I had to do with a case of acute rheumatism. That actual endocarditis existed may be open to doubt, as all the valves of the heart were intact excepting the tricuspids. The "safety valve" function of these valves and the infrequency of trouble (primary) in the right heart might question the diagnosis. But the quick and lasting result from the *glonoine* was very marked.

CYSTITIS.

By JOHN L. MOFFAT, M.D.,
Brooklyn, N. Y.

(Concluded from page 541.)

REPERTORY.

AGGRAVATIONS.

Afternoon : Aloe, natr. s.

Coffee—After : Ign., kobalt.

Coughing : Ant. c., *caust.*, *capsic.*, kreas., natr. m., puls., verat. a., zinc.

Day : Kali. bichr., led., meph.

Desire resisted : Lil. tigr., ruta., sulph. ac.

Dinner—After : Nux m.

Evening : Cann. ind., guarea, lith. c., meph., sabad., thuja.

Every other day : Bar. c.

Exertion—After : Nux m.

Laughing : Natr. m.

Left side : Cepa, par. br.

Lying down : Berb., con., lyc.

Midnight to morning : Par. br.

Morning : Kobalt, lil. tigr., lith. c., meph., phos., senec.

3 to 6 A. M. : Par. br.

Movement : Berb. dig., nux m.

Night : Aloe, am. c., ant. c., bals. peru., cann. sat., carbo. an.,
      chimaph., con., cupr., graph., hyper., kali. bichr., lyc., phos.
      ac., ruta., spig.

Open air : Natr. s.

Presence of other people : Natr. m.

Pressing on the bladder : Berb.

Rest : Rhus.

Right side : *Equiset.*

Sitting, when : Berb., lact., natr. s., puls.

Sneezing : Zinc.

Standing : Canth.

Supper—After : Nux m.

Thinking of micturition : Ox. ac.

Turning over : Lach.

Urination—After : Capsic., kali. bichr., lil. tigr., lith. c., merc. cor.,
      populus, ran. s., sabad., sars.

—— before : Ars., chelid., ipec., sulph.

—— during : Bals. peru, capsic., cham., laur., nitr. ac., squilla.

Walking, after : Calc. o.

—— when : Acon., canth., lith. c., natr. m., natr. s.,[puls.,[ruta., zinc.

Water, sight or drinking of : Canth.

Wind, on passing : Puls.

AMELIORATIONS.

Abdomen, pressing upon : Lyc.

Bending forward : Lactic ac.

Bladder, when there is urine in the : Prunus.

Glands, by pressing on the : Canth.

Horseback riding : Lyc.

Night, at : Led.

Sitting, when : Canth.
Standing, while : Berb.
Urination, by : Carbo. an., lith. c., lyc.
—— during : Raph.

Abdomen, constant desire felt deep in the : Dulc.
—— cutting pains : Canth., sulph.
—— distended and painful to touch : Canth., equiset.
—— drawing in the : Puls.
—— pains, lancinating : Carbo. an.
—— —— in left side : Cepa.
—— rumbling in the : Stram.
—— sensation as of a ball rolling in the : Lach.
—— stitches in the : Carbo. an., nitr. ac.
—— must support the, with both hands : Lyc.
Abdominal muscles, urine can only be voided by bearing down with
        the : Magn. m.
Acid urates, sediment : Ambr. gris., ant. c.
Air passes from the bladder : Sars.
Anæsthesia urethræ : *Caust.*, sars.
Anus, cutting in the : Sumbul.
—— protrudes with tenesmus vesicæ : Mur. ac., valer.
—— stitches in the : Lyc.
Awakened by a desire to urinate : Ant. c., chimaph.
Backache : Equiset., lyc., tanac., tereb.
—— when urinating : Ant. c.
Back, coldness in the : Sumbul.
—— lame and sore : Berb.
—— has to lie on the, to urinate : *Uva u.*
—— shuddering in the : Capsic.
Backward, has to sit bent, to urinate : Zinc.
Belching of wind during urination : Rhus.
Biliverdin in the urine : Chelid.
Bladder, aching in the : Berb., equiset., eup. purp., fl. ac.
—— atony of the : Alum., arg. n., arn., cann. ind., cocc. c., hell.,.
        helon., hepar., mur. ac., plumb., rheum., stann., stram., thuja.
—— ball rolling in the, sensation of : Lach.
—— burning : *Berb.* camph., *canth.*, capsic., nux v., *prunus*, puls.
        rheum, *sep.*
—— crampy pain : Berg., mez.
—— cutting —— : Eup. purp.

Bladder distended : Hell., hyos., kali. iod., sars., tarant.

—— empty : †*Stram.*

—— feels distended : Arn., ars., hell., sep.

—— —— —— as if it would fall out over the pubis : Sep.

—— —— empty : Sumbul.

—— —— full : Cepa, chimaph., *equiset.*, par. br., prunus, ruta., sant., sep., stann.

—— —— —— after urinating : calc. o., dig., †*equiset.*, eup. purp., prunus, ruta.

—— —— —— but none passed : Zinc.

—— —— —— without desire to urinate : Ars., calad., puls.

—— —— paralyzed : Ars., hell., thuja.

—— —— weak : Cepa., stram.

—— fundus of, painful pressure : Raph

—— —— — paralysis of : Op., sec.

—— heaviness in the : Cocc. c., lyc.

—— irritable : Benz. ac., bry., cepa., °ferr. ph., hyos., kali. iod., †sabina.

—— moves up and down (sensation) : Ruta.

—— neck of, heaviness : Kali. iod.

—— —— — inflamed : Hyos., kali. iod.

—— —— — spasm of : Hyos.

—— —— — spasmodic pain : Cocc. c., polyg., puls.

—— —— — stinging : Puls.

—— —— — stitches : Capsic., guaiac., lyc.

—— —— — throbbing pain : Dig.

—— —— — violent cutting and tearing : Kali c.

—— neuralgia of the : Clemat.

—— pain in, if desire be resisted : Sulph. ac.

—— —— before and during urination : Phytol., polyg.

—— —— dull : Cop., *equiset.*, lach.

—— pinching : Mez.

—— region of, drawing : Bar. c., †rhod.

—— —— — violent itching : Sep.

—— —— — soreness, redness and heat : Puls.

—— spasmodic pressure : Con.

—— stitches : Natr. m., thuja.

—— tearing pains : Nux v.

—— tension and heaviness : Cocc. c.

—— ulcers : Merc. bin.

—— unable to empty the : Calc. o., hepar, kali bichr., kali iod., **stram.**

—— uneasiness : Eup. purp., mitchella.

Bladder, warm sensation : Cepa, elat.
—— worm twisting in (sensation of) : Bell.
Blood clots : Acon., cactus, canth., millef.
—— a few drops after urinating : †*Mez.*, puls.
—— — — —— with pain : Hell., thuja.
—— thick black emission of : Sec.
Burning after urination : Capsic., con., ran. s., sabad.
—— before —— : Ipec.
—— —— and after : Apis., canth., fl. ac., rheum.
—— during urination : Clemat., hell., lyc.
—— pain, especially at the beginning of urination : Ars., clemat.
—— worse during the intermissions : Clemat.
—— in neck of bladder when urinating : cham.
—— — —— — —— —— not urinating : †Acon.
—— — —— — —— and urethra : †*Cop.*
—— in urethra after urinating : Kali. bichr., ran. s., sabad.
—— — —— —— and during urination : Ant. tart.
—— — —— when urinating : Ant. c., *berb.*, *camph.*, †cepa.
—— — —— —— not urinating : Graph.
Chest feels congested if desire to urinate is resisted : Lil. tigr.
Chilliness precedes the urging : Senec.
Chlorides diminished : Chelid., dig.
Convulsions from the spasmodic urging : Hell.
—— from the violent pain : Elat.
Coughing, involuntary emission of urine after : Ant. c.
—— —— —— — —— upon : *Caust.* rum.
Crawling in the urethra : Lam., phos. ac., ran. s.
Constriction, sense of : Dig., nux v., puls., stram., thuja.
Cylinder pushed through the urethra, sensation like : Stram.
Desire absent (to urinate) : Ars., bell., calad., hyos., puls., stann.
—— constant : Cact., cann. s., chimaph., dulc., equiset., eup. purp.,
    ham., iod., kali bichr., merc., polyg., sulph., sumbul, tabac.,
    tanac.
—— frequent : Arg. n., bov., cocc. c., euphorb., fagop., magn. m.,
    merc. bin., phos., ran. s., raph., sabin., sumbul, zingib.
—— —— ineffectual : Alum., arg. n., arn., guaiac., nux. v., sumbul.
—— —— emission profuse : Mang. acet.
—— —— —— scanty : Magn. m.
—— immediately after urinating : Bov., chimaph., dig., eup. purp.,
    guaiac., kali carb., merc., mez., nitr. ac., raph., sabad., stann.,
    staph., sumbul.
—— increased : Dig., lactuca.

Desire, painful : Eup. purp., kali carb., nux v., raph., sabin., sulph., tanac.
—— resisted, chest feels congested : Lil. tigr.
—— —— emission impossible : Ruta.
—— —— pain in bladder : Sulph. ac.
Drawing sensations : Bar. c., capsic., kali bichr., puls. rhod., sabad.
Dribbling of urine : Agar., caust., iod.
Dripping after urination : Calc. o., cann. i., caust., clemat.
Drop, sensation as of a, left behind : Kali bichr.
—— —— — — — running through the urethra : Lactuca, lam.,
    sep., thuja.
Emission burning : Aloe, ant. c., ant. tart., apis, arg. n., berb., cact.,
    camph., cann. s., hell., gamb., kali c., *kreas.*, lach,, merc.,
    natr. s., nitr.
—— delayed : Alum., arn., cann. i., *caust.*, kali c., lyc., mur. ac.,
    natr. m., sep.
—— difficult : Alum., ant. tart., arg. n., camph., cann. i., cann. s.,
    caust., lyc., magn. m., meph., nitr., op., *par. br.*, phos., prun.,
    stram., sulph., thuja.
—— drop by drop : Acon., am. m., ant. c., ant. t., apis, arn., cact.,
    camph., cann. s., *canth.*, colch., cop., dros., dulc., eup. purp.,
    euphorb., gamb., hell., merc., merc. cor., nux v., *par. br.*,
    plumb., puls., ratan., rhus., sabad., sars., staph., stram., tarant.
—— impossible beyond the fossa navicularis : Prunus.
—— —— if the desire be resisted : Ruta.
—— —— except when bearing down with the abdominal muscles : Magn. m.
—— —— —— —— on hands and knees : *Par. br.*
—— —— —— —— lying on the back : *Uva. u.*
—— —— —— —— sitting bent backward : Zinc.
—— intermits : Carbo an., *caust.*, clemat., con., gamb., kali c., led.,
    meph., natr. m., op., stram.
—— involuntary : Acon., ant. c., ars., caust., guarea., ph. ac., puls., spig.
—— —— after the bladder seems to be emptied : Clem.,
    helon., fagop., ran. s.
—— —— —— coughing : Ant. c.
—— —— upon coughing : *Caust.*, puls., verat. a.
—— —— on passing wind : puls.
—— jerky : Clem., stram.
—— —— of last few drops : Clem., helon.
—— difficult of last few drops : Cann. i., fagop.
—— painful : *Acon.*, arg. n., bell., borax, con., cop., erig., kali c.,
    lith. c., merc. cor., nitr., nux v., *par. br.*

Emission painful, scanty : *Acon.*, am. c., bar. c., chelid., cop., dig., dulc., nux v., sant.

—— slow : Camph., hepar., kali c., laur., mur. ac., op., plat., rhus.

—— spurting on coughing : Kreas., natr. c.

Enuresis : Acon., ant. c., arn., ars., caust., dulc., °ferr. phos., guarea, gels., *kreas.*, laur., merc., mur. ac., natr. c., nitr. ac., op., petrol., puls., rhus., rum., ruta., spig., spong., zinc.

—— while asleep : †Arn., kali bichr.

Fears wetting the bed : Alum.

Film on the urine : Sulph. ac.

—— greasy : Hepar, kobalt., lact. ac., paris, rum., sulph., sumbul.

—— iridescent : Cepa., hepar, iod.

—— white : Kali bichr., sep.

Fossa navicularis, unable to void urine beyond the : Prunus.

Gasping for breath during urination : Laur.

Glans penis, drawing in : Asar.

—— —— pressing on, relieves the pain in the ureters : Canth.

—— —— violent pain in the : Par. br.

Groins, pains in the : Carbo. an., natr. s.

Head, heat in the, during and after urination : Sep.

Heels, pains down the legs to the : Par. br.

Hippuric acid in the urine : Benz. ac.

Hips, pains in the : Berb.

Hunger with the urination : Verat. a.

Hypogastrium, distended feeling : Sep.

—— pain, dull ; prevents urination : Phos.

—— —— pressive : Raph.

—— —— stinging, deep in the : Calad., canth.

—— painful drawing : Bar. c.

—— sensitive to touch : *Bell.*, calad., canth., cepa., †equiset., lact. ac., merc., sant., sars., tereb.

Indican, excess of : Ant. tart.

Irritation at neck of bladder : Apis., °ferr. phos., hell., mitch.

—— violent, in the bladder : Sep.

—— in the urethra : Lyc., petrol.

Kidneys, aching in the : Zingib.

—— burning in : Rheum.

—— cutting and downward pressure : Graph.

—— soreness during urination : Arg. n.

—— tearing pains : Nux v.

Knees, has to get down upon hands and, to urinate : Par. br.

Legs, pains down the : Par. br.

Loins, pains in the : Berb., carbo. an., Nux v., raph.

Meatus urinarius, burning in : Puls.

—— —— itching : Petrol.

—— —— tickling, crawling : Ran. s.

Mucus plugs the urethra : Sep.

—— abundant : Ant. c., aur. met., cann. i., chelid., chimaph., coloc., *equiset.*, lach., natr. m., *par. br.*, plat., popul., *sep.*, uva u.

—— discharge of : *Sars.*, sep.

Odor Ammoniacal : Asa., aur. met., calc. o., iod., par. br., sumbul., tabac.

—— as if decomposed : Hydr.

—— fetid : Carbo. an., dulc., guaiac., natr. c., petrol., plumb., *sep.*, sulph., tanac., tarant.

—— horsey : Benz. ac., natr. c., nitr. ac.

—— musty : Camph.

—— offensive : Arn., calc. o., kali iod., kreas., lach., lyc., nitr. ac., rhod., sep., tabac.

—— penetrating : Benz. ac.

—— pungent : Ambra gris., ant. tart., asa., borax, kobalt, merc., stram.

—— putrid : Calc. o.

—— sour : *Ambra gris.*, colch., graph., merc., natr. c.

—— strong : Benz. ac., dros., erig., kali bichr., kobalt, nitr. ac., zingib.

—— sweet : Tereb.

—— of violets : Cop., lactuca, nux m., tereb.

Pain, aching : Equiset., eup. purp.

—— after urination : Berb., canth., con., lith. c., lyc.

—— before urination : Berb., borax, canth., carbo an., chelid., lith. c., lyc.

—— burning : *Acon.*, ant. c., apis., ant. tart., *ars.*, *berb.*, cactus, camph., cann. i., canth., capsic., con., nux v., ran. s.

—— constrictive : Dig.

—— cutting : Am. c., berb., canth., con., eup. purp., lyc., mang. ac., par. br., polyg., prunus, puls., sulph.

—— —— during urination : Ant. c., bals. peru., con., polyg.

—— —— violent, in bladder and urethra : Berb., canth., kali c.

—— dragging in ureters like labor pains : Cham.

—— drawing : Asar., capsic., kali bichr., nux v., par. br., puls.

—— dull : *Equiset.*, phos., tanac.

—— in bladder, flashes before urinating : Lith. c.

—— — —— fleeting, when not urinating : Benz. ac.

—— lancinating : Carbo an.

—— piercing : Natr. s.

Pain, pressing : Canth.
—— shooting : Calc. ph., canth., lyc.
—— spasmodic : Canth., cocc. c., puls.
—— sticking : Arg. n., bals. peru.
—— stinging : Calad., canth.
—— stitching : Apis, berb., capsic., carbo an., carbo veg., guaiac., lyc., nitr. ac., thuja.
—— tearing : Kali c., lyc., nux v., par. br., prunus.
—— throbbing : Dig.
—— violent : °Calc. phos., cepa, chelid., elat., lyc., nux v., par. br., tarant.
Palpitation of the heart during urination : Laur.
Paralysis of the bladder : Caust., dulc., hell., laur., nux v., op., tabac.
—— —— —— ——, the fundus : Op., sec., thuja.
—— —— —— sphincter : Eup. purp., gels.
—— —— —— —— momentary : Acon.
Perineum, painful drawing : Kali bichr.
—— spasmodic pains : Canth.
Perspires during urination : Merc.
Phosphates, excess of : Bell.
—— sediment : Benz. ac.
Pinching sensation : Mez., natr. s.
Pressure in the bladder : Am. m., ars., asar., *berb.*, cepa, cop., kali c., lach., lyc., nux v., †*sep.*, sumbul, zinc.
—— —— —— —— continuous : Am. c., lil. tigr., puls., ruta., squilla.
—— —— —— cardiac region : Lith. c.
—— —— —— kidneys : Graph.
—— painful in the bladder : Squilla.
—— —— —— —— —— and urethra : Dulc.
—— to urinate in fore part of urethra, when not urinating : Cann. s.
Priapism : Kali iod.
Rectum to bladder, stitches : Thuja.
—— prolapse of : Valer.
Retention of urine : °Arn., aur., bell., cactus, camph., cann. s., canth., caust., cop., dig., dulc., erig., hell., hyos., laur., merc. cor., °magn. phos., op., plumb., puls., rhus., sabin., sars., sec., sep., sulph., tarant., tereb., zingib.
—— painful : Aur., canth., cop., dig., lact. ac., nitr. ac., sars.
—— with pressure in the bladder : Acon., aur., camph.
Sacrum, pain in the : Graph., polyg.
Sciatic nerve, aching pain down the : Equiset.
Screams with pain : Lyc., par. br., sars.

Sediment, acid urates : Ambr. gris., ant. c.
—— adheres to the vessel : *Par. br.*, puls., sumbul.
—— black : Tereb.
—— blood : Ars., canth., chimaph., merc., puls., sulph. ac., tereb.
—— —— coagulated : Acon., cactus, canth., millef., uva u.
—— bloody mucus : Canth., dulc., merc., phos. ac.
—— bran-like : Aloe, berb.
—— brown : Thuja, sumbul.
—— cheesy : Sec.
—— clay-like : Am. m., berb.
—— coats the vessel white : *Sep.*
—— coffee grounds : Hell., lith. c.
—— curdled milk : Phos.
—— earthy : Mang. acet.
—— filaments (shreddy) : Merc., merc. cor., sumbul.
—— floculent : Cham., cyclam., laur., merc., merc. cor., mez., rum.,
    sars., zinc.
—— gelatinous : Berb., canth., coloc., dulc., laur., *par. br.*, phos. ac.,
    puls.
—— granular : Canth.
—— gravel-like : Tarant.
—— gray : Canth., con., kali iod., spong.
—— greenish yellow : China, °kali mur.
—— lime-like : Canth., kali iod.
—— —— salts : Ant. tart., benz. ac., berb., kreas.
—— mealy : Berb.
—— mucus : Benz. ac., berb., cann. i., coloc., dulc., hydr., kali bichr.,
    °kali mur., °kali phos., lach., lith. c., merc., merc. cor., natr c.,
    °natr. m., nitr.. puls., sumbul, tabac., thuja, uva u.
—— muco-purulent : Benz. ac., chimaph., dulc., ham., hyos.
—— muddy : Sumbul, tereb.
—— pasty : Sep.
—— phosphates : Benz. ac.
—— pinkish : China, sep., sumbul.
—— purplish : Fl. ac.
—— purulent : Arg. n., ars., clemat., ham., kali c., led., lyc., merc.,
    nux v., popul., puls., uva u.
—— red : Acon., berb., bov., carbo veg., cupr., graph., kali c., kreas.,
    laur., mez, natr. s., nitrum., paris, phos., plat., puls., sep..
    sumbul, valer.
—— —— sand : Ars., china, dig., hyos., *lyc.*, merc. cor., natr. m.,
    nux v., par. br., rum., *sep.*, sil.

Sediment, ropy : Chimaph., coloc., hydr.
—— sandy : Sars., zinc.
—— slimy : Aloe, cann. i., hell., kali c., par. br., puls., tereb.
—— stains the vessel : Bals., peru., cupr.
—— tenacious : Sumbul, uva u.
—— tough : *Par. br.*, puls.
—— triple phosphates : Ant. tart., kali iod., kreas.
—— urates : Berb., chelid., dig., kreas., sep., tabac.
—— urate of ammonia : Benz. ac., colch.
—— violet colored : Ant. tart., bov., mang. acet.
—— white : Colc. o., canth., china, colch., con., graph., euphorb., fl. ac., °kali mur., kreas., mitch., natr. s., sec., *sep.*, spig., sumbul, valer, zinc.
—— yellow : Cham., china, kali iod., natr. s., *sep.*, sil., spong.
Shuddering on micturition : *Capsic.*, nitr. ac., stram.
Sides, pain in the : Raph.
Smarting : Apis., capsic., con., lil. tigr., natr. m.
Soreness : Arg. n., berb., cann. s., natr. m.
Spasm of the bladder : †*Arn.*, bell., bry., calad., capsic., cocc. c., colch., dig., eup. purp., gels.
—— — — —— during and after urination : Asa.
—— — — sphincter : Ant. tart., arg. n., arn., cact., kali iod., op., polyg., ruta.
Spasmodic sensation in neck of bladder : Alum, polyg., puls.
Spermatic cord, neuralgia of the : Clemat.
—— —— pain extends into, after urinating : Lith. c.
—— —— painful drawing, when urinating : Capsic.
Stains the clothes yellow : Sant.
—— — urinal red : Bals. peru. cupr., *sep.*
Stomach, pain in the, during urination : Laur.
Stool, involuntary, when urinating : Squilla.
—— following the urging. Urine flows freely with the : Am. m.
—— while straining at, can urinate only : Alum.
Strangury : Camph., cann. s., *cann.k.* capsic., con., cop., dulc., euphorb., hell., helon , kreas., lyc., merc. cor., nux m., *nux v.*, *par. br.*, plumb. sabina, sant., *tereb.*, *uva u.*
—— with vertigo : Con.
Stream divided : Rhus.
—— falls from the end of the penis : Cocc. c.
—— feeble : Cocc. c., prunus, sars.
—— slender : Camph., merc., nitr. ac., op., sars., staph.
Swashing sensation in the bladder : Acon.

Tenesmus : Acon., am. c., am. m., arg. n., †arn., bar. c., bell., benz. ac., berb., camph., *canth.*, capsic., coloc., dig., hedeoma, lil. tigr., lith. c., *merc. cor.*, mur. ac., nux m., *par. br.*, popul., puls., rhus., senec., valer., viola tri.

—— after urination : Lil. tigr., merc. cor., popul.

—— agonizing : Canth., hell.

—— arouses him from sleep at night : Ant. c., chimaph.

—— in the bladder : Am. m., bar. c.

—— —— neck of the bladder : †Acon., am. m., arg. n., †arn., camph., dig.

—— and burning in the urethra : Colch., lil. tigr.

—— rectal : Alum, merc. cor., nux m., par. br., phos., sumbul, valer.

—— violent : Canth., merc. cor., natr. m., tarant.

Testes, painful drawing in, when urinating : Capsic.

—— retracted : Canth., par. br.

—— spasmodic pains in the : Canth.

Thighs, pains in the : Carbo an., par. br., puls.

Thirst while urinating : Terat. a.

Triple phosphates, sediment : Ant. art., kali iod., kreas.

Ulcers in the bladder : Merc. bin.

Umbilicus, constriction around the : Puls.

—— pinching around the : Natr. s.

Urates in excess : Chelid.

—— sediment : Ambr. gris., ant. c., benz. ac., berb., chelid., colch., dig., kreas., sep., tabac.

Ureters to bladder, cutting, pressing : Berb., canth.

—— dragging down the, like labor pains : Cham.

—— sharp stitches : Berb.

—— violent pain before discharge of turbid urine : Chelid.

Urethra, anæsthesia of the : Caust., sars.

—— burning in the : Ant. c., ant. tart., *berb.*, *camph.*, †cepa., cop., graph., kali bichr., natr. m., nitr. ac., nux v., phos., prunus, puls., ran. s., sabad.

—— crawling in the : Lam., phos. ac., ran. s.

—— cutting in : Mang. acet., natr. m.

—— cylinder were pushed through the, sensation as if a : Stram.

—— drawing in the : Asar., kali bichr., nux v., sabad.

—— itching in the : Lyc., petrol.

—— feels too narrow, unable to expand : Stram.

—— —— very sore : Cann. s.

—— neuralgia of the : Clemat.

—— sensation as of a drop running through it : Lactuca, lam.

Urethra, sensitive pain in middle of the : Lith. c.
—— smarting in the : Natr. m.
—— spasmodic pains along the : Canth.
—— sticking pain : Arg. n., bals. peru.
—— stitching —— : Apis, euphorb., natr. m., thuja.
—— tearing —— : Nux v.
—— tickling in the : Ran. s.
—— twitching : Phos.
—— violent cutting and tearing : Kali carb., lyc.
—— sense of warmth : Cepa.
—— —— — weakness : Cepa.
Urgent desire to urinate : †*Acon.*, agar., aloe, alum., ambr. gris., am. c.,
    am. m., bar. c., bell., benz. ac., berb., borax, bry., cann. s.,
    canth., *caust.*, cepa., chimaph., cycl., euphorb., graph., guaiac.,
    ipec., led., mitch., natr. m., petrol., phytol., ruta., sabad.,
    senec., sep., stram.
—— —— with scanty emission : Acon., agar., am. c., am. m., ant.
    tart., bry., graph., hedeoma, lil. tigr., puls., ratan., ruta., sil.,
    staph., uva u.
Urging constant : Arn., asar., aur. met., bar. c., berb., cann. s.,
    chimaph., dig., guaiac., lil. tigr., *par. br.*, phos. ac., ruta., sil.,
    thuja, verat a., viola tri.
—— —— almost : Acon., led., raph.
—— forces him to retain the urine : Lyc.
—— frequent : Aloe, bry., calc. o., calc. ph., camph., caust., coloc.,
    guarea, hell., lam., lil. tigr., lyc., merc., mez., natr. c., phos.,
    ratan., rhod., rhus., spig., spong., squilla, staph., uva u.
—— —— ineffectual : Borax, camph., capsic., carbo an., cop.,
    puls.
—— —— painful : Am. c., *am. m.*, berb., borax, carbo an., cham.,
    chelid., hedeoma, hell., kali iod., nux v., phos., puls., raph.,
    saut., thuja.
—— —— emission profuse : Merc., natr. m., sabina, thuja.
—— ineffectual : Camph., cann. s., cann. i., *canth.*, dig., *ipec.*, lach.,
    nux v., sars., sec., *stram.*
—— sudden : Rum.
—— —— irresistible : Ign., kreas., merc., merc. bin., natr. m.
—— violent : Alum, ant. tart., borax, *canth.*, capsic., cepa., con., cop.,
    dig., dulc., hell., *kreas.*, merc., sabad., sabina.
—— with vertigo : Con., hyper.
Uric acid : Ars., china, dig., hyos., lith. c., *lyc.*, merc. cor., natr. m.,
    nux v., par. br., rum., *sep.*, sil.

Urination dribbling : Agar., caust., cocc. c., nux v., petrol., plumb., spig., stram.

—— frequent : Ant. c., apis., bar. c., borax, †cepa, chimaph., cyclam., erig., eup. purp., fl. ac., ham., lact. ac., led., meph., mur. ac., nitrum, paris, plat., *sep.*, verat. a., zinc.

—— —— at night : Aloe, ambr. gris., bals. peru., cann. i., carbo an., con., graph., kali bichr.

—— —— profuse : *Iod.*, †*kreas.*, natr. m., oxal. ac.

—— —— scanty : Apis, cann. i., china, clemat., dros., eup. purp., gamb., hyos., ipec., kali c., kobalt., petrol., phos.

—— scanty : Acon., agar., ambr. gris., am. c., am. m., bar. c., cocc. c., coloc., cycl., dig., dulc., euphorb., ham., lam., magn. m., ran. s., ratan., squilla.

—— seldom : Cycl., *gamb.*

Urine acid : Colch., cop., cupr.

—— acrid : Asa., erig., hepar., iod., laur., lith. c., paris, sars.

—— alkaline : Fl. ac.

—— bloody : Acon., aloe, apis, ant. tart., arn., ars., berb., cact., calc. o., cann. s., *canth.*, *carbo veg.*, colch., cop., hell., hepar., hyper., lyc., merc., merc. cor., mez., *millef.*, natr. m., nitr. ac., nux v., puls., rhus, sabina, sant., senec., squilla, sulph.

—— —— the last drops : Ant. tart., puls.

—— bright : Fl. ac., sars.

—— brown : Calc. o., graph., kreas., merc. cor., petrol., stann., tarant.

—— dark brown : Ant. tart., bar. c., benz. ac., caust., nitr. ac., zingib.

—— reddish brown : Camph., kreas., puls.

—— like brown beer : Coloc.

—— — buttermilk : Asar.

—— clay-colored : Cham., guarea., sabad., *sep.*

—— clear : Agar., calc. o., fagop., lact. ac., lyc., meph., ox. ac., phos. ac., sars.

—— cloudy : Kreas., nitrum, plat., *sep.*, sumbul.

—— —— on standing : Caust.

—— cold when it passes : Nitr. ac.

—— concentrated : Acon., am. m., ant. c., arg. n., canth., colch., nitrum, senec., sep.

—— dark : Ant. c., ars., asa., bals. peru., colch., dros., fl. ac., hepar., iod., lil. tigr., lith. c., merc. bin., sabad., *sep.*, stram.

—— very dark : Dig., hedeoma, lach., natr. m.

—— decomposes rapidly : Aur., kali iod., phos. ac.

—— frothy : Cop., lach., lyc., spong.

—— greenish : Berb., *carbol. ac.*, rhod., ruta., *sant.*

Urine high colored : Bell.,lact. ac., mitch., nux m.,plumb.,senec., tanac.

—— hot : Acon., am. m., apis, asa., benz. ac., borax, kali c., lil. tigr., merc. cor., mez.

—— increased : Calc o., carbo an., cop., ham., lil. tigr.

—— light colored : Agar., fagop., oxal. ac., ran. s.

—— loam colored in the morning : Zinc.

—— milky : Iod., lil. tigr., lyc., mur. ac., phos., †*phos. ac.*, stann.

—— oily on standing : Dulc.

—— pale : Con., ham., nitrum, nux v., phos., plat., staph., zinc.

—— profuse : Agar., ant. tart., calc. o., erig., guaiac., ham., †*kreas.*, lact. ac., lactuca, mang. acet., nitrum, phos., phos. ac., polyg., rhod., sars., staph.

—— red : Acon., agar., apis., benz. ac., bov., camph., carbo veg., cepa, chimaph., cycl., ipec., kreas., merc. bin., mur. ac., nux v., plat., rhus, rum., squilla, tabac.

—— dark red : Acon., benz. ac., cycl., lyc., merc., paris, tarant.

—— syrupy : *Equiset.*

—— scanty : Acon., agar., ambr. gris., am. c., am. m., ant. c., ant., tart., apis, arg. n., arn., ars., bell., cann. i., canth., cham., china, clemat., cocc. c., colch., cupr., cyclam., dig., dros., dulc., *equiset.*, fl. ac., hedeoma, hyper., ipec., lact. ac., lil. tigr., lith. c., lyc., merc. cor., mez., natr. s., nitr. ac., nux m., popul., prunus, puls., ratan., rum., sars., senec., spong., stann., sumbul.

—— thick : Chimaph., ˉdig., iod., lact. ac., merc. bin., nux v., sep., stram., zingib.

—— —— soon after passing : Cham.

—— turbid : Ambr. gris., am. c., am. m., ant. tart., ars., aur. met., *berb.*, canth., carbo veg., caust., cham., chelid., china, colch., coloc., dig., dulc., hyos., hyper., lyc., meph., merc., nitr. ac., *par. br.*, phos., plat., rum., sabad., *sant.*, *sep.*, sil., stram., zinc.

—— —— on standing : Bell., caust., cupr., graph., ratan.

—— violet : Mur. ac.

—— viscid : Coloc., sars., sep.

—— watery : Ant. tart., cocc. c., kali bichr., kreas., phos., phos. ac., plat., staph.

—— white : Lact. ac.

—— yellowish green : Berb., bov., camph., iod.

—— deep yellow : Am. m., cop., natr. c.

Vertigo with the urging : Con., hyper.

Vulva, smarting and soreness in the : Natr. m.

Walk about, has to, although motion aggravates the desire : Dig.

Weakness, feeling of, in bladder and genitals : †*Alum.*, stram.
—— of sphincter vesicæ : Agar., bell., °ferr. phos.
Wind, belches, when urinating : Rhus.
—— enuresis, —— passing : Puls.

AUTHORITIES CONSULTED.

LEBERT, in Ziemssen's Cyclopædia, Vol. VIII.
SIR H. THOMPSON, in Reynolds' System of Medicine, Vol. III.
NIEMEYER, Text Book of Medicine, Vol. II.
VAN BUREN & KEYES, Genito-Urinary Diseases.
BEALE, L. S., Kidney Diseases and Urinary Deposits.
AUSTIN FLINT, JR., Physiology, Vol. III.
DA COSTA, Diagnosis.
TYSON, Examination of the Urine.
H. C. WOOD, Therapeutics.
BARTHOLOW, Materia Medica and Therapeutics.
DUNCAN, T. C., Diseases of Children.
HELMUTH, Surgery.
GUERNSEY, Obstetrics.
LILIENTHAL, "Therapeutics"; also, "Clinical Medicine."
HAHNEMANN, Materia Medica Pura.
ALLEN, Encyclopedia of Materia Medica.
HERING, Condensed Materia Medica.
HEINICKE, Materia Medica.
LIPPE, Materia Medica.
HALE, "New Remedies."
HULL's Jahr.
SCHUESSLER, Twelve Tissue Remedies.
E. WAGNER, Manual of General Pathology.

ORIGINAL ARTICLES IN SURGERY

TREATMENT OF FIBROID TUMORS BY ELECTROLYSIS.
DR. APOSTOLI'S METHOD.*

By WM. H. KING, M.D.,
New York City.

MR. PRESIDENT, Ladies and Gentlemen—My object in presenting this subject to you is : First, to give a full account of the
various steps of the operation, so that any physician possessing a good
knowledge of gynæcology and but a limited knowledge of electro-
physics, can safely and effectually treat a case; second, to give the

---

* Read before the New York State Homœopathic Medical Society.

result of observations both in my practice and at Dr. Apostoli's Clinic, of Paris, which I attended during a part of last July and August.

The apparatus needed should have a careful consideration.

A galvanic battery capable of generating 250 milli-amperès, with a selector that will introduce any number of cells without interrupting the circuit, must be chosen. Of course, some form of a cabinet battery is to be preferred, as there is no acid to corrode the connections, and it is always in order; but an ordinary zinc-carbon battery may answer the purpose, if it is kept in good condition.

The external electrode should be large enough to cover all the available space of the abdomen, thus reducing the resistance to a minimum.

You will hear many say that any large electrode will answer. I wish to disabuse your minds on this point. The large mesh electrode, covered with absorbent cotton, which is so highly recommended and so much used in this city, I consider useless for this purpose, for I have been unable, when using it, to pass a current of 250 or even 200 milli-amperès without causing excruciating pain, and, in most cases, blistering the abdomen. The one used by Dr. Apostoli is made of potter's clay. It is not elegant, but is very effectual; and, if properly made, can be used without soiling the patient's linen or abdomen. The best material to be obtained here for making it is the finely ground clay used by artists for modeling, which can be obtained at stores dealing in art materials. A piece of ordinary muslin may be used; but I prefer a towel which has been worn until it has become smooth and soft. This should be so cut that, when folded upon itself, it will be of the required shape and size. The edges are sewed together, leaving a space large enough for the hand to enter. The clay, well moistened, is packed carefully in the sack from one to one and one-half inches in thickness. A brass plate, soldered to one end of a copper wire, with a connector on the other end, should now be imbedded in the clay and the opening in the sack closed around the wire. This electrode must be kept moist, which can be easily done by keeping it in a little water in an ordinary dripping pan. It will then always be ready for use, and is certainly the most effectual one I have ever seen. Two hundred and fifty milli-amperès can be passed through it without causing pain or any perceptible redness of the skin.

The internal electrode used by Dr. Apostoli is a small bar, twelve inches long and the size of a number eight French sound. One end is made of platinum and iridium, and shaped like an ordinary uterine sound. The other end is made of steel and has a trocar point; this is used for making punctures.

THE BAR.

THE HARD RUBBER SHIELD.

THE ELECTRODE COMPLETE.

A mille-amperè meter is absolutely necessary to success. It is not my purpose to dwell on its construction. It is simply an instrument by which the intensity of the current can be told at any time, *thus* making the electric current mathematically "doseable."

THE OPERATION.—There should be a distinction made here between the hemorrhagic and non-hemorrhagic, for one requires just the opposite kind of treatment to the other. With the former, the positive pole of the battery should be attached to the internal electrode, with the latter the negative. Please bear in mind these distinctions, for a treatment might prove most disastrous if you introduced the negative electrode into a uterus containing a hemorrhagic fibroid.

The patient is placed on her back, the thighs flexed in position for a bivalve speculum. The abdominal electrode is first placed in position, so that the skin of the abdomen may become moist, before the current is allowed to pass. The platinum end of the internal electrode is then inserted into the cavity of the uterus and a celluloid or hard rubber shield passed over it until it reaches the os; this is done to protect the vagina and external parts. After this, a handle, which also serves as a connector, is passed over the steel end of the sound until it reaches the insulating shield and is made firm by a set screw. The current is then turned on. At the first treatment not more than twenty to thirty milli-amperès should be allowed to pass until the patient becomes accustomed to it, when fifty to one hundred may be used.

At each treatment you will be able to increase the current; but this increase will differ with different patients. With some not more than 150 to 200 can be used; but with the majority, if carefully handled, you will be able to pass 250 to 300 milli-amperès through the tumor.

This must be done without causing any severe pain to the patient, for if the operation is too painful, you will not be successful.

These very powerful currents are the secret of success in this form of treatment of fibroid tumors, and, unless you can pass 150 milli-amperès through the tumor, you will not be successful. Dr. Apostoli attributes nearly all his failures to an inability on part of the patient to bear a strong current. This may be due to pelvic inflammation, but more frequently to a hysterical tendency.

The directions given above are those to be followed when there is no obstruction to the passage of a sound into the uterine canal. When such obstruction exists, a puncture should be made, if possible, through the cervix, but never more than one and a half to two inches, with the trocar end of the electrode and the negative pole always attached. This generally requires an anæsthetic, although it is not unbearable without it. The external electrode is placed the same as before, to which is attached the positive pole, and a current of about 150 milli-amperès allowed to pass for ten minutes. This opening will remain for some time, and is used for the introduction of the sound in after treatments.

Another method of treatment which has been employed by Dr. Apostoli is to puncture the tumor in its most prominent part, if possible, through the vagina, if not through the abdominal wall, with a needle insulated to within an inch of the end and connected with the negative pole of the battery.

Many seem to be particularly afraid of puncturing the peritoneum; but I believe it can be done in most cases, with proper precautions, with impunity, for I have punctured it a number of times with a large electric needle, and only saw the least bad effect once, when the insulation of the needle was at fault. The time of which I speak a strong current was used, and, from the exposed surface of the needle, the peritoneum must have been considerably disturbed. The only result of this was soreness over a circumscribed area of four inches for a few days, no fever accompanying it.

The precaution I would urge upon you, aside from thorough anti-sepsis, is to have the needle thoroughly insulated with hard rubber and not trust the patent varnish insulators of different manufacturers. There is another precaution which should be mentioned. In punctur-ing a fibroid tumor with insulated needles, the current should not be long enough or of sufficient intensity to induce suppuration.

With all these operations, the law of antisepsis should be thoroughly observed. The vagina should be washed with an anti-septic solution before and after each treatment, and when a puncture is made, the patient should have a pledget of antiseptic gauze continually in the vagina.

Exactly the way this treatment reduces a fibroid tumor, I do not profess to know   Nearly all agree that the cauterizing, hardening and contracting effect of the positive pole is the process by which the tumor is reduced, when that pole is used.   There is more speculation regarding the effect of the negative; but all agree that it reduces a tumor more rapidly than the positive.

Dr. Apostoli thinks its effects are due to an over congestion and consequent destruction of the molecules.   Others believe the tumor is composed of certain electrolytes, which are decomposed by the current and are then absorbed.

If I digress further on this point, I would be losing sight of the second object of this paper, the results which are obtained.

These may be divided into two classes.   First, the changes noted in the pathology; and second, the change in the symptoms and the general condition of the patient.   One of the first changes in the pathology is the breaking up of the adhesions.   The tumor which was before immovable, becomes movable.   I have also noticed this as one of the first changes when treating an ovarian tumor by electrolysis. The tumor also begins to decrease in size, which will be recognizable both by external manipulation and internal measurements.   The retrogression will continue for some months after the treatment is discontinued.

I was much surprised on my return to this city this month, on examining a patient I had treated last spring, and who had had no treatment for two months, to find that the tumor, so far as I could perceive, had decreased in size just as fast while I was away as when under active treatment.

Dr. Apostoli has noted the fact that, under treatment, the tumor tends to partially separate from the uterus and become pedunculated. This I noticed in two cases in his clinic, and one in my practice, a ring of depression at the attachment of the tumor to the uterine wall being distinctly felt through the vagina.

We have much more marked changes in the symptoms and general condition of the patient than in the pathology.   If it be a hemorrhagic fibroid, the hemorrhage will almost immediately stop if the positive pole is used internally and the patient be able to bear a very strong current.

Striking as this may be, it is not more so than the improvement in the general health and constitutional symptoms.   The appetite improves, the patient sleeps well, gains flesh, and feels much better in every respect. Fat accumulates in the abdominal wall, the local symptoms one by one disappear, and this same good effect will continue, under proper treatment, until the cure is effected.

Although I have never seen a fibroid tumor entirely removed by electrolysis, I have yet to see a single case that has been under treatment a sufficient length of time in which every symptom that could be traced to the tumor did not disappear, and this relief, so far as I know, has been permanent.

I saw cases in Paris treated by Dr. Apostoli two, three and four years ago which were as well as when discharged from the clinic.

That there are cases which are but slightly or partially relieved, I know; there must be many, only I have never seen one.

I will not tax your patience longer. I wish to say, in conclusion, that success will not be obtained by careless treatment, but only by strict adherence to all the minor details and a careful study of each case.

RADICAL CURE OF HERNIA.*

By J. G. GILCHRIST, M.D.,

Iowa State University.

THE text-books and periodicals, for many years, have had much to say of hernia abdominalis. The general interest felt in this subject is easily explained and understood when we recall the very serious nature of the condition. Whether hernia is recent or ancient, acquired or congenital, every movement is one of danger to the sufferer. Accordingly, for many years, surgeons have been busy devising operations for its cure, so that the number of "radical cures" is very large. Some of them had a very brief life; others survived, in spite of portentous failures, for a generation or two. Most of them have dropped out of sight entirely, but now and then an old method will be revived, modified and "improved," but it quickly goes back to oblivion (again).

The earlier idea was that the canal was to be closed up, either by invagination, or in some manner by reducing its dimensions, and among the majority of operators to-day, the same ends are sought. The operation usually results in failure, no matter what the particular method be, from a failure to recognize or appreciate the import-

---

*Read before the New York State Homœopathic Medical Society.

ance of certain predisposing conditions, and for the want of proper medicinal treatment of the case after an operation has been made. It may be stated as roughly a fact, that the cause of hernia is not, by any means, to be looked for in the patency of the vaginal process, or an unusual size of the abdominal rings. Certainly these conditions are important factors in the causation, but are rarely, if ever, of such importance that other and more potent ones are to be ignored. The chief cause is found to be an elongation of the mesentery, practically producing such augmentation in bulk of the contents of the abdomen, that the capacity of that cavity is insufficient. It is true that the loss of support, when the canal or its rings are too capacious, favors such traction on the mesentery, that elongation is, sooner or later, produced; but with these outlets *intact*, if the mesentery, from any cause, becomes elongated, a hernia will, nevertheless, appear. There can be no question that a radical cure of hernia cannot be secured without closing the canal; but if this is the sole treatment, my experience leads me to state most confidently, few patients will remain cured.

It has been my fortune to make very many operations, probably all the legitimate ones, even to the very doubtfully "legitimate" Heatonian. I am of the opinion that my success has been probably as good as others, but the number of positive *cures* has been very small until quite recently. For the past year or two the successful cases so far outnumber the unsuccessful that I confidently expect, if not an absolute cure, at least a marked improvement on the former state. The procedure, as far as the instrumental part is concerned, varies slightly in different cases, but is generally as follows:

The part is shaved quite closely, and a fold of the integument pinched up over the external ring and transfixed with a curved bistoury, making an incision of from an inch to an inch and a half in length. The fat which now appears is broken through with the finger or the handle of a scalpel, or incised, if necessary, and the incision deepened until the ring is brought into view. Now if the sac is not too voluminous, or too much thickened, it is pushed up into the canal until the lower portion, at least, is fairly filled with it. A needle armed with catgut—carbolized or not is a matter of utter indifference—is entered into the mass of the sac and brought out well beyond the pillar on either side; the needle is unarmed and armed again with the other end of the catgut, and used in the same way on the other side. The ligature is then drawn tight, knotted, and the ends cut off, bringing the pillars together, and retaining the plug formed by the sac in the canal. This stitch is taken in about the middle of the pillars. Should the ring be very large I freshen the edges with scissors or knife, and insert two or even more stitches. Should the sac be voluminous and too vascular, *after* stitching it in the canal it is ligatured by transfixion and cut off. Up to this point there is little, if anything, peculiar or novel in the operation, nor in the closure of the external wound, which is by means of interrupted sutures of silk. Over the wound I place a compress of absorbent cotton, saturated with a solution of *hypericum*, about ten drops of tincture to two or three ounces of water, securing it in place, as well as furnishing support to the parts by a snugly applied spica bandage. The patient is then put to bed, cautioned to apply the hand over the wound in coughing or vomiting, as well as in urinating or going to stool. The compress is not to be wet with the *hypericum* again, but the remedy is given in any dilution, the thirtieth preferable, about once an hour. After twenty-four hours have elapsed, the bandage and compress are removed, a dry compress applied and a new bandage put on ; the hypericum is to be continued for two or three days longer. When the external wound is fairly healed a light truss is to be applied, one with a flat pad, with either a very weak spring or elastic straps, and the patient permitted to go about the house. In fact, he can usually leave the bed for a chair about the fourth or fifth day, but must be careful to apply the hand over the wound while moving from chair to bed. About the tenth day he may leave the house, never without the truss, which should be worn until the parts are evidently healed. The truss is to be worn during the day, and *after lying down at night* must be removed. In the morning it must be replaced *before rising*. These rules are imperative. After the third or fourth day, as soon as the hypericum is discontinued, commence giving lycopodium 30 three times a day for two weeks, then twice a day for two weeks, afterwards once a day until there is evidently no disposition to a reappearance of the hernia. This item in the treatment I esteem *sine qua non*. I was led to employ this remedy on the authority of the late Dr. Holt, of Massachusetts, the first case being as follows :

A young man had a large inguinal hernia on the left side, which came down into the scrotum whenever the truss was removed. It had never been strangulated, but his truss not being comfortable, he applied for a radical cure. The operation was made, as above, and for a time all seemed well. After about six weeks a bubonocele appeared on the right side. Recalling Dr. Holt's experience, I gave *lycopodium* 30, purposing to make a second operation at a later period. *The bubonocele disappeared*, and during the two or three years I had him under observation, did not return.

A second case was one of double inguinal hernia, that on the left side being double the volume of the right. A double operation was made. The left hernia did not again appear, but after a time that on the right became prominent. Lycopodium was given as above, and all trouble pased away.

There are many such cases in my case-book, and finally the question naturally arose, Why wait for the reappearance of the hernia? Accordingly it became a habit to give lycopodium as a matter of course, and the result in about forty cases seems to justify the practice. In my last fifty cases, as far as I have been able to learn, there has not been one that has not been vastly improved, and the large majority (thirty-four) may properly be claimed cured.

There can be no doubt that the desirable shortening of the mesentery is secured by giving the lycopodium.

THE CAPILLARY CATHETER IN RETENTION OF URINE FROM STRICTURE. —Dr. Jno. Ward Cousins writes to the *Brit. Med. Jour.*, that during the last two years he has made an extended trial of the capillary catheter in troublesome cases of retention of urine from urethral stricture. From his experience he recommends a trial of the method at the very onset of the treatment. The operation is painless and generally requires no anæsthetic. The capilary catheter used by Dr. Cousins consists of a fine catheter and filiform bougie, very carefully prepared with woven web and gum elastic, and possessing great flexibility and toughness, together with a smooth and highly polished surface. The combination is about eighteen inches in length, and it can be used for pneumatic aspiration by slipping over it an india-rubber tube, connected with a glass bottle fitted with a two way cork and a hand ball air exhauster. After injecting the urethra with warm oil and covering the patient with blankets, the penis is drawn forward with the left hand and the catheter gently passed down to the stricture. As soon as its progress is arrested it must be withdrawn two or three inches, rotated between the thumb and finger, and again twisted down upon the obstruction. During these manipulations its easy movement in the urethra and the sensations of the patient indicate that the stricture has been overcome. Following the discharge of a little urine, the catheter may be attached to the aspirating bottle and the flow of urine accelerated thereby.

EDITORIAL DEPARTMENT.

EDITORS

GEORGE M. DILLOW, M.D.,	. . . .	Editor-in-Chief, Editorial and Book Reviews
CLARENCE E. BEEBE, M.D.,	. . . .	Original Papers in Medicine.
SIDNEY F. WILCOX, M.D.,	. . . .	Original Papers in Surgery.
MALCOLM LEAL, M.D.,	. . . .	Progress of Medicine.
EUGENE H. PORTER, M.D.,	. . . .	Comments and News.
HENRY M. DEARBORN, M.D.,	. . . .	Correspondence.
FRED S. FULTON, M.D.,	. . . .	Reports of Societies and Hospitals.

A B. NORTON, M.D., ... Business Manager.

The Editors individually assume full responsibility for and are to be credited with all connected with the collection and presentation of matter in their respective departments, but are not responsible for the opinions of contributors.

It is understood that manuscripts sent for consideration have not been previously published, and that after notice of acceptance has been given, will not appear elsewhere except in abstract and with credit to THE NORTH AMERICAN. All rejected manuscripts will be returned to writers. No anonymous or discourteous communications will be printed.

Contributors are respectfully requested to send manuscripts and communicate respecting them directly with the Editors, according to subject, as follows: *Concerning Medicine, 21 West 37th Street; concerning Surgery, 256 West 57th Street; concerning Societies and Hospitals, 111 East 70th Street; concerning News, Personals and Original Miscellany, 161 West 71st Street; concerning Correspondence, 152 West 57th Street.*

Communications to the Editor-in-Chief, *Exchanges* and *New Books* for notice should be addressed to *102 West 43d Street.*

ON THE VAUNTING OF FAITH IN INDECENCY.

THE editorial in our issue for August appears to have precipitated an attack of acute satyriacal fury in the September number of *The Medical Advance.* We confess to some astonishment at the sudden outbreak, so inexplicable and violent. For some unknown reason, the writer's malevolence had seemingly been accumulating to bursting, until, pent up within itself like a mud-volcano, it could no longer contain its vast store of filthy fizz and splutter. The pseudo-correspondent, who would have been at once recognized from his indecency alone, without the vanity of an open *nom de plûme,* rages through six pages of brevier type about "The Crank of an Organ." As nearly as we can pick out the main delusion from its companion host of libidinous fancies, it would seem that the NORTH AMERICAN was imagined to be an organ, "bought by a medical college," whose "faculty—from its own alumni—selected seven to work the new crank," the editor-in-chief being conceived to be a "conscienceless machine" of "wood and leather," and his six associates, supernumeraries, "dummies," "wax figures" and "*simulacra.*" The organ loomed up "very little" before the writer's vision, and was therefore inferred to be worth reviling in an obscene frenzy of insult. So the "wood and leather automaton-editorial-apparatus," was savagely assaulted as if it were a thing of "flesh and blood;" its "wood and leather rhetoric" was then clawed into imaginary shreds, and the "very large crank" challenged, in a final burst of tip-toe stultiloquence, to measure the folly of nastiness with him who wrote about "The Crank of an Organ." Now, assuming that the organ-charger was sane, this was a remarkable tribute to a "debilitated organ," and to a "thing" accustomed to be kicked by a "combination that beats the devil," especially when the "it," the "thing," did not write the editorial in question, and was enjoying its vacation amazingly for an "infernal," "wood and leather " " device," "pretense," "sham," "libeller," " apparatus," " automaton," "fabrication " and " phenomenon."*

The said Editor-in-chief, being now back in his wood and leather so-called Easy Chair, and reassuming labor which, in the meantime, kind friends have undertaken for him, has no desire to evade his ultimate responsibility for all that has appeared in the JOURNAL during his absence. The editorial, so indecently made the occasion of personal abuse, was written by a gentleman to whom we should look for an example in good writing as well as understanding of the principles and history of homœopathy. We have no further explanation to offer, except to him for the slips in proof-reading to whose ill-spiced stew the ravenous contributor of *The Advance* is abundantly welcome. So, too, the malicious straining after captious misinterpretation, indulged in by the defiler, should be left to the penetration of fair minded readers, and surely the interests of decency demand that we should leave his insulting spirit of salacity to sport its own degradation in seclusion. We must, however, deplore the fact—the evident fact— that the editor of *The Advance* has permitted the columns of his journal to be made a mire and a stench to gentlemen in journalism. We await his disavowal in the hope that his confidence has been betrayed.

As for the wanton misstatements concerning the NORTH AMERICAN, we are content with restating facts known to all men, or, if not known, easy to have been learned by any one solicitous to speak the

---

*The light cannot be placed near the nastier extravaganzas.

truth. The NORTH AMERICAN has never been bought by any medical college. The membership of the Journal Publishing Club was in the beginning, and is now, made up from physicians, in and outside of New York, and inside and outside of staffs and faculties. Our present Editors were not, either singly or collectively, selected by any faculty, or, as a body, from the *alumni* of any college; the Editor-in-chief enjoys freedom from dictation, and has thus far been honored with unrestricted trust; his associate Editors, far from being supernumeraries or dummies, he is thankful to say, deserve the credit for all the good selection and work connected with their respective departments. Nor is, nor has been, the NORTH AMERICAN an organ of any faction, or institution; all homœopathic institutions existing, and, in particular, all the homœopathic institutions of New York, have had, and will have, its cordial support. It certainly has not, from personal malice, decried institutions with which its editors have not had the honor of being connected, and of the institutions by which some of us have been honored, too little rather than too much has been said lest our motives might be misinterpreted.

And now, to the author of "The Grounds of a Homœopath's Faith," and likewise of "The Crank of an Organ," we would frankly address a few words in his own interest and in that of clean literature. We regret that we cannot touch his glove: no fair knightly spirit could have thrown such a dirty challenge. It is pitiable, we think, that one who has proven talents, and both literary and scientific culture, whose measurement and weight, in comparison with those of other men, are no concern of ours, should squander his time of usefulness in the indulgence of ignoble feelings, brawling like Thersites, "clamorous of tongue," and smutching the regard, which otherwise might be fully his, with obscene wit and ribald railings. Insult, surely, cannot be the path to honor or persuasion, nor is there any martyr worth burning who pads lewd gibes with canting rhapsodies in parody of Carlyle. If that rugged despiser of nastiness were here, we can imagine that he would instantaneously cover up his "whimsically strutting" "little Brotherkin," within his "largest imaginable Glass bell," leaving the brotherkin in silence to meditate upon the philosophy of wearing clothes enough, at least to cultivate a decent sense of shame. And as "for thy very Hatred, thy very Envy, those foolish Lies thou tellest of me in thy splenetic humor," let them pass by, remembering what Fluellen said of Alexander: "Alexander, God knows and you know, in his rages, and his furies, and his wraths, and his cholers, and his moods, and his displeasures, and his indignations, and also being a little intoxicates in his prains, did, in his ales and his angers, look you, kill his best friend, Cleitus." It were better than attempting to kill Cleitus, if, using "your right wits and good judgments," you should follow the example of Harry of Monmouth in turning "away the fat knight with the great belly doublet." You will then no longer need to betray your consciousness of the dirt in which you have trodden your knightly standing by pleading, "Do not disdain to pick up the glove because it is flung at your feet by him who wrote 'The Grounds of a Homœopath's Faith.'" Let your glove lie in the ditch to rot with your castaway tatters of indecency. It would be far more useful to the cause you claim to have so much at heart if you would go on demonstrating the grounds of your confidence in homœopathy by serious constructive work, instead of exhibiting the irritability of an obscene imagination, vain in its purpose and stirred by ill-will.

THE NEW YORK STATE SOCIETY.

THE semi-annual meeting of the New York State Homœopathic Medical Society indicated that, while a moderate number could fill out an instructive session, something needs to be devised to stir individual interest in the welfare of the Society. With New York for a place of meeting at the time of year when the country, as well as the city, practitioner is presumably least occupied, it was expected that members would flock in in unusual numbers. There was the promise of good papers, and for this occasion the gory locks of the potency question had engaged not to appear, even at the complimentary collation. Yet for some reason the programme failed to draw. There were present less than one-quarter of the number practicing homœopathy in New York City alone, to say nothing of Kings County just across the river, while the great area of the State sent but a meagre sprinkle.

What the reasons were we do not propose to inquire at length. That there is a sufficient explanation not behind this year's attendance alone, but for a long series of years back when the members have done no better, every wiseacre says. But it is not the potency question ; it is not the question of alternation ; it is not the predominance of this or that faction ; nor is it any one question in particular. There certainly is no question but that the great majority of the members systematically shirk the journey and the expense, comforting themselves with the reflection that some one else will look after the cause, and that if it isn't looked after, it doesn't matter very much to them one way or another. That it does matter, the State Society has failed to impress upon its members in their individual relations to it. The interests of the Society as a whole are not brought home to and made the interest of every homœopathic physician of the State. This is not the fault of the officers, present or past, who have faithfully fulfilled their duties, according to the regulations and traditions of the Society. May it not be that an organization and methods of work, effective during other conditions, are ill adapted to present needs, have lapsed, in fact, into "innocuous desuetude?" It is usually true that, as any society grows older and more complex, it must grow likewise in the science of organization, or it is likely to fall asunder of its own weight. We hope that some of our younger men will investigate the problem from this point of view and move accordingly.

Beyond the instruction from papers and discussions, which are elsewhere fully reported, there are two things worthy of note : First— the resolution, passed last February, forbidding the publication of papers elsewhere than in the transactions, was wisely frustrated ; second—the position taken by the President in his address, in which he declared that "so long as the dominant school refuses to accept the homœopathic principle as the leading one in the domain of therapeutics, and places us and our school under a ban because we hold such a tenet, and so long as non-homœopathists refuse to teach their own students the benign truths of homœopathy, it is incumbent upon us to hold our position, to maintain a separate organized existence, and, above all, *to retain the distinctive name,*" and he significantly added, "If we give up our name, who, and what, and where are we?"

THE NINTH MEDICAL CONGRESS.

THE Ninth International Medical Congress has passed without unusual distinction, having been surpassed by previous sessions in numbers, and, more noticeably, in the value of scientific contributions. About one hundred foreign guests and less than three thousand members from the United States were present. There was of course a bewildering number of papers read, none marking a great discovery, but mainly creditable from the standpoint of the general average of medical literature. The Congress, if distinguished at all, could be characterized as a meeting of average practitioners, with an organization reflecting credit upon the executive talents of its officers. The most eminent men both of Europe and America were conspicuously absent. For this homœopathy has been indirectly blamed. It will be remembered that the organization of the Congress was finally wrangled out upon the Code question, the new Codists originally in control having been dispossessed by the old Codists of the American Medical Association. The quarrel was so momentous that it seemed for a long time as if the Congress might not meet at all; but, after the withdrawal of the more eminent men, especially in the East, and the creation of a feeling of distrust in Europe, the Congress did meet, not failing in one sense, but signally failing in another—it was not what it ought to have been, a signal honor to the United States. Yet homœopathy did not lay a straw in the way of the success of the Congress; it acted by its mere existence. In fact, it was not homœopathy but disagreement about how homœopathy could be best annihilated that impaired the full usefulness of the Congress to medicine. In other words, it was the so-called Code of Ethics of the American Medical Association, or, more properly speaking, the code of rules for the suppression of the principles and practice of homœopathic therapeutics. Perhaps, by the time another Congress meets in America, the Code itself, not homœopathy, will be suppressed, and "homœopaths" will be invited to participate not only in the individual sense, as they were exceptionally in this Congress, but in the actual organization, being invited to their fair share in the official representation of American Medicine. Homœopathic physicians are as much interested in the progress of the various sciences of medicine as the physicians of the old school who would hold them aloof. If they should be admitted in full faith to their representative rights, one thing may surely be counted on—the papers presented in the Section in Therapeutics and Materia Medica will not be so barren of curative knowledge as have been the papers in 1887.

A CORRECTION.

WE would ask our readers' indulgence for some relaxation in the supervision of the JOURNAL during the past two months. New York in the hot season necessarily involves a separation of our editors, who have performed their duties under many disadvantages. If there have been some typographical errors we would ask that they be attributed to the stress of mingled heat and vacation. The errors which have crept in, or rather been overlooked, will in the main correct themselves. One, however, in the September number, needs mention. The author of Haschisch (Thorold King) is not Charles Galchell, as stated, but Dr. Charles Gatchell, the versatile editor of *The Medical Era.* He carries his pen with such penetrating skill into the heart of his subject as well as the good graces of his readers, that he deserves full credit for all that he has written.

COMMENTS.

THE PHYSICIAN'S LIBRARY.—"Will you go and gossip with your housemaid or your stable-boy, when you may talk with kings and queens, while this eternal court is open to you, with its society wide as the world, multitudinous as its days, the chosen and the mighty of every place and time? Into that you may enter always, in that you may take fellowship and rank according to your wish; from that, once entered into it, you can never be outcast but by your own fault." How shall this question of Ruskin's, so direct and so searching, be answered? Few, perhaps, would choose to reply affirmatively and acknowledge that association with the vulgar was more congenial than the society of the refined and wise; that the smoking-room was preferable to the library, or the scandal of the present superior to the wit and wisdom of the past. But the half indignant tone of the question tells plainly that the interrogator felt that there were many who turned away from the fellowship of the noble and chosen, and walked willfully in the blindness of ignorance. And while his appeal is made to an audience so vast that it includes all sorts and conditions of men, yet it sounds in the ears of the physician with peculiar significance. For old manners and customs have passed away. A pair of saddle-bags and two or three musty volumes are no longer accepted as satisfactory testimonials to the learning and ability of the physician. The steady advance of the profession has brought it in the van, and the doctor of the nineteenth century cannot be considered as thoroughly equipped unless he possesses a well selected library. The popular opinion of physicians is indicated by Robert Louis Stevenson in the preface to his new book, "Underwoods:" "There are men and classes of men that stand above the common herd—the soldier, the sailor, the shepherd, not unfrequently; the artist, rarely; the clergyman, still more rarely; the physician, almost as a rule. He is the flower (such as it is) of our civilization, and when that stage of man is done with, and only remembered to be marveled at in history, he will be thought to have shared as little as any in the defects of the period, and most notably exhibited the virtues of the race." A physician without books is a soldier without weapons. Public sentiment demands that a professional man procure and read the literature of his profession, and he who neither buys nor reads sinks to a lower plane in the estimation of his associates. Says Beecher: "Flowers about a rich man's house may signify only that he has a good gardener, or that he has refined neighbors and does what he sees them do. But men are not accustomed to buy *books* unless they want them. If, on visiting the dwelling of a man of slender means, we find that he contents himself with cheap carpets and very plain furniture, in order that he may buy books, he rises at once in our esteem. Books are not made for furniture, but there is nothing else that so beautifully furnishes a house. A house without books is like a room without windows. It is a man's duty to have books. A library is not a luxury—it is a necessity." The library of a medical man will naturally show a preponderance of medical books. But the preponderance should not be so great as to be overwhelming. The physician should be a many-sided man, knowing something of many things besides medicine. His sympathies should not be allowed to grow only in one direction. A troublesome question to decide sometimes is what to buy. It is a good rule never to buy a book until you feel the need of it. Haphazard buying will inevitably load the shelves with trash. The presses teem with new works, new editions are a burden, and the canvassers go about the streets. Do not buy a book because it is cheap or can be purchased on the installment plan, unless the need of it has been experienced—unless it is *wanted.* In reading books remember the advice of Bacon, "Read not to contradict and confute, nor to believe and take for granted, nor to find talk and discourse, but to weigh and consider." Read with a purpose, and beware of cultivating a desultory habit of reading. "Every book taken up without a purpose," says Mr. Frederick Harrison, "is an opportunity lost of taking up a book with a purpose. Every bit of stray information which we cram into our heads, without any sense of its importance, is, for the most part, a bit of the most useful information driven out of our heads and choked out of our minds." And as our libraries increase, and the volumes elbow each other for standing room, may we all be able to say, with Petrarch, "I have friends whose society is extremely agreeable to me; they are of all ages and of every country. They have distinguished themselves both in the cabinet and in the field, and obtained high honors for their knowledge of the sciences. It is easy to gain access to them, for they are always at my service, and I admit them to my company and dismiss them from it whenever I please. They are never troublesome, but immediately answer every question I ask them, Some relate to me the events of past ages, while others reveal to me the secrets of nature. Some teach me how to live and others how to die. Some, by their vivacity, drive away my cares and exhilarate my spirits, while others give fortitude to my mind, and teach me the important lesson how to restrain my desires and depend wholly on myself."

BOOK REVIEWS.

A CYCLOPÆDIA OF DRUG PATHOGENESY. PART V. Cantharis —Chromium.

Every student of the Materia Medica hails with joy the appearance of each successive part of this work, which is published with commendable regularity. It is certainly true, as we have been frequently told by teachers, that the real thorough study of the Materia Medica must be done by a painstaking analysis of the provings, poisonings and experiments on animals. This publication affords an opportunity for this study, such as we never before have had, for in it these data are logically and compactly presented. Original records have been diligently sought out and careful analyses made of provings and cases of poisoning; useless and untrustworthy observations have been discarded, and the remainder presented in a clear and concise manner. The scope of the work is very large, embracing not only provings and poisonings on mankind, but experiments on animals, so that the student might have all needful information at hand in one work. The idea is a grand one, but, from the nature of the labor to be done, the compilations must be extremely difficult. Very few works on Toxicology or Pharmacology are complete enough for all purposes, even aside from the study of provings. To review a work of this sort is not an easy matter; critics have attacked the manner of condensation, alleging that in many instances, the finer shades of symptomatology have been brushed away, leaving only general statements of fact, and we are forced to believe that in some instances these complaints are well founded. Others complain that their "favorite" provings have been omitted altogether; and here, also, there is room for almost endless criticism. As a symptomatology, this work will not take rank as entirely satisfactory; the only thoroughly satisfactory symptomatology is the Materia Medica Pura of Hahnemann, here, and in the valuable monographs published by our English friends, each symptom is fully and clearly given, with all of its conditions and concomitants; from such data one can prescribe better, and if we are not mistaken, a reaction will take place in our school toward the earliest methods of Hahnemann.

As we look over this part, we are impressed by the bulk of Chelidonium, by the leanness of Carb. veg. and of China, and by the union of Kali bichrom. with Chromium. In the latter case, the editors follow their plan to group under the most active (supposed) ingredient all of its compounds — all of the Bromides under Bromine, the Iodides under Iodine, the Chromates under Chromium. It must be puzzling sometimes to carry this out; why not all the sulphates under sulphuric acid, all the nitrates under nitric acid? The properties of Kali bichrom. are not so surely those of chromic acid chiefly; Potash is a potent thing, and an opinion may reasonably be held that Potash determines most of the symptomatology of its bichromate. At any rate, it would have been convenient to look for Kali bichrom. under Kali

The first drug treated of is *Cantharides.* More knowledge of the effects of Cantharides comes to us from poisonings and experiments on animals than in any other way; we turn then from the presentation of provings, from any review of the admission or rejection of provings, from the condensation of symptoms, to see how the editors have digested the valuable observations concerning its pathology, which have been given us, particularly by the French. While, no doubt, confusion has existed between the symptoms of acute inflammation of the genital organs and those of true erotic mania, it would have been wise to present some of the most wonderful cases of poisoning characterized by this mania, especially as experiments on animals have developed the same insatiate desire for coition, and even fierce masturbation (in dogs). These have been omitted; but more than this, the editors have entirely overlooked the most important features of cantharis—pathology.

No drug in the whole materia medica so well illustrates the similarity of drug action to disease, through the whole scale, from symptom to post-mortem appearance, as Cantharis. Its occasional homœopathicity to pneumonia, pleurisy, pericarditis, gastro-enteritis, cystitis, et cetera, as well as to the familiar nephritis, might have been vividly illustrated by a few selected cases. The inflammation of both peri- and endo-cardium is characterized by ecchymoses; the pleuritis by ecchymoses, the pneumonia by hæmorrhages, the ulcerations of the stomach and intestines by ecchymoses and hæmorrhage, cystitis by hæmorrhage, and so on. Here we find not only guides, but additional justification for its occasional use in all of these diseases. The experiments of Dr. Voisin at the Salpétriere, the classical work of Dr. Carradi on Aphrodisiacs, and the thorough treatise of over 200 pages on Cantharidine and preparations of Cantharis, with experiments, by Dr. Galippe, have been entirely overlooked. This should not have been done. We hope the editors will not hurry their work, and confine their gatherings to material easily at hand, but have more help, and give us a work which will be in reality, as in name, a Cyclopædia.

These editors need a corps of paid assistants ; the work will not be done over again (unless some supplement be prepared, to include the "apocryphal" matter, by some who believe in it), and it should be slowly and thoroughly done now. Let some one start a fund for it.   * * *

A MANUAL OF THE PHYSICAL DIAGNOSIS OF THORACIC DISEASES. By E. DARWIN HUDSON, JR., A.M., M.D., late Professor of General Medicine and Diseases of the Chest in the New York Polyclinic ; Physician to Bellevue Hospital etc. One volume. Octavo. 162 pages. 93 illustrations. Price, $1.50. New York: Wm. Wood & Co.

The utility of this addition to the many excellent works already published upon its subject lies in the fact that it was the outgrowth of enthusiastic teaching by one who had sifted his reading and extensive clinical study by intelligent effort to make others expert like himself. The result is a thoroughly digested work, arranged to catch and fix attention, with no more in matter and in exposition than is necessary to make it the simple manual that it is for those who would study physical diagnosis as they would learn the practice of music upon an instrument. Accordingly, we have under notice a really serviceable book that will be sure to be well-thumbed by every one who owns it. We should ourselves prefer it for elementary study to any that we have seen.

Topography and regional anatomy, percussion of the healthy and abnormal chest, auscultation, the acoustics of normal and abnormal chest sounds, are presented with precise method and practical brevity, and are followed by synoptical tables, condensing the rational and physical signs essential for the diagnosis of the special diseases of the thoracic organs. The work is abundantly full upon the acoustic phenomena of chest diseases; it is, however, defective in the use of the microscope and sphygmograph as applied to their investigation. In his synoptical tables it would have been better had he omitted all reference to treatment. We notice also that special attention is not directed towards kidney lesions as a common cause of hypertrophy of the heart. For its special purpose, however, the work calls for little criticism, being admirably adapted to make the young physician conversant in the art of eliciting and interpreting the physical indications of the thorax. We are pleased to see that the author advocates Corson's positions of the patient during percussion, and calls attention to the importance of the examination of the interscapular and lateral regions of the chest, too commonly omitted. He also properly directs attention to muscular sussurus as a common source of error, and to the crepitant and subcrepitant rales as often indicative of pleurisy.

It is to be lamented that so excellent a teacher and writer should not have survived to supervise the publication of his work, and to continue the use of the art which it is evident he had mastered.

INDEX CATALOGUE OF THE LIBRARY OF THE SURGEON GENERAL'S OFFICE, UNITED STATES ARMY. AUTHORS AND SUBJECTS. Vol. VIII. *Legier-Medicine* (Naval). Washington, 1887. Pp. 1078.

"This volume includes 13,405 author-titles, representing 5,307 volumes and 13,205 pamphlets. It also includes 12,642 subject-titles of separate books and pamphlets, and 24,174 titles of articles in periodicals." Leprosy has 11 pages; lithotomy and lithotrity, 43 ; liver, 72 ; lungs, 43; malaria, 7; materia medica, 28; medicine (in part), 280. The latter is catalogued under MEDICINE, (Abuses and errors of, satires on), (Anecdotes, curiosities facetiæ, poetry of), (Aphorisms in). (Certainty of), (Collected works of single authors on), (Collections of works by different authors on), (Dictionaries, encyclopædias, and terminology of), (Essays and miscellanies in), (History of), (History of Ancient), (History of mediæval), (History of modern), (History and condition of, by nations and countries), (Legislation relating to. by Countries), (Manuals and vademecums of), (Practice of, systems and manuals of), (Prehistoric), (Systems, theories and principles of). (Botanic and physio-medical), (Chrono-thermal), (Clinical), (Clinical, Cases of), (Clinical, Lectures on), (Clinical, Statistical Reports of), (by localities), (Dosimetric), (Eclectic, etc.), (Magical, mystic, spagyric), (Military), (Military, Cases and statistics of), (Military, History of), (Miltary and Naval, Journals of), (Military and Naval, Schools of), (Naval). Medicine as related to homœopathy, homœopathic societies, institutions, journals, authors, books, etc., is not catalogued in this, but in another volume under homœopathy, we presume for purposes of convenience. The Index Catalogue is a monument to Surgeon-General Billings and his assistants, and serves not only as a clue to the contents of the vast National Medical and Surgical Library, but to medical literature in general, although necessarily incomplete.

REPORTS OF SOCIETIES AND HOSPITALS.

STATE SOCIETY.

THE thirty-sixth semi-annual meeting of the State Society was held in New York City, September 20th and 21st, 1887, at Lyric Hall. There was a good attendance from the beginning. The meeting was called to order by the President, Dr. H. M. Paine, of Albany. Dr. A. S. Ball offered prayer. A message was sent to the Homœopathic Medical Society of Pennsylvania, in session at Pittsburgh, congratulating it on the fiftieth anniversary of the introduction of homœopathy into that city. A return message of greeting was received. The President, Dr. H. M. Paine, of Albany, then gave a short address as follows :

Gentlemen of the Society:—It becomes my pleasant task to announce that the hour has arrived for the beginning of the sessions to be held in connection with the thirty-sixth semi-annual convocation of this Society, and to declare that the meeting is open for business.

In connection with the exercise of this official prerogative, I may be permitted, briefly at least, to grapple with Father Time, and compel him to retrace his hurried steps, in order that we may rescue from oblivion a few of the items of personal history which he, in his impetuous forward career, is steadily endeavoring to cover with the cobwebs of the ages.

I well remember attending the first meeting of this Society, and some of the incidents connected therewith. The records state that:

"In accordance with previous notice, a number of homœopathic physicians, from different parts of the State of New York, assembled in the Common Council room of the city hall, in the City of Albany, at ten o'clock in the forenoon of May 15th, 1850, for the purpose of devising such measures as the condition and interests of homœopathy in this State should render expedient."

I think there were about twenty physicians present. Prominent among the names of these worthies are those of Drs. John F. Gray, I. M. Ward, S. R. Kirby, Jacob Beakley, Henry D. Paine, E. D. Jones, J. W. Metcalf, R. S. Bryan, A. S. Ball and Alonzo Hall.

Of these, as far as I am able to ascertain only five or six remain. These are: Drs. I. M. Ward, H. D. Paine, E. D. Jones, A. S. Ball and H. M. Paine.

At the first meeting, on proceeding to an election of officers, a spontaneous erruption of personal fellowship was strikingly brought out in the election of Dr. I. M. Ward to the presidency. There had been no previous canvassing. There was no apparent motive for the selection of one candidate in preference to another, other than the strength of personal friendship.

Dr. Ward had resided in Albany seven years. A few months prior to the meeting he had removed to New Jersey, and for that reason his eligibility was questioned. He was almost unanimously elected, however, on the ground that it was his intention to spend two months each summer at Saratoga.

Dr. Ward's election was unquestionably owing to his suavity, agreeable manners, and an intimate personal acquaintance with all the members who were present.

Dr. Kirby was the talker for the whole school. He could talk against time on any subject connected with medicine that might be brought up. His great unwieldy body ; his portly bearing; his astonishing mobility of countenance; his peculiar lisp ; his earnestness of manner when interested in any subject under discussion, combined to constitute a character and person the like of whom has not since been seen in our midst.

Dr. J. F. Gray, it seemed to me, ought to have been honored by the presidency. He had even then attained eminence in his profession. His great learning; his recognized skill as a diagnostician; his frequent contributions to the medical literature of the day, ought not, it would seem, even at that early day, to have been overlooked. Twenty-one years afterward, however, his profound erudition and great ability were duly recognized by the Society by his election to the presidency, the nineteenth on the list.

I became intimately acquainted with Dr. Gray during the later years of his life, and learned to admire his good qualtities, and to have great respect for his opinions and wishes regarding many of the practical medical questions of the day.

Dr. Metcalf would, had he lived longer, have become one of the shining lights in our school. He possessed a clear logical mind. His writnigs have enriched our materia medica. His quiet, reserved manner, and his forcible and timely utterances, are still deeply impressed on my memory.

Dr. Ball, whose flowing locks are whitened by more than fourscore and eight winters, is still here with us. His venerable and stately form has been seldom seen at the meetings of the Society.   His life work has been that of a faithful adherent to homœopathic principles, and an honest endeavor to apply them in the treatment of disease.

The last of these founders of the Society whose name I will mention in these brief notes is that of the versatile Beakley.

I do not think that Professor Beakley was present at the first meeting; he was, however, a frequent attendant at the sessions of the Society subsequently.   He always related interesting cases, and was always a great stickler for a strict observance of parliamentary rules.

At the first meeting of the Society he was appointed chairman of a committee to prepare an address to the homœopathic physicians of the State "urging united and harmonious action."   Thus early, at the very beginning of the organization, his tact and fostering services were made instrumental in laying the foundation of permanence, development and substantial progress, by which we, his survivors, have been profited, and have richly enjoyed.

But how does it happen that at the very start, thirty-seven years ago, effort was needed to secure the desirable qualities represented by unity of sentiment and harmony of action?   One would suppose that, having kindred purposes and interests, the homœopathists, of whom at that time there were about two hundred in the State, would instinctively coalesce, and that no special effort for promoting unity and harmony would be required.

These essential qualities were needed at the inception of this organization, in order the better to maintain a defensive position against an opposing school and system; and from that time to the present the reasons for putting forth effort with a view of promoting unity and harmony among homœopathists, have been just as cogent and forcible as they ever were.

Organized opposition to homœopathic truth, although of late years, from motives of policy, is less pronounced, covertly is as earnest and active as at any time in the history of this Society.

What these reasons are; why we allow ourselves to be recognized by a distinctive name; why we are continually planning to maintain our distinct organizations, to develop our resources, and make more rapid advances in future, I must make the subject of an address at the next annual meeting.   Suffice it for the present to say, that so long as the dominant school refuses to accept the homœopathic principle as the leading one in the domain of therapeutics, and places us and our school under a ban because we hold such a tenet; and so long as non-homœopathists refuse to teach their own students the benign truths of homœopathy, it is incumbent upon us to hold our position; to maintain a separate organized existence; and above all, to *retain the distinctive name;* for, if we give up our name, who, and what, and where are we?

The distinctive name is our birthright; it is ours by inheritance; it is ours by conquest; it is ours, and ever will be ours, in spite of ourselves, so long as homœopathy is known as a recognized method of cure.

The committee to whom the President's address was referred, presented the following resolution, which was unanimously adopted:

Resolved, That so long as the dominant school of medicine refuses to accept the homœopathic principle as the leading one in the domain of therapeutics and places homœopathic physicians and the homœopathic school under a ban; and so long as non-homœopathists refuse to teach their own students the benign truths of homœopathy, it is incumbent upon the homœopathic schools to hold its position, to maintain its separate organizations, and to retain its distinctive name.

In the absence of Dr. E. H. Walcott, Chairman of the Bureau of

Materia Medica, Dr. M. W. Van Denberg presented the report of the bureau.

A paper by the chairman, upon "The Single Remedy," was read, in which Dr. Walcott advocated the use of one remedy at a time, claiming much better action and quicker results than where more than one is given. Several cases were cited, showing the beneficent action of our drugs when carefully prescribed according to the strict Hahnemannian method. Dr. B. S. Partridge presented a paper upon the "Medium of Drug Action." The bureau was then closed temporarily to allow that upon Laryngology to present its papers. The first one read was by Dr. Malcolm Leal, upon "Conditions of the Larynx requiring Local Treatment."

Dr. J. M. Schley then read a paper upon the "Local Treatment of Laryngeal Phthisis," in which he held that tuberculosis of the larynx was akin to a wound situated elsewhere in the body and should be treated upon the same broad principles. The diagnosis between phthisis laryngea, acute or chronic laryngitis, in some of its stages, primary lupus, carcinoma or syphilis of the larynx, was at times extremely difficult. In his experience, phthisis of the larynx was never met disassociated from tubercular lesions in some part of the lung. To differentiate, we must observe the congestion (often localized), infiltration, œdema, spots selected by preference, and the erosion. If there are no evidences of pulmonary lesions, there should always be a grave suspicion that the case is syphilitic. The doctor cited a case in which, eight years ago, there were present the congested and inflamed epiglottis and trachea, together with marked infiltration of the upper lobe of the right lung. It appeared to be phthisical; but a month's sojourn in the mountains effected an entire cure, which has been permanent until now. An accurate diagnosis is absolutely essential to a trustworthy prognosis. True tuberculosis of the larynx is an incurable disease. When the diagnosis of laryngeal phthisis is certain, the prognosis is most unfavorable. About five (5) per cent. of consumptives suffer from involvement of the larynx. While treatment is not curative, it relieves the agonizing pain. The medicaments, used in the form of a spray, powder or liquid, are morphia, atropine, iodoform, iodol, cocaine, lactic acid, oily solution of menthol, the balsams, galvano-cautery, submucus injections of lactic acid, peroxide of hydrogen and boracic acid. Local treatment, in order to be effective, must be applied daily. The homœopathic remedies, Apis, bell., lach., merc., caust. phos. and calc. phos., are most useful.

The discussion which followed these papers gradually wandered to the discussion of the treatment of pulmonary phthisis.

Dr. Edwin Fancher cited a case in which a woman had had a very sharp hemorrhage from the lungs, followed by evidences of phthisis. The iodide of ars. was administered till an aggravation was obtained, when sac. lac. was substituted. Later this was followed by phos. acid, which completed the cure, the woman remaining perfectly well at present.

Dr. L. A. Bull:—We do not look sufficiently into the pathological condition of the parts. All the cases which have been reported as cures of phthisis have borne a most striking resemblance to bronchitis.

Dr. Geo. E. Gorham believed that true phthisis of the larynx was an incurable affection.

Dr. J. M. Schley:—In considering the treatment and cure of phthisis, we must maintain the distinction between the two branches of this disease, catarrhal and fibroid phthisis. Their course is entirely different. The latter may run an indefinite length of time, and for years may not seriously disturb the general health of the individual, and in many cases does not materially hasten the death of the patient, while in the former, or catarrhal variety, there is a rapidly destructive process going on, to which the patient must sooner or later succumb. It has been fully shown by Dr. Flint that phthisis is a self-limited disease. Many cases are cured by change of air or locatian.

Dr. Robert Boocock:—For cleansing the larynx he preferred a mixture of equal parts of turpentine and coal tar. This was burned and the smoke inhaled.

The report of the Bureau of Materia Medica was then resumed. Dr. M. W. Van Denberg read a paper upon the "Order of Arrangement of the Symptoms in our Materia Medica Pura." The discovery of the law of similars is ample glory for one man. After such service, it is no disparagement that his methods were not as we would wish. His philosophical works have nearly disappeared and will eventually be lost. He did not go far enough. Much of his philosophy has been outstripped by time. Hahnemann's works may be considered under the following heads: His observation of drug phenomena, recording of symptoms, and method of arranging. Regarding the first, there can be no question but that his ability to observe drug phenomena was pre-eminent. His method of recording them individualized different symptoms of the same disease; it was a process of isolation and separated the concomitant from the main symptoms. It was thus impossible to get a picture of the totality of symptoms. In the method of arrangement of the symptoms there has been no change since Hahnemann's time. All are arranged upon a purely anatomical basis. It makes a confused picture. We need a *physiological* arrangement. The symptoms should be classified under such as the following heads: Mental, Moral, Nervous, Respiratory, Circulatory, Digestive, Genital, Skin, Glandular, etc. We could then obtain a good picture of the disease and would be more servicable. A suitable materia medica would greatly aid in hastening the amalgamation of the schools.

The Bureau of Ophthalmology, Dr. A. B. Norton, Chairman, next reported. Dr. E. H. Linnell read a paper upon "Extracts from Case Book." He first cited a case of irido-choroiditis, caused by using a hairwash made from the oily juice of the bitter apple. There was an acute inflammation of the choroid and iris, with serous effusion. He regarded it as a case of colocynth poisoning, as the abdominal symptoms of the drug were present. It was cured by bry., kali iod. and sulph.

The second case was one of traumatic rupture of the iris, which occurred in a boy who was struck in the eye with a stone. When seen, there was no rupture of the choroid or cornea, but the iris was dilated *ad maximum* and a small slit could be detected in its substance. Atropine was first used, but later eserine. The latter contracted it for a short time, but the effect was soon lost. The wound healed, but the iris was still greatly dilated and did not contract. It was a complete rupture of the iris, with no external wound. The third case was one of retinitis following nephritis, which did not present the full symptomatology of retinitis albumenurica. There was great impairment of vision, with obscuration of the optic disc. He was passing about five gills of urine, the specific gravity of which was 1018. The urine contained pus, renal epithelia, fatty and granular casts, with a slight amount of albumen. He had constant, dull pain in the limbs, with pain across the back and a sensation as if a band constricted the forehead. Helonias was given. Very great improvement in the eyesight resulted. The retinæ became normal and vision was only slightly impaired, although the general health and renal disease gradually grew worse.

Dr. Jno. Moffat:—Many neuralgic remedies, *e. g.,* cedron and prunus, have been of great service, even in inflammatory iritis.

Dr. M. W. Van Denberg cited the case of a lady who suffered from excruciating, stabbing pain in the right side of the face and eye, which was induced by the slightest touch, motion or jar. She could not move the face in eating, talking or laughing, without the greatest pain resulting. Colocy. 3 was prescribed, but the pain became very much worse. He then made a higher dilution and gave it to her. The relief was immediate and lasting.

Dr. Geo. S. Norton:—Kali iod., first decimal, is one of our best remedies in iritis with effusion. He doubted if colocy. would be of much service if the effusion were large or plastic in character. The potash in this form acts much better than either a higher or lower preparation.

Dr. Chas. Deady then read a most practical paper on "Spectacles." He spoke of the harm which opticians and itinerant peddlers of glasses did. In no case of myopia, hyperopia or astigmatism was any one but an oculist capable of fitting a glass. Eyeglasses are not as reliable as spectacles in the majority of cases; as the focal distance is constantly varied, different angles are used; the pressure on the nose is often the source of pain, and they are not in any case as steady as the spectacle. At times, as in cases of a high degree of myopia or hyperopia, eyeglasses are preferable, as the patient might wear the glass too much if others were given. The frame should be heavy enough to hold the lenses at a constant angle. They should incline slightly inwards, even when worn all the time, and should be far enough from the eye to just escape the lashes.

Dr. F. H. Boynton would like to express his thanks to Dr. Deady for the practical paper he has just read. We should not purchase glasses of opticians without first consulting an oculist. The upper rim of a glass should tilt slightly, even for constant use.

Dr. Geo. S. Norton:—All ophthalmologists agree with Dr. Deady. In myopia, especially, we should select a glass only after having the eye tested by a competent oculist. In far-sighted people, the danger of selecting their own glasses was much less, often none; but if any astigmatism existed, harm would result.

Dr. Jno. Moffat:—In purchasing an eyeglass, one should get a case which does not fold the glasses, as the spring becomes weakened and the angles are changed.

Dr. S. Hasbrouck:—In England a recent examination of 1,000 pupils showed that 703 had errors in refraction. It made evident the necessity of an examination of the eye by an experienced oculist.

Dr. Chas. C. Boyle then presented a paper on the "Curative Effects of "Gelsemium in Diseases of the Uveal Tract." One case in which it proved curative was in a gentleman whose retina was detached; vitrious, cloudy; and vision necessarily greatly affected. He had been under the best allopathic treatment, with rest in bed and bandaging of the eye. He was placed in the hospital, his eye bandaged, and restricted to the dorsal decubitus. Gels. was given internally. In six weeks the disease was cured and vision restored. A second case was similar. Gels. here also proved curative.

Dr. E. H. Linnell has used gels. in cases of detached retina, but not with such happy results as those detailed by Dr. Boyle. He had never gone lower than the first decimal, which would, perhaps, account for his failure to achieve favorable results.

Dr. Geo. S. Norton:—In serous effusion of the eye, kali iod. and merc. cor. were most valuable remedies. Dr. Boynton in 1878 first called attention to the curative effects of gels. in detached retina. Since then it has been more commonly used. In the late International Congress held at Washington, one eminent German specialist reported 703 cases which he had treated with seven cures, showing the very low percentage of cures under purely allopathic treatment. With homœopathic remedies we can do much more than that.

Dr. F. H. Boynton:—In order to accomplish much in detachment of the retina, we must enforce rest, bandaging, and the prone position. When he first wrote the article referred to by Dr. Norton, he was very sanguine of most favorable results. Since then he had become less hopeful, but even now he believed that some cases—especially if treated early—could be cured. He had effected a favorable termination even in some cases of traumatic detachment.

Dr. S. Hasbrouck:—In detachment of the retina has never seen a reapplication under gels.

Dr. Jno. L. Moffat then read a paper, "A Clinical Case," in which he detailed the history of a patient who had had diplopia which yielded readily to treatment the first time. About two years afterwards the patient again applied for relief. This time the trouble was variable and would disappear in one spot to appear in some other form. Finally, by means of cedron, kalmia, gels., faradization and galvanism, causticum and giving him proper glasses, the diplopia was cured.

Dr. E. H. Linnell:—In his experience, varying diplopia, which yields to treatment, particularly if a second or third attack presents more complicated features and is more difficult to cure, is very suggestive of sclerotic changes in the upper part of the cord or lower portion of the brain. He had had several cases with such attacks, who subsequently died from sclerotic changes of the cerebro-spinal centres.

TUESDAY EVENING.

The Bureau of Otology, Dr. Ed. J. Pratt, Chairman, reported. Dr. Sayre Hasbrouck read the first paper upon a "Description of an Improved Artificial Membrana Tympani." He was led to perfect this little instrument, because the one in common use had the wire for the adjustment of the disc in the centre, and so pulled it out of place by its weight. The instrument Dr. H. exhibited had a disc of rubber, which was to serve as the drum. To the lower part of this was attached, by a V-shaped bending of the wire, a small wire, which was to serve for the ready adjustment of the disc. This V-shaped piece was included between the layers of the rubber disc which were cemented together, thus avoiding the rivet, which often causes much pain. Practically, he had found this disc to give much more satisfactory results than the old style. It should first be placed in position by an aurist. The best results were, of course, obtained when the ossicles were left.

Dr. M. O. Terry asked what results followed its use in cases of deafness due to scarlatina.

Dr. Hasbrouck said that if the ossicles were left most excellent results followed, and that it was in just such cases that the drum was of the most service.

Dr. H. C. Houghton then read his paper upon a "Practical Modification of Valsalva's Experiment." The doctor said that Politzer's method is the best and simplest way of inflating the middle ear. This may result in harm, if too frequently or persistently used. The object of inflation should be to secure the patency of the tube and to allow the air to adjust the ossicles. Dr. H.'s modification of Valsalva's experiment is to close the external meatus of both ears with the thumbs in order to protect the drums. The anterior nares are closed with the index fingers. The mouth is shut tightly, and an attempt made, as before, to expel the air. In this way the air enters the middle ear most easily without a heavy strain upon the drums. Much good has resulted from this method when others have failed.

Dr. Geo. S. Norton regards this as a wise suggestion. In ordinary cases he does not consider that much damage can result from employing

Politzer's method. Until a year ago, did not think that there was any danger. At this time a lady came to him with partial deafness. He used Politzer's method, and noticed that afterwards the drum was much injected. Probably in acute or sub-acute middle ear disease there is danger of rupture of some of the blood vessels of the drum.

Dr. S. Hasbrouck has been familiar with the modification as applied to the well ear when it was desirable to inflate the other. Had seen it used a great deal in the Dublin hospitals.

Dr. H. C. Houghton:—Dr. Liebold showed that there was danger in the Politzer method in acute cases; but it is in old chronic cases that the lay use of inflation has resulted in the greatest harm. Here the tube has lost its elasticity and is unusually open, and the force being great, there is danger of rupture of the drum.

Dr. Chas. C. Boyle read a paper upon "Aural Mucous Polypi." These are composed of a loose structure of mucous tissue, filled with blood vessels. These growths are about the size of a bean. There is little pain connected with them, but gradual deafness and an irritating discharge results. The polypus may grow and dam back the discharge, causing necrosis of the temporal bone and consequent meningitis. They should be removed with the snare, scraped with the curette, and Munsel's salt applied with calc., thuja, etc., internally. All traces of the growth must be removed or it will reappear. The canal should be cleansed with the peroxide of hydrogen, boracic acid, etc.

Dr. Jno. C. Moffat in a few cases has used the bichromate of potash with good results.

Dr. H. C. Houghton has seen them subside under the administration of the kali muriaticum 12.

Dr. F. H. Boynton:—The dried juice of the melon fig, by its power to digest fibrine, will at times cause the gradual disappearance of the growth, Two or three grains of the dried juice is dissolved in a little water and poured into the ear.

There being no report from the Bureau of Vital Statistics or from Pædology, the Society adjourned to a most enjoyable collation, which had been provided by the New York County Society.

WEDNESDAY MORNING.

The Bureau of Surgery, through its Chairman, Dr. J. M. Lee, reported a number of papers.

The first was by Prof. J. Gilchrist, upon the "Radical Cure of Hernia." His method of operating was as follows: The part is shaved, the skin pinched up and transfixed, making an incision one or one and a half inches long. The tissues are dissected down to the sac. If this is not too much thickened, it is pushed up into the abdomen with the bowel. It is held between the pillars of the ring, a needle entered through the lower pillar, carried through the sac and out through the opposite pillar. In this way the pillars are stitched together, holding between themselves a plug of peritoneum consisting of the sac. If the ring is very large, the edges are freshened and stitched as above. The skin is then brought together and stitched. The whole is covered with a pad wet with hypericum, which is also given internally, preferably in the 30th attenuation. The patient is allowed to leave his bed on the fifth or eighth day. A truss should be worn during the day and be removed at night until the ring is perfectly solid. The hypericum is given for about three or four days, when lyc. 30 is administered for about two weeks. He was led to prescribe lyc. from the effect it had on several cases in which the hernia reappeared. It seems to shorten the mesentary and make the hernia much less liable to reappear. In his last fifty cases thirty-four were cured and all were benefited.

Dr. Boocock :—Dr. Thomas experimented and found that the medicinal property of lyc. was only developed above the sixth potency.   Has cured one patient of hernia by lyc.

Dr. M. W. Van Denberg has had good results from lyc. 3.

Dr. S. F. Wilcox :—When the sac is large he removes it and stitches the edges together with catgut.   The stump is then stitched to the pillars of the ring by deep silver wire sutures.   He believes strongly in antiseptic precautions and dressings.   The latter he allows to remain at least a week before removal.

Dr. S. F. Wilcox then read his paper upon "Wiring the Patella." The knee-joint is very tolerant of operations, if only antiseptic precautions are observed.   Both operator and assistants must be antiseptic.

The cases suitable for the operation are where the bone is comminuted and cannot be drawn together ; where the overlaying tissues are very greatly bruised, or where only ligamentous union has resulted and the functional power of the joint is destroyed.

In a recent fracture the surfaces of the bones and the intervening tissues are covered with a layer of lymph and blood clot.   In such a case, if a primary operation be done, the fragments are best wired without disturbing this lymph deposit.   The production of bone will be more rapid.   If a secondary operation is performed this lymph layer has made a floor between the joint cavity and the ligamentous union, which is of the greatest assistance in preventing the operator from entering the joint cavity.   He then detailed a case in which he had successfully operated upon both patellas.   Everything was antiseptic.   A semi-lunar incision was made below the lower fragment.   The skin was dissected up, uncovering the bones.   A small section was sawn from each of the fragments.   These were detached from the underlying tissue, which consisted of the pseudo-membrane formed from the lymph deposit.   This was left.   The joint was not entered.   Three holes were bored in each fragment and the bones drawn together by heavy silver wire.   The skin and tissues were then sewed together and the leg placed in a plaster of Paris splint, and dressed with antiseptic dressings, which were not removed until the sixteenth day.   The splint was kept on for six weeks.   Both patellas united completely and good motion of the joint resulted.   He would call attention to the false union or pseudo-membrane and to the value of antiseptics.

Dr. J. M. Lee is bitterly opposed to antiseptics ; considers them a mere fashion, which is prevalent at present, but which will pass away soon.   Has opened the knee-joint three times during the last year, twice without antiseptics.   In one case had a sharp fever, with suppuration, but it later recovered with a perfect joint.   We do not know anything about germs or what causes disease.   The only value of Listerism is to teach cleanliness.   At present Listerism is dead and antiseptics harmful.

The Bureau of Surgery here gave place to that of Mental and Nervous Diseases, in order that Dr. B. M. Butler might present his paper on "Neurasthenia."   Dr. Butler considered that persons who were bright, sprightly, high-keyed, were the ones to suffer from neurasthenia.   Precocious children also are liable to it.   No class, however, is exempt.   The main causes are sexual excesses, acute diseases which do not yield to treatment, too frequent pregnancies, miscarriages, leucorrhœa, etc.   The symptoms are legion and occur in every part of the body.   The following are some of the main ones : morbid fears, which they know are foolish; dizziness in all forms, all sorts of head symptoms, entire sleeplessness, or unrefreshing sleep; sensation of suffocation on lying down, cardiac pains, nausea, diarrhœa, constipation, all sorts of gastric pains, most capricious appetite, numbness, pricking of the skin, exhaustion, seminal emissions, great flooding, and inflammation of the toes.   Neurasthenia is apt to be confounded with organic disease of the cord, hysteria and anæmia.   The prognosis, under good treatment, is favorable, but the recovery is necessarily slow.   In treatment no routine plan can be laid down.   Must individualize and treat the disease according to its cause and symptoms. With some, isolation is necessary; with others, the regular routine duties do better.   The physician must gain the supremacy over the patient's mind. Massage and electricity will, at times, prove of great benefit. In prescribing, must consider only the leading symptoms, and not mind the many fancies and freaks of the patient.

The report of the Bureau of Surgery was resumed.

Dr. M. O. Terry stated that he had employed the plain treatment of Dr. Lee, but his experience had not been as successful as the doctor's. He could not agree with him.   It made little difference whether Iodoform, Eucalyptus, Bichloride of Mercury, or some other antiseptic dressing were used, the results would be good, but a plain dressing would lead to suppuration.

Dr. Fred. S. Fulton had had such favorable results with the use of antiseptics that he would not be willing to discontinue them.   He cited the case of a boy who was admitted to the Laura Franklin Hospital with pyo-arthritis of the knee-joint, with all its characteristic symptoms.   The joint was opened freely, a counter opening for drainage made, all the pus washed from the joint cavity with a 1 to 2,000 solution of corrosive mercury, a drainage-tube inserted, and the whole dressed with corrosive mercury gauze.   The fever immediately subsided and the case progressed uninterruptedly to a complete recovery, with a movable joint.   It spoke well for antiseptic treatment.

Dr. S. F. Wilcox :—If antiseptics were not employed, and the case progressed unfavorably, he should consider himself criminally responsible. With antiseptic treatment we can do now, with impunity, what we would not dare to do before.

Dr. J. M. Lee :—The antiseptic treatment is a mere style, of which we will hear no more in a short time.   It a few years it will all pass away. If he had a case of mercurial poisoning, the way very many surgeons have, he should regard himself as criminally responsible.

Dr. S. F. Wilcox :—In his experience he has never seen such a case, although the mercurial irrigation and dressing has been in constant use. The solutions are not so strong as they were formerly used; a 1 to 2,000 solution is all that is necessary.

Parturient women appear to be very susceptible to the action of the mercurial, but other cases are not so.

A paper upon "Cæsarian Section," by Dr. Biggar, was then read.   In this the doctor detailed a case of a lady who was in her fourth pregnancy, None of her previous children had been born alive, owing to deformities in the pelvic canal.   As they were very anxious to have a living child. Cæsarian section was performed.   An incision from the symphysis pubis to the umbilicus was made ; the uterine incision was about six inches in length.   The child and afterbirth was delivered ; the uterus stitched with catgut.   A drainage tube was carried through the os into the vagina and the skin incision stitched.   The wound was dressed with calendula and glycerine dressings.   Ars. was administered internally.   Both patient and child are doing well.

Dr. H. I. Ostrom read a paper on, "The Before and After Treatment of Laparotomy."   Before the operation we must build up the patient, to prevent shock; examine the kidneys carefully to see that no disease is there which might kill the patient, and unload the bowels with a cathartic. The anæsthetic should be ether if there is no counter-indication from the kidneys.   The anæsthetic should be adapted to the individual.

After the operation the patient should have absolute rest of the abdominal organs for the first day.   Barley water, with one-third cream, should then be given. At the end of the first week the patient can commence on more solid food, and gradually return to normal diet. Interference with the bowels is uncalled for. The patient takes but little food and does not need to have a full movement. If the abdomen needs draining it is better done through the drainage tube than through the bowel. If peritonitis, with flatulence, ensues, calomel, as a purge, will often do good. If the bowels do not move, after a week or ten days give an enema. For the first forty-eight hours the patient should drink hot water. It relieves flatulence and prevents the stomach from being empty. The patient can be allowed to assume any position that is most comfortable. Bell. calc., nux, colocy., enemata, the rectal tube, have proven of the greatest benefit in flatulence. If patient has the ability to urinate, let her do so ; if not, catheterize. In his experience much nausea and vomiting is caused by the slow giving of ether or the ligation of adhesions. The ligation of the pedicle will often cause it. The actual cautery will control hæmorrhage and does not cause nausea. The vomiting has been best controlled by a two per cent. solution of cocaine. Morphine should not be given unless it is absolutely essential that the patient have rest and sleep. Its action is depressant and must be avoided. Ac. and Hypericum will usually quiet the patient and relieve the pain, which is not usually severe.

Dr. J. M. Lee has had most excellent results from the abdominal use of hot water in cases of profound shock. In such a case he fills the abdominal cavity with hot water. The use of poisonous antiseptics within the abdominal cavity is the most silly thing in the world.

Dr. H. I. Ostrom always uses antiseptics, and he used hot water in one case of profound shock following laparotomy. He filled the abdominal cavity, and by that means thinks he saved the patient's life.

Dr. S. H. Knight:—At the Helmuth House and at other hospitals with which he has been connected, it has always been the practice to give just as little ether as possible, allowing the patient to partially come from under its influence at times. They are given ice on being first put to bed. Then diluted milk or rice-water. They have no animal food before the seventh day. Abdominal flatulence is always best controlled by lyc., which he finds works best in the fifteenth trituration. For vomiting, ars., verat., alb., hot water or tea is given. The last has been found especially useful. The bowels are not disturbed till the seventh or ninth day, when an injection is given. If that is not sufficient, a gluten suppository is given at night and an enema in the morning. The stitches are usually removed on the twelfth day. Will often get vomiting after the use of the clamp in hysterectomy. The rubber ligation which is tied around the pedicle, below the clamp, will control all hæmorrhage. He has used the corrosive mercury, 1 to 25,000, in the abdominal cavity ; also hot water. The effects from both are about the same. The instruments are always put in a one to forty solution of carbolic acid. The antiseptic treatment is very important.

Dr. M. O. Terry then read a paper on, " Bromine in the Treatment of Septic Wounds." For all septic wounds coming from cutting one's self while operating or dissecting, or from infection from erysipelas or gangrene, he uses the following preparation, which has been of the greatest value: Into an eight-ounce bottle he puts one drachm of the iodide or bromide of potash, one ounce of pure bromine, and then fills it with water. When necessary to use this he pours about one drachm into a glass and fills it one-third full of water. Into this solution he inserts the finger some distance beyond the wound. It has always stopped the poisonous effects.

Dr. Wm. H. King then read a paper upon " Electrolysis in Fibro-myomata." The paper appears in full on page 608.

Dr. Geo. E. Gorham read a paper on "Cases of Nervous Exhaustion." The causes are predisposing and exciting, mental and bodily.

They are mainly found in the pelvic region. The treatment consists in rest, food, discontinuance of tonics and stimulants, and the removal of causes of local irritation. He detailed several cases of profound neurasthenia. In one, the removal of an internal hemorrhoid; in another, circumcision; in a third, the passage of graded sounds to relieve the prostatic inflammation; in a fourth, rest, ignatia, massage, electricity, and in a fifth, silicia, 6 x, effected complete and permanent cures.

Dr. S. H. Talcott presented the case of a lady whose bodily weight was reduced to sixty-five pounds by her fanciful illusions. She was entirely relieved by medication. When her body was sound her mental strength returned. The body is very important. When that is sound the mind will act well. " In sano corpore sana mens."

Dr. Boocock was glad to see that alcohol was being much less used now than formerly. He believes that it retards nutrition and undermines the health, until neurasthenia and allied diseases result.

Dr. J. W. Dowling:—The stoppage of alcohol in chronic cases is most valuable. It is an absolute detriment in all cases. He cited the case of a physician who had just come to him for treatment, who had worked very hard, eaten heartily, and taken little exercise. As a result he had a paralytic stroke, and has developed a systolic aortic murmur. In such a case as this less nitrogenous food should be eaten and no liquor drunk.

Dr. Fred. S. Fulton, Chairman of the Bureau of Histology, then presented the report of their bureau.

A paper by Dr. A. Wilson Dods, upon the " Microscopic Characteristics of Carcinoma," was read. It was profusely illustrated with micro-photographs of the various varieties of cancer.

Dr. Fred. S. Fulton then read a paper on the "Local Origin of Cancer," in which he held that the development of cancer was through the means of local irritation, resulting in inflammatory action of a subacute type. Several cases, and a number of illustrations taken from his sections, showing the gradual development of the malignant growth, through inflammatory action, were presented.

After some discussion on business topics the Society adjourned, to meet at Albany, February 14th and 15th, 1888.

NEWS.

ALL news or matter relating to "Notes and Comments" should be sent to 161 West Seventy-first Street.

VACANCY.—Dr. E. H. Olmstead, of Brooklyn Homœopathic Hospital, soon resign his position and settle at Sayre, Penn.

A DESIRABLE POSITION.—There is a vacancy in the resident staff of the Pittsburgh Homœopathic Hospital. Apply to Dr. J. H. McClelland, 411 Penn. Ave., Pittsburgh.

NEW SOCIETY.—The first Homœopathic Medical Society in the State of Arkansas was organized last summer. Its name is the Pulaski County Homœopathic Medical Society. The President is Dr. W. E. Green.

SOUTHERN ASSOCIATION.—The Fourth Annual Session of the Southern Homœopathic Medical Association will be held in the city of New Orleans, December 14th to 16th, 1887. C. G. Fellows, M.D., Secretary, New Orleans, La.

NEW YORK MEDICAL COLLEGE FOR WOMEN.—The regular winter term of this institution began Tuesday, October 4th, and will continue twenty-six weeks. A reunion was held at the College on Monday evening, October 3d.

INDECENCY IN MEDICAL LITERATURE.—The following pungent extract is taken from the pages of the *New England Medical Gazette.* It is the protest of an earnest and honorable journal against indecency and vulgarism. "The subject of Indecency in Medical Literature was briefly commented upon in the issue of the *Gazette* for February last. In that comment it was said, as it seemed only just to say, that offenses against decency of phrase were, while fortunately not common in the journals of either school, noticeably less common in the journals of the new school than in those of the old. An instance which would seem to go far to proving the contrary is afforded by an article appearing semi-anonymously in the department of 'Comment and Criticism,' in the September number of the *Medical Advance.* So flagrant an example does this communication afford of the indecency referred to, and of the pernicious inappropriateness of its appearance in the councils of those who claim to be not only scientists, but gentlemen, one feels that to let the matter pass in silence were in some measure to soil one's self by tacit acquiescence in the use of methods and phrases abhorrent alike to scientists and to gentlemen of whatever school of professional thought. So nearly as it is possible to catch a drift of meaning through the whirl of illogical and wordy incoherence, the writer in question aims to attack, through attacking our honored contemporary, the NORTH AMERICAN JOURNAL OF HOMŒOPATHY, a gentleman well known to homœopathic practice and literature, whose suggested name, though suggested only in coarsest vituperation, lends to the communication in question the only dignity to which it can lay claim. With this attack we have at present nothing to do. No greater compliment can be offered a writer or a journal, than such evidence as is afforded in the present instance, that his logic and its character disarm adversaries of all weapons, save that of clamorous abuse. What we do wish at this moment to protest against, with such force of protest as in us lies, is the utter indecency of the similies and metaphors employed in the course of his tirade, not once nor twice, but openly, gleefully and continually, by the correspondent of the *Advance.* In this connection quotation is obviously impossible, though quotation alone could bear adequate testimony to the heinousness of the offense. The language is of a sort, that, used on the public street, would speedily relegate the speaker to the safe retirement of the nearest police station, and used in the public print, should condemn a writer, and that permanently, to an analogous fate. Physiological metaphor, undignified and unnecessary at best, in the present connection is sunk to the level of filthy Billingsgate, by the motive of its employment—such Billingsgate as that in which the society of the slums clothes its personal malice, and which society above the slums never employs at all. The appearance of such language in a medical journal, where one takes for granted that personal animosity must at least wear the garments of decent courtesy, is utterly intolerable, and a shame to be cried out against without ceasing. Adam Badeau tells us that once, in the presence of Gen. Grant, a young officer began to tell, as a 'good story,' some anecdote of doubtful savor. The General's uplifted hand silenced him. 'Why, General,' he said in some confusion, 'there are no ladies present' —— 'No,' said Grant with quiet sternness, 'but there are *gentlemen* present.' It is to be hoped that a general expression of protest against entirely gratuitous indecency of speech will make the semi-anonymous vituperator of the September *Advance* conscious, at least, that in the journalistic councils of homœopathic physicians, there are not only ladies but gentlemen present."

Vol. XXXV.   *NOVEMBER, 1887.*   (Volume II, Third Series.)   No. 11.

NORTH AMERICAN

JOURNAL OF HOMŒOPATHY.

ORIGINAL ARTICLES IN MEDICINE.

OUTLINES OF A SYSTEMATIC STUDY OF THE MATERIA MEDICA.

By T. F. ALLEN, M.D.,

New York.

(Continued from Page 518.)

THE study of the whole hitrogen series from nitrogen itself, nitrous oxide gas, and the different oxygen compounds up to *nitric acid*, is of interest chiefly from the great uniformity of general effects. The study of *nitric acid* is of more practical importance, for it has been in use a long time, and has been tolerably well proved, or at least its general characteristics are well known.

The symptoms produced by *nitric acid* must be separated into two fairly well defined groups : (1) those resulting from the ingestion or inhalation of minute quantities, and (2) those due to its chemical action on the tissues. In the latter group we find most prominent, violent inflammations of epidermoid tissue, and ulcerations, with their accompanying symptoms. In the former group we see the pure effects of the substance as a remedial agent. To these we will first direct our attention.

The familiar symptoms of the *amyl nitrite* group again confront us, as among the first and most prominent effects of minute quantities of this agent ; a feeling of warmth and fullness in the chest and head, headache more or less violent, or even pulsating even to a feeling of bursting, followed by a feeling as if the head were in a vise ; frequent micturitions, urine hot ; nose bleed ; salivation, etc. The general character of these symptoms is unmistakable, and their affinity with the group under consideration undoubted. The salivation, however, is a distinguishing feature. All of the mineral acids (with scarcely an exception) augment the secretions of saliva, bile, urine, sweat, intestinal fluid, and bronchial mucus. They diminish, however, the secretion of the gastric juice (which is in general increased by alkalies). One of the most persistent characters of the *nitric acid* pathogenesis is *salivation* ; but of this more hereafter. These symptoms of disordered circulation appear in the later stages of acute poisoning, and hemorrhages from the nose, bowels or lungs may occur without the pre-existence of any ulceration. Another marked symptom is an eruption of (dark) red pimples on the skin, and a general sensation, quite marked, is *sharp stinging pain*. With these pure drug effects, without any regard to the symptoms of destruction of tissue produced by large doses, we are prepared to look over the symptomatology, as given by Hahnemann in his Chronic Diseases, and supplemented by more recent provings. The head symptoms first call for mention, and no doubt the sensation of a *tight band about the head* (reminding one of the chest symptoms of *cactus*) is most characteristic. In the cases requiring *nitric acid* for this symptom, I have noticed the accompanying symptoms of fullness, pressure or even pulsating, and this pulsation seems most on the left side (unlike that of *glonoine*). This symptom, observed by Hahnemann and also Dr. Berridge, has, I believe, been repeatedly confirmed. In all of these neuralgias the disposition of the patient must be taken into account, chiefly nervous irritability and "*vexed at the least trifle.*" The next feature of importance in this group is the fullness and oppression of the chest, especially on lying down at night ; the feeling of rush of blood to the chest, and so on. These symptoms have been too much neglected, for they are extremely valuable in pointing to the use of the drug in asthma, and in acute congestions of phthisis. I have repeatedly relieved sudden oppression of the chest in chronic phthisis, with or without sharp pains, but usually with the heart symptoms given by Hahnemann (strikingly similar to those of *cactus*), with *nitric acid*. For nocturnal asthma it is valuable (though if a staple preparation of *nitrous acid* could be made, I would prefer to use it), and partly bears up the reputation of the nitrites (and especially of saltpetre) in this disease.

The symptoms of exhaustion given by Hahnemann are universal, all *nitric acid* patients are " tired ;" they sleep badly, have hot hands and feet, the latter especially are prone to perspire offensively ; all are worse at night. One striking distinction from *sulphur* is the easy perspiration of the acid : very many other symptoms are similar.

Let us now turn to the symptoms of tissue change which still furnish the chief indications for the use of the acid by a majority of homœopathists. Inflammations, ulcerations, hæmorrhages and sharp stinging pains from the nose to the anus, with free discharges which are generally excoriating.

In the nose, ulcerations, ozæna, bleeding, splinter-like pains, offensive and corroding discharges, *discharges through the posterior nares into the throat.*

In the mouth, ulcerations on the inner side of the cheek with splinter-like pains, corners of mouth ulcerated, gums sore, tongue sore and ulcerated, *profuse salivation.*

In the throat, ulceration, " mucous patches," all with splinter-like pains.

In the stomach and bowels, symptoms of gastro-enteritis of various sorts, but most marked is the action of the acid on the rectum, where the symptoms of violent and deep seated inflammation with ulceration with terrible splinter-like or tearing pains are indeed severe and abundantly verified.

In the urinary apparatus, symptoms of inflammation from kidney to glans penis are abundant, and are supported by clinical testimony. *Nitric acid* is one of the few remedies which presents any similarity to the primary lesion of venereal ulcer (which *mercury* does not), always characterized by splinter-like pains worse at night, with great weakness and easy perspiration.

All of these "chemical" (if I may be allowed to use the term to designate lesions that seem to be caused only by the local action of the drug in appreciable quantity) effects are, curiously enough, just as valuable indications for the internal exhibition of the drug as those symptoms produced only by the action of minute portions on the nerve centres. It may, however, be said that *nitric acid* will not cure inflammations, ulcerations and hemorrhages unless the peculiar conditions of the drug co-exist ; and these peculiarities, splinter-like pains, increased secretions, nightly exacerbations and the like, are all produced by non-chemically acting doses. *Nitric acid* is a frequently indicated remedy in rectal diseases, but rarely in dysentery, rather in the sequelæ of badly treated (with local applications) dysentery ; frequently indicated in the hemorrhage and other complications following typhoid fever, rarely during the fever itself. The conditions requiring it seldom co-exist with a febrile state, rather in the stage of asthenia following such a state.

In these respects it is like *mercury*, which indeed it resembles in its symptomatology, except the splinter-like pains. For *rapidly-spreading* ulcerations with nocturnal aggravation, sweating and with splinter-like pains give *mercurius-nitrate*, a valuable compound for venereal sores of the chancroid type, and in mucous patches in the mouth and on the palate.

While on the subject of *mercury* we may as well look into the nature of this old enemy of mankind a moment, for it is one of the curiosities of the materia medica.

Mercury is thoroughly proved, through and through. It has been mined for hundreds of years and thousands upon thousands have fallen victims to its destructive power.

One of the curiosities about the drug is its almost absolutely *protective* power against syphilis and its almost complete inability to cure syphilis. There is one parallel to this—namely, the power of *quinine* to prevent the development of marsh malaria and its general inability to cure it.

Mercury is supposed to produce symptoms similar to those of syphilis, but in reality the resemblance is very superficial ; it does not attack the same bones, it never was known to cause an iritis nor a sore on the genitals, only some of the contingent symptoms have some resemblance. And yet the workers in *mercury* are perfectly protected against syphilis.

In the action of these two substances, *mercury* and *quinine* are problems yet to be solved. In some way not now known they prevent the development of the poisons of those diseases, but after the disease has developed they can only arrest the progress of it (or not !) but never (or rarely) seem able to help the system to expel the enemy.

The nervous phenomena of mercurial poison are wonderful ; wonderful, that these helpless people with chorea of the most aggravated type and with tremors like a palsy; without a definite pathology, should escape the destruction of mucous membrane and bone that their fellows have, who have no palsy : and that none of them can be infected with syphilis. Most horrible of all are the cases of syphilis which have lost the bones and other tissues, liable to the ravages of that disease, and have been saturated with *mercury* till the remaining tissues and bones, which syphilis left, have been in turn destroyed by *mercury* ; the two diseases going on side by side ; dissimilar, in essence. Perhaps quite as sad is it to witness in one individual the ravages of marsh malaria which has destroyed the *red* corpuscles of the blood, supplemented by the destructive effects of *quinine* on the *white* corpuscles, the poor patient meanwhile trying to get along with little more than his blood plasma.

Nothing will be gained by attempting to group the acids, they do not form a natural group and need not be associated in our minds ; *phosphoric acid* belongs with *phosphorus, sulphuric acid* with *sulphur, etc.*

It would be an easy step in our pathogenetic study to enter the domain of the alkalies and their relations by taking up the consideration of the hydrogen compounds of nitrogen, which would at once open the study of the *ammonias* (those great stimulants to the circulation) : but it is better, in following our plan, to study now a group of drugs which is in a general way characterized by *contraction* of the arterioles, by paleness and coldness of the surface of the body, a group typified by *ergot* and its botanical relatives, and which may include, by symptomatic comparison, such widely separated drugs as *camphor* and *tobacco.*

These studies are not intended to be complete, as regards any single remedy, but only suggestive and helpful, and are perforce quite general in their character, though it is necessary to attend to the individual characteristics of each drug.

Ergot. No fact in pharmacodynamics is better known than that *ergot* produces contraction of the smaller arteries and that this contraction is apt to persist for a long time ; it is not rhythmical but persistent, and may indeed (as in chronic poisoning) be so persistent as to deprive portions of the body, for example the feet, of their proper amount of blood and nutrition and give rise to slow death (gangrene). This power to cause contraction is not confined to the arterioles, but exerts itself upon smooth muscle fibre in other parts, especially in the gravid uterus. Large doses, and, when individuals are susceptible, small doses, will also induce spasms of voluntary muscles; this may be frequently witnessed during the parturition of women who suffer from albuminuria. When a woman is in this state, it is extremely dangerous to give ergot even in the smallest doses, for it is almost certain to precipitate convulsions.

While under the action of *ergot,* the arterioles are contracted, blood accumulates in the veins and hæmorrhages are frequently produced of dark venous blood. It seems to be true that *ergot* will check hæmorrhage in two ways ; physiologically it will check bright "arterial" hæmorrhage by its power to force contractions of the blood vessels, curatively (homœopathically) it will stop venous hæmorrhage by its power to relax the spasm of the blood vessels and facilitate the flow of blood from the veins. The former method need rarely if ever be resorted to. The writer has never found it necessary in over twenty-five years' practice to administer a ponderable dose of *ergot* at any period of parturition, nor has he been convinced of the superiority of *ergot* as an hæmostatic in any other form of hæmorrhage that had to be controlled by medicines.

The peculiar features of ergotismus are:

1. Coldness of the surface of the body with *dryness, intolerance of heat or covering*, general venous enlargement of internal organs with hæmorrhages from them, nose, stomach, bowels, uterus, kidneys and lungs; sighing respiration, great anxiety (or in some cases perfect indifference), and ravenous hunger and thirst. With this state there may be dark, olive-green discharges from the bowels, more or less bloody ; greenish offensive uterine discharges *et cetera.*

2. Formication and loss of sensation in the extremities, especially in the legs, excessive prostration; cramps or drawing pains; gradually increasing paralysis and gangrene of the limb.

3. More rarely convulsions.

From the collapse of *veratrum album*, which presents the similar feature of excessive thirst, we distinguish *ergot* by the dryness of the surface, the intolerance of covering (or warmth), the general absence of vomiting and by the character of the evacuations, which in *veratrum* are profuse and watery, in *ergot* dark olive green and slimy or bloody.

In a terrible epidemic of dysentery many years since several cases died in three or four days in a state of collapse, but when *ergot* was administered, on the first indications of collapse others were saved, the peculiarities of cold dry skin, insatiable thirst and *canine hunger*, perfect apathy and perfect consciousness, involuntary dark olive green or black discharges were present in every case.

In the last stages of puerperal metro-peritonitis, with collapsed abdomen, sunken features, cold skin, thready pulse, offensive olive green discharge from the genitals, *ergot* has changed the whole complexion of the case and brought about convalescence. I am firmly convinced that a large proportion of the cases of puerperal fever, so prevalent in the practice of some physicians (who ought not to be criminally reckless), is due to the free administration of *ergot*, either to check hæmorrhage or to prevent a possible occurrence of one. At least ten lives are sacrificed to one saved by this powerful drug !

Closely allied to the ergot of rye, is the ergot of corn, *ustilago maydis*. Though no cases of poisoning have been reported from the abuse of this medicine the provings show many symptoms similar to those of ergot of rye. Clinically it has been found serviceable in hæmorrhages of the uterus characterized by an "oozing of dark, offensive blood with small clots," particularly if the patient complain of a persistent aching referred to the mouth of the womb, or pain, swelling, and soreness in the left ovary, *and a seated pain in the left anterior spine of the ilium.*

(*To be continued.*)

CAN HEADACHE AND ASTHENOPIA BE PRODUCED BY SMALL DEGREES OF ASTIGMATISM (0.25 D.)?*

By GEO. S. NORTON, M.D.,

New York.

THE frequency with which errors of refraction produce head-aches and various nervous disturbances, is becoming more and more generally acknowledged by the medical profession. Still, even among ophthalmologists, there is a tendency to ignore small deviations from perfect symmetry of the organ of vision. Thus many, without personal examination, follow the teachings of Donders† over twenty years ago, when he says:

"So long as astigmatism does not essentially diminish the acuteness of vision, we call it normal. It is abnormal so soon as disturbance occurs. If it amounts to $\frac{1}{12}$ or more it must be considered as abnormal."

A review of all the chief text books upon Ophthalmology and the special works upon refraction shows hardly a reference to the advisability of correcting an astigmatism of less than 0.5 D. Even Burnett in his recent "Treatise on Astigmatism," page 49, says, *"We feel justified in considering only those degrees of astigmatism abnormal which exceed 0.25 D. ($\frac{1}{100}$),"* though on page 170 he further remarks that, "It occasionally happens, too, that the correction of astigmatism as low as 0.25 D. is found very beneficial. Such cases are usually found in persons whose nervous systems are below par, and on restoration to health the glasses can be laid aside."

This paper has, therefore, been prepared for the purpose of bringing this subject more forcibly before specialists in ophthalmology, and at the same time to prove that an astigmatism of 0.25 D. may produce very marked symptoms in the eyes and head, which may be relieved by the correction of the abnormal curvature by proper glasses; but it is not claimed that so low a degree must or usually should be neutralized by cylindrical lenses.

In the preparation of this article it was my intention to utilize a large amount of material from my clinic at the New York Ophthalmic Hospital, but an examination of the records showed that my assistants had not given sufficient attention to recording the lowest degrees of

---

*Read at the Ninth International Medical Congress held in Washington, D. C., September, 1887.

†Accommodation and Refraction of the Eye, p. 456.

astigmatism (o.25 D.) to make them valuable in drawing conclusions. I have, therefore, only taken my private records of over 2,000 cases of errors of refraction tested by myself and assistant during the past four and one-half years, when more careful attention was given to the lowest grades of astigmatism. During which time there were examined 177 cases in which the astigmatism was 0.5 D., and 147 in which the astigmatism was 0.25 D. in one or both eyes. In only a small proportion of these was the error corrected, as it was often combined with more or less hyperopia or myopia, the neutralization of which was sufficient to relieve the asthenopic symptoms.

From the above, the following ten cases have been selected to illustrate the various symptoms which may arise and the benefit which may be derived from the correction of these low degrees of astigmatism :

CASE I.—Lucy E———, about seventeen years old, came to my office in November, 1882. For one year had had much pain in the eyes on reading. The eyes were weak, sensitive to light, especially gaslight, which caused redness of the eyes the following day. The lids felt heavy and she desired to close them. On reading even five minutes a blur would come before the vision, to be followed by headache over the eyes. Nearly every afternoon had pain through the temples coming and going quickly. V. $\frac{20}{20}$, slight difficulty; + 0.25^c., ax. 90°, made vision $\frac{20}{20}$ and corrected the slight blurring of vertical lines. These glasses were at once given for both distant and near vision. Immediate relief from headache and all eye symptoms was experienced. October, 1884, she wrote that she was still using the glasses and could not read an hour with comfort without them. No pain in the eyes or headache unless she neglected to wear her glasses.

CASE II.—Mr. H———, twenty-one years of age, in September, 1885, had been suffering for one or two years from his eyes. On reading one-half hour the conjunctiva would become injected, with increased flow of tears and moderate secretion of mucus, often aggravated the following morning. Accompanying the above objective symptoms would be dull aching in the eyes after use. R. V. $\frac{20}{20}$, L. V. $\frac{20}{20}$; + 0.5^c., ax., 90°, R. V. $\frac{20}{20}$. After instillation of atropine the test showed, R. V. $\frac{20}{20}$, L. V. $\frac{20}{20}$, difficulty; + 0.5^c., ax. 80°, R. V. $\frac{20}{20}$, difficulty; + 0.25^c., ax. 100°, L. V. $\frac{20}{20}$, difficulty, and lines corrected in both eyes. These glasses were, therefore, prescribed. August 15th, 1887, he writes me as follows : "I used the glasses for both distant and near vision for about three or four weeks. Since then I have used them constantly for near vision only, and am not able to read or write for any length of time without them. With the aid of the glasses I have been able to use my eyes as much as I wish, often eight or ten hours a day."

CASE III.—Alice T———, age 8
weeks of severe headache after 8
1884, + 0.63⁸., were prescribed,
in September, 1884, the headaches
under atropine was made, which
+ 0.63⁸., R. V. 1⁸, + 0.25ᶜ., a1
rect in each eye. These glasses w
enced relief and has since been able

CASE IV.—Anna K———, about
1884, complained of the vision blu
minutes or less ; also some blurring
experienced as in use for music. I
present. An examination both witl
O. U., but the lines were not seen di
ax. 180°, cleared the vision and ᴄ
These lenses were prescribed. In
she was wearing the glasses with coi
out them. In October, 1885, she ᴠ
return of the headaches, though the ᴠ
glasses for both distant and near visiᴄ
tion, relieved in a few days.

CASE V.—P. S———, eighteen yᴄ
University, came to me in February,
had complained of burning in the
nausea after reading two hours or sᴄ
severely from most intense pain in th
throbbing pain in them as if they
noise or exposure to light, and accc
on attempting to rise. Marked ᴄ
especially right, was the only pronᴄ
1⁸, O. U. The ophthalmoscope shᴄ
the pain in the head had been co
As only temporary benefit was oᴋ
atropine, with the following result :
ax. 90°, V. 1⁸, and lines correct in
0.25ᶜ., ax. 90°, were recommendec
Later the spherical was increased to
he wrote that he could read with
without tiring the eyes.

CASE VI.—Mrs. S———, about
years complained of severe attacks ᴄ
the temples as often as once or twi
reading or being in a bright light. A
ing of the eyes, with photophobia,
were present. The examinations we
V. 1⁸, O. U., slight difficulty, both
0.25ᶜ., ax. 20° ⊃—0.25ᶜ., ax. 110°
ax. 150° ⊃—0.25ᶜ., ax. 60°, L. V.

in both eyes. As the above glasses were comfortable to the eyes they were prescribed. August 11th, 1887, she writes as follows: "I have faithfully worn the glasses you prescribed. My eyes are some better. I do not wear them constantly about the house, as I did the first year. I use them for sewing, reading, or riding and walking; it is the only help for the severe pain in head and eyes."

CASE VII.—Alice K———, age seventeen, was seen in November, 1886, on account of blurring of the vision and desire to rub the eyes, with dull feeling in them after reading an hour or so, especially at night. The vision was ⁴⁴ in both eyes, though clearer in the right. No Hm. As general treatment did not benefit, an examination under atropine was made February 19th, 1887, when the right eye was found Em.; while in the left eye was a hyperopic astigmatism of 0.25 D. in the vertical meridian. A prescription for plane. O. D. + 0.25ᶜ., ax. 180°, O. S. was given, as these glasses made the vision equal in the two eyes. They have since been worn for near vision with comfort.

CASE VIII.—Hessie S———, thirteen years old, was brought to me March 3d, 1886, not being able to use the eyes at all without pain in them and letters running together. V. ⁴⁴, difficulty, O. U. The next day, after two instillations of atropine, V. ⁴⁴ O. U., clearer in the right eye. + 0.25ᶜ., ax. 180°, R. V. ⁴⁴; + 0.25ᶜ., ax., 60°, L V. ⁴⁴, difficulty. These glasses were advised. On June 22d, 1886, she reported that she had worn the glasses and had been relieved from the pain in the eyes and blurring of the vision.

CASE IX.—Florence C———, fourteen years of age, consulted me December 18th, 1886. She had been compelled to leave school, as on reading five minutes there would be watering of the eyes and pain in them, with twitching of the lids and headache over the eyes. V. ⁴⁴, slight difficulty, O. U. No Hm. Under atropine, R. V. ⁴⁴, L V. ⁴⁴; + 0.25ᶜ., ax. 180°, R. V. ⁴⁴; + 0.5ᶜ., ax. 180°, L V. ⁴⁴, and lines corrected in both eyes. January 5th, 1887, the above glasses were given, when she was able to return to her work in school, with relief of all the asthenopic symptoms before experienced.

CASE X.—Mr. A———, about thirty years of age, has for four years complained of asthenopic symptoms and chronic inflammation of the margins of the lids. His vision was ⁴⁴ and no error of refraction could be detected. Atropine was, however, instilled, when a very careful test revealed a very low degree of astigmatism, corrected by + 0.25ᶜ., ax. 95°, O. D.;—0.25ᶜ., ax. 45°, O. S. On July 12th, 1887, these glasses were prescribed. Since then his eyes have been steadily improving in all respects. It is too soon to report a perfect cure.

From a study of the above cases and many others which have come under my observation, the following conclusions have been drawn: First—that an astigmatism of 0.25 D. *may*, and not unfrequently does, *produce headache and various asthenopic symptoms,* and that these disturbances may be relieved by the correction of this low degree of abnormal curvature.

The question now arises under what conditions does an astigmatism of 0.25 D. cause "eye strain" sufficient to call for its correction? In the first place, *age* has a very marked influence, as it is more often found in children, particularly in young girls from twelve to eighteen years old. It is very rare that we are compelled to correct so small an error of refraction in adults, as the ciliary muscle has, by constant use, adapted itself to the abnormal curvature, thus practically neutralizing it. This can be readily understood when we remember how often we find it impossible to fully correct a high degree of astigmatism in adults, as the ciliary muscle will not adjust itself to regular work, irregular action having become its normal action. Furthermore, when asthenopia occurs in adults, even though there is an astigmatism of 0.25 D., we usually find more or less hyperopia or myopia (compound astigmatism), in which case it is only necessary to prescribe spherical glasses. It may, however, be advisable to correct an astigmatism of 0.25 D. in adults, as has been shown in Cases VI. and X., especially when other methods of treatment have failed to relieve, or when no other cause can be ascribed for the asthenopia.

Again, this low degree of astigmatism may not unfrequently give rise to eye strain in delicate, nervous individuals, particularly young people and women, also in those who, from one cause or another, are in poor general health. In these cases the glasses may be needed only temporarily and then dispensed with as the patient becomes stronger.

Another most important cause of asthenopia is anisometropia, even though the anomaly of refraction is no greater than the one now under consideration, for when the predisposition to muscular weakness is present, any difference in the refraction of the two eyes is sometimes sufficient to call forth most annoying symptoms.

In compound astigmatism, when the hyperopia or myopia is less than 0.75 D., with an astigmatism of 0.25 D., it is my practice at first to correct the astigmatism only, then later a portion of the hyperopia or myopia, if the asthenopic symptoms are not relieved by the first prescription. If, however, the hyperopia or myopia is of a high degree, it is better to first endeavor to relieve by spherical lenses before having recourse to cylinders.

No ironclad rules can, however, be laid down for the prescription of glasses in anomalies of refraction, as we must take carefully into account the relative power of the recti and ciliary muscles and their influence upon convergence and accommodation, besides the general condition of the patient. How often are we surprised at the relative strength or weakness of the accommodative apparatus when we find the highest form of ametropia present, without the slightest inconvenience having been experienced, while upon the other hand, the lowest degrees will sometimes call out a serious train of symptoms.

With our present knowlege of the muscular apparatus of the eye, it is therefore not difficult for us to realize how in young persons, or in delicate, nervous individuals, who have over-used the eyes, the power of accommodation may be upon the border line between weakness and strength, when slight irregular action may be all that is necessary to exercise a strain, which, though little, may be sufficient to cause pronounced disturbances. Just as a trifling injury will in one person give rise to intense suffering, which in another would hardly be noticed, so an eye strain which the majority of people would not observe, will in some produce headache or marked asthenopic symptoms.

In conclusion let me again say, that no claim is made in this paper that an astigmatism of 0.25 D. should usually be corrected by cylindrical lenses, only that not unfrequently càses will be found in which the only relief we can give will be obtained by its correction, and that if we, as oculists, desire to secure the best results with our patients, we must take into consideration these low forms of astigmatism.

NEURASTHENIA.*

By Wm. M. BUTLER, M.D.,

Brooklyn, N. Y.

NEURASTHENIA or Nervous Exhaustion is a disease characterized by a general derangement and disturbance of the functions of the nervous system.

This disease was first classified and minutely described by the late Dr. Geo. M. Beard, in a paper read in 1868 before the New York Medical Journal Association, and published in the first edition of Beard and Rockwell's Electricity. Previous to this publication, although frequently encountered, it was regarded by the profession as

---

* Read at the Semi-Annual Meeting of the Homœopathic Medical Society, State of New York, September 21st, 1887.

one of the phases of Hysteria, or scoffed at as merely the product of the patient's overwrought imagination. Since this first publication, Beard's elaborate monograph upon this subject, and descriptions of the disease by Dr. Hugh Campbell, of England, Profs. Erb, of Heidelberg, Grasset, of Paris, and Rosenthal, of Vienna, and articles by less noted writers, have verified its existence and given it an established place among the disorders of the nervous system.

Etiology.—Arising from a deficiency of that mysterious power we call nerve force, it may be caused by any one of a multitude of agencies which exhaust the nervous system.

Although liable to occur in either sex and at any period of life, certain persons seem naturally susceptible to its invasion. These individuals always attract by their brightness and keen wit. Favorites in the circle in which they move, their nervous systems seem continually keyed above concert pitch. Extremely sensitive and utterly regardless of their natural resources, in work or recreation they invariably go beyond their strength. Precocious children, the pride of ambitious teachers and foolish parents, are found in this class, and too frequently is their life's work ruined by their school and college honors achieved in hours stolen from rest and sleep. Many a beautiful girl, with the plaudits of her teachers and friends over her valedictory essay ringing in her ears, steps from her graduating stage down into a life of pain and chronic invalidism, produced by this disease.

While these highly strung, sensitive organizations are especially liable, none are exempt from this disease.

Constant work and worry, whether over the intricate schemes and combinations of the counting-room and Stock Exchange, or the endless cares of the household, may in time prostrate the man or woman of iron nerve.

Sexual excess, in either sex, is one of the commonest causes.

Constant seminal drain, whether from masturbation or too frequent intercourse, renders the male especially liable to the disease.

Any acute disease, which exhausts the general system and does not yield to treatment, may plunge the patient into the depths of Neurasthenia, and leave him for months or years a sufferer from this dread disorder.

In addition to the causes mentioned, woman may fall an easy prey to this disease from too frequent labors and miscarriages, profuse floodings, prolonged leucorrhœas and chronic uterine troubles. Exhausted by any of these predisposing causes, the slightest shock or over-exertion may act as an exciting cause, and produce in their full development any or all of the symptoms of Neurasthenia.

Symptomatology.—To describe the totality of the sym
to be encountered in this disease, would be to reverse e\
sensation which the nervous system is capable of pro
well might you attempt to describe the changes of a kale
paint the fleeting tints of the chameleon.

From the top of the head to the tips of the toes, where
is distributed, abnormal sensations may arise singly or
puzzling combinations.

For convenience of description we shall mention, in
order, a few of the common symptoms liable to be encou

Mind.—A peculiar mental feature, often observed, is t
of a variety of morbid fears, differing from insane delusio
fact that the patient admits their foolishness, but cannot
off. As an example, I would cite a recent case of a frien
a lady—who was afraid to go into her parlor. An exam
Dr. Beard calls ''Mysophobia or fear of contamination,'
tered in a patient of my own, some months ago. This
walking near any other person, unless she brought her re
upon it, would involuntarily brush off her clothing. In
cases these symptoms disappeared with improved health.
greatly depressed and fear constantly some incurable di
pending insanity, but the depression usually stops short
insanity.

Head.—Dizzinness of every form is of common occurre

A volume could scarcely describe all the head sympto
the sufferers complain. General and circumscribed hea
bands about the head—opening and shutting of the skul
of the brain—drawings and pullings up and down—in
conceivable sensation which an active imagination ca
liable to be encountered.

In nearly every case sleep is more or less disturbed.
are almost absolutely sleepless, others only sleep in the
hours of the night. In all, even if they get an apparentl
quantity, the sleep fails to afford the needed rest and re
When a drowsy state obtains, as sometimes occurs, we
tient in the morning fatigued and unrefreshed. One of t
couraging and reliable signs of permanent improvement
sleep becomes continuous and refreshing, even if the nor
is not obtained.

Chest.—Of the chest symptoms, the most troublesome
tion of suffocation upon lying down, and numerous fu
rangements of the heart—palpitations, jumping of the hea

as if the heart stopped—and cardiac pains, often closely simulating those of angina pectoris.

Digestive Organs.—The symptoms of the digestive tract are numerous and often among the most difficult to overcome. Possessed of a ravenous appetite, or utterly devoid of all desire and loathing the sight of any food, it is at times almost impossible to get the patient to take and retain the nourishment which is absolutely necessary for the preservation of life, to say nothing of the recuperation of their greatly weakened powers.

In addition to their nausea, vomiting, flatulency, obstinate constipation or diarrhœa—any or all of which, at times, we meet in the same patient—complaints are made of burnings or coldness in the stomach, trembling, faintness, drawings or a general relaxedness. Some have cravings for the most indigestible substances ; others obstinately insist upon their inability to take fluids ; others strenuously oppose solids. However tractable upon other points, in regard to the matter of diet the physician can rest assured that sooner or later he will meet with trouble and opposition.

In addition to the multitude of symptoms already enumerated, we may have tenderness of the whole or portions of the spine—burning in the spine—nervous chills—dull pain and aching in different parts of the back—ataxic pains in the limbs—numbness and pricking in the extremities—coldness or burning of the feet—and a feeling of general exhaustion upon the least exertion. Many are troubled with the most profuse sweatings of the hands and feet, or of the whole body. In men, frequent emissions and deficient virility, and in women, leucorrhœa, and almost every form of uterine disorder, are liable to occur. Profuse menstruation is another frequent accompaniment. One lady at present under my treatment has often fainted from her excessive flooding.

Neuralgias of every variety torment the sufferers. A recent case of mine for days was subject to the most excruciating agony from attacks of intercostal neuralgia, producing the sensation of an ever-tightening hoop around the chest.

Many peculiar symptoms are also met with. I have now under my care a young lady who has been greatly troubled with swelling and inflammation about the nails of the great toes. Before coming into my hands she had undergone a very severe course of treatment at the hands of a chiropodist for what he supposed to be ingrowing toe nails. Upon close examination I was convinced that the nails were not ingrowing, and the inflammation of the toes was but another one of the numerous symptoms of her disease, and, aside from keeping them scrupulously clean, have paid no attention to them. The sequel has proven the correctness of my opinion, and the toes have ever served as a reliable index of her general condition, the inflammation increasing or subsiding with the fluctuations of the disease ; and now, with approaching restoration to health, all signs of inflammation are disappearing.

Such, in brief, is an outline of the most prominent symptoms of Neurasthenia.

Diagnosis.—The diseases with which Neurasthenia is most liable to be confounded are organic diseases of the cord, hysteria and anæmia.

Upon a casual and imperfect examination it may be difficult to differentiate Neurasthenia from some of the organic diseases of the spinal cord.

The shooting pains in the limbs and the paralytic symptoms, may suggest locomotor ataxy. The ability to stand with the eyes shut ; the presence of the normal knee jerk and the absence of the Argyle Robertson pupil—or reflex iridoplegia, as it is sometimes called— and the absence of the girdle sensation about the waist, soon dispel all doubts upon this point.

In general, the changeable character of the symptoms distinguishes it from those of organic nervous disease, which are usually fixed and stable.

Its increased activity of the reflexes, in contradistinction from the diminished reflexes of organic disease of the cord, is another pathognomonic sign.

Hysteria.—The absence of convulsions and the Globus Hystericus, and the less common occurrence of ovarian tenderness and anæsthesia; its more frequent occurrence in males ; the great physical debility, and the course of the disease, will usually distinguish it from Hysteria. In some instances, however, hysterical symptoms are combined with those pathognomonic of the disease, and in these cases the diagnosis is more difficult.

Anæmia.—The nervous diathesis ; the usual occurrence between the ages of fifteen and sixty ; the character of the pulse, often full or normal, instead of weak and compressible ; the absence of cardiac and venous murmurs ; the usual absence of facial pallor ; its almost universal disturbance of sleep ; more frequent occurrence in men, and more chronic character, render it unliable to be confounded with anæmia.

Prognosis.—The prognosis of the disease, under proper treatment, is usually favorable. The course, however, is ordinarily long and tedious—months and years often being passed before complete recovery is obtained. One great cause of the usual prolonged course of the disease arises from the conduct of the patients themselves, who, discouraged by their slow progress, are continually transferred from one physician to another, giving to no one a fair chance—the last one getting all the credit of the cure.

Treatment.—The all-important question in reference to Neurasthenia is that of Treatment. How are we to cure our cases? In considering this question we must recognize the fact that no mere routine treatment can be successful. No iron-sided rules can be laid down, applicable to all cases.

Each case must be studied by itself in its entirety. The individual characteristics, the mental and physical symptoms, the surrounding moral atmosphere of the patient, the influence of any agencies which may have acted as predisposing or exciting causes of the malady—everything which can in any way affect the future course of the disease must be considered before we decide upon a settled mode of treatment.

If we find the patient exhausted by slight exertion and worried by over-sympathetic friends, we must insist upon isolation and absolute rest in bed, the physician and nurse alone being allowed access to the sick-room. Yet this much-lauded *rest cure* will not succeed with every case, and if not indicated will prove an obstacle to recovery.

Many cases will improve more rapidly in their own homes, surrounded by friends, and while engaged in the routine of their daily duties.

Some cases can be indulged in a generous general diet, while others must be limited to the articles most easily digested.

All these questions must be decided by each individual practitioner, and the decision must be made anew with each fresh case, as no previous experience is certain to be of value in the case in hand.

In every case the physician must acquire the patient's confidence and gain supremacy over her mind, or his treatment will be of little avail.

Massage and electricity will be found the most reliable adjuvants in a large majority of ·cases, especially when the *rest cure* is in progress ; nor should they be discontinued until the patient is far upon the road to recovery, or entirely restored.

When the physical strength is sufficiently recuperated, great aid will be obtained by judicious outdoor exercise and enjoyable mental diversion.

Yet, assisted by every external adjuvant which he can bring to his aid, the physician must apply his highest medical skill or he will fail in making a perfect cure.

In the face of an endless multitude of ever-changing symptoms, it the Homœopathist seeks to find a *similimum* which will cover them all, he will soon find himself in a darker than Cretan labyrinth, with no Ariadne thread to guide his wandering steps. In choosing his drug, the physician must eliminate many symptoms, the mere fruit of the patient's overwrought imagination, and only consider those absolutely essential in the causation and continuance of the disease.

When this has been done, the most painstaking research of the Materia Medica will be required for the discovery of the correct remedy; but when the drug is discovered it must be allowed sufficient time to accomplish its work, and not be superseded by another, to meet each passing whim of the patient.

The list required by different patients is only limited by Allen's Index. No one can successfully combat Neurasthenia who is content with an armamentarium more limited than the Homœopathic Materia Medica itself.

EXTRACTS FROM CASE BOOK. *

By E. H. LINNELL, M.D.,

Norwich, Conn.

CASE I.—*Colocynth* in *Irido-choroiditis.* On the 5th of January, 1887, I was called to see Mrs. W. in consultation with Dr. B. I found her suffering with Irido-choroiditis serosa of the left eye. She had been sick five weeks. The condition of the eye, at the time of my visit, was as follows : Iris discolored and pupil contracted. Slight peri-corneal injection, especially in lower portion of eye-ball. Slight cutting pains. Eye very sensitive to touch or motion. T + 1, vitreous filled with fine opacities preventing a view of the fundus with the ophthalmoscope. Vision reduced to counting fingers at three feet. I advised the use of a one per cent. solution of atropin sufficiently often to keep the pupil well dilated, and the use of *bryonia* internally, and the case was left in the hands of the family physician.

One week later I again saw the case in consultation. The pupil was then dilated ad max. above, but not quite as much below, and the iris was still of a greenish hue, instead of the natural blue of the other eye. The subjective symptoms were entirely relieved, but the condition of the fundus and the vision were unchanged, and the

* Read at the Semi-annual Meeting of the Homœopathic Medical Society, State of New York, September 21st, 1887.

tension was still a little increased. *Iod. potass.* 1 x was advised, together with the instillation of atropin one grain to ounce, n. and m.

At my next visit, one week later, the iris was of normal color and lustre and there was no epi-scleral injection. The vitreous was less cloudy, so that the optic disc and the retinal vessels could be dimly made out, and there was a corresponding improvement of vision. The same treatment was continued.

One week later there was still further improvement in the appearance of the fundus and of the vision, although there was again some sensitiveness of the eye, which I attributed to an unfavorable change in the weather. The same treatment was continued, with the addition of a single dose of *sulph.* 30 every second day.

Two days later there was a severe aggravation of the disease, and the case was placed in my hands. Without apparent cause, there was renewed iritis with severe pain and tenderness, increased cloudiness of vitreous and obscuration of vision. In fact, the condition was as bad, if not worse, than at any time previously. I was at a loss to account for this sudden relapse, as the patient's general health was good, and she had not, to my knowledge, been imprudent in any way. The mystery was solved a few days later, when she confessed to having used a solution of *colocynth* (or bitter-apple) in rum as a hair wash just previous to the aggravation of the eye trouble. She had been in the habit of using it frequently for a year or more, and I learned that she had been subject to frequent attacks of colic, which presented the well known characteristics of *colocynth*, and were controlled by that remedy. I will not weary you with a further detailed report of the case. Suffice it to say, the hair wash was not used again and she made a complete recovery in a reasonable time, and with no other remedies than those previously used. *Bryonia* gave relief in the acute stage, and *iod. potass.* and later *sulph.* cleared up the opacity of the vitreous and restored normal vision.

I think we may fairly consider this case as aggravated, if not primarily caused, by *colocynth.* The drug is readily absorbed through the skin, producing its specific effect upon the alimentary canal just as when it is taken by the mouth. In the accounts of poisoning by this drug we find that it produced obscuration of vision in one person, and others report twitching of the upper lid of the right eye, and painfulness of the eyes increased by stooping. In the pathogenesis of the drug we have developed the cutting and burning pains in the eye, and the tearing and boring pains in the temple and side of the head, and in the face. Dr. Watzke, of Vienna, who made a thorough proving of the drug, says: "The hemi-craniæ and persopalgiæ which *colocynth* will cure are in all cases purely functional derangements of the trifacial nerve." Does experience bear out the truth of this statement? ·

If my assumption is correct, that *colocynth* caused in the case narrated actual inflammation of the iris and choroid, it should be curative in similar inflammatory conditions, if there is any truth in

our therapeutic tenets.   The following case is the only one that I can
find recorded, where an organic affection of the eyes was cured by
colocynth.   The case is so imperfectly recorded as to leave us quite
in the dark as to the real nature of the disease, but it evidently was
something more than trigemilal neuralgia.

"The patient had been afflicted for a considerable time with an almost permanently existing headache, after which the eye became inflamed.   When Dr. S. was called the patient had already lost his
sight.   In the right eye, the sight of which was still preserved, the
patient complained of burning, cutting pains.   Congestion of blood
to the head and discharge of acrid tears from both eyes troubled the
patient.   Two drops of the tincture of *colocynth* every three hours removed the headache in twenty-four hours and effected a considerable
abatement of the pains in the eyes.   The continued use of *colocynth*
restored the sight of both eyes completely in eight days, and effected
a perfect cure."

The pulp and seeds of the bitter apple contain a large amount of
mucilaginous matter which I suppose is the quality that recommends
it as a hair wash.   I did not know that it was ever used for such a
purpose until Mrs. W. spoke of so using it, but I have since found it
in another family where I have frequently been called of late to prescribe for attacks of colic.   I do not know how commonly it is used
in this way, but I think we should do well to warn our patients of its.
poisonous properties as opportunity occurs.

CASE II.—Traumatic Rupture of Iris and permanent Mydriasis,
without external wound.
November 8th, 1886.   Harry P——— was struck in the right eye
four days previously.   The lids were closed for three days.   Now
there is no external sign of injury either to lids or ball, but the pupil
is dilated nearly ad max. and there is a small rent in the pupillary
border of the iris at the temporal side.   T,—1, no pain ; vision either
eye $\frac{10}{10}$; that of left made $\frac{10}{8}$ + with —$\frac{1}{10}$, but glasses do not improve
vision of injured eye.   The ophthalmoscope shows a little hyper-
æmia of the retina, but no lesion is discoverable at the bottom of the
eye-ball.   Prescribed *arnica* internally and a solution of atropin, one
grain to the ounce, to be instilled night and morning to still further
dilate the pupil, and prevent, if possible, the formation of adhesions
between the torn edges of the iris and the anterior surface of the lens.
November 15th.   Vision increased to $\frac{10}{8}$.   Retinal veins a little
swollen and retina in vicinity of disc a little hazy.   Discontinue atropin, continue *arnica.*
November 27th.   Vision perfect.   Outlines of disc now for the
first time clearly defined, though there still remains a little retinal
hyperæmia.   Iris dilated ad max. in vicinity of coloboma, not so

much so on inner side. No reaction to light. Slight crescent at inner edge of disc, and choroid pale around it for a distance of one disc diameter. ℞ Eserine one per cent. solution three times a day.

December 28th. Has been using eserine since last date. It contracts the pupil temporarily but the effect passes off in about two hours, when the pupil becomes as large and immovable as before. Discontinue eserine and take *duboisin 3x* once in three hours.

April 22d, 1887. At this date the condition remains as previously, except that two small synechiæ have formed at the edges of the coloboma. Sight is perfect.

This case interested me because of its uniqueness. I do not remember to have read of a similar case of traumatic rupture of the iris without an external wound. I at first considered the above mentioned crescent at the edge of the optic disc as a post-staphyloma, but subsequent examinations proved the eye to be entirely emmetropic, and I concluded that it was a choroidal coloboma produced by the injury. Did I treat the case judiciously? Would the wound in the iris have been more likely to heal if I had used eserine at first, instead of atropin? Adhesions would most likely have formed, but these might have been broken up by a subsequent use of atropin.

CASE III.—*Helonias dioica* in Inflammation of the Optic Nerve.

I find nothing in the pathogenesis of *helonias* to suggest its applicability in any ocular affection, nor is there any reference to it in Norton's "Ophthalmic Therapeutics." In the following case the improvement following its administration was prompt, decided and permanent. It is, therefore, in the hope of adding another drug to the list of those useful in the affections of the optic nerve and retina, and especially when associated with renal disease, that this case is reported.

Mr. M———, sixty-two years old, consulted me first August 9th, 1886. He said that he formerly had had keen sight, but that it had been gradually failing for the past six months. It was then only $\frac{10}{100}$ with either eye. The field of vision was not accurately tested, but it was markedly contracted, for with strongly magnifying glasses he could only see a portion of a printed word at once. The peripheral field was, however, not entirely wanting, as he noticed the movement of my hand in all directions. With the ophthalmoscope the optic disc in each eye had lost its transparency and presented a blurred hazy appearance with indistinct outlines. The retinal veins were somewhat swollen and the arteries upon the disc were small and somewhat veiled by an apparently serous infiltration. The fundus in other respects presented a natural appearance. The gentleman was anæmic and feeble, and his eyelids were œdematous. An examination of the urine gave the following results: Quantity in twenty-four hours five gills, turbid, reaction acid, and specific gravity 1018, and containing a trace of albumin. Under the microscope numerous pus corpuscles, a few epithelia from the tubules of the kidney, and some fatty and granular casts were seen. Under treatment his general health improved, and with it the vision, until the record October 16th was: V. O. U. as before = $\frac{10}{100}$, but + 16 makes it $\frac{16}{40}$. The urine increased in amount and became less turbid and the albumin disappeared, but there was no material change in the microscopical appearance. The next record was October 23d. Vision $\frac{16}{40}$, but only $\frac{16}{40}$ with glasses. This was the only time that vision without glasses was more than $\frac{10}{100}$, and there was no further improvement with glasses. November 22d the condition was as follows: Vision as it has been for the past five weeks, viz., $\frac{10}{100}$ without glasses, and $\frac{16}{40}$ with + 16. The retinal veins somewhat swollen and a faint cloudiness of the disc and of the retina immediately surrounding it. Outlines of disc better defined and less veiling of the arteries. He has gained nearly twenty pounds in weight since he first consulted me, had a better color, but was still weak, though able to walk a mile and a half to my office as he had done all the while. He complained of a constant dull pain in the lumbar region extending around the hips and down the legs, and also of a sensation as if the forehead were encircled by a tight band. These symptoms suggested *helonias*, which I prescribed in the 1 x, two drops four times daily. It was followed by surprising improvement in vision. In one week the vision rose to $\frac{16}{40}$ without glasses, and $\frac{16}{40}$ with + 16. In one month it was $\frac{16}{40}$ without and $\frac{16}{40}$ with glasses, and he was able to read 0.6 of Snellen's test types with some hesitancy. Previously he had not been able to read even large type. *Helonias* was continued uninterruptedly until February 9th, 1887, with the exception of ten days in January, when *rhus* was given for constitutional symptoms. At this date, February 9th, vision was $\frac{16}{40}$ without glasses and $\frac{16}{40}$ with + 16, and it has continued perfect until the present time. He is able to read the finest print without discomfort seven or eight hours a day, although his general health gradually fails and the urine contains pus cells in increasing quantities. During much of the time while taking *helonias* he also took bovinine after meals, but no other medicine, so that I think the improvement in vision may fairly be ascribed to the *helonias*. The last time that I examined his eyes the fundus appeared absolutely normal in every respect, aside from a slight pallor of the disc. One peculiar feature of the case was that he always maintained that he could see very much better in the twilight. I found this symptom under *china, ferrum, hellebore* and *phosphorus*, but none of these remedies, given in the early history of the case, relieved the symptom.

MICROSCOPIC ANATOMY OF THE CARCINOMATA.*

By A. WILSON DODS, M.D.,

Fredonia, N. Y.

WHEN Dr. Fulton invited me to contribute a paper on the above subject, I felt that, although I could offer nothing new in regard to the histology of the carcinomata, yet I might possibly be able, by presenting in compact form those points of structure which characterize this group of tumors, to save to some one a portion of the labor I have gone through with in order to become familiar with their histology, and at any rate I should be doing the work assigned me by the chairman of the bureau. It is therefore with a full appreciation of the fact that I may be, and very probably am, "carrying coals to Newcastle," that I present this paper to the society.

As other members of the bureau will consider the Etiology and Clinical history of these new growths, this paper will be confined as closely as may be to a description of their appearance as seen in the pathological laboratory, and an endeavor to illustrate this by the aid of photo-micrographs.

As a means of conserving your time as much as possible, I shall omit the detail of the preparation of the tissues for microscopic examination, referring to Dr. Geo. Sims Woodhead on Practical Pathology, and a paper of my own, "Practical Hints for the Examination of New Growths," which I had the honor to read before the Homœopathic Medical Society of Western New York last January, and which was published in the March number of THE NORTH AMERICAN JOURNAL OF HOMŒOPATHY, for a full description of all the steps necessary to be gone through before the tissue is ready for the microscope.

Before entering upon the subject matter proper, it will be well to mention that there are no new tissue elements introduced into the system with which to build up the new growths, but that these formations are composed of elements which are normally found in the body at some period of its development. This statement would appear to be superfluous ; but one so often hears of "cancer cells" that it is well to combat the error on every occasion, for it would be absolutely impossible to say on a microscopic examination alone, whether the epitheliform cells found in "cancer juice" were "cancer cells" or not. It is the tissue elements, taken together, of which a tumor is composed ; their amount, proportion and arrangement which deter-

---

* Read at the Semi-Annual Meeting of the Homœopathic Medical Society, State of New York, September 21st, 1887.

mine its classification, and not the presence of any one particular form of cell. What I wish to make clear is, that although the true nature of a tumor is always better known *after* a microscopic examination, it would be folly to assert that its nature and proper classification could *always* be determined by such an examination alone and unaided. It is always wise—and in some cases absolutely essential—that the clinical history be known, e. g., in the case of simple granulation tissue and round celled or mixed sarcomas; without the clinical history it would many times be impossible to distinguish them, as both are made up of young connective tissue cells, embryonic blood vessels, and so on.

The Carcinomata, or epithelial tumors, may be defined as new formations, made up of cells of epithelial type, with little or no intercellular substance, situated, in irregular masses, in the alveoli of a connective tissue stroma, which last has well developed blood-vessels running through and supported by it. If it be further understood that these elements are in excess of the normal amount found in the tissue; are of high vegetative power and great malignancy, we will have a sufficiently clear conception of their nature for our purpose.

There are four varieties of Carcinomata, viz. : Scirrhus, Encephaloid, Colloid and Epithelioma. I have adopted this classification rather than that given by Ziegler, which has, in addition to the above, Simple carcinoma, Carcinoma myxomatodes, Cylindroma C., Giant-celled (or mycloid) and Melano-carcinoma, as these latter seem to be mere modifications of one or other of the former, depending on rapidity of growth or degenerative changes rather than any real difference in structure, and also because a multiplication of names only leads to confusion. The above objection might be urged against making a separate variety of colloid, and with some show of reason; but as all authorities class it as a separate variety, and as it is so often found as a distinct tumor, I have thought best to speak of it separately.

The first three—scirrhus, encephaloid and colloid—are alike in their general characteristics, their differences being in the proportion which the stroma and cell elements bear to each other; in the character of the epithelioid cells, and also in the condition of the stroma.

Take a section from the advancing edge of a scirrhus cancer and the following may be noted : The infiltration of the adjacent tissues with small, round cells; indifferent tissue; then the characteristic stroma, surrounding the alveoli, which in this part of the tumor contains well-marked connective tissue fibres and nuclei; and lastly, the cells filling the alveoli, which, it will be noticed, are of distinct epithelioid form, and also that some of them have more than one nucleus. Now examine a section from the older part of the tumor, near its centre, and it is at once noticed that there is a large increase in the amount of the stroma, and that the alveoli are smaller and fewer in number. Closer inspection will show that the stroma is not only greater in amount, but has altered in character, having become more fibrous, and also that the epitheliform cells in the alveoli have not only decreased in number, but are in various stages of fatty degeneration.

Let me refer you to photos *I.*, *II.* and *III.*, which accompany this paper, as illustrative of the foregoing.

Encephalọid, or Medullary cancer, differs from scirrhus in the alveoli being much larger and more crowded with cells, and in the stroma being more delicate and more of the connective tissue type, less fibrous. (Photos. *IV.* and *V.*) Under a higher power (Photo. *VI.*) it will be seen that not only is the stroma very delicate and cellular, but that the cells filling the alveoli have lost somewhat their epithelioid character, are smaller, and that there are more free nuclei, all of which points to a more rapid growth.

Colloid cancer is really one of the last mentioned forms in which the cells have shown a tendency to colloid by mucoid degeneration. The points to be noted are the large size of the alveoli and the thinness of their walls ; also that the cells have either undergone or are undergoing colloid degeneration. I am sorry that I cannot show photomicrographs of this variety, as I am not in possession of a slide of colloid from which to get the negatives.

The epitheliomata form a distinct group of cancerous tumors, of which there are two varieties: squamous, and cylindrical, or columnar.

Squamous epithelioma is found growing from the skin and mucous surfaces covered with squamous epithelium, and may be said to be characterized by branching finger-like processes of epithelium, pushing down, between the papillæ, into the subjacent connective tissue; by the so-called cell nests, which appear in the section as round or ovoid bodies, made up of concentric layers of flattened epithelium, the more dense portions of which stain yellow when picrocarmine is the stain used ; and lastly, by the great increase of squamous epithelium at the free margin of the tumor. (Photos. *VII.*, *VIII.*, *IX.*)

At the advancing margin of squamous epithelioma is seen the same infiltration of the adjacent tissues with round cells, as was spoken of under scirrhus. This is well shown in Photos. *X.* and *XI.*

Cylindrical, Columnar or Glandular epithelioma has its origin in the columnar epithelium of glands ; most frequently, perhaps, in those of the intestine, but also in the uterine glands, in the liver, mammæ, etc. If the squamous variety may be said to advance by finger-like processes or columns of epithelium, so in the columnar celled the same mode of growth may be assumed, except that in the latter case the columns are hollow and lined by cubical or columnar epithelium. These in the section (see Photos. *XII.* and *XIII.*) appear as spaces in the connective tissue stroma lined with a single row of columnar cells. Ziegler seems to convey the idea that this lumen. is *usually* filled with epitheliform cells, and although I have only once or twice seen such a specimen, it would seem probable that this is the true appearance, as the cells might easily be washed out in the manipulations of staining, mounting, etc., and so give the section the appearance spoken of above.

HYPERTROPHY OF THE PROSTATE.

Translated from *Berlin. Klin. Wochenschrift.*, 18, 1887. With Original Remarks.

By SAM'L LILIENTHAL, M.D.,

San Francisco, Cal.

IN considering hypertrophy of the prostate and its consequences, Dr. Guyon, "Annales des maladies des organs genito-urinaires," differentiates between clinical relations of this disease and other affections of the "urogenital apparatus." Mechanical disturbances, preventing the flow of urine, fail to explain it entirely. In comparing, *e. g.*, the appearance of cystitis in patients suffering from strictures with that of hypertrophy of the prostate, we meet many weighty differences. The former sets in at a later period and happens more rarely; the latter is more often observed and shows this pathognomonic peculiarity, the prevalence of a desire to urinate during the night, whereas in day-time the patient is very little disturbed by it.

Aetiology points decidedly to the influence of advancing age, while other causes, as excesses in venery, old gonorrhœas, etc., are only of secondary importance, and we have to thank Launois for his anatomico-histological studies in relation to this gland *intra vitam.* He shows that in old age specific changes take place in the whole genito-urinary tract, even up to the kidneys, which are of a sclerotic nature. Being atheromatous or arterio-sclerotic, they attack also the connective tissue of the mucous membranes and of the glands, and lead in the kidneys to the well known, mostly slight senile shrinking—

in the bladder to the "vessie à colonnes," in the prostate to neoplastic fibrous connective tissue, to hypertrophy. With these sclerotic processes there is at the same time a retarded circulation in these organs, which causes malnutrition and a venous stasis. Hence the senile bladder must be a debilitated organ. Though it appears hypertrophic like that of a younger person suffering from stricture, it is in fact only a pseudo-hypertrophy; the muscular wall is diminished at the expense of the connective tissue, it fails to exert a strong pressure and the frequently observed diverticles follow, hence tendency to ectasy and the common insufficiency. When increased action is demanded of such a bladder, a mechanical cause, the enlarged prostate inhibiting the flow of urine, is added to the physiological cause and we have a grave case before us.

At first incomplete, finally complete retention sets in, leading to vesical ectasy with dribbling of urine, but without any voluntary discharge of urine. A cystitis is not a necessary complication, but may set in at any time, either from catching cold, from the use of alcoholic drinks, or what is the most frequent cause, in consequence of catheterism. The catheter is far too often accused as the bearer of septic germs; we blame far more the sudden diminution of pressure in an over-filled bladder, producing hæmaturia and vesical catarrh.

The (natural, not treated) hypertrophy of the prostate shows three stages. At first we deal only with a state of irritable weakness with congestion, where rectal palpation reveals only a slight enlargement of the gland, and urination is free. During the second stage we meet insufficiency; in the last one, ectasy.

In relation to treatment we must consider three things : the subjective symptoms, the local status of the prostate, and the state of the bladder. In relation to the first we must remember the constant nocturnal desire to empty the bladder ; during the second stage the trouble is diurnal as well as nocturnal; during the third, complete retention with detention, all local disturbances are often absent and we consider more the general state of the patient; who, though he felt well for a long time, still shows traces of malnutrition, complains often of thirst, has a dry tongue, gastric disturbances, in fact shows the whole picture of chronic urinary resorption, which too often leads to a fatal end.

The prostate often shows nothing which with certainty would indicate the stage of the disease; it grows in proportion to the progress of the disease, but the growth may take place just as well towards the rectum as towards the urethra and bladder. For the former we use anal palpation, for the latter the introduction of an elastic bougie à boule, which shows the probable elongation of the pars prostatica urethræ, any deviation, etc. Of most importance is the study of the state of the bladder. Here Guyon teaches us a valuable rule, that we ought to try to find out the state of the bladder, whether it is fully emptied or not, without the introduction of the catheter; bimanual palpation in the dorsal position and with the aid of deep respiratory movements of the patient ought to clear up the case satisfactorily. In more advanced cases the suprapubic protrusion of the full bladder is conclusive evidence *per se.*

It is mere nonsense to introduce a catheter during the first stage where the bladder is fully emptied; more still, it is dangerous, for it may lead to severe cystic troubles. Not in every case of urinary disease is the catheter our chief aid, even with all antiseptic precautionary measures. Here dietetic-hygienic treatment suffices, a light and easily digested diet, careful warmth, regular diet, perhaps off and on some quieting balsamic, as ol. santali, ol. terebinthinæ, tea of triticum repens, etc. In this stage we never advise medicinal springs, as they irritate and may produce a sudden retention.

More active measures are indicated when the bladder becomes insufficient. Here the essential indication is a thorough emptying, followed by mild washing out of the bladder. Where the muscular wall still possesses some strength, we may thus bring back again the disease to its first stage; but even where no voluntary discharge takes place any more, we may thus prevent its advance into the third stage. Catheterization, several times a day, is necessary, and we must teach to the patient the use of the catheter, which must be a soft one with the curvature of Merciér.

Our hope increases when we deal with a case of ectasy of the bladder. It seems so natural that we ought rapidly to empty the bladder, but we are afraid of it. It may happen that such a patient feels good enough, though standing at the brink of the grave; but from the moment the bladder is emptied, hæmaturia and cystitis follow, with shaking chills, fever and sudden collapse. We harmed the patient where we intended to benefit him. In all cases of uræmic intoxication, great caution is necessary, and here the rule holds good, never to empty the total contents of the bladder: a few hundred grammes suffice at first, and they must be discharged through a catheter of narrow calibre, and only after a few days' repeated trials the bladder may be emptied thoroughly. A cure is here impossible, and the patient has to use the catheter during his remaining days.

For hypertrophy of the prostate, I find in the second edition of my therapeutics mentioned: *Aloes, baryta carb., cann. sat., merc., nitr. ac., puls.*, *sulf.*, *thuja*, and in a foot-note : *Aurum mur.* and *triticum repens;* and under involuntary urination, drop by drop : *Aloes, arn., bell., dig., mur. ac., petr., puls., sep., staph.*

Aloes: Frequent urging to urinate, *worse at night;* incontinence of urine (in an old man with enlarged prostate, with diarrhœa and the usual urinary symptoms); sensation as if a plug were wedged between symphysis and coccyx, pressing downwards ; stools leaving him with a feeling of extreme weakness and prostration.

Baryta carb. Irritation of the bladder, greatest at night when in bed; passes much urine at night; after urination, renewed straining with dribbling of urine; almost complete incontinence of urine and fæces.

Benzoic acid. Enlarged prostate ; sensibility of bladder with muco-purulent discharge; *dysuria senilis;* urine dark, the urinous odor highly intensified ; inability to hold the water even when urine is normal ; gout.

Causticum. Must urinate every few minutes at night with extremely painful pressing and urging ; involuntary micturition at night when asleep, in walking, when coughing, sneezing; symptoms of paralysis of the bladder from prolonged retention of urine, and over-distension of the bladder ; cannot retain urine and could not feel urine passing through urethra.

Conium. *Dysuria senilis;* enlargement of prostate causes intermittent urination in old people, the urine flows and stops ; frequent micturition at night.

Lycopodium. Pressing on perineum and anus, during and after micturition; urging to urinate, must wait a long time before it passes ; incontinence of urine.

Natrum sulph. Enlarged prostate ; pus and mucus in urine; pinching around navel when sitting, with urging to urinate, pain going into the groin (Schüssler's remedy for sycosis, gout, sandy deposits in urine, gravel).

Oleum sandal. Sensation of pain and uneasiness, deep in perineum; desire to change position to get relief; stream small and passed with hesitation; sensation of a ball pressing against the urethra; pain less when walking, worse when standing some time; heaviness in feet in the morning when first rising from bed; sexual powers weak, erections feeble; urine red and scanty (Farrington).

Petroleum. Constant dribbling of urine; frequent micturition, with scanty, brown, fetid urine; involuntary micturition at night in bed ; chronic inflammation of the prostatic portion of the urethra; passes only a little urine at a time.

Pulsatilla. Prostatic troubles of elderly men; urging and frequent desire to urinate, worse when lying, especially on back; frequent, almost ineffectual urging to urinate, with cutting pains; cannot
retain urine; it is passed in drops, sitting or walking; involuntary
when coughing, passing wind, or during sleep; sediment reddish,
bloody or mucous; jelly-like, sticking to vessel.

Secale corn. Unsuccessful urging to urinate; ischuria paralytica,
retention of urine, enuresis in old age, urine pale, watery, bloody in
old people, paralysis of the rectum; bleeding from the bowels.

Selenium. Enlarged prostate of old people; involuntary urination
when walking, drips after stool or micturition, urine dark, scanty,
red in the evening.

Staphisagria. Frequent urging, with scanty discharge of a thin
stream of red-looking urine; urging as if the bladder was not emptied;
discharge of dark urine by drops; pain extending from the anus along
urethra, coming on after walking or riding.

Sulphur iod. Pain in prostate with insufficient urination; sensation
of torpor in the bladder; incontinence of urine; mucous deposits in the
urine.

Thuja. Rectal tenesmus; stitches from rectum to bladder; bladder
feels paralyzed, has no power to expel urine; involuntary urination at
night and when coughing; stream interrupted several times before
bladder is entirely emptied; frequent desire to urinate; worse when
lying down; deep perineal pains with retention of urine.

Triticum repens. Retention of urine in very old people from enlarged prostate, with a great deal of trouble when urinating (T. F.
Allen).

In the late journals of the old school we read a great deal of the
curability of phthisis pulmonalis, as long as there is something left on
which to work, and great stress is justly laid on diet and hygiene.
We may say the same of hypertrophy of the prostate, and though
senility is a drawback, still our materia medica is so rich, that he who
seeks will find, and even paralysis need not frighten us from giving up
the case, and even where a cure is impossible, a wonderful amelioration
may be achieved and the few declining years of life rendered more
bearable. Let us never forget the good advice of Dr. Guyon that during the first stage the use of the catheter is contraindicated and even
dangerous, and that during the second stage this adjuvant is a
necessity; and we would like to hear from our purists whether in that
second stage they can do without it. True, it is only a mechanical
measure and therefore perhaps allowable, but just in the use of the
catheter, antisepsis is a *sine qua non* and does the cleansing of the

instruments with carbolic acid, permanganate of potassium or any other antiseptic interfere with the action of the remedy? I do not believe it, and especially not when the remedy was given in a high potency. I am not too old to learn, and beg, therefore, for instruction.

INDICATIONS FOR SOME OF THE METALS IN NEURALGIA.

By E. A. FARRINGTON, M.D.,

Philadelphia, Pa.

Aurum is useful in neuralgia after abuse of mercury. The pains are of a stinging and tearing character, and are almost always associated with anxious and hasty movements. The circulation is certain to be involved, and you have that anxiety and dread and haste that belong to heart affections.

In *metallic silver*, the pains gradually increase and suddenly cease. They occur usually in very nervous people who are subject to vertigo. The neuralgia is especially apt to occur in the joints.

The pains of *nitrate of silver* have this character: They gradually increase until they reach their acme, and drive the patients almost mad. Then they radiate in all directions.

Platina has for its characteristic gradually increasing and gradually decreasing pains. We will see presently that *stannum* also has gradually increasing and gradually decreasing pains. The distinction between the two remedies lies in the concomitant symptoms. With *platina*, these pains are followed by numbness or cramp in the affected part. With *stannum*, there is more pure nervousness, the muscles jerk, and the patient is low-spirited and sad.

Plumbum has neuralgic pains, and they are relieved by hard, firm pressure, and they are associated with emaciation of the affected part. You will find it indicated in neuralgia of the abdomen, with pains that almost drive the patient crazy. If these are relieved by pressure, *plumbum* is usually the remedy, whether there is retraction of the abdomen or not.

Cuprum metallicum is indicated in suddenly appearing pains in the involuntary muscles, and usually associated with a great deal of congestion and cramps.

The *arsenite of copper* is a very superior remedy in neuralgia of the abdominal viscera. I do not mean neuralgia of the abdominal walls, but of the viscera themselves. The pains are periodical in their recurrence.

The *ferrum* pains are usually relieved from slow motion: in fact, they compel the patient to get up and move about for relief. They are worse at night and are usually accompanied by false plethora.

Manganum is chemically similar to *ferrum*, and suits similar cases. Like the latter remedy, it produces chlorosis and anæmia. But this chlorosis and anæmia are not so erethistic as in *ferrum*. There is not so much ebullition of blood. In addition, *manganese* seems to produce a sort of periostitis, or if not periostitis, periosteal pains which are worse at night and worse from touch.

Kobalt acts upon the spine and its nerves, particularly upon the lumbar spine, causing intense back-ache, which is worse sitting than it is walking. Such back-ache usually follows sexual excesses and is associated with weakness of the legs. The legs tremble and the knees give out.

Niccolum I do not know much about. It promises very well, however. It is particularly indicated in tearing pains in the head, worse in the left eye and recurring every two weeks. This is a periodical remedy. It has hoarseness occurring every spring. It also has a cough which, I would like to have you remember, is a dry, teazing cough compelling the patient to sit up, it jars the head so.

Mercurius is useful for neuralgia of the face, extremities and back, especially when the pains are rendered intolerable by the warmth of the bed and are worse at night. It is especially indicated in facial neuralgia, starting from decayed teeth.

ORIGINAL ARTICLES IN SURGERY.

SURGICAL DISEASES OF WOMEN.　CLINICAL REFLECTIONS.

By W. J. HUNTER EMORY, M.D., M.C.P.S.,

Toronto, Ontario.

AT a time like the present, when medical literature almost everywhere is surfeited with dissertations and discussions upon the various diseases peculiar to women, which require, or at least receive, the interference of the surgical art, one hesitates to add anything to its already replete pages. I shall not, therefore, take up any of the limited time of this institute in discussing the merits or demerits of any of the popular operations or methods in gynæcology of the day, but proceed at once to state as clearly and concisely as I may be able, some of my own experiences of the past year.

CASE I.—Mrs. G., æt. 26, married eight years, no children, medium height, well developed and robust looking. Ever since puberty a sufferer from dysmenorrhœa, with ever growing severity. Has been treated both locally and constitutionally, by various prominent physicians in Montreal, Ottawa, Toronto and the West without any benefit, but rather as the woman of old "had suffered many things of many physicians," and was none the better, but rather the worse. About a year ago determined that she would never again consult a physician, but live and die a sufferer, which resolution she practically carried out, until knowing of the case which I shall present next (being an intimate acquaintance) she made up her mind to try once more, when I obtained the following history :

The menses are regular as to time but very scanty, consisting of dark brownish clots, and fleshy pieces resembling liver, no red fluid blood, and preceded for from twelve to twenty-four hours by labor-like pains, increasing in severity until they become so excruciating that, the husband informs me, she becomes beside herself at times, sometimes becoming perfectly rigid throughout the whole muscular system, the clots before described being forced away by these uterine contractions and the pains subside, and this has been the history of the catamenial periods for the past ten years, with gradually increasing intensity; also suffering from the ordinary symptoms of uterine displacement, bearing down pain in back and thigh on standing, frequent desire with pain in passing water, obstinate constipation, loss of appetite, and for the past year has been gradually losing flesh, having lost forty pounds within the year, and fears she is going into consumption. Has never been pregnant, very feverish in bed evenings, feet and hands burn. Rises in the morning feeling more wearied than when she went to bed, growing brighter towards evening, frequent rush of blood to the head with vertigo, and suffers much from headache, also a constant heavy leucorrhœa.

Sulphur in the 2 c. attenuation, repeated at long intervals, relieved the constipation, headaches, vertigo, sleeplessness, loss of appetite, etc., etc. But nothing availed for the dysmenorrhœa or direct symptoms of uterine displacement. An examination revealed the womb in a condition of acute ante-flexion in a greater degree than I had ever found it before, or, indeed, even heard or read of.

The face of the cervix was looking towards the supra-pubic region, and the body of the uterus so bent that its fundus almost touched the anterior lip of the cervix. By raising the fundus slightly, the finger could pass between it and the cervix, and follow the continuity of surface down over the anterior surface of the body to the cervix; this no doubt explained the dysmenorrhœa; the blood collecting in and distending the uterine cavity, until by its labor-like contractions it expelled the clots thus formed. How to correct the flexion was the conundrum, for all attempts to introduce any kind of a sound whatever proved futile. Failing in all ordinary methods to correct the displacement, three days before the menses the woman was placed on a suitable table, and fully anæsthetized by means of the "London mixture," the cervix exposed by means of the "Hunter speculum," was secured by means of a loop of stout silk cord through either lip, the same as when operating for lacerations, a strong Nott's dilator was inserted into the os as far as it would go (about half an inch), and by means of the thumb screw the blades were separated half an inch; closing the blades again, I was enabled to introduce the instrument a quarter of an inch further, and so on by repeating this procedure the point of the dilator at last reached the top of the uterine cavity, and of course, straightened out the flexion. A strong steel male catheter with the usual curve was then introduced, and by turning the reverse way to that employed for replacing a retroverted uterus, the uterus was thrown into a state of retroflexion. The woman was then placed comfortably in bed, and I was about taking my departure when the nurse rushed out for me. Returning, I found the patient lying on her right side with arms extended at right angles to the body, apparently in an unconscious condition. I took hold of her arm to turn her over so that I could see her face, when I found her whole body quite rigid; not a joint could be bent, even the muscles of respiration were rigid and respiration had ceased. I immediately pressed with force my fist upwards against the diaphragm, at the same time holding a bottle of liquor am. fort. to the nostrils. A gasp ensued, and the inhalation of the ammonia induced a second, when the respiratiou became regular, and the rigidity gradually passed away. The husband, who happened to be in the room, now informed me that it was a common thing for her to have such a spell just before each menstrual period. Perfect quiet was now maintained, and in three days the monthly flow came on without any pain. The patient was kept pretty quiet in bed for two weeks, lying mostly on her back, when she was allowed to gradually resume her usual activities. Improvement in general health began at once upon the administration of lachesis, which covered the totality of her symptoms well, and in four weeks she became unwell while going about her housework, the first indication of the menses being a flow of bright red fluid blood, unaccompanied by the least sign of pain, continuing for four days and disappearing without any suffering whatever. The patient being so overjoyed at what had never occurred before in her life, that she sent her husband off at once to carry the glad intelligence to me.

CASE II.—Mrs S., widow, æt. 37, mother of five children, the youngest seven years of age. First consulted me on August 27th, 1885, having previously been treated by various old school physicians, for indigestion, ulceration of stomach, ulceration of uterus, chronic metritis, chronic congestion, neuralgia and enlargement of left ovary, etc., etc.

Is a woman of more than ordinary physical development and endurance, as previous acquaintance years ago had proved to me. Naturally of a lively, sanguine, cheerful disposition, and the very opposite to anything like hysteria or hypo in any form.

Her husband was an officer in the British army in India, where she lived for years. Has been very gradually breaking down in health ever since her last confinement, and now for some months has been rapidly growing worse. Suffering mostly as follows: When on her feet much bearing down pain, the dragging being felt from umbilicus and lumbar region towards vulva, as though all the internal organs would escape. Frequently is obliged to stand with her limbs crossed on account of this distress.

Sharp lancinating pain through left ovarian region, sense of fullness and soreness in lower part of abdomen; thinks she has a tumor.

An all-gone feeling in pit of stomach; is sure there is some living animal there; can feel it crawling around, which produces the most deathly sickness. Her complexion has changed from that of a florid brunette to almost that of a mullato. Has been told that she has jaundice. But the most distressing of all her symptoms are those of the mental sphere, there being profound melancholia, bordering on suicidal tendency.

Dares not go near a wharf or bridge for fear of being compelled to take her life by jumping off. Has been frequently obliged to leave the church on account of uncontrollable impulse to jump over the gallery. Was afraid to be alone with her children on account of an insane desire to take their lives. Very much feared that she would lose her reason. Said she was perfectly sure that she would become insane if she did not get relief very soon. Palpation revealed exquisite tenderness to pressure over the whole left side and lower part of the abdomen.

Believing that some uterine lesion lay at the bottom of all her trouble, I advised an early examination. But patient was averse to this and wished me to try internal remedies for a time at least. The above symptoms were elicited in my office, and as I wished to review the case carefully before prescribing, I sent her away with the request that she should call again in two or three days. In the mean time she became much worse, all the above symptoms becoming aggravated, and new ones being added, and I was summoned to her bedside.

She now began to suffer intensely from paroxysms of pain beginning in either hyphchondrium and extending across lower borders of ribs, epigastrium and ensiforn cartilage to the opposite side. These paroxysms would occur from six to eight times in twenty-four hours, gradually reaching a climax in about three-quarters of an hour, when the whole muscular system would become tetanized and remain so for about an hour, with complete loss of consciousness, when relaxation would gradually take place and consciousness return, leaving the patient in a state of extreme prostration. During these paroxysms the whole surface of the body would become cold and clammy and of a dark cyanotic color.

From this time on Dr. E. T. Adams saw her almost every day either in conjunction with myself or each seeing her independently.

Hallucinations now appeared to her in the shape of seeing most horrible accidents happening. These occurred during conscious moments whenever she would close her eyes, and sometimes with the eyes wide open.

She saw regiments of headless horses with headless riders gal-
loping over groups of little children. Scores of bodiless arms contending with each other in the room. At one time saw herself
dead and laid out in her coffin, and she seemed to be standing by
her dead self and sympathizing with herself, saying, "Poor
thing; her sufferings are over at last, and I am glad you are gone."

At another time she saw herself dead, and I, with other physicians, holding a post-mortem examination, and she was very glad
we were doing so, as it might prove a benefit to some other sufferer.

These and many other sights, equally as horrible and revolting,
would haunt her as soon as she would close her eyes and try to
sleep.

There was also a violent pulsation, easily seen heaving up the
bed-clothing when she would lie on her back, extending over the
central portion of the abdomen, arising, I believe, from a relaxed
abdominal aorta.

The case was now becoming desperate; carefully selected remedies seemed only to exert a palliative effect, and the patient was
rapidly growing weaker. No food could be retained on the
stomach.

The patient seemed too weak and nervous to think of making
any examination of the uterus, so I determined to take advantage
of the unconscious tetanic condition to make a digital examination,
which revealed the uterus enlarged to about three times its natural
size, the cervix torn transversely on both sides up to the vaginal
juncture, and the torn surfaces studded with soft papillary excrescences the size of a small pea, which bled easily. In my own mind
I at once exclaimed, "*Eureka!*" The next morning I explained to
the patient her condition and my conviction that an operation
afforded the only hope of recovery, as well as the danger of an
operation in her present condition. By the next morning her mind
was made up to undergo the operation.

But the prospects of success seemed anything but promising in
her present condition, while the prospect of bettering it seemed even
less encouraging, as, in spite of our best efforts, she was daily
becoming weaker. So as a *dernier* resort an immediate operation
was resolved upon, and accordingly, on the 25th of September,
assisted by Drs. Howitt, Adams and G. B. Foster, the operation for
lacerated cervix was performed in the usual way, seven sutures
being required to close up the rent after the purplish suspicious
looking granulations and cicatricial tissue had all been carefully
dissected away.

The patient stood the anæsthetic well, as carefully and judiciously
administered by Dr. W. H. Howitt, and made a fair reaction after
some six or eight hours of almost unremitting use of strongest
liquor ammonia and amyl nitrate, in alternate inhalations. On the
twelfth day the silver sutures were removed and the wound found
to be perfectly healed; the remaining horse-hair sutures were allowed
to remain in until the patient was able to come to my office, where
they were removed. The contour of the cervix was entirely

restored and the sound now gave a measurement of two and three-quarter inches as against four and one-half inches before the operation. From the day of the operation forward the paroxysms of pain came on with less severity and at longer intervals for about a week, when they took their final departure, to the great satisfaction of both physician and patient. She now responded nicely to appropriate remedies, which before seemed to give no satisfactory account of themselves, and inside of four weeks was going about entirely free from pain, in good spirits, her complexion again cleared up, and presenting a youthful glow which made her look, as she said she felt, ten years younger.

The remedies which proved most beneficial in her case were, lycopodium, calc. carb., and thuja, and without these potent agents, I think she would have been in a very similar condition after the operation to that of a ship at sea full of water, after the leak had been stopped up, but without machinery to pump her out. In six weeks she was able to resume her usual occupation, that of professional nurse, which she had been obliged to entirely abandon for eighteen months, and to-day is as healthy a woman as one could find.

The above case seems to establish pretty clearly the following three facts : First—that this lesion is capable of, and did in this case, produce a disturbance of the general nervous system of a grave character.

Second—the pressure of such a lesion as a constantly operating cause, may effectually prevent the properly chosen homœopathic remedy from exerting its legitimate benificent influence, as is evidenced by the fact that subsequently the patient responded most gratifyingly to remedies which previously had given no satisfactory account of themselves, though equally well indicated and prescribed in the same form.

That this operation may be undertaken with comparative safety, when the patient is in a very precarious condition, and was followed by the most salutary effects.

The following is an epitome of the results which have followed this operation, in fifteen cases in which I have performed it in the past two years. In every case the operation has been successful from an anatomical standpoint, restoring completely the contour of the cervix and os externum, as well as restoring the cervical canal to its normal condition. Prominent among the abnormal conditions which have disappeared after the operation are—subinvolution, retroversion, prolapsus, metritis, endo-metritis, and cervicitis, numerous cauliflower excrescences, which were, of course, removed during the operation, chronic cystitis, and in three cases, beginning cancerous development. While prominent among the distressing symptoms

which have been dissipated are—menorrhagia, metrorrhagia, dysmenorrhœa, leucorrhœa, constipation, dysuria, insomnia, extreme
nervousness in many forms, sterility, mental aberration, extremely
painful coition, obstinate neuralgias, marked symptoms of ulcer of
stomach, melancholia, and last, but not the least appreciated by the
husband, excessive irritability and peevishness. In several cases, as
in the one cited, the operation has restored confirmed invalids to
health and strength of both body and mind, enabling them to resume
all former activities, while in many cases it has made life enjoyable,
whereas the multitudinous aches and pains and distressing nervous
troubles, entailed by the lesion, had made life almost intolerable, both
for the patient and those about her.

HYDATIDS IN THE CAVITY AND SUBSTANCE OF THE HEART.—Dr. Wm.
Rushton Parker writes to the *Brit. Med. Jour.* for September 3d, describing the case of a boy five years old, who died suddenly within a few
moments of playing about in almost perfect health. Twice in the last few
weeks of his life he had complained of a slight pain about the heart, but
no notice was taken of it. On the day of his death he made a similar
complaint, and his father imagined he felt the child's heart beating a good
deal [quicker, if not more vigorously, than it should do. However, he
played with his ball and helped his mother at the pump, and then sat playing on the sofa, when he suddenly screamed, turned on one side, and in a
few moments was dead. "On opening the pericardium," says the doctor,
"the front wall of the right ventricle near the base was found bulged out
by an hydatid, giving the appearance of another auricle. An incision
was made into this, passing first through the ventricular wall, then
through a tough, adventitious sac about one-fifth of an inch thick, firmly
adherent to the muscular substance, and rough inside, like pericarditic.
lymph; the delicate mother cyst within this contained fresh blood-clot and
eight or more daughter cysts (mostly pyriform or ovoid in shape, and varying
in size from small currants to small beans), and had evidently attained a
diameter of nearly one inch and a half before rupturing into the right ventricle. About the rupture the endocardium seemed rough and fibrinous."
"On raising the heart and detaching it by cutting through the large vessels,
there flopped out of the left auricle a simple hydatid cyst, measuring an
inch and a half in diameter, which must have occupied almost the entire
space of the auricle."

EDITORIAL DEPARTMENT.

EDITORS.

GEORGE M. DILLOW, M.D.,	Editor-in-Chief, Editorial and Book Reviews
CLARENCE E. BEEBE, M.D.,	Original Papers in Medicine.
SIDNEY F. WILCOX, M.D.,	Original Papers in Surgery.
MALCOLM LEAL, M.D.,	Progress of Medicine.
EUGENE H. PORTER, .D.,	Comments and News.
HENRY M. DEARBORN M.D.,	Correspondence.
FRED S. FULTON, M.D.,	Reports of Societies and Hospitals.

A. B. NORTON, M.D., ... Business Manager.

The Editors individually assume full responsibility for and are to be credited with all connected with the collection and presentation of matter in their respective departments, but are not responsible for the opinions of contributors.

It is understood that manuscripts sent for consideration have not been previously published, and that after notice of acceptance has been given, will not appear elsewhere except in abstract and with credit to THE NORTH AMERICAN. All rejected manuscripts will be returned to writers. No anonymous or discourteous communications will be printed.

Contributors are respectfully requested to send manuscripts and communicate respecting them directly with the Editors, according to subject, as follows: *Concerning Medicine, 81 West 57th Street; concerning Surgery, 256 West 57th Street; concerning Societies and Hospitals, 111 East 70th Street; concerning News, Personals and Original Miscellany, 161 West 71st Street; concerning Correspondence, 152 West 57th Street.*

Communications to the Editor-in-Chief, *Exchanges* and *New Books* for notice should be addressed to *102 West 43d Street.*

A NEW SCHOOL OF ANTI-PRO-SECTARIANISM.

OUR antisectarian contemporary whose Editors regardlessly hold fast to prosectarian trusts, with one foot based on the "regular" school and the other on the homœopathic school, has been attempting to bud out a new leg to plant on a new school gotten up to editorial order. This proceeding is not to be wondered at, for its "regular" and homœopathic pedal extremities have been getting very uncomfortable. Last June its right leg received a paralyzing stroke from the American Institute of Homœopathy ; its left leg is frozen in a mixture of ice and salt that has lost its savor ; and in September, the New York State Homœopathic Medical Society, with a practical denial of sympathy, swept away its last pretense of any following whereon to rest its hopelessly disabled homœopathic underpinning. So one editor who will be recognized by his propensity for picking up private gossip to deck forth his public table, calls for a new code of ethics to punish those who express an opinion concerning "traitors in the camp ;" and the other editor labors to prove that the old name, homœopathic, should vanish in a grand transformation scene, where one school with one name would melt into the same school with another name, which it enjoys interchangeably already. Thus there would be a new footing for that third leg to stand upon. But we apprehend that that third leg is budding forth in vain, growing as it appears to us horizontally outwards, at right angles from the congealed inferior extremity. Its support being in and upon air alone, its weight, so far from the centre of gravity, may topple our neighbor over into the freezing mixture before suggested.

Putting aside anticipation, there is the more serious consideration of the question of amputation of our neighbor's paralyzed right member. It is to be noted that the editor, in his October effusion, identifies himself with, and affects to voice, the great body of homœopathic practitioners whom he insinuatingly charges with insincerity and dishonest professions. Whether they will submit to be so charged and represented is to them a question demanding sober attention. The American Institute of Homœopathy has officially and unanimously disowned our contemporary. Should homœopathic practitioners indvidually get from under our neighbor's rostrum, and cease to give it the standing place which subscriptions and contributions imply? Ought a journal which so assails them, to be severely left to meditate upon its own shortcomings? Ought editors, who ignore the question of their own frankness, sincerity and honesty, as related to the honors and trusts which they have acquired and hold by former and present association with homœopathy, to be encouraged to infer that they will continue to receive the support of the men, whose honesty of motive they at the same time impugn? The answer to these questions we leave to individual readers, who can form their own opinions of what constitutes tacit confession and approval.

In the meantime the latest juggle of our name-objecting, name-substituting, anti-pro-sectarian contemporary affords opportunity for exposing in clear contrast by paraphrase, the positions maintained by homœopathy, and that maintained by its enemies, whether open or delusively friendly. We extract from our neighbor's October editorial, placing in a parallel column the views in controversion and denial, not expressed as we should choose for full and accurate presentation, but following another's language for the purpose of bringing out more definitely points of difference:

" What the Old School
*and what they do, their threats
their promises* are of but littl
portance to us as individu:
societies, but it is of the ut
importance to us that we
stand squarely and honestl̩
fore the public with no other
fessions for our societies, or
selves individually, but si̩
the truth."

" We ask Dr. Paine, in all si̩
ity and earnestness, if the
homœopathic represents the
standing of our societies o:
individual practice of nine-t̩
of their members, and if it
not are we justified simply b̩
law of right and honesty, w
should form the basis of our
fessional action, in clinging
instead of that of *physician* w
covers the whole field and w
needs no explanation ?"

" A similar amalgamation
Old and New School Congṛ
tionalism) is going on in
medical world, with this e̩
tion, the old is absorbing the ̩
not only culling largely fro̩
medical literature, but intro
ing its distinctive views in
therapeutics which is rapidl̩
coming more scientific."

" The action of drugs
studied from the homœop̩
standpoint, and the informa
thus obtained, and from exi̩
homœopathic literature, utilize
a certain extent in the treat̩
of disease."

"As a school we must either absorb or be absorbed. In practice we are catholic; in name sectarian. In practice and in our studies, as was shown by the recent papers and discussions, we recognize no exclusive dogma in medicine, but are thoroughly catholic."

As a school we must revolutionize or be revolutionized. In practice we are not indiscriminately miscellaneous; in name, not sectarian but scientifically designated. In practice and in our studies, as was shown by the recent papers and discussions, we recognize a leading principle in drug therapeutics excluding no principle outside its sphere, and are thoroughly comprehensive in our study of the various sciences of medicine.

"With our societies and colleges recognized as New School organizations, with a bureau for the particular investigation of homœopathy or any other speciality, we should stand before the public without need of further explanations than those that could be made with the utmost frankness."

With our societies and colleges remaining as homœopathic organizations, with homœopathic investigation assigned to every bureau and speciality pertaining to the treatment of disease, we will stand before the public without need of further explanations, which have thus far been made with the utmost frankness.

"Do you not think, Dr. Paine, if we take this position standing before the world not as bound to the wheels of a single dogma, but with a name which honestly and frankly represents us as precisely what we are, we should absorb instead of being absorbed?"

Do you not think, homœopathic physicians, if we maintain our position, standing before the world dominantly devoted to the further progress of the single principle which has blessed medicine with such healing power, and which has far greater benefits in store if we but continue faithful to our trust, with the name which expresses that ruling purpose avowed honestly and frankly, not lurking spuriously under a new name which expresses nothing and still carries offensiveness to the old school, we shall go on growing instead of being absorbed?

Returning from the parallel columns, we would call attention to an extract from the address recently delivered before the British Homœopathic Congress by the President, Arthur C. Clifton, M. D. It will be seen that his statement of the position of the opponents of homœopathy essentially defines the position of our contemporary, which declares that homœopathy is "sectarianism," that "sectarianism" is a sin against "general medicine," that we should drop the name of homœopathy, hide our principles under an unmeaning term, and give no note of what we are and what we follow. It moreover states with admirable candor, far from the double-faced perversions of our neighbor, the honest justification for "the bond of our union and the reason of our separate existence," which should be read by every sincere and insincere homœopathic physician :

"We are men equally educated and legally qualified with the rest of the profession, but live under an unbending official ostracism, and are cast out of the camp as pseudo-scientific lepers by those who happen to be in power. It is true that in some instances, and to an increasing extent, able and catholic-minded men are willing to meet us in consultation, in difficult and obscure cases, so far as they can do this without incurring the danger of professional incivism and the charge of assenting to principles of which they are not fully cognizant. This, however, is only the silver lining to the black cloud, and a cloud that overshadows us, not so much because we are charged with incompetence and intellectual blindness, a charge which the results of our practice are every day disproving, and which, moreover, would readily be forgiven, but we are still further charged with the sin of *sectarianism*—a sin which, in their eyes, is greater than all, and past forgiveness.

"We are continually told that ' "general medicine" is not a sect,' but that we by our designation, our attitude and associations as practitioners of homœopathy are so. Yet our critics ignore the fact that a 'sect' is distinguished *far more* by a refusal to examine and discuss any new principle, and the rigid exclusion thereof, than it is by the rigid adherence to one. No community, indeed, can claim to be catholic which maintains so exclusive a policy, and carries it to the point of such misrepresentation and excommunication as those who assume to be the medical orthodox.

"No, indeed ! the head and front of our offending is *not* that we are 'sectarians ;' it is that having investigated homœopathy, and believing it to be the best method of therapeutics, we base our practice upon it, and openly say so in justice to our art and also to the public, but unfortunately to the annoyance of professional 'sacerdotalism.'

"And further, it is because we see that these principles are either ignored or contemned by the members of the old school, that the only way to ensure them their just place is to make them the bond of our union and the reason of our own separate existence. This is not sectarianism—it is fidelity to truth and principle.

"Therefore, gentlemen, to the haughty ultimatum of those who deem themselves the orthodox party, that we must *drop the name of homœopathy, hide our principles, and give no note of what we are and what we follow,* you will reply in such terms as these : ' That we have not cut ourselves off from general medicine, but are true and faithful exponents of all that is good in it, and claim all its rights, privileges, and sources of knowledge ; that we deprecate the practical schism which exists between the majority and ourselves, and believe that great good would result to the profession and to the general community were an honest and open union effected on the principles of ' Liberty, Equality and Fraternity '—*liberty* for all to practice according to the dictates of conscience without prejudice or ostracism ; *liberty* in the medical officering of public hospitals and like institutions, irrespective of medical creed or opinion ; *liberty* also for the teaching of homœopathic therapeutics in the medical schools, as well as of Materia Medica in its fullest sense—the subsequent adoption of any method of therapeutics being left an open question to each individual. Let this ' Liberty,' this ' Equality,' this ' Fraternity ' in *every way* be granted by the powers that be, and whilst such consummation will be for the good of all, the work committed to our hands by Hahnemann will alike achieve its hour of triumph and its death—*that* work by us as a separate body being virtually accomplished, its further development will be left to the profession as a whole. By such means, and by such alone can the breach be healed.

"This reply, gentlemen, will, I feel sure, command your assent, and you will further agree that as homœopathy has gained the position it has, not only in this country but in every quarter of the globe, that as the principle of *similia* in therapeutics is one that can never die, and that as the word "homœopathy" and all that it represents pervades the greater part of the medical literature of the present day, and is a word that can never become obsolete, that under such circumstances if we could by any means be induced to give up such a distinctive title and landmark in medicine before it has gained the full recognition which I have described, we might rightly be designated "Hahnemann-iacs," and incur the contempt and scorn alike of those who are opposed to us, and of our colleagues everywhere.

"You are, moreover, aware that homœopathy is much stronger in every way in America than it is here. It has over 11,000 fully educated and qualified medical practitioners, fourteen medical collegs in which its principles are taught, fifty-seven homœopathic hospitals with an aggregate of 4,500 beds, besides numerous dispensaries and medical societies, and an extensive medical literature. With this power in the hands of our colleagues in that country, with their enthusiasm and grit, we may rest assured that if we could be found willing to compromise our principles, they indeed would not ; they would never let the beacon in therapeutics be extinguished in so craven a manner ; and they would say that if the breach between general medicine and homœopathy is to be healed, it can only be so on the lines that I have laid down.'

COMMENTS.

RUTS.—If great men think through the same quill, all men tend to pass through life in the same grooves. In business, in politics, in social and family matters there are routine courses in which the world moves along without the trouble of thinking. There are "ruts" on every hand, ruts theological, medical and literary. Ruts may be defined as the lazy man's delight and the stupid man's path of safety. They are alluring, deceptive and eternal. To follow others, to servilely imitate, to narrow the vision so that nothing is seen beyond the limited horizon of a special calling, to cling obstinately to the old because it is old, to reject the new because it is new, to plod mechanically on, learning nothing, originating nothing, this is to be in a rut. Not that change should be made for the mere sake of change, nor that respect for the past and adherence to the time honored is not right. But the past need not overshadow the present. A vigorous resolution is needed to escape from musty superstitions and to resist the increasing pressure of our modern civilization, which tends more and more to cast all men in the same mould. And then it is easy to run in a groove. The entrance is wide, the descent easy, the path for a time at least straight and smooth; no thought is required ; it is but to follow your leader. The medical rut is perhaps the most pernicious of all. It is also the most certainly fatal to professional life and growth. Fashion in medicine means intellectual death to the profession. To follow constituted authorities blindly, without comprehending the principles upon which the directions are based, to adopt a certain method in all cases regardless of varying circumstances, is to transform a physician into an automatic mummy. To guard against ruts, professional or otherwise, let us mix brains with our work, widen our outlook, seek for that which is best, hold to that which is tried and approved, and beat a road so wide and level that any deviation may be made without jarring.

HAHNEMANN'S "COMPLAINT AND RESOLVE."—Procuring professional advice and forgetting to pay for it is a species of fraud which has troubled most physicians. The following letter which Hahnemann caused to be twice inserted in the public press shows how he stopped the annoyance. "Dear Public ! It will scarcely be credited that there are people who seem to think that I am merely a private gentleman with plenty of time on my hands, whom they may pester with letters, many of which have not the postage paid, and are consequently a tax on my purse, containing requests for professional advice, to comply with which would demand much mental labor and occupy precious time, while it never occurs to these inconsiderate correspondents to send any renumeration for the time and trouble I would have to expend on answers by which they would benefit. In consequence of the ever increasing importunity of these persons, I am compelled to announce : 1. That henceforward I shall refuse to take in any letters which are not post-paid, let them come from whence they may. 2. That after reading through even paid letters from distant patients and others seeking advice, I will send them back unless they are accompanied by a sufficient fee (at least a Friedrich's d'Or) in a cheque or in actual money, unless the poverty of the writer is so great that I could not withhold my advice without sinning against humanity.   3. If lottery tickets are sent to me I shall return them without exception; but I shall make the post-office pay for all the expense of remission, and the senders will get them back charged with this payment.—SAMUEL HAHNEMANN, Doctor of Medicine, Altona by Hamburg, November 9th, 1799."

A MODERN PEST HOUSE.—The account recently published concerning the condition of a small-pox hospital not far from New York City reads very much like an extract from ancient history.   If the story be but partially true, should investigation cause the darker shadows of the narrative to fade away, even then pest houses of the thirteenth and fourteenth centuries would compare favorably with it. A wretched frame building through which the wind whistled at pleasure, insufficient and unfit food, straw mattresses spread on the floor for beds, irregular medical attendance, ignorant nurses—these are the items in the indictments.   What a graphic picture of complete misery ! Popular opinion is too apt to amplify rumors of mismanagement in public institutions of this sort, and it is quite possible that the worst features of this melancholy tale may be disproved. It is to be hoped that they will be.   Still public judgment is too often confirmed. Efficient supervision is lacking, physicians overburdened with care become remiss, brutal attendants are employed, a public scandal follows and a popular horror of such places is engendered.   When exposure comes, the medical staff generally has to bear the weight of the storm of wrath that follows. In some instances this may be deserved, but in more it is not. The main reason why so many hospitals for contagious diseases become, instead of places of refuge, localized hells, repulsive and monstrous to the sight, unspeakably foul within, nests of festering corruption, where the devils of disease hold high carnival, is to be found in our vicious system of administering public institutions.   When the factor of politics is eliminated an improvement will follow.

A POINTED SERMON.—The energetic editor of the *Southern Journal of Homœopathy*, moved by a righteous indignation, recently ascended into the editorial pulpit and preached from thence a short but most pithy sermon for the especial benefit of the Southern brethren.   From the facts presented, there can be no question but that the audience sadly needed a discourse to arouse within them a quickening sense of duty unperformed. Says the preacher, '' Of our nearly one thousand subscribers, less than one hundred (eighty-eight) are southern physicians.   Of the four hundred and fifty homœopaths in the South, less than twenty per cent. take the only Southern homœopathic journal published.   Of the eighty-eight who take it less than sixty pay for it. There are three hundred and seventy homœopaths in the South who ought to be ashamed of themselves." Should any erring brother bowing before this sturdy blast hastily raise a kind of moral umbrella to the end that the storm may drip upon his neighbor, he will evince a lamentable lack of discernment. For this is no ordinary storm—it is a gale that drives straight home. The most hardened Southern sinner, even though he be a moral pachyderm, must feel its beatings. A good sermon and excellently delivered. May it have the effect desired!

MEDICAL PAUPERISM.—There is but one way to treat a glaring and impudent evil. To temporize, to compromise, to handle gingerly, is but to lose valuable time. Steady pounding well directed and long enough continued will in the end destroy any abuse. The process of medical pauperization sometimes known as medical charity still goes on, but not quite so complacently and blatantly as before. A partial reform has been effected. Many dispensaries have displayed a commendable determination to no longer allow their charity to be abused by the designing. Investigation of patients is the rule, and the tricky individual who while able to pay comes to the clinic for the poor, and filches from them the treatment that is theirs, is quickly sent about his business. But a partial reformation is not enough. It must be entire. There are dispensaries here in the City of New York treating daily hundreds of patients where no attempt at discrimination is made, and a very large proportion of the persons prescribed for are abundantly able to pay. This is an outrage on both the profession and the people. Is it self-interest that hinders this reform? Or laziness or inefficiency?

THE SAN FRANCISCO HOSPITAL.—The *California Homœopath* for October contains a detailed account of the obstacles met in the establishment of a homœopathic hospital in San Francisco. It appears that after the hospital building was equipped and open for patients, the Board of Supervisors passed an ordinance placing the prohibitory limits (within which no hospital was to be allowed) very remote, but excepting from the action of this law all hospitals established on or before January 1st, 1887. As the homœopathic hospital was the only institution opened since the date fixed, it was evidently designed to crush it out of existence. Legal warfare followed, Dr. Ward, the Superintendent of the Hospital, and Dr. Smith, House Surgeon, being arrested, brought before a Police Court Judge, and ordered either to pay a fine of $100 or go to fail for fifty days. A writ of habeas corpus was sued out, and argued before Judge Toohy. The decision was favorable to the hospital, and the struggle came to an end. We hope there are no more breakers ahead. The medical sky has been overcast for some time on the Pacific slope; it is time for clear weather.

A NEW DRESS.—The *Medical Institute* comes to us again with a new editorial staff and arrayed in a bright and becoming garb. It devotes a long editorial in replying to and refuting the statements of an individual vaguely termed "Ad." We vehemently suspect this personage cursorily dubbed "Ad" to be identical with the gentleman who is said, in the *Medical Era*, to have quite recently instructed Hahnemann in homœopathy. If this be so, then it doth appear that the *Institute* devotes a large space to an indifferent subject. Arguments of this variety should be kindly but firmly relegated to the junk shop.

BOOK REVIEWS.

CHOLERA AND ITS TREATMENT ON HOMŒOPATHIC PRIN-
CIPLES (Based mainly on the results of fourteen years' practice
as a homœopath), by RADHA KANTA GHOSH. Published for the
author by Berigny & Co. 12 Lal Bazaar, Calcutta. Price, 1 shill-
ing threepence.

This little book of less than sixty pages is by far the most clear,
practical and useful treatise that has hitherto come to our notice. It
ought to be in the hands of every physician who may be called upon
to treat Asiatic cholera. The description of the disease in its different
stages bears evidence of having been taken from personal observation of a large number of cases.

The author speaking of the sequelæ says: "Some physicians are
of the opinion that these complications and sequelæ are rare when
homœopathic treatment has been adopted from the commencement. I cannot agree with them; I find that some of these
complications, such as relapse, typhoid symptoms, uræmia,
ulceration of the cornea, vomiting and hiccough, occur even under
judicious homœopathic treatment." Dr. Ghosh finds *camphor* indicated in the stage of invasion " as long as the stools contain fæcal
matter," but if no improvement follows after three doses at intervals
of twenty to thirty minutes, other remedies are to be thought of ;
"also in the stage of collapse when the purging and vomiting have
stopped and reaction does not get in ;" illustrative cases are given.
The next important remedies are veratrum and arsenic, which are
clearly differentiated. The following remark concerning *veratrum* is
doubtless to, be accepted as reliable, " in veratrum there is *no pain* in
the epigastrium or abdomen, nor much restlessness and tossing
about."

The author's experience with *ricinus* has not been satisfactory to
himself, though he has had favorable reports from some of his con-
frères. He gives a case of his own unsuccessfully treated with it,
and remarks, " although in this instance and in several subsequent
ones I met with failure with ricinus, yet from the favorable reports
already spoken of, and from the study of the pathogenetic symptoms
(which, I may say, resemble those of cholera in all its varieties), I
should like to see this agent given an extensive trial in spasmodic
cholera." Speaking of *aconite*, which he always carries and uses in
the tincture, he says, " Now I own, I am not so sanguine about its
efficacy as Dr. Hughes, though I do not deny its usefulness to a considerable extent." His indications for it are "generally in children,
when, in collapse, the stools are yellowish, slimy and mucous." " In
the cholera epidemic at Dacca of 1871, Mr. Pares Náth Mukerja cured
nearly 80 per cent. with drop doses of tinct. of acon. rad. alone."
Cuprum "is more clearly indicated if the extensor muscles of the legs
and hands are affected by the spasms (secale corn., flexor muscles)."
" Now I use almost exclusively cuprum met. (12th potency) (instead
of C. acet.) with better results." *Carbo. veg.* "In India, physicians

are unanimous in their testimony to the *efficacy* of this drug in that stage when the above symptoms are present." *Cantharis*, suppression of urine in stage of reaction, followed well by kali bichrom. or terebinth. *Cina.*, "I generally use the 3d and 30th potencies; where these fail I resort to the 200th, a dose every hour or two (symptoms in imperfect reaction); I do not administer more than three doses of any given potency;" for convulsions, *cicuta.;* speaking of *hydrocyanic acid* he says, "In the early years of my practice I was more sanguine than even Dr. Sircár, about the efficacy of this agent ; though my recent experience with it has led me to moderate my estimate of the drug." A little chapter on auxiliary measures, food and hygiene is very concise and good. Indeed the whole book is so concise, so practical, and evidently so honest, that it ought to receive marked favor. As regards mortality he says, "Under judicious homœopathic treatment adopted from the first, the mortality does not generally seem to exceed 40 per cent., but in the epidemic that broke out in 1884, after the exhibition, the mortality was very great even under homœopathic treatment, being 60 per. cent. at least under my treatment. My personal observation inclines me to think that mortality is less under judicious homœopathic treatment than under the rival system." * * *

THE GUIDING SYMPTOMS OF THE MATERIA MEDICA, by C. HERING, M.D. Vol. V. Philadelphia. Published by the estate of Constantine Hering, 112 and 114 N. 12th Street.

After considerable delay we welcome the present volume of this important work, and hope the editors will be able to continue the undertaking to a successful completion. This plan of arranging the materia medica was Hering's own, and to his memory the book is dedicated by his loving descendants. The plan is too well known, perhaps, to need explanation, but a few words may be said concerning it. The work "is principally a collection of *cured symptoms*," but it includes many symptoms which have never been verified on the sick, and also many symptoms which have been observed *only* in the sick, never in the healthy, from provings. In the introduction to the first volume the author said "the Greek letter 'Pi' stands before symptoms observed only on the sick," by which we presume is meant that symptoms observed in the sick as the result (presumably) of the drug administered, are so designated, for it certainly is not prefixed to symptoms not in any pathogenesis, cured in the sick, and fortunately is not often found anywhere in the book. The idea to present to the profession a book of guiding symptoms is splendid; such a work is of great practical use, and while the scattering of groups of symptoms which are presented by a patient seems even more violent, in theory, than the same treatment of symptoms which occur in provers, still it must be confessed that it affords the prescriber a ready method of finding what he wants.

There are two radical defects in Hering's work as shown in the volume before us—*one, the great inequality of the material;* and the *other,* the lack of any distinguishing mark between *verified* and *cured* symptoms, that is, between symptoms that are pathogenetic and have been verified at the bedside, and symptoms that have simply disappeared from the patient after the administration of the drug.

The inequality apparent all through these five volumes has always been characteristic of Hering's work. Just as much space and even more is given to unimportant (comparatively) drugs as to the most important; thus in this volume, which comprises the remedies from cundurango to helonias inclusive, eight pages are given to daphne odora, nine pages to euphorbium, ten to formica, and so on, and very few of the symptoms of either of these drugs have ever been verified. The work thus seems to attempt too much and to fall short of being a complete materia medica, both pathogenetic and clinical. A purely clinical and *verified* symptomatology is what should have been given us and that only. The second criticism we have to make is that we are unable to judge of the relative value of the symptoms because there is no indication which points to a verification of a pathogenesis. Our attention has been recently called to curare, to its characteristic *heaviness of the extremities* and other paralytic symptoms; these we find properly verified as they have been by cures, but we also find that in a case, reported by Dr. T. F. Allen, in which these symptoms of weakness and paralysis had occurred, they were associated with *soreness of the chest* and other symptoms not in the list given by Houat, from whom the characteristic "heaviness in the arms" was obtained which determined the remedy. Hering gives "soreness of the chest" verified in the same way as the other symptoms, and one might prescribe *curare*, starting with that symptom and with perhaps a few more in Hering but not in the provings, and make a failure. This plan renders the selection of the remedy uncertain where it should be certain. Houat is bad enough, mixing pathogenetic and clinical symptoms, but Hering, starting with a few of Houat's uncertain symptoms, widens the field by including a lot of associated symptoms from a patient, and carries us far, far away from homœopathy; the ground becomes very like a quagmire.

But with even these drawbacks the work possesses a distinct value and will certainly facilitate the finding of a similimum. * * *

PRINCIPIO OBBIETTO E LEGGE DELLA MATERIA MEDICA OMIOPATICA SEGUITA DA UN SAGGIO DI PATOGENESIA (Lavaro letto dall' autore al congresso internazionale omiopatico in Londra, 1881). Dottor Tommaso Cigliano. Napoli, 1887.

RIMEDII INDIVIDUALIZZATE PER SINTOMI E MALATTIE ORVERO GRANDE REPERTORIO CLINICO OMIOPATICO, del Dottor Tommaso Cigliano. Napoli, 1887.

The former of these works is a pamphlet of 114 pages, the first part of which consists of a treatise on the materia medica divided into pharmacopœia, pharmocodynamics, pharmacology and a general summary in which many of the questions that have arisen concerning the action of drugs and the arrangement of symptoms are briefly discussed. As an appendix to this is an arrangement of the symptoms of kali bichromicum after the plan proposed by the author to the American Institute (see transactions for 1883). The rubrics are arranged alphabetically, beginning with abdomen and ending with vomiting. Pustule comes between Pupil and Sacrum, and an attempt is made to render the finding of symptoms as easy as possible. To our mind this method banishes completely the advantages, clearly seen by Hahnemann, of having under one's eye groups of related symptoms, so that if one does not find the identical words of the patient's symptoms one can readily see if the pathogenesis offers similar symptoms; but there are all sorts of ways of looking at it; some like one method, some another.

The second work is a portly volume of 964 pages, and comprises a reproduction of the treatise published in the former work (spoken of above) occupying about 80 pages and an elaborate repertory to the whole materia medica, and to homœopathic therapeutics. The arrangement is alphabetical, beginning with "abbattimento" (despondency) and ending with "zona." It is almost entirely clinical and compiled from a goodly list of repertories which are duly mentioned. It is obviously impossible to give a full list of medicines needed for every disease or that have hitherto been found curative, but we must confess to a feeling of disappointment at the numerous omissions in many rubrics; for instance, under "Peritonitis, puerperal" are found bell., bry., cham., cimic., pul. Such books are after all only hints to beginners, but to them they usually prove to be stumbling blocks, obscuring the right remedy. Homœopathy is to be practiced only by prescribing for the symptoms, and there is little to be gained by giving a list of medicines to be used in any "disease." We presume, however, that this book is needed in Italy, and will meet a want.

Many rubrics are exceedingly good, such as "aggravations," "ameliorations," et cetera. The work is the only one of the kind (we believe) in the Italian language, and will without doubt facilitate the practice and promote the spread of homœopathy in that awakening country.   * * *

HUMANITY, A VISION—A REALITY. A Poem by Wm. Tod Helmuth. New York: E. P. Dutton & Co., 1887.

It is good to be reminded occasionally that medicine is not all science, but touches the humanities of literature, that even a surgeon may indulge in visions of the ideal and embody them in melody. The "Humanity" of Dr. Helmuth is a meditation in the Duomo of Pisa under Galileo's swinging "lamp of bronze" upon

> The first, great, grand absorbing attribute
> Of him who tends the suffering of his race,

and "Reality" is "a simple, touching incident" of the self-sacrifice and death of an army surgeon, told with pathos and dramatic force. The poems have thus an interest to the physician as idealizing the nobler motives of his calling. All readers will enjoy the rhythm, local color and imaginative grasp of the verses, which are sumptuously printed, bound and illustrated.

REPORTS OF SOCIETIES AND HOSPITALS.

PENNSYLVANIA STATE SOCIETY HELD AT PITTSBURGH.*

TUESDAY, September 20th, 1887.

The Society was called to order by the President, Dr. A. R. Thomas, Philadelphia.

J. C. Burgher, M.D., President of the Allegheney County Medical Society, delivered an address of welcome, which was responded to on behalf of the Society by the President.

Dr. J. H. McClelland announced that as the New York State Society was in session in New York City, he moved that the Secretary be instructed to send a telegram of friendly greeting. This motion was carried.

The necrologist, W. R. Childs, M.D., reported the death of H. H. Detwiller of Easton, S. J. Charlton of Harrisburgh, David Cowley, of Pittsburgh, and J. H. May of West Chester.

In the paper by Dr. Wm. B. Trites, of Philadelphia, on Syphilis as an Unrecognized Factor in Disease, Dr. Trites referred to the marked tendency of the late manifestations of syphilis to simulate diseases of the most diverse character and to the fact that this tendency is not sufficiently appreciated by the general practitioner, and as the result patients suffer. To substantiate these statements Dr. Trites read the reports of five cases. 1st. Syphilitic gumma of the lung simulating phthisis. Recovery under suitable treatment. 2d. Cerebral syphilis, paralysis of the trifacial with aphasia. Recovery. 3d. Syphilitic orchitis simulating cancer. One testicle had been removed before the doctor saw it. The other becoming affected the true nature of the disease was discovered and the testicle was saved. 4th. Syphilitic headache, followed by meningitis and death. 5th. Syphilitic disease of the liver simulating in its history and symptoms, cirrhosis. Improvement. Medical schools neglect to give *full* instructions in this subject.

The diagnosis between syphilis and the diseases which it simulates was then considered, and attention called to the fact that it is a much more common disease than is generally supposed. The various characteristic signs of syphilis were then noted, such as nodes, iritis, nocturnal pains, destructive ulcerations, lymphatic enlargement, alopecia and in hereditary syphilis, the history, peculiar facies and the syphilitic teeth of Hutchinson.

The diagnostic signs of syphilitic lung diseases and the affections of the nervous system were considered. The paper concludes with a quotation from Hutchinson: "The first requisite of success in the diagnosis of late syphilis, is a mind constantly awake to suspicion and fully impressed with the all-important fact that diseases of the most diverse character may have their origin in this taint."

The Society adjourned and the discussion postponed until the following morning.

In the afternoon the celebration of the Fiftieth Anniversary of the Introduction of Homœopathy was held at the Grand Opera House.

In the evening a banquet was given the members of the Society by the Alleghany County Society.

WEDNESDAY, SEPTEMBER 21ST—MORNING SESSION.

Dr. Dudley, Philadelphia, was strongly convinced that if there be no tubercular or syphilitic dyscrasia in cases of infantile marasmus the dis-

---

*From notes kindly furnished by Wm. A. Haman, M.D., Reading, Pa.

ease is always due to mismanagement and gross neglect in the matter of diet. In many cases the contents of the intestines are irritating the canal and he always institutes a change of diet. He has often succeeded in curing cases, which had been utterly unaffected by medicine, by changing the diet in toto. Cases with persistent loose green feculent stools and possible enlargement of the mesenteric glands were quickly relieved by completely excluding milk from the diet for a period of three to forty-eight hours, substituting almost anything for it, oyster broth, beef tea, barley water, etc. He enjoyed Dr. Trites' paper very much. A case which he attended illustrated the assertion of Dr. Trites that persistent headache with nightly aggravation is very likely to be syphilitic. The case had been under the treatment of another practitioner, but without any result. It commenced with nightly headache accompanied by blindness, which gradually lasted longer and longer, until permanent blindness was the result. She denied any trace of syphilis ; the husband also denied any such history, but the mother of the lady patient admitted that her daughter had had an eruption, accompanied by falling out of the hair, and that the husband was afflicted in a similar manner at about the same time. He placed her on three grains of the iodide of potassium three times a day for three weeks, when her headaches disappeared. Subsequently she got a numb sensation on one side of her face which spread over one-half of her body. Finally she was taken with coma and died. The autopsy revealed degeneration of cerebral tissue at the base of the brain and involvement of the meninges.

Dr. Mohr, Philadelphia, thinks more highly of diet than the antisyphilitic remedies, and calls attention to the Turkish baths in assisting the elimination of the poison. Dr. Trites said he believed it was better to treat of syphilis in our medical text-books than surgical. It should be thoroughly studied by general physicians and not relegated to specialists. Dr. Mohr then related a case illustrative of syphilis as an etiological factor in chest affections. A man supposed to be rheumatic was treated for a quiet pleurisy with effusion. He became feverish, and when examining him more closely the bared chest revealed nodes upon the clavicles. His personal history gave a complete account of the usual syphilitic manifestations. Iodide of mercury was given, but the patient got worse ; his fever was higher and he went into a typhoid condition with diarrhœa ; his infusion increased in quantity and he became greatly exhausted. After carefully studying the case, Dr. Mohr considered sulphur to be the indicated remedy. It was given him and he immediately improved. But the quantity of effusion remained the same. Ten drop doses of potass. iod. in a saturated solution were then given him and finally changed to the 1x trituration of the same drug, which perfected the cure. Syphilitic diseases are not to be treated only with the antisyphilitic drugs ; others are exceedingly valuable, aurum, sulphur, etc. In a very severe syphilitic headache, without the history of an initial lesion, every physician during a period of eight years treated her for syphilis and although she suffered with the toxic effects of the iodide of potassium, she had no relief from her suffering. Dr. Mohr saw symptoms of apis mellif. and gave it in the 30th dilution and it was astonishing to see how quickly the headache disappeared. While antisyphilic remedies are useful, it must not be forgotten that cases must be individualized and prescribed for accordingly.

Dr. Z. T. Miller, Pittsburgh :—All the cases of cystocele he ever met, were cases directly caused by the syphilitic virus. All the cases did not manifest the syphilitic taint. In two cases the patients confessed to having been infected. In another who denied any history the signs in her children and in her own bones were too clear for misinterpretation. All the children of another patient have the syphilitic teeth. As syphilis is capable of producing paralytic lesions of the cranial nerves, so is it capable, in his opinion, of producing paralysis of the structures supporting the bladder. In men prolapsus of the rectum occurs from the action of the same poison. So far as treatment is concerned, he wishes to state that he never uses the antisyphilitic remedies. He finds that patients always get worse after receiving merc. iod. 3 x. They do better under the influence of sulphur than any other remedy. The iodide of sulphur would probably be still better.

Dr. Smeadley, of Philadelphia, asked whether potentized drugs can cure in secondary and tertiary syphilis? He believes that the iodide of potassium is thoroughly homœopathic to these stages of the disease. He saw a case of a child covered with a mass of sores produced, he thought, by the drug just alluded to. He does not use the drug in ordinary homœopathic doses, but in finely divided states as the saturated watery solution. He always thought that notched incisors of children were indicative of the syphilitic taint. Mr. Hutchinson told him that a peg tooth with the notch was a syphilitic tooth. He had seen many cases of cystocele, but could not trace the relation of cause and effect. He can't see how it can be caused by syphilis. Loss of support to base of bladder is the principal cause.

Dr. Bartlett, Philadelphia, claimed that syphilitic nervous lesions are associated with paralysis of the cranial nerves. The motor oculi is the one most frequently affected. Paraplegia with paralysis of the motor oculi is almost always syphilitic. He remarked that secondary symptoms were frequently mistaken for prickly heat.

Dr. Korndoerfer, Philadelphia, said that no one had yet mentioned the antipsoric drugs. He could not see how any case can be cured without any antipsoric. Almost every case of syphilis is complicated with psora and both classes of drugs will have to be used.

Dr. Trites, Philadelphia: Very many are suffering from modified hereditary or acquired syphilis. We must constantly bear this in mind. His treatment during the primary stage is merc. sol. 1x, gr. j. three times a day, and he continues this well into the second stage. In the later secondary and tertiary stages compounds of mercury and iodine are required. In dangerous brain syphilis he gives the iodide of potassium in massive doses, thirty to forty grains if necessary. He believes that hundreds of people die from the lack of heroic treatment. He called attention to a small work of Hutchinson on syphilis, published in Lee's series of manuals as one of the best on the subject.

Dr. Dudley, Philadelphia, said that all are familiar with the statement that it can be acquired in unusual ways. Can any of the members present confirm these statements?

Dr. Seip, Pittsburgh, said that he lately saw a case which confirmed these assertions. A lady playfully put the cigar of her lover into her mouth and in consequence has a chancer on her lip. The young man with syphilitic mouth lesions is also under his care.

Dr. Korndoerfer, Philadelphia, had two cases in which there was no direct sexual cause. A young lady for a number of weeks prior to coming under notice had no male company and was constantly attended by her mother. The woman who washed her linen also washed the linen of a niece of the patient who had syphilis and had been discharged from the Pennsylvania Hospital as incurable. From the contaminated linen his patient had contracted a chancer on the labia. Another young woman under his care had sore mouth and throat contracted through kissing one who had syphilis of the mouth in a marked manner.

Bureau of Ophthalmology, Otology and Laryngology. Dr. Bigler, Chairman.—Dr. Joseph E. Jones, West Chester. Diseases of the Ductus ad Nasam. Two causes of epiphora were mentioned, excessive production of lachrymal fluid with normal channels which are not capable of carrying away the excess of fluid ; and true epiphora caused by obstruction of the ducts which in consequence cannot drain away the normal amount of fluid. Stricture of this duct can in his opinion occasionally be cured by medical treatment. A lady patient came to him for treatment after suffering for a considerable length of time. Believing that surgical treatment only was likely to benefit her, he subjected the obstruction to a full trial of Bowman's probes, but without doing her any good. Studying the case he selected sulphur, but it effected no change in her condition, Then pulsatil., argen. nitricum and mercurius, were employed with similar negative results. Petroleum was finally selected for the troublesome burning and itching of the lids, swelling and injection of the conjunctiva, etc., and radically cured the patient.

Two cases of dacryo cystitis were detailed with stubborn swelling, occasioning epiphora. These were finally cured with merc. sol., without rupture of the sac.

Another somewhat similar case was accompanied by rashes on the mucous membranes, bronchial and nasal, and believing that the closure of the sac and duct was due to an extension of the trouble from the nasal passages, he cured the disease by medical treatment. The only external treatment used in these cases was arnica oil. In the future he will abandon the oil and trust to his remedies when suitable cases present themselves.

Atrophy of Optic Nerve.—Dr. W. H. Winslow, Pittsburgh, called attention to the benefit of homœopathic treatment in this affection. He drew attention to the use of tobacco as an etiological factor in many cases.

Chromic Acid in the Treatment of Post-Nasal Growths.—Dr. Horace F. Ivins, Philadelphia, used a bent hard rubber tube, with a concealed copper cotton carrier in its interior. The cotton is medicated with the solution of chromic acid. Care must be taken that not too much fluid is contained in it. The contact of the drug with the growth is not painful. It should remain until the parts assume a yellow color. It should be repeated in four or five days. Cocaine was used at one time, but its use has been found unnecessary. The strength of the solution used is not so important as the method of applying it. He uses a solution which is not quite saturated.

Hypertrophic Rhinitis.—Dr. W. H. Neville, Philadelphia: In the majority of cases of hypertrophy of the nasal membrane, had abandoned the scalpel, and since that time gets better results from the use of chromic acid. He does not use it, however, to the exclusion of snares, knives, etc. He described a very interesting case of chronic catarrh, which was cured by applications of chromic acid.

Diagnostic Value of the Various Types of Bulbar Injection.—Dr. W. H. Bigler, Philadelphia, said, that "an absence of any pericorneal injection indicates an entirely superficial hyperæmia or inflammation of the conjunctiva. Intense congestion, especially when attended by chemosis, as in purulent ophthalmia, may mark or entirely conceal a pericorneal injection, indicating a more serious injury. The presence of pericorneal injections may have a different diagnostic significance, according to its several types :

(*a.*) A pink or rose-colored zone (the non-perforating branches of the anterior ciliary arteries), surrounding the cornea, becoming fainter in color away from this, and consisting, on close examination, of fine straight radiating vessels, points to an inflammation of the cornea, or uveal tract, iris, ciliary, body, or choroid.

(*b.*) A similarly placed dark or dusky réd zone, finely reticulated (epischeral venous plexus), is often found in glaucoma, but may occur in other conditions, especially in the aged; the increased tension, impairment of vision, and pains will occur to confirm the diagnosis of glaucoma.

(*c.*) An equally marked congestion of a peculiar lilac tint in the same region points to cyclitis, and will be attended by sensitiveness to pressure on the spot of congestion.

(*d.*) A bright red superficial congestion of small vessels in the same location, often running over on the surface of the cornea, usually shows superficial corneal ulceration.

DISCUSSION.

Dr. Bigler, Philadelphia, referred to one case reported by Dr. Jones, a case of stricture of the nasal duct being cured by medical means. Some forms of treatment established or negatived a diagnosis, and in this case he thinks the treatment proves the obstruction to have been ordinary swelling of submucous tissue, and not a true stricture. He believed that the rubbing caused by itching of the eczematous eyelids caused swelling of the mucous membrane and closure of the duct. In true stricture of this duct he does not believe in any medical treatment.

Dr. Jones, West Chester, thinks we depend too much upon pathology. He doubts that the obstruction, in the case Dr. Bigler referred to, was one of ordinary submucous swelling.

Bureau of Materia Medica.—Dr. Chas. Mohr, Chairman, presented a lengthy report for the bureau, descriptive of the work which is being done by the committee on the new repertory of symptoms based on Hering's Materia Medica.

Dr. Korndoerfer then read a paper entitled, " Exclusion of Irrelevant Symptoms from the Materia Medica."

Hahnemann presented only the schematic arrangement of the symptoms and did not publish his day book. The schematic form of presentation is not the best method. Hahnemann taught that in treating a case, or in making a proving, every symptom and modality must be taken, yet in selecting the drug the most prominent and characteristic symptoms only are taken to represent the individuality of the case. The mental symptoms should be especially considered. A Materia Medica which shall be thoroughly reliable must retain all the symptoms of the day book, and the characteristics must be taken only from reliable provers.

Dr. A. P. Bowie called attention to a remedy which, on account of being used only for one disease and that gonorrhœa, was too little thought of. He referred to copaiba off. Armstrong first called attention to the use of this remedy in diseased mucous membranes. He, Dr. Bowie, found it to be particularly useful in old men who had retention of urine or strangury, and who have borborygmi and mucous discharges from the bowels. He prescribes five drops of 1st dilution. In using the catheter he lubricates the instrument with this balsam. Since he has employed this treatment he does not dread to meet with cases of urinary retention in old men. He has also found the remedy to be of use in bronchorrhœa.

Dr. Z. T. Miller, Pittsburgh, related a verification of a peculiar symptom of staphisagria.

DISCUSSION.

Dr. J. Dake, of Nashville, Tenn., considers all reliable symptoms as important. In order to distinguish the true from the false, we must have a concurrence of evidence of many uninfluenced provers. Repetition of symptoms must be avoided. Positive evidence of provings can only determine the value of symptoms; clinical confirmation then gives the desired results.

Dr. Korndoerfer, Philadelphia, claimed that certain isolated symptoms that had been experienced by one prover only, were occasionally of extreme value. He had had a patient who was suffering from mental alienation and who continually said that if he could only " think with his head " he would be all right. On being questioned in what part of his body his mental processes were performed, he said it was " in his stomach." This symptom occurs not only in the proving of but one drug, but also in the proving of the drug by a single person, and it was never after experienced by the same person, although it was taken for this express purpose. He referred to Von Helmont. Aconite root in water restored the person to mental health, which he retained until his death.

Dr. Dudley, Philadelphia :—Single symptoms, *i. e.*, experienced by but one prover, are of value. But what is to be done with them ?

Dr. Korndoerfer, Philadelphia, would suggest that none but positive symptoms be introduced into our Materia Medica. Symptoms experienced by but one person should not be eliminated completely, but should be kept separate. All common symptoms, *i. e.*, those common to all drugs, under all the common circumstances of life, should be eliminated.

Dr. Trites, Philadelphia :—We don't want abbreviation, but we want substantiation. We want provings and reprovings.

AFTERNOON SESSION.

Bureau of Gynæcology.—The treatment of cervical endometritis must be both local and constitutional. They cannot be separated. The first step is to remove the cause and improve the general health ; forbid alcoholic stimulants, and have a daily movement from the bowels without the use of purgative drugs ; the clothing must be sufficient and must be suspended from the shoulders, not the waist ; gentle active exercise should be enjoined, but too violent exercise must be prohibited ; she should lie down daily for a few hours in either Sim's position or on the abdomen ; if lactation appears to be the cause the child must be weaned. Displacements of the uterus must be rectified with pessaries, lacerations must be repaired, and polypoid growths must be removed. Hot water injections must be perseveringly tried, either plain or medicated with tincture of iodine, calendula or eucalyptus. The plug of tenacious mucus hanging from the os must be frequently removed, or the treatment will be unavailing. If the os be closed it must be opened either with tents or the cutting operation, The best application to the diseased membrane is Churchill's tincture of iodine. The application is to be followed with a tampon of cotton, or, better, sheep's wool. These applications should be made at intervals of four days. Erosions, if present, must be touched with some stimulant. In his hands hydrastis had not accomplished what was expected of it. If the local congestion be well marked local blood-letting by leeches or multiple punctures is admirable, the latter method being preferable.

Bureau of Surgery.—In the absence of the chairman, Dr. Van Lennep, of Philadelphia, Dr. John E. James took his place.

Dr. Wm. Tod Helmuth presented a paper on the " Myo-fibromata of the Uterus." He described the nature of that class of tumor to which they belong, and then proceeded to and gave statistics of the operations myomotony and hysterectomy, and awarded to the Bureaus of America the credit of having performed the first successful operation. In supravaginal hysterectomy the chief mishap to be dreaded is hæmorrhage, either primary or secondary. Success depends upon the method of treating the pedicle and the rapidity of performing the operation. In Dr. Helmuth's opinion, the clamps are to be succeeded by elastic ligatures. The clamps of every noted operator have so far failed to meet the requirements of every case. Dr. Helmuth inserts two steel pins at right angles to each other through the pedicle, as far down as the abdominal wall will allow, and screws bulbous tips to them to prevent slipping of the elastic ligature, which is put well on the stretch and then wound around the pedicle below the needles. The tumor is then removed, the stump seared and left outside the abdomen, and dressed with iodoform. He uses no drainage tube. He believes that hysterectomy will eventually be as successful as ovariotomy.

Dr. J. H. McClelland, of Pittsburgh, read the notes of an aggravated case of general melanotic carcinoma. It had first appeared under one thumb nail. This member was amputated, after which it appeared in the axilla of that side. This was then cleared of its infiltrated glands, when it came out over the whole body. The doctor regretted that the absence of the patient prevented his being shown to the Society.

Dr. C. Bartlett, Philadelphia, read a paper entitled, " Early Paraplegia in Pott's Disease as Affecting the Diagnosis." Paraplegia is not specially related to the deformity. Paralysis may result from pressure, but in the majority of cases it results from extension of the strumous inflammation from the bones and ligaments to the meninges and cord. The symptoms are pain in the back, relieved by lying down, weakness in the limbs, starting and rigidity of limbs, exaggerated cutaneous and tendon reflexes, great wasting, no alteration in the electrical reactions, occasional loss of control over the rectum and bladder, and increased temperature. Five cases were detailed in illustration.

Dr. H. J. Evans, of Altoona, read the notes of a rare case of fracture of the inferior maxilla, the break occurring on the side opposite to that on which the blow was received.

Dr. Willard, of Pittsburgh, read a paper on "Open Section in Orthopædic Surgery." In illustration, he related the results of open section of fascial contractions of fingers and palm of hand. The results were perfect.

EVENING SESSION.

Bureau of Clinical Medicine.—A paper prepared by the Allegheny County Medical Society on "Cystitis" was presented.

Dr. Z. T. Miller made some remarks upon the treatment of this trouble. He related cases cured by the indicated remedies prescribed in high dilutions.

Dr. Thomas, of Philadelphia, then presented the President's address. A vote of thanks was tendered the President for his carefully prepared address.

Dr. R. K. Flemming, of Pittsburgh, read the notes of several very interesting clinical cases.

Constipation of long standing cured with natrum mur., 5000. Chorea cured with cimicifuga I x.

Threatened abortion averted by sabina and patient carried her child to the end of pregnancy. In this case the interest lay in the fact that the os was partly dilated, uterine contractions were strong, and the bleeding profuse.

Dr. Clarence Bartlett, Philadelphia, read a paper entitled, "Some Points in the Treatment of Gastric Disorders." The "points" were the use of water in the treatment of constipation, the description of lavage (washing out of the stomach), and the relation of several cures of hysterical vomiting by this procedure.

The use of hot water was mentioned and attention called to dyspepsia from self-inflicted starvation, and some remarks were made on the form of dyspepsia accompanying the gastric neuroses, and the great difficulty in curing them.

DISCUSSION.

Dr. P. Dudley, Philadelphia, was struck by the statement of Dr. Martin, that in the treatment of his three cases of sciatica each was strictly individualized. Ever since gnaphalium had been recommended as useful in sciatica, he has used it with more success than he had attending the administration of any other drug. The characteristic symptom is burning pain, followed by numbness in the affected part. He is also obliged to use other remedies and with good results. He had a case to treat, but as the pain was not of a burning character, and it was attended with cramps when the pains came on, he resorted to nux vom., bry., sulph., but without effect. At last he gave gnaphalium and cured his patient. It must be given for several days. He once had a very stubborn case, with the pain commencing at the *middle* of the thigh. Nothing he gave had the slightest effect, but at last he succeeded by telling the man to wrap a rag about the thigh where the pain commenced. The history showed the man to be obliged to press his thigh at the spot where the pain commenced against a cold iron support, hence the advice.

Dr. Mohr, Philadelphia, wished to refer to the paper on gastric disorders by Dr. Bartlett. Thought his advice to those who feel bad effects from drinking milk very appropriate. One case was brought into this condition by carrying out the advice of an old school physician. Physical examination revealed nothing abnormal except marked anæmia. He ordered nourishing food in gradually increasing quantities. She had a strong craving for celery and her former physician said it would be sure death for her to eat it. However, he (Dr. Mohr), insisted upon her satisfying the craving, which she did, and in a few months made an excellent recovery.

Dr. Bartlett stated that an ordinary stomach and funnel were the only instruments required. One quart of water was introduced at one time and then allowed to run out. This was repeated until the water ran clear. One gallon of water was used at each sitting and ended with introducing some easily digested fluid into the stomach.

Dr. Mohr asked Dr. Flemming, of Pittsburgh, whether he used anything besides nat. mur., 5000, in the treatment of his case of constipation, either in the way of hygienic or dieted measures.

Dr. Flemming replied that nothing but one dose of natrum mur., 5000, was given his patient and that he did not recommend any change in her mode of living. He tried the remedy in that strength merely as an experiment.

Dr. Korndoerfer referred to atonic dyspepsia. In his own case, which was an aggravated one, rhus tox. of any strength always relieved his symptoms, which were intense pain in the left hypochondriac region; the pain being sharp and weakening, and was relieved by walking. In sciatica gnaphalium acts well, no matter if the pains are burning in character or not; persistent lameness is always present. He prescribes it in tincture or the lower dilutions.

THURSDAY MORNING.

After the report of the Bureau of Pathology and Sanitary Science and the transaction of some business, the Society adjourned.

HOMŒOPATHIC MEDICAL SOCIETY OF THE COUNTY OF NEW YORK.

AT the regular meeting, Thursday, September 8th, at eight P. M., President Beebe in the chair, the Committee on Diseases of Women and Children, Dr. Wm. O. McDonald, Chairman, first reported. Mrs. W. A. Brinkman, M.D., read a paper upon "The Rational Treatment of Uterine Displacements."

Discussion, Dr. Brinkman's paper.

Dr. McMurray :—In the treatment of uterine displacements there are two extremes often advocated—one, the complete dependence on mechanical treatment; the other, its entire exclusion, and the use of medicines alone. Both are unreasonable and neither successful. The study of the individual case, the constitutional condition, the cause and its removal, and the careful adaptation of mechanical support until tone is restored, are the means to be employed in the treatment of these cases. Pessaries may be doing injury by friction, and the patient be unconscious of it. In a patient of mine suffering from antiflexion, I introduced a pessary, relieving all the symptoms she had been suffering from, produced by the pressure of the uterus on the bladder. Some six months later I was called to see her for some other trouble and incidentally asked her if the pessary was still there. She replied that she supposed so. On removing it I found the pessary covered with blood and muco-purulent matter, and the anterior wall of the vagina denuded of its mucous membrane to the extent of half an inch. Here was a case where the patient felt nothing, but still the pessary was doing mischief. There is no pessary of universal application; if they are to be used they must be selected carefully.

Dr. Clark :—I consider pessaries a valuable aid in treating many displacements. If equal care is given in selecting and introducing a pessary, as has been advised in regard to the tampon, I think the result is equally as good. I do not think that the properly fitting pessary interferes with the circulation any more than the tampon does.

Dr. Danforth :—Despite all that is said against pessaries, I often find one or another variety very useful in my practice, and I cannot entirely abandon their use. I know that some women cannot tolerate a pessary in the vagina, no matter how carefully employed, or how much needed; indeed, occasionally a patient will be met with who cannot wear a cotton tampon. Individual peculiarities have something to do with the toleration of foreign bodies in the vagina—there is no doubt of that. Medicated cotton tampons have their uses and cannot be dispensed with. When the cervix uteri is diseased, congested, granular and eroded, medicines applied by some form of tampon effect great good, at the same time that the tampon acts as a comfortable support to the displaced uterus. In uterine disease, marked by great tenderness, as a rule tampons are superior in point of comfort and safety to pessaries. But not all cases which require support present these features. There may not be much tenderness of the uterus, but it is displaced and requires support. The comfort and well-being of the patient demand it. The patient cannot come to the office every two or three days to have a tampon reintroduced. It is in these cases that pessaries find their most useful sphere of application. They are certainly cleaner and more agreeable in many respects than medicated tampons. But pessaries must be selected with care, and applied with strict reference to the features of each individual case. The gynecologist should have a large variety in his office to select from. No one kind will suit all cases. Prof. Thomas frequently reiterated the statement that it required as much skill to fit a pessary properly in the pelvis of a woman, as is necessary to fit a boot to a foot and have it comfortable. Herein, no doubt, lies the success of some and the failure of others in the use of these instruments. Pessaries and tampons will relieve local symptoms, but the constitutional symptoms, and many of the local ones, too, will require the *similimum* before they will get well. In conclusion I would add, that antiseptic wool is superior to absorbent cotton for tampons ; it is more elastic and keeps its place much better.

Dr. Keatinge :—I removed a pessary from a patient of mine some time since, who said she had been pronounced cured by her previous physician, of retroversion and ulceration. I found an abrasion as large as a twenty-five cent piece, which had been caused by the "pessary." The uterus was congested and the patient was in great pain for a week afterwards. I never use pessaries excepting in cases of procidentia. If the parts are anæmic and relaxed it may be tolerated, but if there is inflammation or ulceration, my experience is, it aggravates. I have had many cases where it has taken months to cure the trouble caused by pessaries.

Dr. S. N. Smith :—If we give our time and talent to the selection of remedies for the constitutional condition of the patient, and to the removal of the causes of the uterine trouble, there will be no occasion to use pessaries. In order to cure displacements, we must study to improve the general condition. A diseased uterus comes from a morbid condition of a system below par; if you set it right, the displacement will pass away and the organ resume its normal functions.

Dr. Mossman :—My thoughts are in harmony with Dr. Brinkman against curetting the uterus for slight cause. There is danger of its setting up uterine and pelvic inflammation. Antiseptic wool, I think, is preferable to absorbent cotton as a soft support and to correct uterine deviations, as it has more resiliency after being saturated with a medicated solution or the secretions of the vagina. I regard postural treatment as an important aid in displacements of the uterus posteriorly, the patient in the knee-chest position assists in replacing the organ and the medicated substance can be carried higher and placed more satisfactorily. The hard rubber pessary, if properly adjusted, is sometimes of great benefit. I removed one recently which had been worn over two years with comfort and benefit and no bad results.

The Committee on Public Health, Dr. J. M. Schley, Chairman, then reported. Dr. H. C. Houghton read the first paper on "Adulterations of Food and Liquors, their Prevention."

Dr. Danforth :—The influence of diet on disease is often remarkable. A case of neurasthenia, with dysmenorrhœa, functional disturbance of the heart and allied disturbances, which I have treated lately, is recovering rapidly under proper food when medicines alone utterly failed. The young lady has taken eight bottles of Murdock's liquid food and has progressively improved.

Dr. Berghaus :—I wish to deprecate the extensive use of tea and the idea that it sustains strength. Many poor people hurt their systems and spend their money foolishly by buying tea which is often only such by name. In charitable institutions I have lately recommended cocoa shell tea. It is comparatively inexpensive, and is very nutritious and contains little or no narcotics.

Dr. J. G. Baldwin presented his paper, "Concerning the Necessity of Hospitals in General, and the Proposed Free Homœopathic Hospital in Particular." Dr. J. M. Schley also read a paper on "State Prevention of Alcoholism."

Dr. McMurray :—Dr. Baldwin has treated the subject fairly, but has not had as much experience with these people as myself. If we observe them of a morning we notice a peculiarity in their appearance called the tenement house rot. They are pale and sallow, their tissues are lax and there is a lack of tone to their system. What causes it? They pass their nights in rooms where there is not one-tenth the amount of atmospheric air there should be. If the weather is cool they shut the windows, because they are too sensitive to air. They are compelled to work, and to appear in the best shape they feel the need of a stimulant. Rum shops are to be found on every corner and the habit of drink grows by that it feeds on. They feel its necessity and will get it. There ought to be a law passed to prohibit the building of such tenements as are provided for the use of our poor.

Dr. Houghton :—Dr. Schley has raised a pertinent question, Shall the State control this matter? I think it will not be long before not only the State but the Nation will be compelled to face this matter. Last spring I had the pleasure of hearing Canon Wilberforce on the occasion of his reception in this City, and was impressed with the earnestness of his warning, that Americans must be on their guard lest political power should be captured by. the liquor traffic. We must not only guard the poor man from the dangers of cheap and impure liquors, but the wealthy must practice self-denial for their sake.

Dr. Schley :—It seems to me Dr. McMurray has put the cart before the horse in this instance. I have seen families from time to time occupy a whole floor in a tenement house—consisting of several rooms. I have also seen such families reduced to two rooms, through drunkenness. If liquors were not so easily obtained—at such a low cost—this could not occur.

RECORD OF MEDICAL PROGRESS.

TETANUS (Traumatic) is an infectious disease, due to a specific virus, which exists in the tissue at the seat of infection.—Dr. Shakespeare, in *Boston M. and S. Jour.*

ELEPHANTIASIS FROM POSTURE. — Dr. E. D. Mapother, in *Brit. M. Jour.*, September 17th, 1887, reports case of elephantiasis in a woman, *æt.* 80, who had been kept in a sitting posture for seven years. The left leg measured twenty and one-half inches and the right leg seventeen inches just above the ankle fissure.

STENOCARPINE—A NEW LOCAL ANÆSTHETIC.—Dr. Claiborne, in the *Medical Record* of October 1st, gives further researches on the stenocarpine of Mr. Goodman, obtained from a plant which he identifies with the *Gleditschia triacanthos*, or honey locust. It is a mydriatic, and produces anæsthesia of conjunctiva and cornea, and of mucosa of nose and throat, together with other effects not as yet established.

ASCENDING PARALYSIS AFTER WHOOPING COUGH.—Dr. Möbius, in the *Centralblatt für Nervenheilkunde*, reports case of a child *æt.* three years, who was brought to the hospital in November, 1886, on account of loss of power to stand or walk. The child had had whooping cough, which began six weeks previously, and was then replaced by a simple cough. As the whooping cough subsided, the loss of power came on.

BERGER'S AMPUTATION.—The *Brit. Med. Jour.* of August 13th announces the successful performance of Berger's Amputation in the case of a woman with a large ossifying periosteal sarcoma of the head of the humerus, with secondary lymphatic tumors in the axilla and supra-clavicular region. The hemorrhage was unimportant, and primary union resulted throughout the greater portion of the extensive wound.

HYDROCELE IN THE FEMALE.—Mr. Hirst reports in the *Brit. Med. Journal,* September 3d, a case of a woman who, during her third pregnancy, gradually developed a swelling in the left labium. The tumor was translucent, fluctuating and distinctly circumscribed, with no impulse on coughing or other indications of hernia. Six ounces of fluid were drawn off and the tumor collapsed. Subsequent treatment was deferred on account of the patient's condition.

FLUORHYDRIC ACID IN TUBERCULOSIS.—Dr. Garcin presents to the *Académie de Médicine* (see *Jour. des Soc. Sciéntif.*, September 21st, 1887), the results obtained by the treatment of eighty-eight patients, supposably suffering from tuberculosis, by inhalations, in a cabinet, of air charged with hydrofluoric acid. He varies the dose according to the patient, and his results are as follows: Stationary, eleven; ameliorated, thirty-eight; cured, twenty-nine; died, nine.

WEIGHT OF THE BRAIN IN DEMENTIA.—Bartels discussed the above subject at the twenty-first reunion of the *Médecins Aliénistes*, held at Hanover in May last. His conclusions (see *Jour. des Soc. Scientifiques*, September 7th, 1887), were as follows: 1st. All mental diseases result in a diminished weight of the brain, 2d. This diminution in weight depends (*a*) on the age of the patient; (*b*) on the duration of the disease; (*c*) on the intensity of the disease. He gives the details in the original article.

NATRUM MURIATICUM IN HEMICRANIA.—Dr. Rabow has treated successfully several cases of hemicrania with chloride of sodium. The first case was that of a young man, whose attacks of hemicrania were preceded by a well marked aura. Upon the manifestation of the aura, the patient swallowed a teaspoonful of kitchen salt; the effect was excellent. Six other patients who suffered from hemicrania, preceded by gastric disturbances, were successfully treated in the same manner.—*Paris Letter to Brit. Med. Journal,* September 3d, 1887.

THE LAW AND THE LANDLORD.—"At present, in Scotland at least, and I believe in England and Ireland also, a landlord who knowingly lets an ill-drained house, or who, being informed by a tenant of the bad sanitary state of a house, neglects to put it in right, is liable for damages to health. This was shown in a case which was tried at Glasgow on May 13th last, £150 being awarded to the tenant; in addition to this, the tenant was allowed to leave the house, and the rent which he had paid was ordered to be returned to him."—T. Churbon, M.D., in the *Brit. Med. Jour.*, August 13th, 1887.

CHRONIC POISONING AS A RESULT OF SYPHILIS.—Dr. Rumpf, of Bonn, in considering this question, considers the view of Strümpell concerning the character of the connection between tabes dorsalis and dementia paralytica, and syphilis. He cannot agree with Strümpell that both diseases result from the action of a chemical toxic agent resulting from previous syphilitic infection, and having a selective action upon different systems of fibres; he thinks rather that the cause of syphilitic affections of the nervous system is a pathologico-anatomical one.—*Berlin. Klin. Wochens.*, No. 29, 1887. O'C.

UNUSUAL RELAXATION OF FEMALE URETHRA.—Married woman, æt. 42, nullipara; had retroflexion of uterus, and I had introduced ring pessary into the vagina. "At a subsequent visit I was much embarrassed by the following appearances : Unusual smoothness of vagina, which projected very much anteriorly, and contained no pessary; uterus entirely retroverted, the os pointing upward and beyond my reach; an obscure movable tumor, which I had not previously noticed, lying along the sacrum.

"I determined on trying a still larger ring, and only then discovered that my obscure tumor was the original instrument occupying its proper situation. I had been exploring the cavity of the bladder. The urethra was sufficiently dilated to admit two fingers quite easily. The posterior lip of the orifice was enormously hypertrophied and stretched like a valve across the vagina."—H. DAVIS, in *Brit. M. J.*, September 17th.

THE ETIOLOGICAL SIGNIFICANCE OF THE TETANUS BACILLUS.—Dr. Beumer considers this subject in a lecture delivered before the Griefswald Medical Society, on July 2d, 1887, and gives the results of experimental researches. The details will not bear abstracting, but among his conclusions, the following is of great interest : My investigations upon the etiology of the two forms of tetanus bring up the question, how will the bacillary etiology stand in relation to a form of disease held by many to be distinct from traumatic tetanus, but which in many respects is closely related thereto—that is, trismus and tetanus neonatorum. I will simply say that according to my investigations the same etiological cause is here existing and that tetanus neonatorum depends upon the introduction through the wound at the umbilicus of tetanus bacilli, the apparently widely distributed bacteria being planted, so to say, by means of unclean hands or unclean bandages, and after a short incubation the disease appears.—*Berlin. Klin. Wochens.*, No. 31, 1887.   O'C.

AMAUROSIS DUE TO EXHAUSTION.—Prof. Immermann, of Basle, reports a case of a boy aged 14½, received into the Basle clinic with typhoid and at the same time totally blind. He had received in the beginning of March, for the abdominal condition, calomel and jalap, which caused a severe diarrhœa lasting for two days. Having the notion that he was afflicted with a tape worm, the patient took also ten grams of ethereal extract of male fern, following which was a renewal of the diarrhœa and great prostration. On the following night there resulted complete amaurosis, which still existed at the time of the report. By the beginning of May there were evidences of double optic nerve atrophy. Immermann considers the affection to have been in the beginning a solely functional affection of the nervous visual aparatus, of diffuse nature, similar to amaurosis following severe hæmorrhage. This patient was in consequence of the profuse diarrhœas, the typhoid condition and febrile inanition, etc., in a state of severe exhaustion.—*Berlin. Klin. Wochens.*, 1887, No. 29.

THE GENESIS OF CHRONIC INTERSTITIAL PHOSPHORHEPATITIS.—Herr Kronig says : While the nature of acute phosphorus poisoning has been more completely brought within our knowledge by the work of prominent investigators, the same cannot be said in equal degree of *chronic* poisoning by phosphorus. Wegener, indeed, showed the changes in growing bone in this with great exactness, but gave less consideration to changes in the glandular organs, especially the liver. He declared the objective point of acute phosphorus poisoning to be the hepatic cell, that of chronic poisoning by phosphorus being the interstitial connective tissue. Kronig's conclusions read : That the anatomical changes in chronic phosphorus poisoning are : (I.) In a chronic necrotic process in the hepatic cell and probably also in the nucleus. (II.) In a hyaline degeneration occurring at the same time with this in the larger and smaller vessels. (III.) In a secondary proliferation of the interstitial tissue, which is to be considered as a simple reactive connective tissue hyperplasia not inflammatory in character.—*Berlin. Klin. Wochens.*, No. 31, 1887. O'C.

DIPHTHERIA CIRCUMSCRIPTA.—Mr. Alfred E. Barrett, in the *Brit. Med. Jour.*, of July 23d, writes that he has observed a "class of cases having all the essential characters of diphtheria, rapid and extreme exhaustion, and death by asthenia, preceded by convulsions." In cases of recovery the characteristic paralyses occur during convalescence from the throat affection. The local manifestation, however, instead of being an exudation, with a tendency to spread over the surface of the fauces, "is rather a circumscribed and ash colored slough on one or both tonsils. This slough remains stationary; forms a center from which the surrounding structures are invaded by a low form of inflammation, with swelling but no suppuration." He says the last case he saw was in a boy aged thirteen years. "In this case there was the circumscribed slough on one side only, and after its separation, a distinct pit or sulcus remained; convalescence was gradual but continuous for a fortnight or three weeks, when diplopia occurred, and the tongue, palate and the extremities were subsequently affected by paralysis, which came on while the patient was in the country, where he had gone to recruit his health."

DISTENSION OF TRANSVERSE NASAL VEIN IN CHILDREN.—Spicer, *Brit. Med. Jour.*, August 27th, 1887, refers to this condition shown by the black distended vein at the root of the nose, and overfilling of neighboring superficial veins, as being an accompaniment of an obstinate naso-pharyngeal catarrh, often with swollen middle turbinated bodies and rhinorrhœa, and chronic congestion or hypertrophy of the post-nasal mucosa, and frequently post-nasal vegetations. The condition is produced by obstruction to the venous outlet, through the spheno-palatine foramina and pharyngeal collaterals. It is a sign of disease of the post-nasal space, and leads to disease of the nasal turbinated bodies, impairment of nutrition of the bony and cartilaginous framework of the nose (causing the latter to remain sunken and ill shaped), to headache, drowsiness and a heavy appearance. The condition is often cured by removing the post-nasal vegetations or scraping off the hypertrophied post-nasal mucosa, especially in the region of the spheno-palatine foramina, this treatment being followed up by local application of some astringent pigment to the post-nasal space. Hygiene and good diet are important.—*Jour. of Laryngology and Rhinology*, September, 1887.

LUMINOUS MICRO-ORGANISMS.—Dr. C. B. Tilanus, who has been working in Prof. Forster's laboratory in Amsterdam, on culture preparations of luminous micro-organisms, gives an account of his researches in the *Weekblad van het Nederlandsch Tigdschrift voor Geneeskunke* of August 13th. He prepared a flat culture from luminous mucus, obtained from the exterior of fish, with fish broth peptone jelly, to which two per cent. common salt had been added as a medium. This became speckled with numerous cultures, some of the jelly, but not the greater part, becoming liquefied. In the dark this flat culture emitted a distinct light, and appeared as if strewn with stars. From this a stripe culture was prepared, and after successive preparations had been made, Dr. Tilanus believed he had obtained a pure culture of the phosphorescent organisms. They stained well with methyl violet or methylene blue. With a power of 1,000 diameters they appeared of ovoid form, with numerous clear, colorless points. A low temperature ($4°$ C.) was found to be most suitable for these cultures. Besides fish broth, potatoes sprinkled with salt were found to serve as a medium, but blood serum gave very unsatisfactory results.—*Brit. M. Jour.*, September 17th, 1887.

ORIGIN OF VERTIGO PARALYSANS.—Gerlier has described (*Revue Med. de la Suisse Romande*, No. 1, 1887) a new disease consisting of vertigo with a peculiar paralysis. In No. 5 of the same journal, Gerlier reports having met two cases, last winter, of slight degree, the hands becoming paretic only while milking, with transitory ptosis and amblyopia. The patients were cowherds who fell sick fourteen days after beginning to work in a cow-stall in which during the preceding summer five men were attacked by the same illness ; the individuals slept also in this stall. As the patients so far affected by the disease were cowherds, or those caring for their own cows, exclusively, Gerlier holds that the exciting cause of the disease must have existed in the stall. Dr. Haltenhoff, in *Progres Médical*, No. 26, 1887, reports nine cases of Gerlier's disease observed between 1874 and 1886, of which the first three came at the same time to the same house, the other cases being solitary both in time and location. The patients complained of dullness of the head, weakness of the whole body and showed lessened acuteness of vision ; single cases had double vision at different times. Ptosis, paresis of the flexors of the fingers, vertigo and falling, consciousness being retained, with peculiar turning of the head and trunk, and dysphagia, were other symptoms. Hysteria and malarial poisoning were excluded, and Haltenhoff agrees with Gerlier as to the cause being in some *materia peccans ;* he considers it to be a functional trouble which disappears upon change of residence and proper rest and are.—*Neurolog. Centralb.*, No. 14, 1887.   O'C.

PREVENTION OF LACERATED PERINEUM.—Dr. L. M. Bossi, (in the *Annali di Ostetricia et Ginacologia*) after reviewing the methods recommended to prevent laceration of the vulvar ring during labor, gives the results obtained by him by the following methods: The method used was that of manual extension of the fœtal head, and this can, according to the author, be managed in two equally advantageous ways. The woman is placed in dorsal decubitus, the pelvis being slightly raised. When the fœtal head appears at the vulva, the left hand of the accoucheur is applied to the vertex and presses back the fœtal part in such a manner as to obtain a gradual distension of the vulvo-vaginal strait. This Bossi denominates the period of *counter pressure.* When the posterior angle of the anterior fontanel is first felt by the index finger of the left hand, the right hand intervenes to perform *rectal expression,* as has been recommended by Olshausen and Ahlfeld, for deflexing the head. To this end one or two fingers are introduced into the rectum and caught wherever the forehead, mouth or chin of the fœtus can be felt through the recto-vaginal partition, thus serving to aid in the deflection of the head by pressing it upward and forward, while the left hand opposes the strong contractions. This manœuvre is ordinarily made in the interval between the contractions; but if the woman is instructed not to bear down much, or at all if expulsion is imminent, the manipulation may be resorted to during the pains. The objections to this method are its painfulness and the danger of lacerating the rectum, etc. To obviate these inconveniences, the method of *extra rectal expression,* as advocated by Ritken, may be substituted. In this, instead of introducing the fingers into the rectum, three fingers of the right hand are placed against that region lying between the anus and coccyx, and upward (*sic*) pressure is made against the fœtal forehead, which is easily felt in this region. The author's observations were made entirely on *primipara,* and in only two cases, where he used rectal expression, was the fourchette torn, and in these the laceration resulted not from the passage of the head, though the diameters in both were above normal, but from the passage of the shoulders. The necessity, therefore, for protection of the perineum during the expulsion of the shoulders and chest would seem to be apparent. By extra rectal expression only one case was lacerated, and that was the first time the method was used. In all other cases the perineum and vulvo-vaginal ring remained intact. A slight œdema of the fourchette was observed during the first few days following delivery in some cases.—*Gas. Méd. de Paris*, September 17th, 1887.

NEWS.

PERSONAL.—Dr. F. Parke Lewis, of Buffalo, N. Y., has been spending a week in New York City.

ALL news or matter relating to "Notes and Comments," should be sent to 161 West Seventy-first Street.

APPOINTMENT.—Dr. C. C. Huff, of Huron, Dakota, a prominent homœopathic physician, has been appointed President of the Territorial Health Board.

COLLEGE NEWS.—Dr. Philo L. Hatch, Dean of the Minnesota Homœopathic College, has resigned his position because of serious illness in his family necessitating removal. Dr. D. M. Goodwin has been elected in his stead.

AN obstinate pain in the back is often relived by oxalic acid. Ammon. carb. is said to be excellent for loss of voice. A paste made of bismuth subnitrate and water is claimed to be one of the best applications to swollen testicles.

PROPHYLAXIS OF CROUP.—Dr. Dumas believes that iodine given internally in quantities not exceeding eight drops daily, in orange flower water, sweetened with syrup, with a little iodide of potassium, prevents attacks of croup.—*Med. Reg.*

AN EXCUSABLE MISTAKE.—The four-year-old daughter of a Boston druggist was prepared to recite in Sabbath-school the " Search the Scriptures." When the teacher asked for her verse, however, she hesitated, then bravely uttered the verses " Hunt for the Prescription."—*Ex.*

MARRIAGES.—Clarence N. Payne, M.D., '85, married to Miss Eugenia McLean, daughter of Dr. D. C. McLean, Brooklyn, N. Y., on Wednesday, November 16th, 1887.—Miss Belle Middleton to Daniel R. Atwell, M.D., '85, Thursday Evening, October 26th, 1887, in First M. E. Church, Hoboken, N. J.

OBITUARY—DR. C. G. DAVIS.—Charles G. Davis, M.D., Class of '82, New York Homœopathic Medical College, died September 18th, 1887. Dr. Davis had established an excellent practice in Harlem and stood well in the profession. He was a member of the Alumni Association of the College, and also belonged to the Homœopathic County Medical Society.

IOWA UNIVERSITY.—Two additional full chairs have been created in the homœopathic department of the Iowa State University—a chair of surgery and a chair of obstetrics. Prof. J. G. Gilchrist has been selected to fill the first, and Dr. C. H. Cogswell the second. It is stated that arrangements are being made for a separate hospital distinctively homœopathic.

HOLMES ON ALLOPATHY.—" Now look at medicine by wigs, gold headed canes, Latin prescriptions, shops full of abominations, recipes a

yard long, 'curing' patients by drugging as sailors bring a wind by whist-
ling, selling lies at a guinea apiece—a routine, in short, of giving unfortunate sick people a mass of things either too odious to swallow or too acid
to hold; or if that were possible, both at once." (Professor at the
Breakfast Table)—*H. W.*

ON THE STUDY OF ANATOMY.—"I must no less commend the study
of anatomy, which whoever considers, I believe will never be an atheist;
the frame of man's body and coherence of his parts being so strange and
paradoxical, that I hold it to be the greatest marvel of nature; though when
all is done, I do not find that she hath made it so much as proof against
one disease, lest it should be thought to have made it no less than a
poison to the soul."—Lord Herbert of Cherbury (about 1630), *Homœopathic
World.*

OBITUARY—DR. C. O. NORTON.—Died at Bainbridge, N. Y., August
30th, 1887, Charles O. Norton, M.D., in the twenty-sixth year of his age.
The doctor was a graduate of Bellevue, and also of the New York Homœopathic Medical College, receiving his diploma from the latter institution
in 1885. At the time of his death he was assistant surgeon at the New
York Ophthalmic Hospital. Of a kindly, genial nature, not only will his
classmates of '85 deplore his loss, but a host of other friends will be sad-
dened by the intelligence of his death.

MARRIAGES—Miss Helen M. Cox, daughter of the Rev. Samuel Cox,
Rector of St. James' Protestant Episcopal Church at Newton, L. I., was
married on September 3d in St. Agnes Catholic Church, this city, to Dr.
Joseph T. O'Connor, of West Forty-sixth Street.—Mrs. Ellen L. Jackson an-
nounces the marriage of her daughter Lora to Dr. William W. Black-
man, Wednesday, September 14th, 1887, at Philadelphia.—Miss Helen S.
Hurd was married on September 21st to Dr. James A. Freer, Gilbertsville,
N. Y.—At Ironton, Ohio, September 26th, 1887, Miss Rosalie Hamilton to Dr.
N. L. MacBride.

PERSONAL.—Dr. Samuel Worcester left New England on August 16th
for his new home in El Cajou, San Diego County, Cal., where he proposes
to engage in the practice of his profession, and also interest himself
actively in fruit growing. He will have an office for consultation in the
City of San Diego. Dr. Worcester is well known to the profession as the
author of a standard work on Insanity and Nervous Disorders, and also as
the lecturer on Insanity in the Boston University School of Medicine for
several years past. The best wishes of his Eastern colleagues will follow
him to his new home.

OBITUARY—DR. BROWN.—Intelligence has been received of the death
of Titus L. Brown, M.D., of Binghamton, N. Y. Dr. Brown graduated at
Hahnemann Medical College of Philadelphia in 1853, and soon attained
prominence as a skillful practitioner. For many years he has been well
known not only at his chosen home, but in the profession at large. He
was a leading member of the State Homœopathic Society, and was also a
member of the American Institute of Homœopathy. A hard worker, an
earnest student of homœopathy, a public spirited citizen, a kind friend,
his death will be mourned by many.

SOCIETY ITEM.—At the regular quarterly meeting of the Albany County
Homœopathic Medical Society, held at Dr. Paine's office, Dr. Pratt described the main characteristics of a large morbid growth that had lately
come under his observation. Dr. Gorham reported the main features of
a similar case. Dr. Walde related in detail the history of a remarkable

case of typhoid fever complicated with pneumonia. Dr. Paine presented an extremely rare specimen of a degenerated ovary which he had recently obtained at a *post mortem*, the person having died of abdominal cancer. The next meeting will be held on the second Tuesday in January, 1888.

OPENING LECTURE.—The Introductory Lecture of the regular winter session at the New York Homœopathic Medical College, was delivered on Tuesday evening, October 4th, at eight P. M.. by Prof. Malcolm Leal, President of the Faculty, to a large and interested audience. His subject was "The Study of Medicine." At the close of the lecture, Dr. Allen, Dean of the Faculty, exhibited the plans for the new college buildings, and gave a brief account of the progress made during the summer. Great interest was manifested by those present in the plans of the new buildings and the progress of the work. The entering class is large and of good quality.

NEW JERSEY STATE SOCIETY.—The semi-annual meeting of the New Jersey State Homœopathic Medical Society will be held at the Winsor Hotel, Atlantic City, N. J., Wednesday and Thursday, October 5th and 6th, commencing at 11.30 A. M. Clarence W. Butler, of Montclair, is President of the Society, and an interesting session may be expected. Among the papers promised are "The Diagnostic Significance of the Epithelia," by Drs. Youngman and Baily, Atlantic City; "Diagnosis of Typhoid Fever," by E. M. Howard, M.D., Camden; "Homœopathy and Intermittent Fever," by Dr. Samuel Long, New Brunswick; and "The Contamination and Analysis of Drinking Water," by Ch. F. Adams, M.D., Hackensack.

THE STATE SOCIETY.—The papers presented at the recent meeting of the Homœopathic Medical Society of the State of New York were of exceptional interest and the discussions pointed and vigorous. Dr. Paine's administration seemed to have given general satisfaction. On Tuesday evening a collation was served, and when the cigars were reached, Dr. Paine, after a neat little prologue, called upon some of the veterans present to give some of their experiences. Drs. Ball, McMurray and Moffat responded, and portrayed the practice of medicine when homœopathy was in its earliest infancy. Quite a number of applications for membership were received, and on Wednesday the Society adjourned, after a most pleasant and successful session.

THE BRITISH HOMŒOPATHIC CONGRESS.—The meeting of the Congress this year was of special interest because of the opening of the new Hahnemann Hospital, the gift of Mr. Tate to the citizens of Liverpool. The attendance was satisfactory and the papers presented of exceptional value. The President's address was upon "Therapeutic Changes in General Medicine During the Victorian Era; Their Meaning and Lesson for Homœopaths." Dr. J. G. Hayward read a paper on "The Use of Drugs in Surgical Practice," and Dr. Proctor gave some "Practical Observations on Ammonia." The Congress elected Dr. Dyce Brown President for 1888, and selected Birmingham as the place of meeting. On the 23d of September the Hospital was formally opened in the presence of a large audience.

SANTONIN.—In order to obtain its vermicidal effect it must be administered in such a form that it will not be acted upon by the gastric juice. It has been proved by experiment that santonin, when given in an oily solution, is not at all absorbed in the stomach, the entire quantity passing into the intestine; and Küchenmeister has shown that while ascarides are not affected by santonin crystals floating in water, they are killed when brought in contact with an oily solution of the drug. In such a solution any form of oil may be used, and the best effect is obtained by three grains of santonin dissolved in two ounces of oil, to be taken in four doses. It is good practice to add one drop of wormseed oil to each dose, all volatile oils being poisonous to the lower organisms. If movement of the bowels is desired, castor oil will be suitable, although in not too large a dose, because with too strong peristalsis the santonin does not remain long enough in the intestine to produce the desired effect. About two drachms of the oil to each dose will be sufficient.—*Practitioner.*

ONE THOUSAND POUNDS REWARD.—It is stated in the *Homœopathic World* that the "Grocers' Company" have offered a thousand pounds reward for the discovery of " a method by which the vaccine contagion may be cultivated apart from the animal body, in some medium or media not otherwise zymotic; the method to be such, that the contagion may by means of it be multiplied to an indefinite extent in successive generations and that the product, after any number of such generations, shall prove itself of identical potency with standard vaccine lymph." A correspondent claims that the question is not an open one, as an artificial vaccine lymph prepared by dissolving tartarized antimony or tartar emetic in glycerine fulfills all the conditions laid down by the Grocers' Company. He supports his assertion by quotations from eminent authorities. However, this may be the action of the "Grocers' Company " in offering a substantial reward as an encentive to original investigation cannot but be approved. It is an example that may be followed with profit and honor by other bodies organized not on a commercial but on a scientific basis.

TOBACCO POISONING.—For the treatment of chronic nicotism, Favarger recommends as prophylactic means: (1) Never to smoke when the stomach is empty, but always after a meal. In this way the number of cigars smoked will be limited, the nicotine will be made to act on a full stomach, loss of appetite will be prevented, and the antidotal action of the tannin, contained in the wine, coffee or tea, will be obtained. (2) Smokers should avoid holding their cigars long in their mouths. (3) Cigar holders should be frequently renewed and regularly cleaned. Smokers should smoke the milder cigars occasionally instead of always choosing the strongest. According to Erlenmeyer, smoking cigars is vastly more injurious than smoking a pipe, because the preparation of tobacco for the latter purpose destroys as much as two-thirds of its nicotine, while the former loses but little of its active principle in the manufacture. More than twenty-five years ago Dr. Richardson presented the following conclusions as the result of an exhaustive study of the effects of tobacco poisoning: (1) The effects produced are very transitory. (2) The evils of smoking are functional in their character and statements that it causes insanity, epilepsy, chorea, apoplexy, organic disease of the heart, and consumption, are devoid of fact. (3) The habit of smoking is deleterious to the young. (4) Tobacco is a luxury, but probably the least hurtful of luxuries. Stillé, in commenting on these propositions, remarks that there are several diseases not enumerated by Dr. Richardson, which excessive smoking unquestionably develops. One of them is amaurosis, many cases of which have been traced to tobacco smoking by no less competent authorities than Mackenzie and Sichel. The former, not many years ago, hinted his suspicion that it is a frequent cause of amaurosis, and the latter is now of the opinion that there are few persons who have smoked during a long period more than five drachms of tobacco per diem without having vision, and frequently memory, impaired.—*Medical Record.*

OPENING OF AN INTRACRANIAL ABSCESS, WITH CURE.—At a Society Meeting in Berlin, Köhler presented a patient, aged eighteen, who went through an attack of measles in January of the present year. This was followed by abscess of the middle ear, which was relieved by spontaneous rupture of the drum membrane, but no alleviation of the patient's symptoms, or lowering of temperature, resulted, and when, after some days, opening of the mastoid bone was determined on, a sudden change for the better seemed to make it undesirable. For fourteen days the patient was without fever, had only slight headache, and his general condition was greatly bettered. In the next week there was increase of temperature, and a small swelling was noticed on the mastoid process. Violent headache returned, and a new symptom, vertigo, was observed. Incision was now made into the mastoid process, and the neighboring bony parts were laid bare as well. A small amount of pus was found, four centimetres behind the posterior border of the meatus auditorius, thus beyond the process itself. After cleansing, a small hole, the size of a pin's head, was found in the external table, from which the pus came. With hammer and chisel the opening was enlarged at this part, and the pus evacuated from the intracranial abscess, to the amount of a tablespoonful. The trephining had to be done wiih great care, as the site of the opening corresponded to that of the transverse sinus. The abscess lay between the dura mater and the bone and had encroached upon the sinus. A communication between it and the external ear was demonstrated by injection into the pus cavity of antiseptic fluid, which ran out of the external meatus. Hemorrhage was considerable and was stopped by antiseptic tamponade. Headache and vertigo disappeared after the evacuation, as also did the fever. Within fourteen days after the operation the wound had closed, and within three weeks there was only a linear scar to be seen as the evidence of surgical interference.—*Berlin Klin. Wochens*, No. 33, 1887. O'C.

New Homœopathic Hospital at Leipzig.—For an account of the dedication of this new hospital we are indebted to Dr. W. Y. Cowl, who writes as follows : " In answer to your request for some news from this quarter, allow me to send you the following extract from the *Leipsiger Tageblatt*, which will give you an idea of one of the most interesting occurrences of late with reference to homœopathy on this side of the water. The date above, as many of your readers may be aware, is the anniversary of Hahnemann's graduation dissertation, and upon it each year the Central Homœopathic Society holds its annual meeting in one of the cities of Germany, Austro-Hungary or Switzerland." " In the presence of many homœopathic physicians as well as delegates from homœopathic societies in different parts of Germany, was held this morning (August 10th), the dedicating exercises of the newly founded Homœopathic Hospital." "We say newly founded, for it is not the first institution of its kind which Leipzig has seen within its walls, and it may be pointed out in this place that the first homœopathic institution of relief in Leipzig (as well as in Germany) was established in 1833, but because of various exigencies closed its existence in 1837." "What, beyond a doubt, the inaugural festivities of the new Homæopathic Hospital import, is the addition of a lasting medical institution to our city, and they form thus an occasion of importance. After the singing of the choral ' *Nun danket Alle Gott*,' speeches were made by several gentlemen. The principal address was delivered by Dr. von Weber, of Cologne. He closed as follows : ' But all these expectations, hopes and wishes are suppositions, and it remains with the medical faculty here in Leipzig to carry out their victorious emulation in the clinic. As for us, we entertain no doubt but that this emulation will result happily; the results of which will rest upon competent supervision, and should also be laid openly before the studying physician of all schools by a well informed and apprehensive arrangement. We therefore bespeak the greatest attention to management, which in the arrangement of the hospital should conform to the furthest warrantable claims of the present time with reference to health therein.' "

OURSELVES AS OTHERS SEE US.—The New York *Commercial Advertiser* lately published the following article : " The International Medical Congress, now in session at Washington, is composed of unusually learned, able and intelligent men. They have dived deeply into the hidden nature of things ; they have studied hard ; they have investigated closely substances that are too infinitesimal to be apprehended by the unassisted senses ; they are fired by an insatiable ambition to know more and more. Why is it then that they seem to know so little ? They write whole libraries on otology, and gynæcology, and laryngology, and bacteriology, and various other ologies, which the average educated man can neither define nor spell, and can hardly manage to pronounce ; they have more drugs and surgical instruments and healing appliances of all sorts, than there are hairs on a normal head; and still they cannot, except in rare instances, keep a man in normal health, even if the patient does exactly as he is told to do. We do not require the impossible. We must all die and no one will blame the doctors for failing to preserve life indefinitely, or for being unable to avert fatal consequences in the case of a severe accident or disease. The question is not so much ' Why don't we get well ?' as ' Why don't we keep well ?' People are seldom downright ill but they are perpetually ailing. Why cannot the doctors stop this ? It is fair to assume that they cannot because they certainly do not. The preservation of health is largely a matter of personal habits. It depends greatly on our way of eating, drinking and taking care of the body generally. But there is no subject on which the doctors differ more hopelessly than on this. Some recommend tea and coffee; others denounce them as poisons. Some permit tobacco and alcohol in moderation; others forbid them entirely. Some say that pork and ham though hard to digest are still useful foods; others declare that no pig meat or anything derived from the pig is fit to be eaten. Some advise fruit only before breakfast; others only after dinner. Some depreciate the vegetables; others extol them as a main reliance. Some counsel bathing in cold water; others in warm or tepid. Some say we must sleep with the windows open always; others limit this injunction to the summer season. It is scarcely an exaggeration to say that no two doctors will give you the same instruction as to the commonest physical habits of life. Now, messieurs the doctors, it is all very well for you to raise men from the dead, and to cure violent diseases, and to be letter-perfect on sarcoma of the larynx, and the bacteriology of aural furuncle; but what we want to know is what shall we eat ? and what shall we drink ? and wherewithal shall we be clothed ? The Gentiles are seeking after all these things, and they propose to find them out too. It surely ought to be possible for the doctors at this late day, to tell definitely whether coffee is a food or a poison, and how a sleeping apartment ought to be ventilated. It will not do to fall back on the old excuse that what is one man's drink is another man's poison. Constitutions differ doubtless, but not to that extent. Any particular chemical substance—nicotine or alcohol for example—has a certain fixed unvarying effect on every normal mucous membrane, and that effect must be either beneficial or deleterious to the membrane and the system. Which is it, messieurs the doctors ? " *N. Y. Med. Journal, Atlanta Med. and Surg. Journal.*

VOL. XXXV.   *DECEMBER, 1887.*   (Volume II, Third Series.)   No. 12.

NORTH AMERICAN
JOURNAL OF HOMŒOPATHY.

ORIGINAL ARTICLES IN MEDICINE.

MALARIAL COMPLICATIONS OF THE PUERPERAL STATE.*

By L. L. DANFORTH, M.D.,

New York.

I DESIRE to call the attention of this Society to a class of cases not infrequently met with in obstetrical practice, characterized by a peculiar form of febrile disturbance which usually sets in within the first week of the puerperal period, and simulates in some of its manifestations true puerperal septicæmia. So close is the resemblance of this post-partum fever to the true septic fever of child-bed, that experienced practitioners are sometimes in doubt as to the nature of the affection in question, and it is only after the most careful analysis of the local and general symptoms, combined with a knowledge of the history of the patient, and a consideration of all corroborating circumstances, that a true solution of the case can be reached.

Doubtless many members of this Society have seen such cases, for they are not uncommon in this city, where malaria abounds. Notwithstanding its frequency very little has appeared on the subject in current literature, and the entire omission of the subject from the pages of most of the standard text-books on midwifery is surprising.

Nearly all authors speak of malarial complications of pregnancy, which in my experience are very rarely seen, while malarial complications of the puerperal state of vastly more frequent occurrence are almost wholly neglected.

A paper by Fordyce Barker, M.D., entitled " Puerperal Malarial Fever,"† first called attention to the condition as a complication of the puerperium.

Dr. Barker says: " The title of this paper is one not yet adopted in medical literature in the nomenclature of diseases, but it is so sig-

---

*Read before the Hom. Med. Society, County of New York, Nov. 10th, 1887.
†American Journal of Obstetrics, Vol. XIII., 1880, p. 271.

nificant a term, as descriptive of the etiology, pathology and clinical phenomena of a class of affections in late years frequently met with in puerperal women in this city and vicinity, that I have for several years made use of it." * * * * "The occurrence of chills, a high temperature, rapid pulse and great depression of the vital forces in a puerperal woman, must inevitably cause anxiety in the mind of her medical attendant; and this anxiety must be greatly increased if there be also some indications of a local pelvic phlegmasia, or the foregoing phenomena are followed by such grave complications as mania, secondary hemorrhage, and the development some days after parturition of extremely offensive lochia. Hence the great importance of being able to decide whether the symptoms be due to one of the puerperal diseases strictly so-called, such as epidemic puerperal fever, septicæmia, phlebitis or metritis, or whether it be due to constitutional infection from telluric or atmospheric causes, acting upon a system whose physiological condition is modified by the various changes which are taking place during puerperal convalescence."

Playfair is the only author within my knowledge who mentions this form of malarial manifestation. He says, "It is especially apt to be confounded with septicæmia, and is met with in women who have been exposed to malarial poison during their former lives, the recurrence of the fever being probably determined by the puerperal state. The diagnosis is not always easy."

Robert Barnes merely mentions malarious influences as among the conditions that may disturb the orderly course of puerpery.

Emanuel Goth, of Germany, says, "Very frequently women fall ill of malaria in the puerperal condition who were well during pregnancy, and the malaria is often of a severe type. Puerperæ possess a great disposition to malaria, even those who formerly successfully resisted the disease. It even happens that women who never suffer from malaria are affected by it only during their lying-in period." (*Zeit. f. Geb. u. Gyn.*, VI., I.)

The truth of Playfair's statement that the recurrence of the fever is probably determined by the puerperal state, has been abundantly proved to me by numerous instances in practice.

The term "latent malaria" has suggested itself to my mind as an appropriate expression to indicate the fact that the woman has had malaria in the system throughout pregnancy, and that it has remained quiescent until after child-birth. The "latency" of the poison may be, and probably is, accounted for by the fact that in pregnancy there is a state of high nervous and vascular tension; after parturition, in the puerperal state, there is low nervous and vascular tension. As

Robert Barnes has graphically described it, the balance of osmosis in the gravid woman is centrifugal, in the puerperal woman it is centripetal. Hence in the former, the system is fortified against the reception of various infectious diseases, as the malarial poison ; while in the latter, she is especially prone to their influence manifested in their typical or some modified forms.

The majority of the patients that I have seen, who had malarial disease subsequent to confinement, were entirely free from any suspicion of the trouble prior to that event. Occasionally a patient will admit having had malaria at some time previous to pregnancy, but more frequently there is no knowledge of the existence of such a condition of the system. If the woman has ever been subject to the influence of malaria it is apt to make itself felt in the lying-in state.

The occurrence of a sharp chill with high fever at a time when the system of the woman is most likely to be affected by the absorption of putrid material from the genital tract (auto-infection), or by the inception of disease germs from without (hetero-infection), is certainly calculated to produce the most serious apprehensions as to the true nature of the attack.

As an example of malaria manifesting itself in a puerpera the following interesting case is cited :

CASE I.—Mrs. M——, aged 23, second pregnancy. Enjoyed good health during present pregnancy, with the exception of obstinate constipation, and in the latter months, on account of the unusual enlargement of the abdomen. considerable distress in walking and in breathing ; also cold perspirations, coming on at night during sleep. The great enlargement of the abdomen gave rise to the suspicion that twins were present *in utero,* and an examination by palpation and auscultation in the last weeks of gestation revealed unmistakably two fœtal heart sounds, one of 140 and the other of 120 pulsations per minute, the position of the children corresponding to the first vertex, and the first breech presentations, respectively. Labor began on the morning of September 4th, 1887, continuing six hours, and terminating in the birth of two girls, weighing, respectively, seven and eight pounds. The first was a vertex and the second a footling presentation. Two placentas came away entire, with no hemorrhage. Firm contraction of the uterus followed the administration of a half-drachm of the fluid extract of ergot. After the completion of the labor all went well with the exception of severe after pains, and an unnaturally rapid pulse, until the morning of the fourth day at 9 A. M., when a temperature of 101° was observed ; at 10 P. M. it had reached 102⅘°, and the patient was at this time suffering from a severe headache. *Antipyrine,* 10 grains, was then given by the husband of the patient, who is a physician, and who assisted in the treatment throughout. Profuse perspiration followed the administration of the medicine, the fever abated, and the headache was soon entirely relieved.

September 9th.—*Temperature normal,* and continued so throughout the day.

September 10th, 9 A. M.— Temperature 100; intense pain in lower right inguinal region, at times sharp and lancinating, with tenderness on pressure. Vaginal examination reveals a slight puffiness, which is quite sensitive to pressure in the direction of the right broad ligament. Lochia, very scanty, though not offensive. *Bryonia* 1 x was prescribed every half-hour. *10 P. M.*—Temperature 103⅘. Headache severe. Pains in right inguinal region about the same. *Antipyrine* was again administered with relief to the headache, profuse perspiration and lowering of the temperature.

September 11th, 8 A. M.—*Temperature normal.*

September 11th, 10 A. M.—Severe chill, lasting half an hour, with a temperature of 101°. *Lochia scanty and offensive.* Pain in opposite inguinal regions continued, with same dullness and tenderness on pressure as was noticed the preceding day. Vaginal examination shows tenderness to touch in region of both broad ligaments. Uterus now washed out with solution of the bichloride of mercury, 1 to 5,000.

Six grains of the sulphate of quinine were then given and the *bryonia* continued. The quinine was given to antidote the evident malarial complication, which was believed to be present in the case. At this time in the history the diagnosis was not at all satisfactorily defined. The intermission in the fever on the 9th inst. (the fifth day of the disease), and also on the morning of the 11th, was decidedly characteristic of malaria, at the same time the local pelvic symptoms were of such a character as to make the possibility of a septic element in the case exceedingly alarming.

On the evening of this day (the 11th), 10 P. M., the temperature was 103⅘°. Did not deem it advisable to give any more antipyrine, on account of its masking influence on the character of the fever. *Bryonia* was continued in alternation with *veratrum vir.* once in half an hour.

September 12th, *8 A. M.*—Temperature normal. Pains in inguinal region relieved. *Quinia,* grs. xii., given. *Bryonia* continued.

1 P. M.—Temperature 100°. Intra-uterine injection of bichloride solution 1 to 5,000 given.

10 P. M.—Temperature 102°. Medicine continued and a second douche given.

September 13th, *8 A. M.*—Temperature 101°. A circumscribed tumor, about three inches in diameter, discovered in the right inguinal region, above Poupart's ligament.

9 A. M.—Swelling entirely disappeared after the escape of considerable gas per rectum.

1 P. M.—Temperature 102°. Flatulent pains in different parts of abdomen, otherwise better, except extreme thirst. *Bryonia* 1 x continued.

10 P. M.—Temperature 104°. Pains in inguinal region much better. Intra-uterine injection of bichloride solution.

September 14th, 9 A. M.—Temperature normal, and continued so throughout the day. *Quiniæ,* grs. xii. given. Injection of bichloride repeated.

September 15th, 9 A. M.—Temperature normal. Quiniæ, grs. xii.
"   "   1 P. M.—   "   100°.
"   "   10 P. M.—   "   101°.
"   16th, 10 A. M.—   "   normal. Quiniæ, grs. xii.
Temperature did not rise above normal after this date. Throughout the whole course of this fever the flow of milk was not diminished, being sufficient for the nourishment of both children. Diet exclusively liquid throughout. Bovinine, milk, chocolate, beef tea, etc.

There is no doubt that the fever in this case was telluric in origin, as evidenced by the marked intermissions which occurred at first on alternate days, then in the morning of successive days. But in addition to this fever there was a local condition which simulated closely the simplest form of puerperal septicæmia.

It is comparatively easy, now, on reviewing the history of this case, to see that the malarial element predominated. During its daily progress, however, the existence of severe pelvic pain, first in the region of the right broad ligament, then in the left ; suppression of the lochia, and afterward the discharge of foul-smelling muco-sanguinolent material, made the condition appear alarmingly like a septic endometritis of the catarrhal form, with a co-existing parametritis, or lymphangitis. It was to meet the latter phases of the disease that the intra-uterine douche was given, and to this cleansing we attribute in part the gratifying result obtained. It is altogether probable that the local disturbance was due to the influence of a vitiated state of the blood (owing to the presence of miasmatic germs) acting upon organs which were undergoing marked organic changes, retrogressive in character, hence especially liable to take on diseased action, and *not* to the influence of specific disease germs received by absorption through the genital tract.

A case of pernicious remittent fever after parturition, reported by J. Lewis Smith, M.D.,* of this city, is worthy to be cited in connection with this subject.

"Patient was a primipara, æt. twenty years. Delivered on May 22d, 1882, after a labor of thirteen hours, by means of short forceps. No laceration of perineum, and no hemorrhage. Pulse was unnaturally quick during first days after confinement. On second day patient had a discharge of pure fresh blood, not offensive. Vagina washed out with carbolic water. May 24th.—Forty-three hours after labor, lochia normal, patient had a rigor, not severe, and this was followed by more marked evidence of fever. Temperature did not rise above 102°. No abdominal pain, tenderness or headache. In a few hours the moderate febrile movement which followed the rigor diminished, and no unfavorable symptoms were observed the following day (May

*Am. Jour. of Obstetrics, Vol. 16, p. 154.

25th), except the slight fever. But on the 26th another chill occurred, and from this time without any appreciable local cause fever of a remittent type continued. At some time each day the patient experienced a chilly sensation, followed by a febrile exacerbation which continued several hours and ended in a free perspiration. The temperature in the first week did not at any time rise above 101 to 101½°. So mild was the beginning, and so gradual the development of this case, that danger was not suspected until May 28th, when the paroxysm of fever became more pronounced and of longer duration. Professor Lusk was called in consultation, and after a careful examination could discover nothing in the state of the uterus and its appendages. Professor Fordyce Barker saw the patient and concurred in the opinion that the uterine system was not in fault. Notwithstanding the most skillful treatment the chills occurred each day at irregular intervals, and the fever gradually became more intense and prolonged. Sometimes two distinct chills would occur at different times in the course of the same day, as in some cases of undoubted pernicious malarial fever.

"Temperature, during last week, succeeding each chill rose to 103°, 104° or 105°, and toward the close of life to 107°. Finally remissions were shorter, perspiration during abatement of fever was more profuse than at first, drenching the underdress and pillow, and cooling the surface. Patient became despondent toward the close of life, and on the seventeenth day after her confinement *muguet* appeared over the faucial surface, a sure forerunner, in Dr. Smith's opinion, of a fatal ending in febrile and chronic maladies.

"Up to this time there had been no abdominal tenderness or distension, but on this day, and until death, the abdomen was considerably distended, but without tenderness. Overcome by the violence and long continuance of the fever, the patient died on the eighteenth day after confinement."

In discussing the history of this case Dr. Smith says, "In my attendance upon the present case, although having the utmost regard for the opinions of the distinguished consulting physicians, I could not discard the thought that perhaps we were contending against a case of septic poisoning, until the occurrence of another case of genuine malarial disease in a member of the same household removed the doubt." Subsequent to the report of this case a criticism appeared in the same periodical (*American Journal of Obstetrics*) written by a physician who maintained that the case as published presented all the symptoms of septicæmia, except fetor of the lochia, and this he argued was prevented by the use of vaginal injections. The preliminary conditions (inertia, hemorrhage and laceration), the insidious onset, the marked and irregular remissions and exacerbations, the failure of quinine, and the fatal termination, seemed conclusive evidence of the truth of this theory.

That it is possible for such doubts to exist as were raised in the minds of the attending physicians, and by the other physician who ventured to question the diagnosis, only shows that these cases of post-partum fever sometimes require the most careful differentiation to classify them as they deserve.

The following case in my own practice is a more common example of malarial infection complicating the lying-in state:

CASE II.—Mrs. G———; third confinement, labor natural, and no lacerations of soft parts. No unusual symptoms until forty-eight hours after birth of child, when patient was seized with a violent chill, followed by a high fever, the temperature rising to 105½, pulse 130. Accompanying this the patient complained of a severe pain in *left* iliac region. No alteration of the lochia, and no uterine tenderness. *Verat. viride* was given in water every half hour, one teaspoonful at a dose, and in the course of six hours there was a decided improvement. On account of the pelvic pain a suspicion was aroused as to the pelvic origin of the chill, and it was feared that the attack was inflammatory in character. But the marked subsidence of the fever within twelve hours, coming down to 100°, and on the following day to nearly normal, with corresponding diminution of the pelvic pain, indicated that the remedy given had either cut short a sharp inflammatory attack, or else that the pain and local disturbance was resultant from, and not a cause of, the chill. If the latter, it was probable that there might be a recurrence of the attack, as malaria was the most probable cause for such a chill and fever, after the exclusion of local inflammation. Forty-eight hours from the first chill a second chill of equal violence with the first, together with high fever and local pain, occurred. A large dose of quinine (ten grains) was followed by a reduction in all the symptoms. Another dose of quinine was given the following day. On the alternate day a third, but very slight, chill was noticed, with less fever than before. Quinine was again given, and continued daily until complete convalescence was established.

Several cases of this character have come under my personal observation, and could be cited were it necessary to further exemplify this subject.

Symptoms.—Like most febrile attacks in the puerperal state, a sharp chill, or chilly sensations, mark the inception of the disease. Fever, which quickly runs up to a very high point, 104° or 105°, is the immediate sequence of the chill. In some cases there is pelvic pain, and when present it is an added source of anxiety, since it naturally leads one to fear that an inflammatory process in the pelvic system is the origin of the chill and fever. Fortunately our fears are soon allayed, for such an explosion of striking and alarming symptoms is usually followed by a marked remission of the fever within a period of from twelve to twenty-four hours. This feature is quite characteristic of malarial diseases under all circumstances, as is well known, and as a complication of the puerperal state, forms no exception to the rule.

If, after the occurrence of such a remission, there is still any doubt as to the nature of the affection, the repetition of the chill or the increase in the fever will soon dispel the uncertainty, for one or the other of these events generally follows. The succession of phenomena just described only occurs, however, in typical cases. In the first case cited in this paper there was no preliminary chill, and the onset of the fever was gradual. The first and only chill occurred on the seventh day after confinement. In many cases, three or four days before the explosion, the patient complains of malaise, pain in head, back and limbs; sleeplessness, thirst, and loss of appetite. If chills occur they are mild, and the temperature does not run so high, and the pulse is less rapid, and the remission is less marked than in the typical forms of the disease.

In this asthenic and more obstinate febrile disease, the patient is dull, heavy and sleepy, with moderate wandering delirium. If in addition to the above there be diarrhœa, the most experienced observer will wait, as Professor Barker says, for further developments, before he decides whether he has to deal with a case of septicæmia or of puerperal malarial fever. In order to place the differential points between these two affections side by side so that they can be studied more intelligently I have arranged the salient features in parallel columns, as follows:

MALARIAL PUERPERAL FEVER.	PUERPERAL SEPTICÆMIA AND PELVIC INFLAMMATION.
May come on as early as the first day, or as late as the twenty-first day. Instances of both the earliest and latest period of development are recorded.	Attack usually occurs from third to fifth day; rarely after this time. When the disease manifests itself after the sixth day, however closely the symptoms resemble septicæmia, the fear of this may with considerable degree of certainty be dismissed, since by this time the placental site and all lacerated surfaces are covered by protective granulations.
Usually sets in with a chill or chilly sensations, followed by fever, often with a temperature one or two degrees higher than is found in the beginning of any other puerperal disease.	Chills followed by fever, which in nearly all the forms of puerperal fever does not reach its height until the evening of the second to fourth day.

Onset is often preceded or marked by pain in back, head and limbs.	Onset is free from these symptoms.
It matters not how high the temperature, or rapid the pulse, or seemingly grave the condition of the patient at the onset, the symptoms under malarial causation rapidly improve in from twelve to twenty-four hours; the remission or intermission becomes decided.	There may be a remission, but the course of the fever is pretty steadily upward until the highest point is reached, and the decline to normal is quite as gradual. In septicæmia the temperature may rapidly decline, but the pulse will increase in frequency, and the general condition of the patient grow more serious.
Sensibilities morbidly acute.	Sensibilities blunted.
Pelvic pain is exceptional in uncomplicated malarial puerperal fever.	Uterine tenderness and sensitiveness in broad ligaments always present.
Lochia not offensive, and free as usual ; or if diminished not offensive.	Lochia suppressed, or offensive discharges from uterus.
Lacteal secretion unaltered.	Lactation suppressed.

In addition to the symptoms which have been given, the occurrence of secondary hemorrhage, apparently as a result of the fever, was noted in five cases seen by Professor Barker. The first case reported in this paper suffered a hemorrhage moderate in degree.

Two of the cases alluded to by Professor Barker had alarming hemorrhage, in the other three it was slight only for several days.

Treatment.—The treatment may be well described as symptomatic and specific. For the former such remedies as meet individual symptoms will be called for, such as *bryonia, belladonna, baptisia, arsenic, nux vomica, ipecac, veratrum alb.* and *viride.* These theoretically ought to be sufficient to cure the whole disease, but practically they modify symptomatic conditions, while the febrile paroxysm usually continues, or the fever recurs, if it has for an interval disappeared, until quinine is administered in decided doses. In all the cases, which I have seen, quinine has been the remedy that I have relied upon to break the paroxysm. The system of the puerperal woman seems to be especially sensitive to the action of quinine, and its effects here have been more gratifying than in any other class of malarial affections for which I have ever given the drug. In proportion as the case presents the typical manifestations of malaria, *vis.*, the pronounced chill, high fever and marked remission, or intermission, may we expect a marked effect from quinine.

In those cases which come on gradually with prodromal symptoms, and which eventuate in the low type of fever described, quinine is not so effective, and we have to rely upon *arsenic, baptisia, bryonia, gels.* and other remedies.

My own opinion concerning quinine is, that it is "homœopathic," as we term it, or indicated according to the law of similars, in those marked and typical cases of malarial infection, in the cure of which it so often proves effective. An analysis of the symptoms of the drug as they appear in the "Guiding Symptoms," by Hering, will show their applicability to cases having a marked periodicity in the appearance of the chill, fever and sweat; while we all recognize its usefulness in "cachectic persons who have suffered from loss of blood, or from continued and long prostration." Surely the puerperal woman represents these conditions. If the use of quinine is considered by some as empirical practice, and following too closely in the footsteps of our old-school brethren, the probability that the drug is useful only in proportion to its similarity should be carefully thought of. The quantity of the drug used is a matter of secondary importance.

SOME POINTS IN THE TREATMENT OF GASTRIC DISORDERS.*

By CLARENCE BARTLETT, M.D.,

Philadelphia.

IN the following pages it is my intention to review briefly some points having a practical bearing on the treatment of gastric disorders. No attempt will be made to deal with the subject exhaustively. Were I disposed to do so, such attempt would be futile, as the time of the Society would not permit of such trespass. First, I will speak of the use of water. A more practical point than this I know not. The importance of water in the treatment of the gastro-intestinal troubles of infants was brought very forcibly to my mind in two cases which I treated three years ago. Both patients belonged to the poorer classes; water had been kept from both as an injurious

---

*Read before the Homœopathic Medical Society, State of Pennsylvania, September 21st, 1887.

article ; both were apparently dead when brought under observation ; in both, the administration of water in the form of ice produced marvelous results. In the case of one, who had been vomiting for two or three days, and who, as already intimated, had been reduced to an almost lifeless state, consciousness returned almost immediately, and ultimate recovery took place. In the second case, improvement was also marked, although but temporary.

The drinking of a glass of water immediately on rising in the morning is, in many cases of gastric disease, of inestimable value. As is well known, the mucous membrane of the stomach is well covered with a layer of mucus in the morning. The ingestion of a glass of water serves to remove this and to prepare the way for the ready digestion of the morning meal.

The drinking of a glass of water on retiring at night and another on rising in the morning, is a popular and effectual method of combating the constipation which is a frequent accompaniment of dyspepsia.

Next, I would refer to the use of water in the operation of washing out the stomach, technically known as *lavage*. This is a therapeutic procedure, the full value of which I am satisfied has not yet been fully developed. It has already served me well in two cases. The first of these I reported in detail in the *Hahnemannian Monthly* for April, 1887. Briefly, the points of the case were as follows : A woman aged 43 years has been suffering with uncontrollable vomiting and headache, in association with a high degree of vertigo, for nearly one year. It was suspected that she had a tumor of the brain. Her breath, however, was horribly offensive, her tongue very heavily coated, and the vomited matters had a sour, putrid odor. The bowels were constipated. She had undergone marked emaciation and was unable to get out of bed without assistance. Within ten days after beginning the *lavage*, both headache and vomiting ceased. The operation was continued for some three months, when the patient was considered as cured of her stomach trouble, although she was treated for three or four months longer for atrophy of both optic nerves but without any benefit. It is now nearly ten months since the washing out of the stomach was discontinued in this case and the patient still remains free from headache, vomiting and vertigo. She has gained in weight and is enabled to take long walks without fatigue. The theory that I have always held respecting the origin of the intense headache and vertigo in the above case, is that these symptoms were the direct result of systemic poisoning by the absorption of food decomposing in the stomach by reason of too long detention in that viscus.

The second case in which I have used *lavage* was one of hysterical vomiting. The patient was a young woman of 27 years. Her
symptoms were so numerous that a description of them covered six
pages of foolscap paper. The improvement in this case was also
marked, although by no means as rapid as in the preceding one.
The matters removed from the stomach by the operation had an intensely sour odor.

Lavage is especially indicated in gastric disorders in which food is
forced to remain longer in the stomach than it should normally, and
in cases of chronic gastric catarrh with excessive production of mucus.
Under the first of these heads we may include dilatation of the stomach,
pyloric obstruction from any cause, and cancer of the stomach. It
has also been highly recommended in various forms of vomiting arising from nervous causes, and in the vomiting of pregnancy. In cases
of the latter trouble I have not yet had the opportunity of employing
the operation, and so cannot speak of its use here from personal experience. The quantity of water used at a sitting has been with me
about one gallon. One quart of water was introduced and then
allowed to flow off by siphonage, when the process was repeated
again and again until the water returned from the stomach was perfectly clear. At first the operation was made difficult because of the
vomiting excited by the presence of the tube in the pharynx and
stomach. Toleration of this irritation is soon secured, however, after
which one meets with but little trouble. The patient soon learns to
use the tube himself. Sometimes, while the water is flowing from
the stomach, the tube becomes obstructed. In such cases one must
dislodge the foreign body either by pouring in more water or removing the tube. In some cases I have been able to dislodge the obstruction by the following procedure : Taking the tube in the left hand and
holding it firmly and steadily in position, with the right I closed its
lumen completely, and alternately stretch and relax the tube two or
three times, and then let go. The suction force thus exerted will often
start the flow once more.

In cases in which the production of mucus is excessive, the use of
Vichy instead of ordinary water is advisable. On account of the expense of the former, however, I have employed in its stead the artificial Vichy water, prepared from the granular effervescent Vichy salts
made by well-known chemists.

A few years ago quite a popular furore was excited over the use of
hot water as a remedy for dyspepsia. Everybody tried it, some with
benefit, but many more with failure. Thus the remedy has gone out
of fashion. Still it is one of value in its sphere. In cases associated

with marked flatulence it is a valuable aid in securing relief by exciting eructations of wind. It also seems to do good in cases of atonic
dyspepsia. In gastric catarrh it prepares the stomach for the more
ready digestion of food by the removal of the coat of mucus from the
walls of that organ. It favors normal action of the bowels first by
softening fæcal masses, and secondly by increasing peristaltic action.
My method of using hot water as a remedy has been to order the
patient to take one tumblerful of it in the morning on rising and
repeat the dose at intervals during the day, so that he shall take not
less than three pints in that time.

Next let me refer to a form of dyspepsia not uncommonly met
with, and one, too, the true nature of which is not sufficiently recognized. I refer to dyspepsia brought on in nervous people by too
much dieting, in other words, by self-inflicted starvation. So far as I
know but one medical writer has referred to dyspepsia of this variety
in sufficiently forcible terms. The subject has certainly not received
due attention in our text-books. Dr. J. Earle Jenner, of Pictou, Ontario,
gives a most excellent description of it in the *Journal of Reconstructives*
for January, 1887, under the title of "A Very Common Form of Dyspepsia." Dr. Jenner truly says, the histories of all these cases are
nearly identical. A slight dyspeptic trouble appears in a nervous
person ; a course of dieting is followed with relief. A renewal of the
dyspepsia excites more stringent dietetic regulations than before.
Finally, the patient is reduced to a pitiable condition.

Five years ago I was consulted by Mrs. ———, aged 40 years,
who had been dyspeptic for eighteen months past. Her former
physicians had imposed on her such stringent dietetic rules that she
now partook of little save dry toast and tea. On such a diet her
nutrition was necessarily bad and emaciation marked. Evidence pointing to the existence of any marked degree of actual gastric disease was
wanting. The bowels were constipated. The plan of treatment
adopted was one calculated to improve general nutrition. Abundance
of milk was first ordered taken with Metcalf's *liquor pancreaticus*. As
the patient's strength increased, article by article was added to her
diet list until she had resumed her old eating habits. *Hydrastis* was
the remedy used internally ; occasional doses of *nux vomica* were also
given. In six months the patient was cured and has remained so up
to the present time.

There is a form of dyspepsia, which I believe to be the most difficult of all forms to cure, the true nature of which is seldom recognized,
and that is a true nervous dyspepsia—a gastric neurosis. As in the
case of the form of dyspepsia last mentioned, this occurs in neurotic

subjects. The symptoms are mostly the same as those noted in ordinary dyspepsia, but with these important distinctions : The tongue, as a rule, is not coated ; objective symptoms are rare ; the accumulation of flatus is marked ; but all the symptoms disappear as soon as the patient's attention is drawn from himself. While away from home, traveling and exposed to dietetic irregularities, he is perfectly well; at home with his friends he is a burden to all. What will cure these cases I know not. Diet will not, and few medicines can. On this subject we need more light.

The use of artificial digesting agents, as pepsin and pancreatin, is of importance. The common mistake in practice is, I think, to use too much of the former and too little of the latter. For the artificial digestion of milk nothing is better than the peptonizing tubes of Fairchild Brothers & Foster, of New York. Each of these tubes contains ten grains of pancrein and five grains of bicarbonate of soda, and is sufficient for the peptonizing of one pint of milk. The peptonized milk thus prepared has never failed, in my experience, to agree with the most delicate stomach. If exposed too long to the action of the pancreatin it may become bitter, but otherwise it is relished by the patient.

To aid in the digestion of starchy foods taken into the stomach pancreatin is invaluable. Here the best form for its exhibition is found in the neatly prepared pancreatic tablets of Fairchild Brothers & Foster. These tablets are sugar-coated. One should be taken immediately after the meal and followed by a second one-half an hour later.

The special advantage derivable from the administration of pepsin and pancreatin is found in the fact that they permit of a more extended dietary than would be otherwise allowable, and so secure for the patient better nutrition. In some cases in which the appetite is so completely absent that all food is refused, feeding through the stomach-tube is of value. Articles thus administered should be of a character readily assimilated. It should, moreover, be introduced slowly into the stomach. Thus far I have only used peptonized milk in this manner.

As regards the best diet for dyspeptic patients no hard-and-fast rules can be laid down. The patient's inclinations and appetite should be followed as far as possible. Idiosyncrasies to certain articles of diet should only be accepted by the physician as real when he has proved them to be such. The most important thing is to see that the patient gets sufficient to nourish him. Certain articles of food known to be injurious to the patient should be forbidden. Of more importance than the food, is the manner of eating. On this point, our American habits are so well known that it is unnecessary for me to dwell.

So much time has been occupied in the above remarks, that little remains for me in which to speak of remedies. The indications I have used in practice are the indications of our text-books. I will refer to the use of two remedies, however. One of these is *hydrastis*. This remedy I have employed with very satisfactory results in the sore mouth which is sometimes in association with gastric disorders.

Hepar, which has been so highly recommended in cases of dyspepsia in which the patient complained of a sensation of weakness in the epigastrium, with marked amelioration from stimulating food, has proven very successful in the cases in which I have used it. *Nux vomica, carbo veg., cinchona, pulsatilla, ipecacuanha, bryonia* and *lycopodium* are all remedies which find frequent use in practice.

I now leave the subject in the hands of the Society, trusting that a sufficient number of thoughts have been presented, however inadequately, to lead the way for an interesting discussion. That no organ of the body occupies a more important position in the management of patients will not be contradicted. On its welfare depends nutrition and on nutrition depends the welfare of our patient.

EXPERIENCE IN THE MANAGEMENT AND TREATMENT OF NEURASTHENIA.*

By GEORGE E. GORHAM, M.D.

IF there be a disease, the management of which is trying and tedious to the physician, and discouraging to those seeking relief, it is that generally known as nervous exhaustion. Whether it be named neurasthenia, hypochondriasis, spinal irritation, spinal anæmia, crankism or nothing but nervousness, the symptoms of all have the same general characteristics. I need not take your time to relate them here.

We have all heard them. The pathology of these cases is said to be obscure; but many hypotheses are formed to account for the various symptoms of which these sufferers complain. Perhaps the most prominent theory is exhaustion or anæmia of the nervous centres, and upon this theory so-called nervous tonics, the different

*Read before the Homœopathic Medical Society of the State of New York, September 21st, 1887.

phosphated compounds, are bought and taken in large quantities by nearly all neurasthenic patients, and far too often they get no further advice from their physician than to take Fellows' Hypophosphites, Crosby's Vitalized Phosphates, or some similar mixture ; perhaps are laughed at, as they pour forth their tale of woe, and are told that it is nothing but nervousness : a term which would be nearer a correct diagnosis if it were put : *Something with* nervousness.

To assume that exhaustion is the cause, and tonics and stimulants the treatment for these cases, is as easy as it is common with the busy practitioner, but in my hands it does not cure.

To laugh at and ridicule a patient does not cure, and is often a cruel thing to do. That patient who comes to us filled with morbid fear, is restless in mind and body, is startled by every sound, and cries at trifling things, can be calmed and comforted and perhaps put on the road to recovery at that very visit, by simply admitting to that patient and to our own mind as well, that he *is* sick and not think and try to make him think he is simply nervous, fussy or foolish. There is cause for these conditions of mind and body, and to tell a patient so, and then make intelligent and earnest effort to find and remove it gives them a comfort, and a hope that will enable them to bear patiently the flying pains, the palpitating heart, the tormenting fears, or the sad and painful emotions, until we shall have removed or alleviated the exciting cause ; when they will slowly and surely grow into a degree of health, gratifying to us, and surprising to them. The causes would be divided I suppose, after the manner of medical authors, into predisposing and exciting.

I will not mention the former. The latter, the exciting causes, may be divided into two general classes, mental and physical. It is difficult to find the mental cause, for the patient is slow to admit some secret sorrow, or burning anxiety that is constantly harassing his mind ; but they are frequent and often found in some business complication, or among the many trials incident to social life.

Unfortunately the physician can do little to remove these causes, but he can do much by kind words and encouragement to help the patient bear them.

The bodily causes are most frequently found within the pelvic cavity. In man an hypertrophied prostate, a chronic urethritis, a stricture or a phimosis may make him a wretched hypochondriac; a morbid condition of the rectum, piles, fissures, strictures and pockets and papillæ as described by Pratt, are often a constant source of irritation and exhaust the whole nervous system.

The abuse of the sexual function by masturbation or too frequent intercourse is a cause too well known to need mention.

In women, the same conditions of the rectum often prevail, while any or all of the morbid conditions known to the gynæcologist may be the exciting cause of a persistent neurasthenia. The treatment which has been quite successful in my hands has been, removal of the exciting cause when possible ; rest properly prescribed, sometimes an hour each day, sometimes weeks at a time, and sometimes an occasional day or two off from business. Proper food eaten slowly and regularly, sufficient sleep and the discontinuance of nerve tonics and stimulants of all kinds, excepting sometimes tea and tobacco in moderation, when they have been long accustomed to either (never allowing smoking), and the indicated homœopathic remedy.

The ones which have most often served me well are, *nux vom.*, *ignatia, silicia, cal. carb., cal. phos., verat. vir., cactus grand., hypericum, scutellaria, sepia and phos. acid and sulphur.*

The indications for these and many other important remedies may be found in that most excellent article, "Therapeutics in Spinal Irritation," by F. F. Laird, published in the NORTH AMERICAN JOURNAL OF HOMŒOPATHY. The benefit derived from the removal of rectal irritation is shown in the following :

CASE I. Mr. L., aged 64, has for several years complained of being tired, being unable to go through the day without lying down for rest. Sudden noises annoyed and pained him, was emotional, crying without cause, and a firm conviction that he had but a few months to live had settled upon him. His face showed a tired and haggard appearance, and his sleep was unrefreshing, always disturbed by distressing dreams. He said he was worn out. The removal of a large internal hemorrhoid was followed by entire relief of all his trouble. He says it made a new man of him, and so it did. The tired look is gone, the sleep is quiet and refreshing, and the hope and ambition of his earlier manhood have returned, and he has endured a hard, hot summer's work with no return of his trouble.

CASE II. Mr. W., aged 29, unmarried, a banker, sought relief of many doctors, tried rest and change of air and the popular nervous tonics without relief. His palpitating heart, his imaginary consumption, his wild restless feelings when he attempted work at his desk and his great sense of exhaustion about 11 A. M. continued.

Slitting up the foreskin for a congenital phimosis cured this man in one month, and he has had no return of his trouble now for four years.

CASE III. Mr. H., unmarried, an editor, complained of dizziness, inability to do bodily or mental work, constant restlessness, poor sleep, pains in the knees, and pain and soreness in each tuber ischii, occasional nocturnal emissions and a whitish sediment in the urine which he was hourly examining, carrying a bottle in his pocket for the purpose.

The point of irritation in the man was found in the prostatic urethra, which the passage of graded sounds relieved, and his pains and nervous symptoms disappeared. He gained fifteen pounds in three weeks and has remained well for three years.

CASE IV. Mr. M., an excessive smoker, met with business reverses and began to worry. He soon became irritable, nervous and slept but little. He complained of painful emotions, and said nobody could imagine how badly he felt.

His legs felt numb. His sexual power was wanting, and he was very restless. Morbid fears came in to add to his torment, would not sit or ride alone. He became depressed and suicidal. For two years he rode and walked and talked and cried almost constantly.

He was a large red faced man, and looked the picture of health.

Yet his trembling hands, his great restlessness and his rambling conversation, often crying as he talked, told of trouble somewhere. The exciting cause in this case was a mental one, and strange to me, every one of the eminent specialists whom he had consulted, had advised tonics or stimulants or both and exercise. He had exercised until he was a bundle of exhausted and hyper-sensitive nerves without hope or will power, a victim of his ever-changing emotions.

At this stage he took the case in his own hands by an attempt at suicide.

I was then called, and prescribed continued rest in bed, which the patient said he *could not* take. It was enforced for three days, and *veral. vir. 3x* given and stimulants taken away which soon changed our patient to a quiet, tired, sleepy man. He lay quietly in bed for three weeks, eating and sleeping well, when he was allowed to go to the sea-side, where his improvement went steadily on for a month. He spent the summer on a farm, and then returned to the city, where he has been in business for two years. *Ignatia* 3x did more to quiet this man than all the bromide, chloral and other hypnotics he had ever taken.

Unfortunately we can not locate and remove the cause in all cases as successfully as in those just cited.

We then have to call to our aid massage, electricity, diet, rest, exercise and homœopathic medication. The following case will show what can be done with the true similimum :

CASE V. Mrs. V. consulted me in May, 1887, after having been under treatment six months for nervousness.

I copy from my case book : Mrs. V., aged 63. mother of six children, ceased menstruating at 56, is fat, and apparently well nourished, digestion good, bowels regular. Not an ache or a pain

Pulse and urine normal, but complains of great weakness. If she reads, cannot remember what she is reading. A walk of two blocks tires her Visiting fatigues her so she must leave the room. Sleeps badly and has a fear night and day that something will happen to her family. A fat woman with muscular and nervous prostration. Failing to find any cause, I give her *silicia* 6x trit. four times a day. Reported in a week, better. Continued. The next week much better. Continued medicine. In one month's time she could read, visit and walk a fair amount for one of her age and enjoy it.

She counted herself well and the little powders a wonder. *Silicia* will cure sweating feet. *Silicia* will control too rapid formation of pus. It cures also some forms of bone trouble, and it does it, I believe, by its power to correct that weakened or depraved condition of system which tends to development of such troubles. It cured Mrs V. in the same way.

It is often indicated in cases of neurasthenia and muscular weakness, when it is more valuable than all the stimulants, nerve tonics and phosphorous compounds made.

SYPHILIS—AN UNRECOGNIZED FACTOR IN DISEASE.*

By W. B. TRITES, M.D.

THE peculiar tendency of syphilis to simulate diseases of the most diverse character is not, we think, sufficiently appreciated. We are certain that mistakes in diagnosis often occur from a failure to bear this tendency in mind, mistakes detrimental to the patient and the cause of chagrin to the physician, especially if he sees what he has diagnosed as incurable rapidly improving in the hands of some one else. Allow me to present a few cases of syphilitic affections which seem to substantiate the above statements :

CASE I.—*Syphilitic gumma of the left lung, simulating consumption. — Recovery.*—Mrs. X., æt. 35. in the winter of 1885 began to rapidly decline in flesh, and to feel weary upon the least exertion. Had a constant pain in the left lung of a sharp, stabbing character, seeming to be deep in and localized. She had dysyncœa and a short hacking cough, with free expectoration of a white tasteless phlegm. From time to time she had had hæmoptysis and night sweats. Her appetite was fitful; there was circumscribed dullness over the left lung, but the right lung appeared healthy. She had consulted a number of physicians, and they had united in pronouncing her disease phthisis, and given a corresponding prognosis. Struck with the perfectly healthy condition of the right lung and noticing some scars upon the chest and a bronzed look of the face, I asked for a syphilitic history, but this she stoutly denied. She admitted that in 1887 she had lost her hair, had had sore throat and general eruptions, but did not know the cause of these symptoms. From her husband I afterward learned that he had communicated syphilis to her about this time. I gave her a

---

* Read before the Homœopathic Medical Society, State of Pennsylvania, September 20th.

hopeful prognosis, which, under appropriate treatment, a nourishing diet, and a prolonged visit by the sea, was fully confirmed, and to-day she is in fair health, without cough, pain or expectoration, has been recently confined and attends to her household duties.

CASE II.—*Cerebral Syphilis, with Paralysis of the Facial, and Aphasia.* —*Recovery.*—Was called June 21st, 1885, at noon, to see Mr. K., æt. 30, whom the messenger stated had been stricken with paralysis during the night. Found the patient in bed in a deep sleep, breathing not stertorous, the conjunctivæ of both eyes deeply injected, the pupils unaffected, responding promptly to light; his tongue heavily furred, and when protruded inclined strongly to the right; speech almost unintelligible, though he talked incessantly when aroused; the saliva ran from his mouth constantly. He was unable to swallow anything but liquids and these only in the smallest quantities. Even then he would choke and part would return through the nose. He slept most of the time, and when aroused would quickly and awkwardly assume a sitting posture, rub his head violently, especially over the right eye and at the back of the head, would yawn incessantly, complain of being cold, wrap the clothing about him and in a moment toss it off again, swinging his legs and arms from side to side. All his motions were rapid and impatient. His mind seemed dull, but when addressed gave proper answers, writing them on a slate. The writing was cramped and unnatural looking, and words and letters were often omitted. He would spell brandy "bandy," and when told of his error would rub it out and spell it again in the same way. His mental action was extremely slow, halting and thinking, writing and erasing over and over again, in composing an answer of half a dozen words to such a question as "How do you feel to-day?" I could get no history from the patient, owing to his mental condition, but his wife told me that this was his third attack, his first one being on December 18th, 1885. In the other instances the paralysis had been slight. Each attack had been proceded by severe and prolonged attacks of headache and pains in feet. He had feared this attack; for several days had had headache, dribbling of saliva, inability to apply his mind, and a distortion of his face to the left side. Went to bed as well as usual; got awake at one o'clock in the wildest excitement; leaped out of bed; rushed up and down; gave his wife his pistol, telling her to hide it, as he was impelled to kill both himself and her. (Afterwards he told me that a great negro man seemed to stand beside him and urge him constantly to commit the deed, and that it was with the greatest difficulty he could control his actions.) Soon afterwards she noticed his words were unintelligible; she then sent for a physician, who pronounced his disease paralysis.

From the slow advent of the paralysis, from its confinement to the muscles of the face and throat, from the history of previous attacks from which he recovered, I was led to diagnose a paralysis of the seventh nerve, of syphilitic origin, and treated him accordingly, and by the 10th of July had the satisfaction of seeing him in sound mind, able to talk well, and soon after took charge of his business. Afterward learned that he had a chancre nine years before, had lost his hair and had had general eruptions.

CASE III.—*Syphilitic Disease of the Testicles simulating Cancer.— One testicle removed, the other becoming affected; true history discovered and testicle saved.*—McI., æt. 40. In the spring of 1884 struck his right testicle while trimming a grape vine; it began to swell, became very large and hard; went to a hospital, where it was diagnosed as cancer and removed. I was called to see him in June, 1885; the left testicle was then greatly enlarged, painless, irregular in shape, and quite hard. His lower limbs were dropsical, had rheumatic pains, and was extremely weak and anæmic. Positively denied that he had ever had syphilis. Had left his wife some three years before because she had been unfaithful to him ; remembered that his hair came out, but could not remember having had any skin manifestations; recollected that after the testicle had been removed at hospital he heard one of the house doctors say to the surgeon that they had examined the removed organ and that it was not cancerous. From the fact of his wife's infidelity, his loss of hair, and the overheard conversation at the hospital, syphilitic orchitis was diagnosed, and in six weeks the testicle was in a perfectly normal state, and in another month the patient was at work.

CASE IV.—*Syphilitic headache, followed by severe brain disease and death.*—Mr. M., æt. 40, consulted me for a violent and long standing headache; the pain he described as being intense, located in the frontal region and extending from temple to temple; for the past two weeks had been very dizzy, and this continued even when his eyes were shut and when he was lying down. The dizziness was so great that he had been excused from going up a ladder, which was a part of his daily work, feeling certain that he would fall if he did so. He had also noticed a numbness in his left arm and so affecting his fingers of the left hand that he could not hold a cigar between them. I immediately suspected syphilis and on inquiry he admitted that he had had a hard sore eighteen years before followed by general manifestations, but that for years he had been clear of it. Had been treated by his family physician for the headache without improvement, who did not know of his syphilitic history. Under appropriate treatment he improved, but neglecting himself, not taking medicine, he relapsed, but again improved. Lost sight of him and afterward heard that he had died from inflammation of the brain. I feel sure that this man's life could have been saved if his physician had recognized the syphilitic character of the meningitis from which he died.

CASE V.—*Syphilitic disease of liver simulating in history and symptoms cirrhosis—improvement.*—Col. W., æt. 50, consulted me in 1882. He had been ill for some weeks, had tenderness in the hepatic region, ascites, jaundice, and had had repeated hemorrhages from the nose and bowels. He was emaciated, weak and without appetite, often rejecting his food after eating it. His mind was considerably affected, comprehension being dull and his mental action slow, could not make change, would get lost in parts of the city with which he was perfectly familiar. Had served throughout the war, being greatly exposed

in south and west. Since war, had traveled constantly in the extreme
south and south-west, had suffered again and again from malaria, was
an habitual dram drinker, taking ten or a dozen drinks of brandy or
whisky a day. First diagnosed cirrhosis with contraction of the liver, but
finding later that he had had a chancre some fifteen years before, tried
specific treatment. In a few weeks ascites diminished, intellect cleared
up and within six months was back at business, though his jaundice
still remained when I last saw him in 1884 and his mind lacked that
veracity it once had shown.

These cases are not given with the thought that they contain anything new, but merely to call attention to the errors of diagnosis and
the direful results of these mistakes to at least two of the patients, one
losing a testicle and the other his life.

Many mistakes, of the kind recorded above, are due to an imperfect acquaintance with the nature, course and tendency of syphilis.
Says one of the most eminent of English syphilographers: "The
power of recognizing syphilitic disease, when brought under notice, is
one of the most valuable gifts which the physician can possess.
These diseases meet us at every turn in practice and present a most
bewildering variety of external aspect."

Bewildering as the variety is, there are certain positive signs which
mark syphilitic diseases, and these should be understood by every
physician.

There are several reasons why syphilitic diseases are not more
readily recognized and one of these finds its origin in the delicacy of
the questions which the physician must put to the patient. Indeed
this difficulty is almost insurmountable, for in some quarters to suggest syphilis or any other venereal disease, would give unpardonable
offense. Here we can have recourse to the iodide of potassium, a
wizard's wand in the solution of such questions. In many cases, however, questioning is well borne and the fear lies entirely on the side of
the physician, who for fear of offending goes on in the dark when a
word might send a flood of light upon some dark corner of disease.

We have noted the fact that a superficial knowledge of syphilis is
a fruitful cause of error. But why this superficial knowledge of a question so important?

It is partially dependent upon the chaotic state of venereal medicine in the past, but this difficulty is rapidly passing away; but the
traditional chaos still exists and turns many from the study of these
conditions. Venereal medicine of to-day approaches nearer to perfection than does any other branch of the science.

The medical schools of the past are also blamable for part of
this general inattention to syphilis.

It is only recently that full instructions could be had by students in colleges or hospitals on this important subject. But now everywhere its importance is recognized and instruction given. We think that better work could be done in this field of medicine, if the study of syphilis could be separated from the chair of surgery and placed where it properly belongs, in general medicine. For ninety-nine cases of syphilis out of a hundred are purely medical and receive only medical attention.

The prolonged course of syphilis and the comparatively insignificant appearance of its initial lesion are both points which render the recognition of its late manifestations difficult. Owing to the prolonged course years and years may have elapsed between the primary sore and the development of the disease, and during this time the patient may have forgotten the trivial sore or the sparsely scattered eruption, and hence be utterly unaware that he has ever had syphilis. Again, such patients are prone to deny a syphilitic history, even when they know of its existence. We cannot hope to reform the race, but we can impress upon the minds of our syphilitic patient the necessity to himself of always informing his physician of his disease. This tendency to deceive is often due to a desire to protect one's own character, being ignorant of the important truth they are hiding from the medical attendant.

I shall not mention that often heard reason for ignorance in matters pertaining to syphilis, to wit: "I do not attend syphilitic cases; they are distasteful to me." I hope no physician in this assembly, feeling the importance of his office and the responsibilities which it brings with it, gives any such excuse for ignorance of this subject.

Upon this subject, your knowledge of this question, may depend the life of your next patient, the welfare of an unborn family, or the happiness of your own household. No man can successfully practice who neglects this branch of the art.

This paper will not be complete unless I say something about the diagnosis between syphilitic simulation of diseases and the diseases themselves. In the first place, we should be constantly on the alert for these syphilitic forms of disease. Syphilis is very much more common than we are in the habit of thinking, unless we have investigated the subject carefully. The staid gentleman of to-day may not always have been so, and the errors of a single night in youth may entail this horrible dyscrasia. Nor are we to forget that syphilis is not always venereal in its origin. The great majority of cases are probably acquired during the sexual act; but of all the so-called veneral diseases, this is *the one* which is most frequently acquired innocently.

The mode of invasion in certain visceral diseases is of great value in diagnosis between the type disease and its syphilitic simulation. Visceral affections are usually preceded by certain prodromata, and affect certain ages, sexes and conditions of men. Often they are the sequelæ of other diseases. If we find these diseases existing, having developed suddenly, without the forerunners, we should remember that syphilis has this power of simulation, and carefully examine for signs of that disease.

In doing this we must carefully review the life of the patient to see if we can detect anything which might indicate syphilis. In prosecuting such a search we must be guarded in what we accept. We must remember that, in common parlance, all sores on the penis are chancres; hence nothing can be deduced from the name given the disease by the patient. Again, if the patient has had a sore followed by a suppurating bubo he will certainly call it a chancre, but the chances are that *that* sore was positively not syphilitic.

But if we obtain the history of a sore followed, after an interval, by general eruptions, sore throat and falling of the hair, we may be certain that the patient has had syphilis. This certainly may be often reached without so complete a history, for it is not uncommon to find truthful persons denying syphilis when the evidences of tertiary disease are clear.

Forgetfulness, inattention to symptoms and unacquaintance with syphilitic diseases will account for many of these incomplete forms.

The presence of periosteal nodes upon the long bones is also a suspicious symptom, and would lead us almost certainly to declare that syphilis was present. Scars about the nose, upon the forehead, symmetrical scars on the trunk and limbs, signs of destructive ulcerations in the throat, an adherent iris in either eye, nocturnal pains or pains exacerbated at night are symptoms pointing strongly toward syphilis.

In every case a careful examination of the lymphatics should be instituted, for years after the original infection, the inguinal, the epitrochlear and the glands of the neck have been found hardened, painless and freely movable, the three characteristics of syphilitic glandular affection.

Nor must we forget that syphilis may be acquired by heredity, and, late in adult life, develop, retaining the power of simulation which is so marked in the acquired form. In the diagnosis of hereditary syphilis we must depend upon the history not only of the patient but also his parents. The face of the patient and the shape of the head are often diagnostic in this form of the disease, and in all suspected cases the mouth should be examined for the peculiarly formed syphilitic teeth described by Hutchinson, a sure indication of the venereal taint.

The site of development of syphilitic disease is often of value in diagnosis.

In the lung the middle lobe is the one most frequently affected and it is seldom that both are affected.

As compared with tubercular phthisis, the disease with which syphilis of the lung is most apt to be confounded, the process of syphilis is more rapid, the expectoration abundant, but without signs of softening of the pulmonary tissue. The patient is weak and debilitated, but often without the marked emaciation of phthisis.

Later in the course of syphilis we have a flattening of the chest over the affected locality, with dullness on percussion and a prolonged and harsh inspiratory and expiratory murmur, with a decided intermission between the two.

Years ago, at the Pennsylvania Hospital, I remember to have heard Forsyth Meigs say that tenderness on pressure over the sternum was a characteristic symptom of constitutional syphilis. In a recent paper by Dr. Porter, of New York, this symptom is again brought forward and its importance in diagnosis urged. He says that it is a very strong pathognomonic sign of syphilis, and describes it as a peculiar pain and *œdema* of the sternum and of the tibial crests elicited by pressure. The recoil of the patient when pressure is made its characteristic, and the pain is described as being intense. A noticeable feature is that when the sternum is excessively sensitive the tibial crests are less so, and *vice versa.*

The nervous system is especially liable to suffer from late syphilis, and results in the production of a variety of nervous affections, such as eclampsia, chorea, epilepsy, paralysis, locomotor-ataxia and even insanity. In many of these affections, if the syphilitic taint is recognized, health can be restored; in others, notably in locomotor-ataxia, the syphilitic form seems as incurable as when the disease is dependent upon other causes.

Headache is one of the most common and usually the earliest symptom of meningeal syphilis; it is peculiar in being very persistent, apparently causeless and shows a decided tendency to nocturnal exacerbation.

Such a headache should always be regarded with suspicion and nervous diseases in patients with a history of such headaches should be carefully examined for other signs of syphilis. If such a headache is accompanied by slight spells of giddiness its syphilitic origin is still more probable.

Paralysis, so frequently accompanying diseases of the nervous system, often has its origin in syphilis. The early forms are transient and repeated; for instance, the patient has noticed several attacks, lasting for a few hours, perhaps, in which his toe dragged, or has had momentary weakness of one arm, a slight drawing of the face, a partial aphasia, which appears and disappears. These transient, incomplete forms of paralysis have their origin in syphilis, and Wood thinks they result from intense congestion about certain parts of the brain or from stoppages in the circulation.

Gummata may develop at almost any point, but they especially affect the base of the brain, and hence are apt to impinge upon the nerves originating there.

If a paralysis involve only one nervous trunk, especially if only one cranial nerve be involved, it is almost sure to be syphilitic.

Hutchinson estimates that a full half of the cases of paralysis of the third, fourth, fifth and sixth nerves, when such paralysis affects only one nerve, are due to syphilis.

Most cases of rapidly, but not abruptly, appearing strabismus, ptosis, dilated pupil, or any paralytic eye symptom in the adult, are due to syphilis and can be cured if this cause is recognized.

Aphasia is another very common symptom of brain syphilis, and when occurring the patient should be carefully examined for other signs of syphilis.

Fournier has noticed that epilepsy occurring after thirty years of age in persons otherwise healthy, is almost invariably due to syphilis.

Other pathognomonic signs of syphilis might be mentioned, but the paper is already too long. Allow me to close it with the following quotation from one of the most celebrated of English syphilographers.

"The first requisite to success in the diagnosis of late syphilis is a mind constantly awake to suspicion and fully impressed with the all-important fact that diseases of the most diverse character may have their origin in this taint, and if so, they will prove to be curable only by treatment directed against it."

A CASE OF NEURO-RETINITIS.*

By N. L. MACBRIDE, M.D., O. ET A. CHIR.

Surgeon to the N. Y. Ophthalmic Hospital.

ON the 1st of last March, the following interesting case was admitted to my clinic at the N. Y. Ophthalmic Hospital. The patient, Sarah Blank, aged 18 years, complained of slight discomfort when reading. Upon examination, vision of the right eye was found to be $\frac{20}{20}$, and that of the left eye $\frac{20}{100}$; that is, the acuteness of vision in the right eye was normal, while the left eye had $\frac{1}{5}$ of the normal acuteness of vision. Vision was not improved by lenses, and the refraction was apparently emmetropic. An ophthalmoscopic examination revealed the following appearances of the fundus : In the right eye the retina and disc were hyperæmic. The left eye, in addition to the hyperæmia of the retina and disc, exhibited slight swelling and haziness of the retina. The dioptric media were clear in both eyes. The general appearance of the patient was good, she being muscular and of large build, but her face was very pale and waxy-looking. Advice was given for the patient to enter the hospital the next day, prepared to stay, and to bring a specimen of her urine. She did not report again until May 1st, at which time she was taken into the hospital. An examination of the eyes, at this time, showed that vision was practically lost, the mere perception of light alone remaining. Upon ophthalmoscopic examination, the fundus of the eye revealed all the appearances of the retinitis of Bright's disease. The retinal arteries and veins were enlarged and tortuous, the optic disc swollen, and masses of whitish exudation were scattered throughout the retina, being more marked in a zone surrounding the optic disc and giving rise to the appearance of the so-called mound, which is said to be characteristic of retinitis albuminurica. In addition to this there were numerous hæmorrhages scattered over the fundus ; there were numerous stellate spots in the macula lutea, and a general cloudiness of the retina. The ophthalmoscopic appearances were almost identical in the two eyes. The patient had no pain, either in the eyes or in the head. The urine was examined, but neither albumin nor sugar was found. Repeated examinations, both chemical and microscopical, were made by Drs. Helfrich, Hart and myself, all failing to find any trace of albumin. A specimen (of 24 hours) was sent to Dr. Heitzmann, who reported that it contained no albumin, and gave it as his opinion that "no nephritis existed or ever had existed in this case."

Numerous ophthalmoscopic examinations were made from time to time, and revealed the fact that the inflammatory symptoms were gradually disappearing. Symptoms of atrophy of the optic disc and retina began to appear, the stellate exudation in the macula lutea being the last of the inflammatory products to be absorbed. An ophthalmoscopic examination made upon July 16th revealed a well

---

* Read before the Homœopathic Medical Society of the County of New York, October 13th, 1887.

marked atrophy of the optic disc and retina, the retinal arteries being
unusually small even for a case of advanced atrophy.   At the present
time, atrophy of the optic disc and retina is well marked, but there is
slight improvement in the patient's vision, she being able to distinguish the form of large objects.

My reason for reporting this case is its marked resemblance to that
form of retinitis which accompanies Bright's disease. I think we have
established the fact that no Bright's disease existed, neither was the
patient pregnant, and at the present time she is apparently in perfect
health.   Yet the clinical history of the case is almost identical with
that of retinitis albuminurica, with the exception of the marked atrophy of the optic disc and retina.

THE DIAGNOSTIC VALUE OF THE VARIOUS FORMS OF BULBAR INJECTION.*

By W. H. BIGLER, M.D.,

Philadelphia.

THE unreliability of subjective symptoms alone, in the case of
any class of disease, is pretty generally acknowledged at the
present day, but in none with greater justice than with ocular disturbances.

The varying subjective symptoms are here not only so little characteristic in themselves, but are so modified—as, indeed, are most
subjective ones—in the mode of their expression by the habits of life
and thought of the patients, as to be almost useless for purposes of
diagnosis, and consequently, of treatment.

An objective symptom becomes of importance in proportion
as it is unique or characteristic of but one single diseased condition, where its presence serves to establish a differential diagnosis.

The various types of bulbar injection—injection of the eyeball—
while not occupying the first rank as diagnostic symptoms, are yet
sufficiently distinctive to enable us, by close attention to their peculiar features, to place them in certain groups, both for diagnostic
and therapeutic purposes.

In order to obtain a reliable basis for the grouping of the various
forms of congestion of the eye, we must glance at the arrangement of
its vascular system.

---

*Read before the Homœopathc Medical Society, State of Pennsylvania, September
20th, 1887.

As we will, in this short paper, refer only to the external objective symptoms of disease, we need not take into consideration the *arteria centralis retinæ*, which enters the ball through the optic nerve, is destined exclusively for the retina and optic nerve, and forms almost an anastomosis with other vessels. There are then left to be considered three (3) systems of vessels.

1. The vessels proper to the conjunctival (*the posterior conjunctival*), both arteries and veins. They are usually not very conspicuous, but become easily engorged, on account of the looseness of the surrounding tissue and then become plainly visible.

They are then large and form a bright red network by anastomosis, which increases in intensity towards the folds of transmission, and is less distinct near the margin of the cornea. The vessels can be moved with the conjunctiva when it is slid over the globe, and can be momentarily emptied by stroking through the closed lids in a direction radiating from the cornea.

2. The *anterior ciliary* vessels. These lie in the subconjunctival tissue and by their perforating branches supply the sclerotic, iris and ciliary body, and receive blood from Schlemm's canal and the ciliary body. The perforating branches of the arteries are seen in health as several rather large tortuous vessels, extending to within a twelfth or an eighth of an inch of the corneal margin. These vessels join with the branches of the posterior ciliary arteries which perforate the posterior part of the sclerotic, and supply the choroid, the ciliary body and the iris.

The non-perforating episcleral branches of these anterior ciliary arteries are very small and numerous, *invisible in health*, but forming, when distended, a pink zone of fine nearly straight, closely set vessels, radiating all round the margin of the cornea—the so-called "ciliary congestion," "circum- or peri-corneal injection."

3. The *anterior conjunctival* vessels, with their loop plexus on the corneal border. By these numerous vessels, which are proper to the margin of the cornea and the adjacent zone of conjunctiva, the two former systems anastomose.

Thus we have in the zone, immediately around the cornea, a system of vessels which have communication with both the deep and superficial tissues of the eye. This thus becomes the most important region of the eye for purposes of diagnosis, but we see at the same time, from the above, that the vascular phenomena will not, in themselves, be sufficient to decide in doubtful cases.

Applying these facts, let us see what valuable practical points we can derive from them. ·

1. An *absence of any peri-corneal* injection, *i. e.*, of anything but a large meshed network of tortuous bright red vessels, increasing in size and intensity of color away from the cornea, and capable of being moved with the conjunctiva and temporarily emptied by pressure—indicates an entirely superficial hyperæmia, or inflammation of the conjunctiva. This will usually be accompanied with mucous or muco-purulent discharge. Here, if external applications are used, astringents are in place.

We must remember that an intense injection of this type, especially attended with chemosis (as in purulent ophthalmia), may mask or entirely conceal a peri-corneal injection, indicating more serious injury.

2. The *presence of peri-corneal* injection may have a different significance, according to its several types.

a. A pink or rose colored zone (the non-perforating branches of the anterior ciliary arteries) surrounding the cornea, becoming fainter in color away from this, and consisting, on close examination, of fine straight radiating vessels, not moving with the conjunctiva, points to an inflammation of the cornea, or of the renal tract (the iris, ciliary body, or choroid).

b. A similarly placed dark, or dusky red zone, finely reticulated (episcleral venous plexus) is often found in glaucoma; but may occur in other conditions, especially in the aged. The increased tension, impairment of vision, and pains, will serve to confirm a diagnosis of glaucoma.

c. An unequally marked congestion of a peculiar lilac tint in the same region points to cyclitis, and will be attended by sensitiveness to pressure on the spot of congestion (cf. *a*, supra).

d. A bright red superficial congestion of small vessels in the same location, often running over on to the surface of the cornea, usually shows a tendency to superficial corneal ulcerations.

When localized or fasiculated, it points to phlyctenular disease. This symptom, found usually, in fact, almost invariably, with some degree of photophobia, will often enable us to diagnose the approach of a keratitis, even before there are any symptoms to be discovered in the corneal tissues. It will further guard us against mistaking a keratitis for a simple conjunctivitis, which, in the early stages, is quite possible.

e. A congestion of a deep red color, subconjunctival and in patches, usually situated opposite the palpebral fissure, near the outer margin of the cornea, points to episcleritis.

In connection with these several forms of congestion we will have, as we have here and there indicated above, symptoms confirmatory of our diagnosis. For example, in iritis, with its distinguishing peri-corneal injection, the iris will be at first more, and then less, brilliant than normal, and, at times, much altered in color, while its action will be sluggish, or entirely abolished. Vision will also be impaired.

In corneitis the transparency and lustre of the cornea are more or less diminished and photophobia is present.

Further, we may say in general, that in all forms characterized by peri-corneal injection, astringents are to be avoided. In certain complicated forms of eye disease this may have exceptions, but, as a practical rule for the non-specialist, it should be emphasized.

In many severe forms of acute disease of the eyeball several of these types of congestion may exist at once, and be scarcely separable, but enough cases occur where they are met with singly, to make them valuable indications in diagnosis.

CHROMIC ACID IN POST-NASAL TUMORS.*

By HORACE F. IVINS, M.D.,
Philadelphia.

THE writer does not claim any novelty as to the use of this preparation in the treatment of post-nasal tumors, for such applications are by no means new. He wishes simply to state his experience with it in a general way, which is, perhaps, rather more extended than that of some of his colleagues. Thus it has been made available in many cases in which others would have selected operative measures.

Although many complicated applicators may be employed, the writer prefers to use the bent guarded cotton carrier, which he had made of a hard rubber tube bent in a form to pass easily back of the soft palate. Through this tube is passed a piece of moderately pliable copper wire about an inch longer than the tube.

The outer end of the wire is bent in the form of a ring, and serves as a handle for moving it forwards or backwards during its use. The inner end should be roughened so that a piece of cotton may be wound securely upon it.

* Read before the Homœopathic Medical Society, State of Pennsylvania, September 20th, 1887.

The probe thus covered with cotton is dipped into the solution to be used. The saturated absorbent cotton is then drawn within the sheath, which effectually protects it from contact with the soft palate and pharynx, thus preventing the injury which would, most probably, otherwise follow, should a spasmodic action of the muscles supervene. Except in the most tractable throats this muscular contraction is liable to occur ; but with the covered cotton-carrier no harm can result.

Before making the application it is not only very important to see that the cotton is securely fastened to the probe, but that it is not so over-saturated that a drop of the solution may run down the walls of the pharynx, or, still worse, drop directly into the larynx.

The applicator being in readiness, and, if necessary, the tumor thoroughly cleansed either by an atomizer or a post-nasal syringe, the rhinoscopic mirror is introduced, so that a clear view of the parts to be cauterized may be had. The end of the applicator is then brought in light contact with the tumor when the wire is pushed forwards. Very slight pain is occasioned if contact is not continued longer than a half minute. If the pressure be not too suddenly exerted, and only gradually increased until quite firm, but little annoyance is usually occasioned. ˙

The applications—from one to five—should be continued until the parts requiring treatment are coated yellow, thus showing the action of the acid. The treatment may be repeated every four, five or six days. As a rule, a change in the size of the tumor will be noticed after the first or second application ; and in some of the smaller hypertrophies one treatment may be all that is necessary to effect its complete reduction ; but at times it seems impossible to reduce these tumors completely.

At times cocaine has been used prior to the applications of chromic acid, but the patients were indifferent as to its use, alleging that the pain was so light that they would, usually, rather not have the anæsthetic used, as it requires extra introductions of the instruments within the post-nasal space. When used as a spray the taste of the cocaine is often more unpleasant than the pain resulting from the acid applications.

Following the use of the solution there is slight pain for a few minutes only, as a rule, but in exceptional cases sneezing occurs and continues for a short time, considerably to the annoyance of the patient.

The strength of the solution is not as important as the manner of its application. It acts best when quite strong, but not amounting in strength to saturation.

It is found impossible, in some cases, to get the consent of either parent or patient to an operation, and yet it is very evident that there is no way of curing the case within any reasonable time without removing the increased tissue; in such a case the chromic acid may act equally well, so far as the final condition is concerned, but it must not be supposed that the desired object can be speedily attained as with operative measures of a more radical nature. Such experiences as the foregoing are not infrequent.

Again, it may be exceedingly difficult and extremely painful to grasp a tumor by passing the instrument through the nares, so that it is advisable to desist; complicated with this it may be found difficult to continue instrumentation post-orally, owing to greatly thickened tissue, irritability of muscles, difficult respiration, etc., not impossible combinations. In such cases one need have no hesitation in advising the chromic acid treatment as the best. These difficulties could, it is true, be overcome by means of a general anæsthetic, but that is not always advisable, and to this patients will not always consent. Local anæsthesia does not always act satisfactorily.

In most cases of mild hypertrophy of the mucous membrane in the post-nasal region the writer has given up the use of the various snares and cutting forceps, substituting for them the chromic acid, the latter often accomplishing its work less painfully, more thoroughly, with less hemorrhage, and with less annoyance to the operator, particularly where the hypertrophy is small and difficult to grasp, and where we have to deal with an hemorrhagic diathesis.

In singers and speakers these hypertrophies are often a great hindrance to the vocal function, not only interfering with the resonance of the voice, but actually preventing the production of the higher tones. It is a great satisfaction to be able to relieve these defects by the application of the chromic acid solution.

It must not be understood that the writer advocates the use of the chromic acid to the exclusion of the more vigorous operative measures; far from it, for he very often uses the various instruments which have been found so efficient, particularly the snares both hot and cold.

The object of this paper is simply for the purpose of pointing out the efficiency of the solution used and of its great advantage in certain cases. Again, it must not be supposed for an instant that the acid can take the place of the knife, the scissors, and the chisel in the removal of large fibromata or cancerous growths.

In conclusion, it may not be considered superfluous to cite one case bearing upon this subject; an instance which has been the source of much satisfaction to those most interested, not excluding the writer, as it shows in an extreme manner what can be done with the chromic acid in post-nasal tumors.

CASE.—On the 26th January, 1885, Miss C., age 19, called and gave the following history. She had had severe naso-pharyngeal catarrh since quite small, perhaps always. The discharge was thick, profuse, yellow or green and very offensive; it came from both the nose and throat. It necessitated the use of the handkerchief every few minutes, and the effort to clear the throat was exceedingly annoying not only to her friends but to herself. Nasal respiration was rarely possible and then it was accompanied by much effort and dyspnœa. She always slept with her mouth open, and awoke with a dry, parched throat and with thirst.

The voice was usually thick and nasal, but not strictly speaking, hoarse; no cough; occasional headache; appetite and sleep good; general health moderate. Has had several attacks of some cutaneous affection, and has passed through the ordinary diseases incident to childhood. Family history good. Had been treated for a long time for the catarrh and skin affections.

Examination.—The face presented many of the usual appearances present in mouth breathers, viz. : the retracted, wrinkled lips, open mouth, contracted nasal orifices, shrunken alæ, and slightly stupid appearance. It had not existed long enough or to such an alarming degree as to result in all of the deformities sometimes noted in these cases.

The tonsils were sometimes enlarged and the surrounding mucous membrane and submucous structures were much thickened and catarrhal. This latter condition was general in the pharynx and nasal passages.

In the post-nasal space a large growth was found. It filled nearly the whole cavity, leaving a very moderate opening at the lower meatus on the left side, and almost no free space at the lower portion on the right. The tumor apparently sprang from the vault of the pharynx in the region of the pharyngeal tonsil; perhaps a fibro-mucous polypus. There is one objection to this mode of treatment; it is not always possible to be positive of the nature of the tumor, as microscopical investigation is out of the question.

After several applications of the solution were made to the tumor, in the case in question, the young lady was obliged to leave the city. She returned, however, some months later, and after a second series of treatments (in all about twenty) the tumor was reduced to a small projection, when she again abandoned treatment for the same cause as at first; but not until the discharge had nearly ceased; the voice had become quite clear; nasal respiration a permanency ; the stupid appearance had vanished and her condition greatly improved in every respect.

ORIGINAL ARTICLES IN SURGERY.

BROMINE AS AN ANTIDOTE FOR DISSECTING AND SEPTIC WOUNDS.*

By M. O. TERRY, M.D.,

Utica, New York.

I HAVE had poisoned fingers so many times and have been relieved so speedily on these various occasions with the use of *Bromine*, that I feel that I shall be a "Good Samaritan" to the surgeons wherever they may reside, to the unfortunate physician, as well as to the student in the dissecting room, if I reimpress this old remedy on your minds in a not unknown light, namely : its value as a remedy in poisoned wounds. It has been considered valuable and used quite extensively in gangrene and phlegmonous erysipelas. Perhaps one of the most practical articles on the subject referred to, is that of Dr. George Allen, of Waterville, printed in the xviii. volume of the Transactions of this State. But "brevity is the soul of wit," and I wish to make this article so short, yet impressive, that it cannot be forgotten. It was soon after I had been poisoned by operating on a malignant case of diphtheria that I noticed the death of a Brooklyn surgeon, poisoned in the same manner. This case, together with numerous cases of wounds which have come under my notice, directly or indirectly, that were tedious in healing and dangerous in character, has caused me to direct your attention to a remedy of wonderful activity and reliability.

You may theorize as you like in regard to how *bromine* acts and why it is superior to other agents, like carbolic acid, or the cautery. It has seemed to me, however, that its intrinsic worth depends principally on two properties, namely : *its power to penetrate tissues*, and to coagulate albuminoids. It not only, therefore, forms a coating over the poisoned surface of the wound, but destroys the germs of the diseased part. It has another characteristic : It arrests the inflammatory action; the abnormal heat disappears and with it the pain.

Bromine should always be kept in solution in a glass-stoppered bottle in the surgeon's office.

It can be prepared in the following manner : To an eight-ounce bottle, add about a drachm of bromide, or iodide of potash, one ounce of pure bromine, and then fill with water.

---

*Read before the Homœopathic Medical Society of the State of New York.

When necessary to use it for a poisoned finger, for instance, pour about a drachm into a glass and fill one-third with water. Insert finger for some distance beyond the wound for a few moments, and repeat every three or four hours. Occasionally one application is sufficient. No surgical dressing is necessary.

IMPROVED ORTHOPÆDIC APPARATUS.

By SIDNEY F. WILCOX, M.D.,
New York.

A NEW FOOT PIECE FOR TAYLOR'S HIP SPLINT.

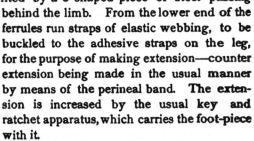

THIS consists of a pair of crutch ferrules with their rubber tips attached to the lower section of an ordinary Taylor's brace. The two ferrules are united by a U-shaped piece of steel passing behind the limb. From the lower end of the ferrules run straps of elastic webbing, to be buckled to the adhesive straps on the leg, for the purpose of making extension—counter extension being made in the usual manner by means of the perineal band. The extension is increased by the usual key and ratchet apparatus, which carries the foot-piece with it.

The advantages of this foot-piece over the ordinary cross-bar are : 1st. It is much easier for the patient to walk, as he does not have to be strung up so high in order to keep him from treading on the cross-bar. 2d. The foot swings free between the ferrules without the danger of the patient's treading on the cross-bar. 3d. The extension is made constant by means of the elastic straps which take up all the slack caused by the stretching of the adhesive plaster. 4th. The rubber cushions at the end of the ferrules diminish the noise made in walking to a great degree. This apparatus was exhibited by me at the meeting of the American Institute of Homœopathy, held in Saratoga, last summer.

GENU VALGUM OR KNOCK KNEE. APPARATUS.

The method of applying pressure to the knee is the peculiar feature of this brace. In most braces the pressure is made by means of straps which pass around the knee and are attached to the outside bar, for the purpose of drawing the knee outward. The trouble is, however, that these straps, passing around the leg, make pressure on

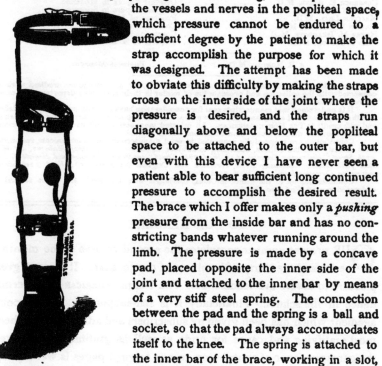

the vessels and nerves in the popliteal space, which pressure cannot be endured to a sufficient degree by the patient to make the strap accomplish the purpose for which it was designed. The attempt has been made to obviate this difficulty by making the straps cross on the inner side of the joint where the pressure is desired, and the straps run diagonally above and below the popliteal space to be attached to the outer bar, but even with this device I have never seen a patient able to bear sufficient long continued pressure to accomplish the desired result. The brace which I offer makes only a *pushing* pressure from the inside bar and has no constricting bands whatever running around the limb. The pressure is made by a concave pad, placed opposite the inner side of the joint and attached to the inner bar by means of a very stiff steel spring. The connection between the pad and the spring is a ball and socket, so that the pad always accommodates itself to the knee. The spring is attached to the inner bar of the brace, working in a slot, so that the pad can lie close up against the bar or projected to some distance from it, as more or less pressure is desired. The pressure is regulated by means of a small screw which, being passed through the bar and spring at a higher or lower hole, increases or · decreases the angle of the spring with the bar.

I have employed both of the above forms of apparatus with excellent results in several cases.

EDITORIAL DEPARTMENT.

EDITORS

GEORGE M. DILLOW, M.D., ...	Editor-in-Chief, Editorial and Book Reviews.
CLARENCE E. BEEBE, M.D., ...	Original Papers in Medicine.
SIDNEY F. WILCOX, M.D., ...	Original Papers in Surgery.
MALCOLM LEAL, M.D., ...	Progress of Medicine.
EUGENE H. PORTER, M.D., ...	Comments and News.
HENRY M. DEARBORN, M.D., ...	Correspondence.
FRED S. FULTON, M.D., ...	Reports of Societies and Hospitals.

A B. NORTON, M.D., ... Business Manager.

The Editors individually assume full responsibility for and are to be credited with all connected with the collection and presentation of matter in their respective departments, but are not responsible for the opinions of contributors.

It is understood that manuscripts sent for consideration have not been previously published, and that after notice of acceptance has been given, will not appear elsewhere except in abstract and with credit to THE NORTH AMERICAN. All rejected manuscripts will be returned to writers. No anonymous or discourteous communications will be printed.

Contributors are respectfully requested to send manuscripts and communicate respecting them directly with the Editors, according to subject, as follows: *Concerning Medicine, 21 West 37th Street; concerning Surgery, 256 West 57th Street; concerning Societies and Hospitals, 111 East 70th Street; concerning News, Personals and Original Miscellany, 161 West 71st Street; concerning Correspondence, 152 West 57th Street.*

Communications to the Editor-in-Chief, *Exchanges* and *New Books* for notice should be addressed to *102 West 43d Street.*

TO OUR · READERS.

OUR present number completes the second volume of the monthly series and the thirty-fifth volume of our JOURNAL. It gives us great pleasure to assure our readers that THE NORTH AMERICAN is a permanence in the school. Financially it is self-supporting. The encouragement which has been given by subscribers and advertisers has been most gratifying and cause for pride as well as gratitude. Moreover, the generous favor of contributors to our original pages is warmly appreciated as furnishing the essential condition of our success.

Yet by no means should it be thought that we have reached the acme of our aspirations. It has been the hope from the beginning to enlarge the JOURNAL as it grew in means, to properly illustrate its articles and to pay for the better class of contributions. With eleven thousand homœopathic practitioners in America alone such a hope ought not to seem extravagant. Surely some one journal of the school should be excellent enough to command sufficient patronage to warrant the publication of a periodical upon the liberal scale to which homœopathy is entitled by reason of its numbers and its talents. It was believed that, if confidence could be made to grow in the motives of the promoters of our enterprise and that if the editors could demonstrate their ability to present a good journal in the infant stages of their experience, support would finally come in such abundance as would realize our reasonable ambition. And that ambition was to furnish a journal that would rival in scholarly editing the best models of medical journalism and be distinctively homœopathic in its purposes. In two years the Monthly has more than quadrupled the subscription list of the Quarterly as we took it, and we believe that we can say, with becoming modesty, that it has equalled in every respect the best of our homœopathic contemporaries. Moreover the signs ahead are such as to lead to the positive expectation of the income that will warrant a larger expenditure in the interests of our subscribers and especially of better journalism.

However, we can make no more definite promises for 1888 than that all profits over and above expenses will be directed toward the improvement of the Journal. The editors receive no compensation and will take none, for in no sense is The North American a commercial enterprise, directly or indirectly. It is entirely independent of all publishing and pharmaceutical firms, of all colleges and all societies, and is backed by a sufficient number of physicians to make it broadly representative of the school, and so variously composed as to put it beyond any single influence that might dominate its policy. The editors have full discretion to edit the Journal without direction, dictation or interference, a freedom undisturbed thus far without a single exception. They have endeavored to sink their individuality or at least their individual interests in their work, which has been divided for its more efficient performance and faithfully done without an exception by every member of our corps. Their harmonious coöperation in the past gives every reason to believe that it will continue.

To our subscribers therefore we would say that we look to them not as endorsing our every opinion or as viewing us without criticism, but as coöperating with us in our endeavor to evolve a journal of ampler scope and a higher standard of excellence. In return we engage to give them, and through them the school, our best efforts to make our pages as scholarly, original, practical and abreast of advances in medicine as the editors can command with increasing means. The policy of publishing no original paper which has appeared elsewhere in print will be adhered to, and as before we shall fill our columns throughout with matter not taken from other journals, except in the abstracts in Medical Progress made expressly for our pages. Padding and scissorial stealing will find no countenance in THE NORTH AMERICAN ; for honesty is believed to be the best policy even in medical journalism.

THE BOARD OF HEALTH AND THE MEDICAL PROFESSION.

IN a recent paper read before the New York Academy of Medicine, Dr. Joseph D. Bryant, in behalf of the Commissioners of Health, of whom he is one, presented a forcible appeal to the members of the profession to co-operate more actively with our city Health Department. He estimated that from fifteen to twenty-five per cent. of the cases of contagious diseases and from twenty-five to thirty per cent. of births were not reported by the physicians of the city. He urged that all forms of contagious diseases should be reported at once so that the Health Department may apply quickly all possible means to prevent their spread, and that patients with contagious diseases be strictly isolated. Where isolation cannot be practiced or where adequate treatment cannot be provided, he recommended immediate reports to the Board, so that patients may be removed to the hospital. He called attention to the facilities for the treatment of contagious diseases in the Willard Parker Hospital at the foot of East Sixteenth Street, and in the buildings on North Brothers' Island. The paper throughout showed a most commendable desire to furnish much needed information relating to the organization of the Health Board and its plans, and to bring about more harmonious action between it and the profession, or at least that portion of it which assumes to comprise the whole profession as limited in the New York Academy of Medicine.

There can be no question but that the recent changes in our Health Board have done much to take this department out of the baneful influence of politics and to make it a more enlightened and efficient organization for the protection of public health and the prevention of disease. In appointing a medical man as one of the Commissioners, a further step was taken in advance, for without the interested co-operation of the physicians of the city the Board will be practically fettered in an important portion of its work. Attention should, however, be called to the fact that the Academy of Medicine is but a portion of the profession of the city, and that while it may furnish the most flattering audience to the medical Commissioner, it is not practically the widest avenue to the ear of the profession, and moreover is but one of many. The Academy of Medicine is comparatively small and exclusive in membership, and is essentially not a body representative of the profession as a whole. If the Board of Health wishes to ally with it the whole profession, it should seek the profession as a whole ; all medical bodies, regardless of distinction as to schools, ought to be appealed to. The Board, especially, should see to it that the Society affiliation of its one medical commissioner should not bring about unwise discrimination within the profession. It should be remembered that the several County Societies of New York are, under the law of the State, the representative societies of the City, and to *all* of these the Commissioners of Health should properly go when communicating with the profession. If the Board limits its appeals to one section of the profession it so far limits its power to restrict and prevent contagious diseases. For contagion utterly ignores the so-called codes of ethics, and will spread as quickly from any focus, whether it be under "regular" or "irregular" observation. The law of the State furnishes the standard of what constitutes the profession, and the Board of Health should treat the profession as broadly and impartially as the law.

There is also a question in regard to the treatment of patients with contagious diseases in hospitals to which the Health Commissioners should give attention. With all due respect to the medical officers of the hospitals for contagious diseases, it should be said that the Health Board has not made full provision for adequate treatment in them, that is, in the belief of a large number of laymen of the city and a very respectable body of physicians. There is not a hospital, public or private, in the city of New York where a person sick of scarlet fever, of diphtheria, of small-pox or of any other serious contagious disease can have homœopathic treatment. If the city assumes the power, in the interests of public health, to compel removal to hospitals, it is bound equally to respect the rights of private judgment in regard to the method of medical treatment upon which the individual may believe that his life will depend. Not only should this be accorded as a matter of right, but also in the interests of the public health. In giving the sick no choice as between methods of treatment there is a direct incentive to the concealment of cases of contagious disease both on the part of physicians and patients, who have an assured confidence in the superiority of the one method over the other. The homœopathic physicians of New York have forborne to push their just claims to a share of the appointments in the control of our Board of Health, but it is questionable whether homœopathic laymen, who are taxpayers as well, should submit to be deprived of a very clear and proper right in obedience to the tantamount dictation of one portion of the medical profession as against the other. The Board of Health has a simple remedy in the appointmeut of one or more homœopathic physicians upon the staffs of the city hospitals for contagious diseases, or in setting aside a small hospital, or even pavilion to be under homœopathic direction. By acting with fairness and impartiality toward believers in homœopathy, the suppression of contagious diseases in the city would be more practically invited than is now the case.

A CYCLOPÆDIA OF PURE DRUG PATHOGENESY.

A T the last meeting of the British Homœopathic Congress (for 1887) Dr. Herbert Nankivell was appointed to edit a companion volume to the Cyclopædia of Drug Pathogenesy, which is to supplement that record of pure drug effects with the pharmacology and therapeutics of our remedies. The work is to appear *pari passu* with the volumes of the Cyclopædia as they are issued, but not to be embodied with them. There is the further good news that Dr. Hughes expects that the Cyclopædia will be completed by 1890, and that the Index will then be proceeded with, most likely in the schematic form.

In the discussion which took place upon the subject of Materia Medica, the Cyclopædia was criticised freely by Dr. Hayward as comparatively useless to the general practitioner in his daily work.

Attention was drawn to the fact that in the hurry of practice "it is simply impossible to find in it whether any particular drug has produced any particular symptom when wanted for comparison in a case of disease." Even with the proposed Index, it was doubted whether any symptom will easily be found. On the other hand, it was contended by Dr. Dudgeon, that its editors had never intended that it should be used as a repertory, but that its value lay in its giving a connected history of medicinal diseases for intelligent study. Dr. Pope showed that the Cyclopædia would prove to be the foundation for commentaries, repertories and clinical guides when the demand comes, and that "if practitioners would make their own indices it would be far better for them, and that they would learn far more than by merely reading the work of other men." The indexing he had found to be easily done.

In the soundness of the conclusion arrived at—to adhere to the original plan so far carried on—every clear-sighted observer of the present needs of homœopathy will concur. The school needs to be led back to systematic study of our fundamental science for its own sake as well as for its application. The pure science of drug-diseases ought to be kept distinct and apart from the art of applying that knowledge to the cure of other diseases. Just as there can be no good practical chemist who has not studied chemistry as a pure science before he has passed on to its applications for useful purposes, so there can be no good therapeutist, who has not studied his Materia Medica systematically apart from its applications to the cure of disease. And as the pure and applied works in all the sciences are kept distinct, so should they be separated in the sciences of the pure and applied Materia Medica, before they can be satisfactorily brought together. Our works upon Materia Medica have been mainly such mixtures of pure and empirical indications that the science of homœopathy has been almost lost as a serious study among its practitioners. We are sincerely glad that in this case there has been no yielding to the pressure of the "general practitioner," whose cry is for a Materia Medica made easy which he can apply without study in a moment. The fact is, no Materia Medica can be made easy for a mind which has never attained intelligent elementary conceptions of the action of drugs upon the healthy human body, clearly outlined apart from their use in disease. Dr. Pope justly observed that, "in such an enormous study as is that of Materia Medica, when rightly viewed, we need, not one, but several works, each looking at it from a different point of view."

The one view and that the most essential view of all—because the fundamental view—has been the one hitherto most neglected. It may or may not be true that the practitioner will not be able to use the Cyclopædia for a ready-reference repertory or symptom-catalogue, but it is certain that it will give him something better—the pure material for working out by himself a coherent view of the general pathogenetic action of each drug, or if not by himself, by some other man, less indolent or more capable.

A COMMENDABLE REFORM.

OUR neighbor, *The Medical Times*, should be applauded for the reform it has instituted upon its editorial pages; the reader can now determine how much is borrowed matter and how much editorial learning and meditation. The reform should be completed by placing copied matter in different type and embracing it with quotation marks.

We notice, however, that as our neighbor advances in one direction it is slipping back in another. Anonymous correspondence, after having been eliminated for a season, is re-appearing, and it may not be long before editor and asterisk will begin the old game of battledore and shuttlecock, in which responsibility is kept so continually flying in the air, as it were, that no one can tell exactly where it should be placed. Anonymous letters, to be sure, have the advantage of affording opportunity for the practice of editorial ventriloquy, and there is, perhaps, a greater sense of security in resorting, on occasion, to the journalistic puppet-show when one would like to escape the consequences of saying all one wishes; but, after all, puppet-shows in medical journalism are pretty certain to be recognized, and the practice of ventriloquy, somehow, takes out the tone of sincerity from the editorial voice, may even render it aphonic. Avowed responsibility is better in the long run for every editor and correspondent.

AN EDITOR'S RESPONSIBILITY.

WE would again call attention to the fact that the editor of a medical journal is responsible for the decency of his columns. While an editor, by publication, does not necessarily endorse the opinions of contributors, he is bound not to permit his pages to be made the medium of malice, reckless misstatements, and obscene suggestions. Especially is this true in the department of controversial correspondence, where vigilant supervision is demanded in order to eliminate the malevolent element in personalities. These remarks are apropos of the Editor of *The Medical Advance,* who has admitted correspondence which would in New York State legitimately claim the censorship of Anthony Comstock. His offense of September is repeated in his November number, and aggravated by an attempt to saddle his editorial responsibility for publication upon the shoulders of the writer of the letter.

As a gentleman in journalism the Editor owes an apology to his readers for a grave offense against the decency of the press. It is not now a question of homœopathy or no homœopathy or of anything else except, what should constitute the tone of a journal and an editor.

COMMENTS.

CHRISTIAN SCIENCE.—Some time ago Rev. Dr. Buckley, editor of the *Christian Advocate,* in an article contributed to the *Century Magazine,* declared that the tendency of faith healing is to produce an effeminate type of character which shrinks from pain and concentrates itself upon self and its sensations. He also gave as his opinion that it destroys the ascendency of reason in the soul, and that it tends to mental derangement. That these conclusions, reached only after prolonged study and experiment, were eminently just there can be no doubt. Accumulating evidence demonstrates clearly their foundation in fact. Many cases have been reported where insanity has followed adherence to the faith cure. Drawing their dupes from the ranks of the ignorant or credulous these new apostles of charlatanism gain rapid mental dominion. The victims, fascinated by the strange and mysterious methods, go again and again, and perhaps essay to learn the wonderful art. The ordinary duties of life are neglected, visions and dreams fill the weak brain, and finally mental aberation results. The doctrines of these so-called Christian scientists are at once pernicious and blasphemous. Should their methods obtain ascendency genuine science would disappear, the light of extended knowledge would be replaced by the cimmerian darkness of superstitious ignorance. That the mental attitude of the patient has much to do with his recovery is well known. In the hands of the thoughtful physician this is sometimes a potent weapon against the power of disease. To employ this marvelous power which the mind wields over its tenement is legitimate. To cheer and encourage the sick, to stimulate the flagging energies, to rouse the sluggish intellect enfeebled by disease, is the province and duty of the doctor. But to traffic in the innocence and simple-mindedness of the weak and unfortunate, to barter and trade upon the miseries of the suffering, this is the province of ghouls, or of the "Christian Scientists" falsely so called.

BOARD OF CHARITIES REPORT.—The Standing Committee on the Insane of the State Board of Charieties, to whom was referred the letter of the Mayor of the city of New York dated June 17th, 1887, and calling attention to certain complaints made to him "that the management of the Lunatic Asylum on Ward's Island is not such as to entitle it to public confidence," and asking that a prompt investigation be made, has submitted a special report. The findings of the Committee as set forth in their report are not especially favorable to the asylum. The buildings are overcrowded and insufficient, the food is not decently cooked and prepared and there is incontestable evidence that the patients are subject to abuse and indignities by the attendants. A suggestive fact brought out during the investigation was that a large proportion of the keepers appointed were or had been bartenders. The Committee mildly aver that while bar-keepers may be suitable persons to place in charge of the insane it is more than probable that they are quite the reverse. It would be interesting to know why the saloon should be so well represented in the matter of appointees. The Committee swing a large club somewhat savagely around, but do not seem to be quite sure whom to hit, so they give everybody a gentle tap. Responsibility is so divided up in the administration of affairs that they cannot succeed in holding any one directly responsible. They state that some blame must attach to the system. They might have said more. They might have said, and truthfully, that the system is an eminently vicious one, honeycombed with saloon politics. When the present system gives place to better methods, then may better results be expected and not till then.

ANNUAL REPORT OF LAURA FRANKLIN HOSPITAL.—The first annual report of this institution for the care and homœopathic treatment of children will shortly be given to the public. It will be of special interest from the fact that the results of the year's work will be at once compared with those attained at the children's hospital in this city controlled by the allopaths. The *Record*, in its spleen and disappointment at seeing the new hospital placed under the charge of homœopaths, gratuitously insulted the generous founder of the noble charity, and feebly sputtered forth that putting homœopaths in control was little less than criminal. Let us see what the "criminal" homœopaths have done. There have been admitted to the hospital since

November 21st, 1887, 153 patients from ten to twelve years of age. Of these there have been discharged cured, 78 ; discharged improved, 30 ; and discharged unimproved, 9 ; not treated, 2 ; transferred, 2 ; died, 7. In the hospital at present, 25. The causes of death were secondary hemorrhage, 1 ; pneumo thorax, 1 ; heart-clot, 1 ; double pneumonia, 1 ; extensive burns, 1 ; pulmonary tuberculosis, 2. The surgical cases have numbered 77, and the medical 76. The number of operations is 26. Percentage of deaths, .045. This would seem to be pretty fair for a "criminal" record. Can our amiable friends of the *Record* produce a report to beat it ?

STRINGENT LAWS.—The laws of Canada applying to physicians coming there from other countries to practice are singularly severe and exclusive. In Ontario, for instance, no physician or surgeon can practice without passing all the examinations held by the Council of the College of Physicians and Surgeons; and he must also attend one or more sessions at one of the medical colleges recognized by the Council. These laws, however, are impartial and apply with equal force to both homœopathic and allopathic practitioners. In educational matters the standard is high, and all students have to pass the same examinations, with the exception of materia medica and practice of medicine. The great difficulty that obstructs the way of homœopathy in Canada seems to be the want of a school where homœopathy is taught. At present there is no chair of homœopathic therapeutics, but students are examined upon them if they desire. This renders the growth of the new school slow.

THE CHIRONIAN.—This bright semi-monthly magazine, edited and published by the students of the New York Homœopathic Medical College, again appears, after the usual summer sleep, upon our table. Its good looks secure it a welcome, and its contents, ranging from clinical reports to poems and college news, ought to bring in a subscription from every alumnus.

BOOK REVIEWS.

THE STUDENT'S GUIDE TO DISEASES OF THE EYE, by EDWARD NETTLESHIP, F.R.C.S. Third American, from the Fourth English Edition. Royal 12mo. Pp. 475. Philadelphia : Lea Brothers & Co. 1887.

This edition of Nettleship's work upon Diseases of the Eye, enlarged by some fifty pages in accordance with the progress of ophthalmology, is a decided improvement over former editions. The high standing of the author as a writer and earnest investigator merits for his work a careful review. The arrangement is somewhat different from the usual text books upon ophthalmology. It is divided into three parts.

Part I., in four chapters, considers, "Optical Outlines," "External Examination of the Eye," "Examination for Color-perception," "Examination of the Eye by Artificial Light." The chapter upon color-perception is a monograph by Wm. Thompson, M.D., upon "Examination of Railway Employees." Though this may be of interest in itself and a good advertisement for the Pennsylvania Railroad, yet it does not briefly give the information a student desires in a text book of this kind. Special mention must be made of the clear explanation of the theory of Retinoscopy and its method of application as given upon page 82. It is concise, yet full, and easy to understand.

In Part II., "Clinical Division," the author describes the various affections of the eye, and gives the appropriate operative and medicinal treatment according to the most improved old school therapeutics. One chapter is devoted to all injuries of the eyeball, and another to all tumors and new growths, both extra- and intra-ocular. Instead of explaining the method of operating for any particular affection along with the treatment of the disease, as is customary, reference is made to Chapter XXIII., in which all operations upon the eye and its appendages are described. This arrangement is more of a disadvantage than otherwise. The anatomy is not given with the exception of a few points now and then which are necessary to intelligently understand disease.

Much credit is due the writer for the clearness and accuracy with which he pictures the diseases under consideration. This, together with many excellent illustrations, make it easy for the student to understand his subject.

In the author's endeavor to condense, he has in some instances passed over with a mere mention, or even omitted entirely, affections which to us seem more important than some which have received a detailed description. This is true in nearly all sections; still in this respect great charity must be allowed an author of so condensed a text book as this, for no two ophthalmologists will agree upon the relative importance of all diseases of the eye.

Part III. pertains to "Diseases of the Eye in Relation to General Diseases," in which will be found the various eye changes which occur as a part of the general disease, those which are symptomatic of some local malady at a distance, and those which share in a local process, affecting the neighboring parts. This will be of interest to the general practitioner.

The book is one in which there is much to commend and much to criticise, but more favorable will be the criticism when one bears in mind the size of the volume. There is no better text book upon ophthalmology in so small a compass, but there are two or three others, larger and a little more expensive, which are far superior and of more value to the student and general practitioner.

The names of the publishers are a sufficient guarantee of the excellence of their work.   G. S. N.

HOW TO STUDY MATERIA MEDICA. Three Lectures by C. WESSELHOEFT, M.D. Boston: Otis Clapp & Son, 1887.

The lectures reprinted, as above, from the *New England Medical Gazette*, have been published at the request of graduates of the Boston University School of Medicine. The method of study recommended is first, self-proving; second, methodical reading of reliable pathogenesies, toxicological essays and experiments, grouping according to botanical, zoological and chemical analogies; third, condensing in writing the long symptom lists and narratives ; fourth, arranging the condensed symptoms in four columns according to their kind, location, time and conditions, with a short summary at the foot of each column of the chief characteristics ; last, comparing the members of a group to bring out points of similarity and difference. For the tedious memorizing of dislocated symptoms he would substitute study of the narratives of provers. especially as embodied in the Cyclopædia of Drug Pathogenesy. He believes that the method proposed, or something akin to it, will result in an actual saving of time and give the student the clue to the "inner meaning that is to be read between the lines of a pathogenesy." He says : "I would urgently advise you to select some practical method of this kind; but not to let things drift along, hoping 'and trusting that, in future practice, your reliance on repertories will in time furnish the experiences and practical routine you need. All you will get by that will be an uncertain habit of groping about; and this, in turn, will surely lead to want of confidence in yourselves, and inability to separate that which is reliable from that which is useless." How truthfully this latter sentence describes a great number of homœopathic prescribers is alas too evident. Whether the author's plan, too briefly indicated in the preceding to present an adequate conception of its practical application, will or should meet with general acceptance we cannot consider, but there can be no question of the need for some better plan of study than is commonly pursued. We doubt, however, whether the author has not overrated the power of the average student to analyze, condense and generalize for himself, and we fear that, while his study of How to Study Materia Medica is practically suggestive, it leaves so much option to the student that he will go on as before. Not only do students need to be methodical in study, but they need to be guided in learning how to be methodical to the best advantage, and moreover, guided in detail. If the author would prepare an outline manual for drug-proving and an outline manual of drug-pathogenesy where the student will be directed specifically what he should do, as he is in a course of laboratory study of chemistry, for example, he would put his valuable suggestions into still more practical form, and perhaps lead a reform in the methods of Materia Medica study in our colleges.

OPERATIVE SURGERY ON THE CADAVER. By JASPER JEWETT GARMANY, A.M., M.D., F.R.C.S. New York, 1887. D. Appleton & Co. 150 pages, with two illustrations.

The preface of this book, dedicated by the author *in memoriam* to his preceptor, the late Prof. James R. Wood, M.D., LL.D., states that his endeavor is "to present a guide to the manipulative procedures of the ordinary surgical operations." The author having modestly promised but little, and there being so many works on the same subject, one naturally expects little that is new ; but he has given in a very small space what many writers describe at great length with far less satisfaction to the reader.

The lack of illustrations gives a first impression that the book is inadequate to fulfill its object, but when one comes to read over the concise, graphic descriptions of operative procedures, he finds that illustration is almost wholly unnecessary. An exception may be made in regard to the descriptions of the various knots and sutures, which are a trifle ambiguous; illustrations in this chapter would have been a great addition. The two colored plates are from Smith and Walsham, giving the collateral circulation after tying arteries at various points.

The author has evidently sought to give only descriptions of the *best* operations, discarding as worthless lumber such methods as have long been handed down, and which have been superseded by better ones. The author has really given more than he promised, for besides what we consider "ordinary operations" he has given the newest methods for performing many operations which are not yet in general use. Intubation of the larynx, the various operations on the abdomen and its contents, shortening of the round ligament, operations on nerves and the circulatory and osseous systems are described at sufficient length, and with remarkable clearness.

We endorse it as among the best and most valuable works on operative surgery.   W.

CYCLOPÆDIA OF OBSTETRICS AND GYNÆCOLOGY, Vol. VII. Operations on the Tubes, Uterus, Broad Ligaments, Round Ligaments, and Vagina. Operations on Urinary Fistulæ. Prolapse Operations. Operations on the Vulva and Perineum. By Dr. A. HEGAR and Dr. R. KALTENBACH. Translated by EGBERT H. GRANDIN, M.D. New York: Wm. Wood & Co., 1887.

This work treats of the various pathological processes and operations, which it discusses in a very able manner. In their advocacy of the vaginal extirpation of the uterus under certain conditions, the authors are certainly in advance of American writers and operators. They present the successful aspect of an operation which is almost universally shunned and feared on this side of the water. While there is much boldness in many of their operations, their technique is not equal to that of American surgeons. The methods in many instances are more crude and less finished. They recommend the use of a 1 to 1,000 solution of bichloride of mercury. In many instances, where we would regard it as essential, they do not employ Sim's speculum, but cling, with German tenacity, to the old-fashioned bivalve. Emmet's operation of trachelorrhaphy does not receive the consideration due it. Their results, after its performance, are not satisfactory, nor do we see how they could be otherwise than poor, with their method of operating. The lips are simply pared and united, leaving all the diseased tissue behind. We should like to have seen rapid dilatation discussed in connection with discission, but the harsher and nearly abandoned method is the only one recommended for the evils for which such treatment is advised. The work represents the heavier style of operative procedures, which is in marked contrast with the more finished technique of our own operations. Every surgeon should be conversant with the various modes of operative procedures, but, in the main, they will do well to follow the methods as laid down in American text books. F.

AMERICAN MEDICINAL PLANTS. By MILLSPAUGH. Boericke and Tafel. Fascicle VI. Nos. 26–30.

This, the concluding number, contains the title pages (one for each volume), the preface, an alphabetical list of remedies, a natural arrangement of the plants illustrated, an appendix of sixty-six pages comprising a glossary, a bibliography, a bibliographical index (very full and valuable), a general index to this work, and notes and corrections, as well as the illustrations and text of the following plants: Aethusa, Anthemis nob., Cannabis, Dioscorea, Epilobium, Erechthites, Erigeron, Eryngium, Euphrasia, Fraxinus, Gnaphalium, Hedeoma, Helleborus vir., Hyoscyamus, Lamium, Lapathum, Lobelia card., Lycopodium, Mentha pip., Nabalus, Prinos, Raphanus, Rumex, Sambucus Can., Scutellaria, Spigelia mar., Stillingia, Tanacetum, Urtica urens and Uva ursi.

Among the most excellent plates we are best pleased with Lycopodium (its accompanying text is fine), Dioscorea (a bold and artistic drawing), Cannabis (a double plate), Urtica, Hyoscyamus (the finest plate in the whole collection perhaps !), Helleborus, and Sambucus. This part seems to comprise the most satisfactorily drawn and colored plates of the whole work ; indeed there is nothing but unstinted praise for every part. The completion of this work should mark a proud day for Millspaugh, who has erected an enduring monument to his skill and learning. * * *

VOL. IX. DISEASES OF THE FEMALE MAMMARY GLANDS, by TH. BILLROTH, M.D. ; and NEW GROWTHS OF THE UTERUS, by A. GUSSEROW, M.D.; edited by EGBERT H. GRANDIN, M.D. New York: Wm. Wood & Co., 1887.

Both divisions of this work we believe to be in advance of corresponding treatises by American authors. The description of tumors of the mamma and uterus is more scientific and exact. While the clinical portion is not curtailed, or its importance slighted, the pathological histology, as established by the microscope, is recognized as the basis of classification in a most practical and thorough manner. Their presentation of the subject is more scientific, as well as practical, than that of authors on this side who, through lack of investigation, are less scientific. The chapters on the pathology, course and symptoms of uterine fibro-myomata are the most complete we have ever seen, while that on uterine fibroids, in their relation to pregnancy, parturition and childbed, fills a most notable lack in the literature of gynæcology and obstetrics, and supplies abundant and reliable information upon that subject, for which many students have searched long and fruitlessly. F.

CORRESPONDENCE.

HOMŒOPATHY IN CANADA.

To the Editors of the NORTH AMERICAN JOURNAL OF HOMŒOPATHY:

Glancing over the past year there certainly has been some advance made in this offshoot of the homœopathic world, but the supreme effort put forward appears almost to have strangled the new growth for the time being, but I am in hopes it is only a passing stroke which will give place to healthy reaction and increased development.

Perchance my language is rather obscure to those unacquainted with the conditions under which homœopathy *exists* in this country; if so I will explain.

The stripling shrub (homœopathy) has remained stunted in growth since the year 1869, at which time the Ontario College of Physicians and Surgeons was incorporated, which absorbed the then existing Homœopathic Board, allowing it instead a representation of five members and an examiner in the homœopathic branches of medicine.

The larger trees of the wood have truly choked the growth of the young sapling in their midst, and although its appearance may be as fresh as any of its neighbors (for the allopathic and homœopathic profession are on an equal footing as regards their recognized medical standing), yet, sad to relate, its proportions are as near as possible similar to those of twenty years ago ; the reason of this I cannot argue now, but will seek to set forth at some future date.

The supreme effort, above referred to, was in the form of establishing a free homœopathic dispensary in February last, the first public institution in Canada under the banner of homœopathy. May it only be the prelude to still greater achievements and secure for this system of medical science the honor it so richly deserves. The institution is supported entirely by public subscriptions and carried on by an association in connection therewith, and though the beginning is small, still it will no doubt in time (if the homœopaths maintain concerted action) lead up to still greater things in the not far distant future. A homœopathic hospital may be the outcome of a few more years, provided our citizens are generous enough to set apart sufficient funds for the carrying out of such a project, but in this respect we are much behind the wealthy citizens of the United States.

Jealousies and hard feelings crept in among the different members of the homœopathic profession during the establishment of the dispensary, unfortunately resulting in splitting up our local Society which had been flourishing for three years, but perchance the smouldering embers may brighten up again before long. Our local society used to meet once a month during the winter session for the reading of medical papers, discussions and the transaction of other business of interest to the profession. For a time harmony existed and much profit ensued to the members and to homœopathy, but eventually antagonistic forces crept in and destroyed our unity with the above stated result.

The Canadian Institute of Homœopathy met in its twelfth annual session on June 20th and 21st of this year, at Toronto.

The session was a very profitable one, though the attendance was not as large as might have been expected; still many good papers were read and discussed, and important business transacted in the line of securing a homœopathic ward in the general hospital for the homœopathic treatment of diseases. This Institute of Homœopathy is now the only cementing link between the different members of the profession throughout Canada, and we may hope that it will yet raise our system of medicine out of the obscurity into which it has fallen during the past fifteen years.

Our union with the College of Physicians and Surgeons has raised our standing as medical men in the eyes of the public, but nevertheless, I believe, it has lowered the standard of homœopathy very materially and given us somewhat of an eclectic system,

The Canadians are more conservative in their views than the Americans and slower in the progress of reform, which facts may account in some measure for our feeble strides. Still good seed sown will bear fruit in course of time if properly tended and fostered.

R. HEARN, M.D.

TORONTO, November, 1887.

REPORTS OF SOCIETIES AND HOSPITALS.

HOMŒOPATHIC MEDICAL SOCIETY, COUNTY OF NEW YORK.

STATED meeting, October 8th, 1887, President Beebe in the chair. Bureau of Ophthalmology and Otology, Dr. George S. Norton, Chairman. The first paper presented was by Charles C. Boyle, M.D., upon "The Treatment of Convergent Strabismus."

Dr. G. S. Norton admires the confidence of the writer in correcting squint, but cannot agree with Dr. Boyle in all points. The use of convex glasses, atropine and systematic exercises are most important. In relation to the operation, some ten or twelve years ago, he advocated operating both eyes at once, and was especially enthusiastic upon the subject, writing an article upon it for the New York State Society, but he found that the results were not always permanent. In a few cases slight divergence occurred, or symptoms of muscular asthenopia some time after the operation. Of late years he does not consider the operation for squint so easily and certainly curative as he did in his early experience. At the International Congress,'just held in Washington, Dr. Henry Power seemed to voice the experience of the oldest operators when he said that he was not near as certain of a positive cure of squint as formerly, and that he now took a great deal more care of his cases before operation. Landolt usually advances the external rectus at the same time that he makes tenotomy of the internal. This operation Dr. Norton does not consider so simple that it will be universally adopted. He further believes that it is usually better to operate one eye at a time, being careful to tell the parents that two operations will probably be required. He would not operate until the child is six or seven years of age, if the vision can be retained by exercise and the strabismus is not excessive; for a perfect correction of squint at four years of age is liable to result in weakness of the internal recti after the child begins the use of eyes for reading.

Dr. Deady feels that the operation for squint requires as much or more care and judgment than that for cataract. Has had none that turned outwards, but has always exercised great caution to avoid doing too much, and in some cases has had them still turn in somewhat after the operation.

Dr. John L. Moffat :—The best surgery is that which succeeds without operating. While in many cases the operation is unavoidable, doubtless a large percentage of the failures is because the cause was not thoroughly removed before resorting to the knife.

Dr. Boyle, in closing the discussion, stated that in the cases he had operated none had turned outwards. That formerly, while Dr. Norton's assistant, he had been taught to divide the operation between the two eyes, but that lately he had operated both eyes at once, and would continue doing so until he saw the eyes operated on turning outwards.

Dr. Charles Deady read a paper upon " Progressive Myopia."

Dr. George S. Norton :—There is one point that the general practitioner should bear in mind, *viz.:* that *all* cases of myopia are progressive, or tend to become so, between the ages of ten and eighteen, while the eyes are constantly used in study. Therefore, during this period, all cases should be frequently tested and the results recorded, so that any tendency to increase may at once be detected.

Dr. Deady, in closing the discussion, said that he agreed with Dr. Boynton as to the use of atropine, as he has seen cases where trouble has followed from its use, but believes that in this disease it is a necessity and must be used. Has never seen bad results where a perfectly pure preparation has been used with proper precaution, unless instilled with much greater frequency than is necessary in this variety of trouble.

Dr. N. L. McBride read a paper on " A Case of Neuro-retinitis."

Dr. George S. Norton thought that the case was one of interest. A similar case of neuro-retinitis simulating retinitis albuminurca was reported in *Graefe's Archives* many years ago, and in the Ophthalmological and Otological Societies' Transactions for 1879, the doctor had recorded another case with same characteristics. In both cases the autopsy had revealed a glio-sarcoma in the brain.

Dr. Boyle said that Gower, in his work, speaks of appearances in the retina in every way similar to those found in Bright's disease, resulting from tumor of the brain.

Dr. F. H. Boynton read his paper on "Cerebral Gumma, Paralysis of the Ocular Muscles—Cure."

Dr. John L. Moffat asked his method of administering the iodide of potash, because in one of his cases the patient stopped short of as large doses as were desired because of sore throat, burning and gas in the stomach, resulting whenever the drug was taken.

Dr. Houghton spoke of a case of retinitis that he had watched at the Manhattan Hospital, where the iodide of potassium was given in doses of one hundred and eighty grains, three times a day in milk, with no apparent effect upon the system. The disease was checked.

Dr. F. H. Boynton then read a second paper upon cases illustrating t e influence of small degrees of astigmatism in producing nervous disorders.

Dr. George S. Norton read a paper upon "Can Headache and Asthenope be produced by small degrees of Astigmatism ? "

Dr. George S. Norton said that at Washington he was surprised to find so few eminent ophthalmologists who never corrected their small errors—some of whom doubted if their small errors could be detected. This was probably due to their using too large lines in the examination. Your radiating lines must be small or you will not discover an error of 0.25 D.

Dr. Schley:—Mr. President: I do not think we can let the ophthalmologists go uncontradicted in the brilliant results claimed to be obtained by them in cases of cephalalgia and nervous troubles, due to ocular abnormalities. I have seen a goodly number of my own patients accurately fitted by oculists with glasses, such as would remedy their eye trouble. In most of these their abnormal refraction, etc., was claimed to be the *fons et origo mali*. They were subjects of migraine, etc. I have found in a great many of these cases that at first they were often much relieved by their glasses, and then, later, the symptoms would return as bad as ever. In cases of migraine, where it has been asserted that a cure followed the adjustment of proper glasses, I maintain, in some, that such is not a fact. One case in especial I should like to mention of a gentleman—a member ·of the Produce Exchange, overworked and of an exceedingly nervous temperament—was advised by a Dr. S—— to have both of his internal recti cut, as the sole means of a cure for his many small ailments. . He consulted me about it. I advised adversely, and urged a three-months' trip to Europe. The patient since his return is better than ever.

In relation to large doses of iodide of potash, as mentioned by Dr. Boynton, I would cite some observation of Dr. E. Hurry Fenwick, in which he states that it may be administered in very large doses if kola (sterculia acuminata) in half ounce or one ounce quantity be given at the same time.

Dr. Norton did not wish to be considered as believing that *all* headaches, even of a special type, result from refractive anomalies, as disturbances in any organ may produce pain in the head. But he does believe that many more headaches are dependent upon the eyes than is usually imagined. Therefore, in all obstinate cases of headache, especially if the cause is at all obscure, the eyes should be examined carefully to find if they are at fault. The doctor has also met cases which have only been relieved temporarily, but many of these have been again improved by a re-adjustment of glasses. In most of the cases he reported in his paper, the results two years afterward were given.

Dr. H. C. Houghton presented a paper upon "Clinical Cases of Disease of the Middle Ear."

Adjournment, 11 P.M.

RECORD OF MEDICAL PROGRESS.

CREOLIN V. CARBOLIC ACID.—Dr. E. von Esmach, assistant in the Royal Hygienic Institute of Berlin, has made a series of experiments with creolin, a new disinfectant, which has been highly spoken of by Professor Fröhner, of the new Veterinary School of Berlin. Dr. von Esmach made a number of comparative observations with carbolic acid on the disinfecting, deodorizing and antiseptic properties of creolin. Amongst other observations he noted the effects of the two substances on fluids containing cholera, typhus and anthrax bacilli. As a rule, creolin appeared to be much the more active. Similarly, the offensive smell of various putrefying liquids was controlled much more readily by creolin than by carbolic acid. Creolin soap, too, showed itself more active as a disinfectant than corrosive sublimate soap.—*London Lancet*, October 15th, 1887.

CONCERNING LACERATED CERVIX.—Noegerrath, in a paper read before the Gynæcological Section of the meeting of German Naturalists and Physicians, summed up his conclusions as follows: 1. Women with diseased uteri conceive more readily when the cervix is torn than when uninjured. 2. The position of the uterus is uninfluenced by laceration of the cervix. 3. The uterine axis undergoes no lengthening as a result of a lacerated cervix. 4. Erosions and ulcerations occur just as frequently in the injured cervix as in the uninjured, and the cervical tissue is not found to be more diseased in torn cervices than when intact. 5. Cervical laceration has no influence upon the development of uterine disease whether considered as to intensity or frequency. 6. Eversion of the lips is not the immediate result of a laceration.   O'C.

EBSTEIN ON DIABETES.—Prof. W. Ebstein gives, in a monograph of 231 pages, his theories concerning diabetes mellitus, a *résumé* of which (by Lohnstein) appears in *Berliner Klinische Wochenschrift*, No. 42, 1887: Diabetes mellitus is not a symptom of different morbid conditions, but is an independent disease traceable to some faulty property of protoplasm in consequence of which there is a too small production of carbonic acid within the tissues. One consequence of this anomaly is the abnormally strong action of the diastatic ferment contained within the organism, both upon the glycogen existing in different organs, which becomes changed into readily diffusible kinds of sugar that is resorbed and partly excreted, as well as, in severe cases, upon the albuminous principles that likewise are changed into more fluid forms. The carbonic acid has the property, as the author has shown by a long series of experiments, of checking the influence of diastatic ferments, especially upon glycogen. If the protoplasm loses from any cause the property of directing in sufficient degree the production of carbonic acid, the glycogen contained in the organism is exposed unprotected to the action of the saccharifying ferment, and thus result hyperglycæmia and glycosuria. While thus in the normal organism the sugar formation and sugar consumption correspond with tolerable exactness, there exists in the organism of diabetics a loss of this sugar equilibrium of such kind that too much readily diffusible sugar is formed, the unconsumed portion passing out as an excretion. Now, in one series of cases (light form of diabetes), the deficit can be compensated for by increased ingestion of highly albuminous food which also determines an increase of CO_2. There is another series in which the disturbance of the oxidation processes of the protoplasm is so great that the carbonic acid from non-nitrogenous food is no longer sufficient to protect the glycogen sufficiently, so that the albumen of the body is now drawn upon to supply the deficit always existing in the amount of CO_2. One consequence of the lessened formation of carbonic acid, as Voit and Pettenkofer, among others, have shown, is a lessened need for oxygen, and from this in turn results a decrease of body temperature, an extremely unfavorable prognostic symptom. Albuminuria, which is in severe cases the most important symptom next to the glycosuria, is explained by the author as depending on the failure of protoplasm to form carbonic acid in sufficient amount. For carbonic acid also protects the difficultly diffusible globulin and prevents this albuminous body from being changed under the action of ferments existing in the organism into readily diffusible albumens. Thus albuminuria is the result of the increased transformation of globulin. Concerning the unquenchable thirst of diabetics the author accepts, in the main, the hypothesis of Bouchard that the sugar circulating in the blood exerts its dehydrating power upon the tissues. A second dehydrating influence is, according to Ebstein, that the glycogen is not, as in the normal organism, burnt up into CO_2 and H_2O, under which condition the water of the tissues is retained by them, but leaves the organism as carbohydrate, and in this way a certain portion of the water necessary for the preservation of the organism is lost. The pathogenesis of diabetes is probably, then, a congenital weakness of the protoplasm, an innate diathesis whose symptoms become manifest through different exciting causes. The author is very sceptical concerning the etiological importance of the brain affections, whose causal connection with diabetes is not nearly so sure as it seems to be considered. The brain affections may with far better right be considered the result rather than the cause of diabetes; similarly, the changes in the solar ganglia, affections of the pancreas, etc., to which have been ascribed an excessive influence in the causation of diabetes. These theoretical views of the nature of diabetes have led the author not only to allow to diabetic patients the use of fatty foods, but even to urgently recommend them, as fats are burnt up in the organism into CO_2 and H_2O without any intermediate stage of sugar-formation. He does not limit his diabetic patients to a strict meat diet, but allows them from 60 to 100 grams of bread per day. Further, he endeavors to increase in them the production of carbonic acid through muscular activity by gymnastics or massage.   O'C.

NOTES ON METHYLAL.—At a meeting of the Medical Society of London, held on October 24th, Dr. B. W. Richardson read some notes on Methylal and advanced the following conclusions : 1. Methylal is hypnotic and antispasmodic. 2. Its action lies between methylic alcohol and ethylic ether ; it may be looked on as a volatile alcohol, and resembles closely pure methylic alcohol in action. 3. It can be administered by inhalation as vapor, by hypodermic injection, and by the mouth in aqueous solution. 4. It reduces arterial tension, and by local action excites glandular activity. 5. The sleep it induces is not profound unless the dose be excessive ; it is quickly eliminated, and leaves no serious effects ; it causes no vomiting or stomachic disturbance. 6. A fatal dose by inhalation kills by complete relaxation of the muscular fibres of the heart, leaving the heart distended with blood and the vascular organs intensely congested. 7. It combines with ether, alcohol, amyl nitrite, and many other remedial agents with which it acts in concert, and equalizes their action by reason of its own solubility. 8. Its tendency is to maintain the fluidity of the blood, and it may therefore be of service in combination with ammonia. 9. It promises to yield a safe and effective anæsthetic mixture in combination with ether. 10. It reduces the animal temperature, but not to the same degree as common alcohol. 11. Used as an anodyne it passes out of the body without producing organic injury, when not often repeated. 12. But, like all bodies of its class, it must be given in increasing quantities, in order to keep up its effects, and it would soon yield evil as well as good by its habitual use in the community at large.—*London Lancet*, October 29th, 1887.

NEURALGIA OF STUMPS AFTER AMPUTATIONS.—Witzel reports three cases from the clinic at Bonn with some remarks concerning the nature of the affection, which he decides to be a pure neuralgia only in the beginning, the later stage being chronic neuritis. When the motor nerves are implicated there occur fibrillary twitchings and spasmodic contractions. How long after the amputation the trouble begins is as yet undetermined. In one case, an amputation in the lower arm, neuralgia appeared five years later and was cured by extirpation of a large piece of the radial nerve ; the nerve was found to be adherent to the bone, and higher up a neuroma had formed. After the extirpation the neuralgia ceased at once. In a second case there was found after extirpation of the nerve, marked increase of the interstitial connective tissue of the nerve; and in a third case, neuralgia of the tibial after a Pirogoff's operation, where simple section of the nerve was of no avail and in consequence amputation of the thigh was done, the nerve was found to be in a condition of endo- and peri-neuritis for a long distance. The so-called end-neuroma is often present without causing the symptoms of neuritis, and for the avoiding of the latter result it is recommended in all operations to cut out the nerve as high as possible. Simple neuralgia should be treated by cutting out the nerve or perhaps by nerve stretching.—*Berliner Klinische Wochenschrift*, No. 40, 1887.   O'C.

MORRHUOL.—There has just been published in Paris, by G. Steinheil, an interesting clinical study upon Morrhuol, the extract of cod liver oil, by E. Chazeaud, and the chief conclusions at which he has arrived are as follows: Clinical observation has demonstrated in a conclusive fashion the high therapeutic value of morrhuol. It increases the appetite and regulates the digestive functions, increases rapidly the weight of the body, and leads to positive *embonpoint*. The urea discharged in the urine is also augmented, the cough is diminished and finally extinguished, whilst the debility disappears. These excellent results are not confined to cases treated at hospitals, but cases in private practice are equally benefited. Besides tuberculosis, anæmia, rickets and scrofula (lymphatism) are equally amenable to its beneficent influence. The small size of the morrhuol capsules enables them to be taken with ease by the patient, and nausea and diarrhœa are also prevented. To so many advantages one slight disadvantage must be added, but even that is of rare occurrence—it is the development of acne-form spots similar to those produced by the iodides. The number of capsules to be taken varies in different cases, from two to eight per day, and eight capsules are equivalent to forty grammes of brown cod liver oil.—*London Lancet*, October 29th, 1887.

IODINE TRICHLORIDE AS AN ANTISEPTIC AND DISINFECTANT.—Dr. Carl Langenbuch, of Berlin, gives in *Berliner Klinische Wochenschrift*, No. 40, 1887, the results of experiments with this compound as follows:
I. Iodine trichloride is in watery solution an active disinfectant, as even in great dilution, 1 to 1,000, its influence on bacillary spores is fatal in a comparatively short time. Its influence on spores far exceeds that of carbolic acid and stands next to that of mercuric chloride as an available disinfectant.
II. In its behavior towards bacilli free from spores and to cocci, iodine trichloride shows, in a solution of 1 to 1,000, equal activity with a carbolic acid solution of 3 to 100. Some experiments gave it a higher power in further dilution.
III. The antiseptic influence in preventing the development of micro-organisms causing septic conditions was shown in the results of a solution of 1 to 1,200 added to culture gelatine. Langenbuch admits that the "trichloride," as he calls it for short, cannot be used for the wiping of metallic instruments, but he employs it as a substitute for the bichloride of mercury in preparatory disinfection of the hands of the operator, as well as of the part of the patient to be operated on. He finds that no danger is to be apprehended from the use of the trichloride in surgical practice; the chlorine is not absorbed by the skin, and the slightly poisonous iodine may give a temporary slight yellow staining which soon disappears or may be readily removed by washing in ammonia water.   O'C.

POSTURE FOR SLEEP AND POSTURE IN SLEEP.—It would seem on the first blush of the matter that the posture for—that is, to favor—sleep must be generally the same as that voluntarily or instinctively assumed during sleep; but a little consideration will make it apparent that this is not correct. It may be granted that, supposing a person to be sleeping lightly and uncomfortably, the posture will be changed half unconsciously to one of comfort. It would be more correct to say that it is changed in the endeavor to avoid distress or discomfort: but even the fact that sleep is quieter in the new position will not suffice to prove that it is a better one, because the sleep may meanwhile have become deeper. It is on the whole impossible to ascertain either by experience or observation which is the posture most conducive to sleep, and attempts to lay down rules for the guidance of bad sleepers are always arbitrary, generally empirical, and rarely of any practical value. Those who think " anæmia of the cerebrum " is the cause of sleep, and those who think that, though not the cause a diminution in the quantity of blood in the vessels of the encephalon is a necessary concomitant of sleep, prefer, and recommend that the head should be higher than the feet; while those who adopt the opposite view, and think that passive congestion causes or promotes somnolence, should have the feet raised and the head lowered. The confounding of stupor with sleep, may, and probably has, something to do with these differences of opinion. Meanwhile a common sense view of the subject would conclude that, as there is evidently some change in the blood state when the brain falls asleep, the best plan must seem to be to place the body in such position that the flow of blood through the vessels of the head and neck may be especially easy and free. The way to secure this is to allow the head to lie in a posture and on a level that cannot offer any obstacle to the free return of blood through the veins of the neck, and does not tend to make the blood flow specially in any particular direction, but leaves Nature at liberty to act as she will.—*London Lancet,* November 5th, 1887.

ANTIFEBRIN FOR LANCINATING PAINS.—Dr. G. Fischer, of Canstatt (*Münchn. Med. Wochenschr.,* No. 23, 1887), has tested antifebrin for lancinating pains, on ten tabetic patients; about ninety trials, in all, were made, In one case only the remedy was without good effect, in the other nine the results were favorable. In three of them attacks of different " crises " were benefited (gastric crises, spasm of the bladder, feeling of constriction in the rectum). Slight cyanosis was the only annoying state produced by the drug. Shortly after taking it there was an agreeable, warm, quieting feeling through the whole body. Typical cases of lancinating pain were most markedly impressed by the remedy. The influence of the drug was felt as a rule in from thirty to ninety minutes after taking the first dose, seven and one-half grains, but was not observed after a dose of three and one-fourth grains. Fischer has employed it with good results in occipital neuralgia (syphilitic) which was not influenced by the inunction cure ; in one case of paralytic dementia (syphilitic) with tearing pains in the legs ; in recurrent anæmic headache and in four cases of hemicrania. O'C.

THE PROGNOSIS IN ALBUMINURIC RETINITIS.—An interesting discussion was raised as a digression at the last meeting of the Ophthalmological Society on the subject of the prognosis of albuminuric retinitis. Dr. Angel Money, who gave the turn to the discussion, said that in his experience the average duration of life was to be measured by months. This view was supported by Dr. J. Anderson, who had instituted an inquiry in the matter, and came to the conclusion that the longest duration was thirteen months and the average six months. Dr. Stephen Mackenzie did not contest the main issue, but narrated some cases which went to show that life might be prolonged even for years. Indeed, he mentioned one case in which considerable progress towards recovery took place, so that after a time the ophthalmoscopic changes were not very noticeable. Mr. Marcus Gunn agreed with the view that the duration of life was not usually long. Mr. Nettleship considered that if the changes in the eyes were associated with renal disease and pregnancy, then, provided a safe delivery was accomplished, the prognosis was much more favorable than in ordinary cases. Mr. McHardy had seen a case in which the patient lived for many years after the detection of the albuminuric retinitis. Dr. W. Y. Collins thought the prognosis more favorable, where mere hemorrhages existed, but less hopeful if other retinal changes had developed.—*London Lancet,* October 29th, 1887.

EPHEDRIN, A NEW MYDRIATIC.—In a preliminary communication to *Ber. Klin. Wochens.,* No. 38, 1887, Kinnosuke Miura, a medical student at the University of Tokio, Japan, calls attention to an alkaloid isolated by Prof. Nagai from *ephedra vulgaris*, rich. var. *helvetica*, Hook et Thomp. The method of production and the chemical constitution are promised in a future publication. Ephedrinum muriaticum is a readily soluble salt, white in color and crystallizing in needles. The solution is not decomposed by light. The first experiments in 1885 gave the following : As the result of a dose of from eight to ten milligrams given to a moderate sized *rana esculenta* the respiration gradually slowed and finally ceased, no stage of acceleration having been observed. The heart's rhythm was interfered with, the organ finally stopping in diastole. The pupils were dilated. In rabbits and dogs the frequency in rate of both pulse and respiration was considerably increased, to be followed later, after a special slowing, by sudden cessation of both. At the same time clonic convulsions occurred with increase of temperature in the rectum. Blood pressure was notably diminished, but during the spasms increased beyond the normal, falling again quickly. The pupils dilated as well by subcutaneous injection as by instillation into the conjunctival sac. Death occurred by respiratory and cardiac paralysis. The lethal dose, given subcutaneously, is for rabbits about four decigrammes per kilo of body weight; in dogs two decigrammes. Clinical experiments were made in 1887. A six or seven per cent. solution gave somewhat unequal results upon the pupil in man; on the other hand, a ten per cent. solution produced tolerably constant ones whether the individual was well or suffering from some eye affection. With a ten per cent. solution there followed, after instillation of one or two drops, in eighteen patients, dilatation of the pupils in from forty to sixty minutes equal in both eyes when the refraction was equal, and no inflammation existed. Dilatation was not absolutely complete but was sufficient to permit examination of the whole retina by the direct method. By strong illumination a slight pupillary reaction could be obtained in all cases. Accommodation was not paralyzed at all, or only in slight degree. Children and old persons were affected more readily than young, vigorous individuals. Upon an inflamed iris no dilating was produced. The duration of dilatation, from the instillation until a return to the normal, varied between five and twenty hours. No conjunctivitis or other annoyance was observable even after fourteen days' use, nor any change in intraocular pressure. Comparative experiments with one per cent. homatropin solution showed that in the latter sixty-nine hours elapsed before the pupil returned to the normal. The drug is especially valuable for examination of the fundus.   O'C.

COMMUNICABILITY OF DISEASE FROM ANIMALS TO MAN.—The transmission from the cow to man of scarlet fever and tuberculosis was the subject of the opening address of Professor Hamilton at Marischal College, Aberdeen, in which the lecturer gave an excellent account of the investigations, conducted by Mr. Power and Dr. Klein, into the relation of a cow malady to scarlet fever in man. He referred also to the observations of Copland, who believed that both the dog and the horse could suffer from the latter affection, and stated that a febrile condition of some kind can be communicated to animals by inoculating them with the blood of persons who are the subjects of scarlet fever. He further expressed the opinion that tubercle could be conveyed to man by means of milk from tuberculous cows. While the possibility of such occurrence cannot be denied, it must be borne in mind that Klein has pointed out that there are certain important differences between bovine and human tuberculosis; and again, Creighton has shown that man occasionally suffers from a form of this disease which resembles the bovine malady, making it probable that by far the greater number of cases are not of bovine origin. Nevertheless the subject deserves much greater investigation, and certainly every effort should be made to prevent the distribution of milk of tubercular cows.—*London Lancet*, October 29th, 1887.

MULTIPLE NEURITIS AFTER INTOXICATION.—In *Berliner Klinische Wochenschrift*, No. 35, 1887, Minkowski contributes to the present knowledge of multiple neuritis, considering its symptomatology, etiology and especially its relation to chronic alcoholism. A noteworthy phenomenon observed by him in one case was the occurrence of peculiar attacks of laryngeal dyspnœa, reminding one of the laryngeal "crises" of tabes and which could be attributed to implication of the laryngeal nerve. In two cases in which there had been a previous syphilitic infection the employment of mercurial inunction had a distinctively unfavorable influence on the course of the disease, and had to be stopped. He was of the opinion that in cases of multiple neuritis in which syphilitic infection appeared to play an etiological *rôle*, antisyphilitic treatment gave as little prospect of good results as in the non-specific diseases of the central nervous system that develop as a result of syphilis, viz., dementia paralytica and tabes. The unfavorable influence of the inunction method upon nutrition appears to have a directly injurious action in multiple neuritis. In one case the question became imperative whether or not the neuritis was not induced by an energetic inunction cure, and hence the result of mercurial poisoning.

THE URINE OF TABES DORSALIS.—The following facts are set forth by MM. Levou and Alezais as the result of a series of researches on the urine of patients affected with an apyrexial disease of the cord—namely, tabes dorsalis. A tendency to diminution of the urea eliminated in the twenty-four hours; a diminution in the total daily discharge of phosphoric acid, with a tendency to proportional augmentation of the discharge of earthy phosphates; a great variation in the elimination of chlorine, with a bias in favor of hyperchloruria. Intravenous injections of tabetic urines appear to be sufficiently toxic in their action, since it has been found that from twelve to twenty-four cubic centimetres of urine per kilogramme of body weight of animals was sufficient to kill dogs.—*London Lancet*, October 15th, 1887.

THE URINE OF MELANCHOLIA.—Dr. Marro finds that in all forms of melancholia, the total quantity of phosphoric acid in the urine is diminished; this is especially the case for the alkaline phosphates which are wanting, while the phosphates of calcium and magnesium may be excreted in unusual amount. The increase of the earthly phosphates stands in direct relation to the presence of a volatile fatty acid. In melancholia anxiosa formic acid is constantly found in the urine. In other forms of melancholia, acetic and carbonic acids are usually increased. In parallel relation to the earthly phosphate, the chlorides also are increased, and the proportion of ethylsulphuric acid increases with the whole amount of sulphuric acid excreted. Marro considers melancholia to be a disturbance of nutrition.—*Neurolog. Centralb.*, No. 15, 1887. O'C.

TREATMENT OF GALL STONES.—Dr. Samuel Morales Pereira, of Puebla, Mexico, gives an account in a Mexican medical journal of a case of "Biliary Calculus Diathesis," with enlargement of the gall bladder, in which he found a decoction of a well-known fern, *Asplenium ceterach*, or *doradilla*, as it is called in Spanish, of great value. The patient was a gentleman of good general constitution, who had suffered for a long time from pain of a more or less periodical character in the hepatic region. His digestion and his temper were considerably affected. He had applied to a number of medical men, but had never derived any benefit from their treatment. On examination, the right hypochondrium was found to measure six centimetres more than the left, the region of the gall bladder being distinctly enlarged and tender to the touch. The hepatic dulness in

the axillary line was of normal breadth, but it extended five or six centimetres beyond the normal in a downward direction in the mammary line.
On changing the patient's position, no alteration in the situation of this abnormal dullness could be detected. The patient, on being asked, said that
his urine deposited a red sediment, and that he had at times passed calculi in his stools. Dr. Pereira, having had experience of the good effects
of ceterach in gravel and urinary calculus, and believing that it exerts an
influence in "calculous diathesis," decided to employ it in this case. A
decoction of half a drachm of the plant in five ounces of water was ordered four times a day. During the first twenty days no effect was
observed. By the end of another twenty days, the symptoms of mental
irritability had disappeared and the pain in the hepatic region had very
greatly diminished. In fifteen days more the tumor in the region of the
gall bladder had become much less perceptible. The patient had been
kept on milk and broth, which he did not at all like. He had passed three
gall stones and some gravelly matter with his stools, there having been
some severe hepatic pain. After this the patient continued to improve,
though it was not easy to convince him that he was doing so. The amount
of ceterach was diminished and capsules of tauren prescribed, belladonna
friction being also applied to the hepatic region. He passed a succession
of gall stones, and the whole of the abnormal physical signs as well as the
subjective symptoms passed away. Dr. Pereira hazards a suggestion that
ceterach may have some effect on calculi already formed, as well as the
"calculous diathesis." He remembers being struck with the appearance
of a stone—he does not say of what kind—which he saw removed from a
young man's bladder, and which, though hard in some parts, was so
friable in others that it could be broken down with the fingers. On questioning the patient, it was found that he had for some time taken ceterach
by the advice of an old native medicine man, and that while he was doing
so he had remarked that he passed more urine and that it contained
gravel. The pain, however, did not diminish, and so he lost faith in the
treatment and gave it up. It is to be remarked that the use of ceterach in
urinary calculi is by no means new. Dr. Pereira does not explain what
relationship he supposes to exist between the "calculous diathesis," which
leads to urinary calculi, and that which produces gall stones, or why a
remedy which is useful in one case should be prescribed in the other; still
his facts, such as they are, are worth noting, and they seem to have interested the members of the Mexican Academy of Medicine, before whom
they were brought, and who had the opportunity of examining the various
gall stones and gravelly matter passed with the fæces, as well as the partly
friable vesical calculus, upon which Dr. Pereira's suggestions were in part
based.—*London Lancet*, October 1st, 1887.

NEWS.

A HOMŒOPATHIC HOSPITAL and dispensary has been recently established at St. Paul.

MARRIED.—Mr. William M. Decker, '79, to Miss Bessie Smith, on
Tuesday, November 22d, at Kingston, N. Y.

HELMUTH HOUSE REPORT.—The summary of the half yearly report of
this private homœopathic institution states the total number of patients
received, 94; cured, 65; improved, 5; unimproved, 4; under treatment,
11; died, 9.

ALUMNI LECTURE.—The third annual lecture lefore the Alumni Association of the New York Homœopathic Medical College was delivered

Wednesday evening, November 30th, 1887, in the lecture room of the New York Ophthalmic Hospital, by Prof. Joseph S. Mitchell, M.D., of Chicago.

WOMEN IN RUSSIA.—Slowly, but surely, old things are passing away in Russia. It has recently been determined to establish a course of medicine for women there. The institution will be limited to simple courses of medicine for women, of which four will be theoretical and the fifth will be devoted to clinical work in the hospitals.

RHUS POISONING.—Anacardium 4x is recommended for the cure of rhus poisoning, together with lotion of grindelia. Frequent and thorough washing of the parts in hot soapsuds and water is said to be sure and speedy in giving relief. Washing soda spread upon a slice of bread, which is kept moist, and applied so the soda comes directly upon the inflamed part, is also highly extolled.

SOUTHERN ASSOCIATION.—The fourth annual meeting of the Southern Homœopathic Medical Association will be held at New Orleans, December 14th, 15th and 16th, 1887. The Secretary of the Association states that there is every prospect of a large and interesting meeting; that the Bureaus and Committees are all in working order and urge Southern homœopathic physicians to be present.

SOCIETY ITEMS.—At the last meeting of the New York Society for Medico-Scientific Investigation, at its rooms at 201 East Twenty-third Street, papers were read by Dr. King on "Dr. Apostoli's Treatment of Uterine Inflammations," by Dr. Bullel on "Otitis Media Hemorrhagica," and by Dr. Shelton on "Cannabis Indica in the Treatment of Alcoholism." Papers of an eminently practical nature, bearing on topics of great interest to the profession, may be expected at an early meeting.

THEREAPEUTIC HINTS.—Prunus spinosa 30 is said to remove the neuralgic pain which so often remains after the eruption of zoster disappears. Eczema attended by intolerable itching is relieved and cured by chloral hydrate. This drug causes an eczematous eruption accompanied with intense and constant irritation. It is claimed that irrigation with a warm antiseptic fluid is an excellent way to treat carbuncles. Use a fountain syringe holding about two quarts of carbolized water, hot. Direct to point of suppuration. Repeat in from two to four hours, as symptoms require.

BUREAU OF GYNÆCOLOGY.—"Uterine Therapeutics" is the general subject selected for discussion at the coming meeting of the Institute. The special topics are "Changes in Form and Position of the Uterus," "Neoplasms of the Uterus" and "Nutritive Disturbances." Among those who will either prepare reports or discuss them are Dr. O. S. Runnels, of Indianapolis; Dr. L. L. Danforth, New York; Dr. T. G. Comstock, St. Louis; Dr. R. Ludlam, Chicago, and Dr. E. M. Hale, Chicago. The Bureau is displaying through its officers a very commendable energy. The members should see to it that the performance does not fall behind the promise.

REMOVALS.—In the change of location made by Drs. F. S. Bradford, and Chas. A. Bacon, the former to Morristown, N. J., and the latter to Washington, D. C., New York loses physicians highly esteemed for their worth and usefulness. It is to be hoped that they will find the health for themselves and families which they seek in new homes. They carry with them the best wishes of a large circle of friends among patients and physicians.

The many friends and former pupils of Dr. O. B. Gause will regret to learn that ill health has compelled his resignation as Professor of Obstetrics in the Hahnemann College of Philadelphia, and removal to a warmer climate (Aiken, S. C.) for the practice of his profession.

A SAD EVENT.—Dr. George M. Smith, Junior Physician at the Five Points Homœopathic Hospital, was found dead in his room on the morning of November 9th. He had retired to his room the preceding evening in unusually good health and spirits. Dr. Smith graduated from the New York Homœopathic Medical College, class of '87. For two years he was the dispensing druggist in the Ophthalmic Hospital. During his last term in college he was Business Manager of *The Chironian*. The funeral services were held in the chapel of the hospital, Pastor Haliday of Plymouth Church officiating. A large number of the students were present, and Prof. Dowling spoke for the college. Dr. Smith was a nephew of Dr. St. Clair Smith, of New York, and of Dr. Hugh M. Smith, of Brooklyn. Dr. Smith was of a genial, social nature and leaves many friends who deplore his untimely death.

OBITUARY.—John K. Lee, M. D., one of the best known physicians in Philadelphia, died suddenly at his residence on November 10th of heart disease. Dr. Lee was born in Allegheny City. After receiving a good academic education in his native town he entered as a student in Allegheny College, from which he graduated with the highest honors of the institution in 1849. On leaving college he came to Philadelphia and began the study of medicine under the instruction of Dr. Williamson. He entered the Homœopathic Medical College of Pennsylvania, and graduated on March 4th, 1851. Dr. Lee was distinguished as a thoroughly well equipped physician, a close scholar and a man of dignity, honor and integrity. He was a humanitarian and much of his time was spent in deeds of quiet charity. He was a fluent, polished and forcible writer. He was a member of the State Board of Charities.

THE BULL OPTOMETER.—There has recently been presented to the profession a very ingenious optometer devised by George J. Bull, a young American doctor, who has made a series of studies at the laboratory of ophthalmology at the Sorbonne. The optometer permits of a quick determination of the value of the amplitude of accommodation in dioptrics. It consists of a light wooden rule about twenty-four inches long by one and one-fourth inches wide, that can easily be held in the hand by means of a handle fixed at right angles with the flat part. At one extremity there is a square thin piece of metal of the width of the rule, and at right angles with the latter, but on the side opposite the handle. This piece of metal contains a circular aperture a few hundredths of an inch in diameter. Toward this aperture may be moved either a converging lens of five dioptrics or a diverging lens of the same diameter, but of six dioptrics. On holding the apparatus by the handle and putting the eye to the aperture, provided or not with a lens, we see a series of dominoes extending along the rule, from the double ace, which occupies the extremity most distant from the eye, to the double six, which is very near the eye. The numbers from ten to twelve are indicated, and it is very important to fix the attention upon them, since they are arranged at distances expressed in dioptrics and shown by the number of spots. The use of the optometer is simple. If we wish to express in dioptrics the myopia of a person, we put the apparatus in his hand, and ask him to place his eye very near the aperture and note the number of spots in the most distant domino that he sees distinctly. This is the number sought. If the observation be made through the upper lens, it will be necessary to subtract five from the number obtained; if, on the contrary, the other lens is used, it will be necessary to add six. Upon the whole, Dr. Bull's optometer permits of measuring the amplitude of accommodation, and, consequently, of obtaining the approximate age of people, of knowing the extreme distance of the accommodation, and of quickly finding the number of the glass necessary for each one.—*La Nature.*

Lightning Source UK Ltd.
Milton Keynes UK
UKHW041106141218
333981UK00015B/1725/P